Psychiatric Epidemiology

Psychiatric Epidemiology

Searching for the Causes of Mental Disorders

Ezra Susser
Sharon Schwartz
Alfredo Morabia
Evelyn J. Bromet

with

Melissa D. Begg (Statistics)
Jack M. Gorman (Biological Studies)
and Mary-Claire King (Genetic Studies)

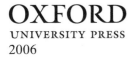

UNIVERSITY PRESS
2006

OXFORD
UNIVERSITY PRESS

Oxford University Press, Inc., publishes works that further
Oxford University's objective of excellence
in research, scholarship, and education.

Oxford   New York
Auckland Cape Town Dar es Salaam Hong Kong Karachi
Kuala Lumpur Madrid Melbourne Mexico City Nairobi
New Delhi Shanghai Taipei Toronto

With offices in
Argentina Austria Brazil Chile Czech Republic France Greece
Guatemala Hungary Italy Japan Poland Portugal Singapore
South Korea Switzerland Thailand Turkey Ukraine Vietnam

Copyright © 2006 by Oxford University Press, Inc.

Published by Oxford University Press, Inc.
198 Madison Avenue, New York, New York 10016

www.oup.com

Oxford is a registered trademark of Oxford University Press.

Library of Congress Cataloging-in-Publication Data
Psychiatric epidemiology : searching for the causes of mental disorders /
Ezra Susser . . . [et al.].
      p. ; cm.
   Includes bibliographical references and index.
   ISBN-13: 978-0-19-510181-2
   ISBN 0-19-510181-2
   1. Psychiatric epidemiology.   2. Mental illness–Etiology.
   [DNLM: 1. Mental Disorders–epidemiology.   2. Mental Disorders–etiology.
3. Epidemiologic Methods.   WM 140 P97412 2006]   I. Susser, Ezra S., 1952–
   RC455.2.E64P79   2006
   362.2′0422–dc22
                                                                2005015870

9 8 7 6 5 4 3 2 1
Printed in the United States of America on acid-free paper

Epidemiologists are not free of the prejudices and oversights of their times. In retrospect, it is evident that some of the landmark discoveries of previous eras depended upon experiments that would today be considered unethical, even if well within the norms of the period. Psychiatric patients were subjects in some particularly important experiments, which led to great advances in human health, such as the work leading to the discovery of vitamin deficiencies causing beriberi and pellagra. We believe it is the duty of every scientific discipline to be knowledgeable about its past practices and recognize the debt owed to the participants. Thus, this book is dedicated to all psychiatric patients who have knowingly or unknowingly contributed to our understanding of the causes and prevention of disease. Our society is much indebted to them and to their families.

Foreword

It is a dull week in which there is not a new claim that some putative risk factor, such as diet, hormone replacement therapy (HRT), drugs, toxins, or immunization, "causes" some undesirable outcome, such as cancer, heart disease, autism, or schizophrenia. Professionals, science writers for the media, and the general public are full of uncertainties about what to make of the findings. Many of the claims seem impressive because they are based on epidemiological analyses of large samples. The problem is that the results of one study are contradicted by the next one. "HRT *protects* against heart disease" becomes "HRT *increases* the risk of heart disease." Which claim should anyone believe? The consequence has been a rise in public and professional skepticism about the value of epidemiological studies. If the risks are relatively small (which usually they are), and the findings are contradictory, maybe none of the claims is to be trusted.

This splendid book provides the much needed counter to the destructive cynicism about the value of epidemiology. It is not, however, an evangelistic defense of epidemiology. Rather, it is an immensely readable and interesting account of how epidemiology can provide rigorous tests of causal hypotheses. The preface is at pains to note what the book does not do, so let me use the foreword to indicate what it does do, and does supremely well. Anyone who wishes to understand modern concepts and findings in medicine, including concepts in psychiatry, must appreciate what is meant by *risk factors*, why it is usual for there to be multiple causal pathways, why most risk factors have relatively small effects, and why such small effects truly matter. This is the place for clinicians and researchers, and dare I add science writers, to gain the necessary understanding. The language used is largely nontechnical, the concepts are very clearly explained, and there are numerous fascinating, and telling, examples of epidemiological research successes. Good textbooks are fine sources of knowledge but they are rarely a good read. This book is a wonderful exception because it holds the attention throughout, and because the examples make the whole research enterprise come to life in a riveting fashion. There is no other book quite like it.

The preface notes, honestly, that it does not provide a review of all that is known in epidemiology or a comprehensive account of general epidemiology, or a manual on how to conduct an epidemiological study. All that is true, but what the book does extremely well is provide an understanding of how it is possible to make the journey from a statistically significant association to an inference about probable causal processes and how the risks are mediated. The book outlines some of the key statistical considerations, but it emphasizes that research design considerations, including the use of "natural experiments," are at least as important. Also, it is made explicit throughout that the search for causal mechanisms must involve a range of research strategies that bring together genetics, social and physical risk factors, and developmental considerations—all of which are part of biology. In the past, there was a tendency to consider that these various influences acted in parallel, but it is now evident that it is common for there to be a synergistic interplay. This synergy complicates the research challenges, but it is open to rigorous testing.

Anyone, whether clinician, researcher, or science writer, who makes use of epidemiology will find this book invaluable as a guide on how to think about epidemiology. But, in addition, it is likely that reading the book will leave him or her with an excitement about what epidemiology can do and, at its best, does do. The necessary cautions and concerns are all presented, but so, too, are the solutions to the research problems. All together, the book is a remarkable accomplishment from which all of us will benefit.

Professor Sir Michael Rutter, M.D.
Professor of Developmental Psychopathology
Institute of Psychiatry
Kings College, London

Preface

This book distills concepts and methods from epidemiology in devising a strategy to search for the causes of mental disorders. Searching for these causes is as exciting as it is complex. The discovery of a cause means meeting an intellectual challenge, unraveling a mystery of mental life, and ultimately helping to reduce human suffering. But these causes are elusive. One reason is that the relationship between pathophysiology and its overt manifestations in mental life is exceedingly intricate. It is our good fortune that because of rapid advances in genetics, neuroscience, and other disciplines the causes of mental disorders increasingly fall within the reach of epidemiologic investigations.

Readers will differ somewhat in the uses to which they put this book. For trainees in psychiatric epidemiology—and for their teachers—we try to produce a volume that can be used as a textbook alongside primary scientific material. For clinical researchers, we try to show how epidemiologic thinking will improve investigations of any type, be they biological, genetic, or psychosocial. For academic epidemiologists, we offer a unified perspective on the discipline, one that we hope will help to integrate epidemiology for "mental" and "physical" disorders, and to advance epidemiologic concepts toward the future. Although the book is directed primarily toward researchers, we believe that it is both relevant and valuable for clinicians and public health practitioners. We also hope that interested readers with no specifically relevant professional training will be equally intrigued and engaged.

In the first book to articulate the uses of epidemiology in the modern era, Morris (1957) identified seven central domains of investigation, summarized as follows:

1. The rise and fall of diseases in the population
2. The presence, nature, and distribution of health and disease among the population
3. The workings of health services
4. The individual's chances and risks of disease
5. The clinical picture, including all types of cases and the relation of clinical disease to the subclinical
6. Syndromes identifiable from the distribution of clinical phenomena in the population

7. The causes of health in relation to ways of living among populations[1]

Our focus on causes of disorders does not mean that we attach little importance to the other uses of epidemiology. Rather, it reflects our perspective on the present state of psychiatric epidemiology. The discipline has grown exponentially in the recognition it receives, as well as in its substantive findings, but at the same time it has lagged in the search for causes. We are now poised to find them, but to do so we need to take up the advances that have been made in modern epidemiology and to incorporate developments in related fields. We also need to preserve and solidify the strengths of psychiatric epidemiology. As we hope to demonstrate, psychiatric epidemiology has much to offer other rapidly developing fields of epidemiology, such as social epidemiology, life course epidemiology, and genetic epidemiology.

What We Mean by "Mental Disorders"

Our concern is mainly with the conditions defined and delineated by the *Diagnostic and Statistical Manual of Mental Disorders* (*DSM*) and the *International Statistical Classification of Diseases and Related Health Problems* (*ICD*) *Classification of Mental and Behavioural Disorders.*[2] A distinctive feature of these disorders is that their diagnosis generally depends on thoughts, behaviors, and feelings. We use the terms "mental," "psychiatric," and "neuropsychiatric" interchangeably to refer to this entire class of disorders.

We do not find it helpful, however, to draw any rigid line between mental and physical disorders. The *DSM* and *ICD* nosologies include many disorders that might not always be considered "mental" in common parlance, such as substance use disorders, neurodevelopmental disorders, and dementias. Mental disorders frequently have physical manifestations and vice versa. Like other disorders, mental ones have biological underpinnings in the brain or other organs. As neuroscience advances, the boundary between mental (or psychiatric) and physical (or neurologic) brain disorders is increasingly blurred. Thus, in the following chapters we sometimes use examples of brain disorders classified as neurologic or neurodevelopmental, such as epilepsy and neural tube defects.

---

[1] See Davey Smith (2001) for a contemporary perspective on Morris's book.

[2] The *DSM-IV* states as follows: "In *DSM-IV*, each of the mental disorders is conceptualized as a clinically significant behavior or psychological syndrome or pattern that occurs in an individual and that is associated with present distress (e.g., a painful symptom) or disability (i.e., impairment in one or more important areas of functioning) or with a significantly increased risk of suffering death, pain, disability, or an important loss of freedom" (American Psychiatric Association 1994, pp. xxi–xxii). The *ICD-10* states as follows: "The term 'disorder' is used throughout the classification, so as to avoid even greater problems inherent in the use of terms such as 'disease' and 'illness.' 'Disorder' is not an exact term, but is used here to imply the existence of a clinically recognizable set of symptoms or behaviour associated in most cases with distress and interference with personal functions. Social deviance or conflict alone, without personal dysfunction, should not be included in mental disorder as defined here" (World Health Organization 1992, p. 5).

Organization of the Book

The book has eight parts. The first introduces our ways of thinking about the causes of mental disorders, and traces their origin in epidemiology and psychiatric epidemiology. The second presents the concept of a risk factor and the logical foundation for using cohort and case control designs to identify risk factors. Parts III and IV cover the methods of cohort and case-control studies in psychiatric epidemiology, and part V shows how to adapt the case-control design to biological psychiatry. Part VI describes statistical procedures for analyzing data from case-control and cohort study designs. Part VII extends the discussion to the study of genetic causes, showing the potential of epidemiologic designs to contribute to genetic research and vice versa, as well as the adaptations required to incorporate gene biology into our designs. In part VIII, we make the transition from identifying causes to explaining causal processes. We also present still developing concepts and methods that we believe may play an important role in the future of epidemiology.

This book is written as a single piece and is meant to be read as a whole. For readers who cannot do so, the following suggestions may provide some guidance. Those unfamiliar with epidemiology might begin with parts I–IV and then read other parts according to their specific interests. Those with substantial knowledge of epidemiology may find parts VII and VIII to be of most interest. Readers engaged in biological studies might focus on parts IV and V, and readers mainly involved in genetic studies might focus on part VII, although a full understanding depends upon the concepts introduced in previous parts of the book.

In addition to the main text, the book includes a glossary and two appendixes. The glossary comprises definitions of the key terms that appear in **bold font** in the text. The first appendix discusses in more depth our conceptual approach to studying causes and is intended mainly for readers well versed in epidemiology.

What This Book Is Not

We hasten to warn that this book is not suited for certain purposes. First, we do not summarize the current and past findings of psychiatric epidemiology. Our purpose is rather to set out a logical framework that can be used for future studies of the causes of mental disorders. We do, however, offer a historical perspective on the field and use some of the landmark studies as examples. For current and past findings, interested readers can consult the following sources: for key publications from 1900 to 1950, see Gruenberg (1950); for early textbooks on psychiatric epidemiology, see Susser (1968) and Cooper and Morgan (1973); for landmark studies and selected publications from the World Health Organization, see Reid (1960), Lin and Standley (1962), de Girolamo and Reich (1993), and Henderson (1994); for overviews and collected writings, see Weissman et al. (1986), Henderson and Burrows (1988), Mezzich et al. (1994), and Anthony et al. (1995); for epidemiologic findings on key psychiatric disorders, see Tsuang and Tohen (2002); for epidemiologic findings on child and adolescent psychiatric disorders, see Verhulst and Koot (1995); for epidemiologic findings on late life psychiatric disorders, see Mayeux and Christen (1999), Blazer et al. (2004), and Skoog (2004); for an application of epidemiology to understanding recovery from mental disorders, see Warner (2003); and for a broad synopsis, see the Surgeon General's reports on mental health (U.S. Department of Health and Human Services 1999; National Institute of Mental Health 2001).

Second, this book is not meant to replace the many excellent textbooks on general epidemiology, but rather to complement them. For introductory epidemiology, readers may consult Giesecke (2002), Aschengrau and Seage (2003), Friis and Sellers (2004), or Gordis (2004); and for more advanced epidemiology, Kelsey et al. (1986), Rothman and Greenland (1998), or Szklo and Nieto (2000). These represent only a small fraction of the books now available on the methods of general epidemiology.

Third, the book is not a manual for conducting epidemiologic studies of mental disorders. Our strategy is to introduce a small number of principles and show how they can be adapted to a wide variety of contexts. Readers seeking a more "how to" book may consult Prince et al. (2003) and Blazer and Hays (1998).

Finally, because most studies of mental disorders have been conducted in high-income countries, readers will find relatively few examples from other countries. However, in our collective experiences conducting studies in low- and middle-income countries, we have found the framework we present to be adaptable for use in these countries.

Ezra Susser, M.D., Dr.P.H.

Sharon Schwartz, Ph.D.

Alfredo Morabia, M.D., Ph.D.

Evelyn J. Bromet, Ph.D.

References

American Psychiatric Association (1994). *Diagnostic and Statistical Manual of Mental Disorders*, 4th ed. Washington, D.C.: American Psychiatric Association.

Anthony JC and Eaton WE, eds. (1995). Psychiatric Epidemiology. *Epidemiol. Rev.* 17:1–242.

Aschengrau A and Seage GR (2003). *Essentials of Epidemiology in Public Health*. Sudbury, Mass.: Jones and Bartlett.

Blazer DG and Hays JC (1998). *An Introduction to Clinical Research in Psychiatry*. New York: Oxford University Press.

Blazer DG, Steffens DC, and Busse EW, eds. (2004). *The American Psychiatric Publishing Textbook of Geriatric Psychiatry*, 3rd ed. Washington, D.C.: American Psychiatric Publishing.

Cooper B and Morgan HG (1973). *Epidemiological Psychiatry*. Springfield, Ill.: Thomas.

Davey Smith G (2001). The Uses of "Uses of Epidemiology." *Int. J. Epidemiol.* 30: 1146–1155.

de Girolamo G and Reich JH, eds. (1993). *Epidemiology of Mental Disorders and Psychosocial Problems: Personality Disorders*. Geneva, Switzerland: World Health Organization.

Friis RH and Sellers TA (2004). *Epidemiology for Public Health Practice*, 3rd ed. Sudbury, Mass.: Jones and Bartlett.

Giesecke J (2002). *Modern Infectious Disease Epidemiology*, 2nd ed. London: Arnold.

Gordis L (2004). *Epidemiology*, 3rd ed. Philadelphia: Saunders.

Gruenberg EM (1950). *Review of Available Material on Patterns of Occurrence of Mental Disorders: Major Disorders*. New York: Milbank Memorial Fund.

Henderson AS (1994). *Epidemiology of Mental Disorders and Psychosocial Problems: Dementia*. Geneva, Switzerland: World Health Organization.

Henderson AS and Burrows GD, eds. (1988). *Handbook of Social Psychiatry*. Amsterdam: Elsevier.

Kelsey JL, Thompson WD, and Evans AS (1986). *Methods in Observational Epidemiology*. New York: Oxford University Press.

Lin T and Standley C (1962). *The Scope of Epidemiology in Psychiatry*. Geneva, Switzerland: World Health Organization.

Mayeux R and Christen Y, eds. (1999). *Epidemiology of Alzheimer's Disease: From Gene to Prevention*. Berlin, Germany: Springer.

Mezzich JE and Jorge MR, eds. (1994). *Psychiatric Epidemiology: Assessment of Concepts and Methods*. Baltimore: Johns Hopkins University Press.

Morris JN (1957). *Uses of Epidemiology*. Edinburgh, Scotland: Livingstone.

National Institute of Mental Health (2001). *Mental Health: Culture, Race, and Ethnicity. A Supplement to Mental Health: A Report of the Surgeon General*. Rockville, Md.: National Institute of Mental Health.

Prince M, Stewart R, Ford T, and Hotopf M, eds. (2003). *Practical Psychiatric Epidemiology*. Oxford: Oxford University Press.

Reid DD (1960). *Epidemiological Methods in the Study of Mental Disorders*. Geneva, Switzerland: World Health Organization.

Rothman KJ and Greenland S (1998). *Modern Epidemiology*, 2nd ed. Philadelphia: Lippincott-Raven.

Skoog I (2004). Psychiatric Epidemiology of Old Age: The H70 Study—the NAPE Lecture 2003. *Acta Psychiatr. Scand.* 109:4–18.

Susser M (1968). *Community Psychiatry: Epidemiology and Social Themes*. New York: Random House.

Szklo M and Nieto FJ (2000). *Epidemiology: Beyond the Basics*. Gaithersburg, Md.: Aspen Publishing.

Tsuang M and Tohen M, eds. (2002). *Textbook in Psychiatric Epidemiology*, 2nd ed. New York: Wiley.

U. S. Department of Health and Human Services (1999). *Mental Health: A Report of the Surgeon General*. Rockville, Md.: U. S. Department of Health and Human Services.

Verhulst FC and Koot HM, eds. (1995). *The Epidemiology of Child and Adolescent Psychopathology*. Oxford: Oxford University Press.

Warner R (2003). *Recovery from Schizophrenia*, 3rd ed. New York: Brunner-Routledge.

Weissman MM, Myers JK, and Ross CE (1986). *Community Surveys of Psychiatric Disorders*. New Brunswick, N.J.: Rutgers University Press.

World Health Organization (1992). *ICD-10 Classification of Mental and Behavioural Disorders: Clinical Descriptions and Diagnostic Guidelines*. Geneva, Switzerland: World Health Organization.

Acknowledgments

Many generations of colleagues and students in the Department of Epidemiology at Columbia University (Mailman School of Public Health) and the neighboring New York State Psychiatric Institute contributed directly or indirectly to this volume. Columbia University has a strong tradition of research in psychiatric epidemiology, dating back to the influence of Joseph Zubin, Ernest Gruenberg, Zena Stein, Mervyn Susser, and Bruce Dohrenwend in the 1960s. Acknowledging this tradition, we offer a multidisciplinary and multi-institutional perspective.

We were fortunate to have three extraordinary contributions to the book from Melissa D. Begg (biostatistics), Jack M. Gorman (biological psychiatry), and Mary-Claire King (genetics and genomics). We are also grateful to current and former colleagues from Columbia who contributed expertise as coauthors of one or more chapters: Habibul Ahsan, Michaeline Bresnahan, Ana V. Diez Roux, Gary A. Heiman, Susan E. Hodge, Nancy Sohler, Regina Zimmerman.

Sir Michael Rutter served as a role model and inspiration for our work. He graciously contributed the Foreword. In addition, his critique significantly influenced the shape of the book.

Many other people read drafts and made insightful comments during the writing of the book. Sander Greenland and Myrna Weissman gave us detailed critiques of key segments of the book. Ongoing dialogue with George Davey Smith influenced our thinking in many areas. Pam Factor-Litvak, Ramin Mojtabai, and Carole Mosco reviewed numerous drafts and were extremely helpful in fashioning some of the chapters, and Michaeline Bresnahan made careful and judicious contributions to the entire text, well beyond the chapters she coauthored. We are also indebted to many others who challenged our thinking: Ulka Campbell, Katherine Chen, Pamela Collins, Sarah Conover, Linda Cottler, William Eaton, Sandro Galea, Nicolle Gatto, Madelyn Gould, Steve Hamilton, Per Magnus, Cheryl Merzel, Landon Myer, Gerald Oppenheimer, Ruth Ottman, Deb Pal, Megan Perrin, Shaun Purcell, Marcus Richards, David Rosner, Natasha Schull, Sam Shapiro, Sara Shostak, Zena Stein, Camilla Stoltenberg, Mervyn Susser, Mary Beth Terry, and Lydia Zablotska. The comments of all these people vastly improved the manuscript.

We thank Jeffrey House, our now-retired Oxford University Press editor, for nurturing this project through many drafts, never wavering in his enthusiasm.

Our most special thanks go to Kim Fader, who oversaw the preparation of the book, while at the same time providing both intellectual and moral support.

Contents

Contributors

HABIBUL AHSAN, MBBS, MMEDSC
Associate Professor of Epidemiology
  and Director, Center for Genetics in
  Epidemiology
Mailman School of Public Health
Columbia University
New York, New York

MELISSA D. BEGG, ScD
Professor of Clinical Biostatistics
Mailman School of Public Health
Columbia University
New York, New York

MICHAELINE BRESNAHAN, PhD,
  MPH
Assistant Professor of Clinical
  Epidemiology (in Psychiatry)
Mailman School of Public Health
Columbia University
New York, New York

EVELYN J. BROMET, PhD
Professor of Psychiatry and Preventive
  Medicine
Departments of Psychiatry and
  Behavioral Science and Preventive
  Medicine
State University of New York at Stony
  Brook
Stony Brook, New York

ANA V. DIEZ ROUX, MD, PhD
Associate Professor of Epidemiology
University of Michigan School of
  Public Health
Ann Arbor, Michigan

JACK M. GORMAN, MD
President and Psychiatrist-in-Chief,
  McLean Hospital
Chair, Partners Psychiatry and Mental
  Health
Professor of Psychiatry, Harvard
  Medical School
Boston, Massachusetts

GARY A. HEIMAN, PhD
Assistant Professor of Epidemiology
Mailman School of Public Health
Columbia University
New York, New York

SUSAN E. HODGE, DSc
Professor of Clinical Biostatistics (in
  Psychiatry),
Mailman School of Public Health
Columbia University
New York, New York

MARY-CLAIRE KING, PhD
American Cancer Society Professor
Departments of Medicine and Genome
  Sciences
University of Washington, Seattle
Seattle, Washington

ALFREDO MORABIA, MD, PhD
Professor and Head of the Division of
    Clinical Epidemiology
University Hospitals of Geneva
Geneva, Switzerland
Professor of Clinical Epidemiology
Mailman School of Public Health
Columbia University
New York, New York

SHARON SCHWARTZ, PhD
Associate Professor of Clinical
    Epidemiology
Mailman School of Public Health
Columbia University
New York, New York

NANCY SOHLER, PhD
Assistant Medical Professor
Department of Community Health and
    Social Medicine
City College Medical School
City University of New York
New York, New York

EZRA SUSSER, MD, DrPH
Anna Cheskis Gelman and Murray
    Charles Gelman Professor and Chair
Department of Epidemiology
Mailman School of Public Health
Columbia University
Professor of Psychiatry and
    Department Head
Epidemiology of Brain Disorders
New York State Psychiatric Institute
New York, New York

REGINA ZIMMERMAN, PhD, MPH
Director, Office of Vital Statistics
New York City Department of Health
    and Mental Hygiene
New York, New York

Psychiatric Epidemiology

PSYCHIATRIC EPIDEMIOLOGY, THEN AND NOW

I

The Burden of Mental Illness

Evelyn J. Bromet and Ezra Susser

1

We write this book at a pivotal moment in psychiatric epidemiology, the central science of public mental health. Mental disorders are now understood to be important to public health in societies of all kinds, in large part because of the findings from psychiatric epidemiology. Signifying the shift, just as the 21st century began, the World Health Organization (WHO) for the first time ranked psychiatric disorders among the leading contributors to the global burden of disease (WHO 2001). Thus, the legitimacy and importance of the public mental health mission—namely, to reduce the incidence of psychiatric disorders and improve the mental well-being of the population—have been firmly established.

The scientific developments that helped bring about this recognition of mental disorders have taken place over the past 50 years and include the development of systematic classification systems for mental disorders, evidence that mental disorders are pervasive in ordinary communities, and compelling findings about the contributions of mental disorders to the onset and course of physical diseases. This progress in psychiatric epidemiology has been influenced by—and has contributed to—progress in the treatment of mental disorders. It has also occurred in parallel with breakthroughs in basic research on the biological underpinnings of thoughts, behaviors, and feelings. Now that scientists are able to visualize and measure brain structure and function, as well as study the cellular processes that sustain them, we are beginning to illuminate the interrelationships between physiology and mental life that lie at the heart of these complex disorders (Kandel 1998).

Inspired by these developments, the authors joined together to articulate a vision for advancing psychiatric epidemiology toward discovery of the causes of mental disorders. In this and the next two chapters, we set the stage for this effort. This chapter traces the roots of psychiatric epidemiology in medical sociology and the emergence of the community survey as its predominant research design, especially in the United States. We also follow the steps taken in psychiatric epidemiology to document the burden of disease due to mental disorders. Chapter 2 shifts the focus to the evolution of causal research in epidemiology and how it influenced and was influenced by studies of psychiatric disorders. Chapter 3 introduces an integrative approach to studying causes in the present era, which will be elaborated throughout the book.

Roots in Sociology

Psychiatric epidemiology has roots in the work of early 20th century sociologists in Europe and the United States (Eaton 2001). In Europe, Emile Durkheim, one of the founders of sociology, conducted the first cross-national investigation of suicide (Durkheim 1987/1897), showing that suicide rates were higher in Protestant than in Catholic countries, and proposing that the explanation resided in differences in the countries' social structure and the individual's place within it. In the United States, the Chicago School of Social Ecology conducted a series of studies in the early 20th century on the geographic patterns of mental disorders. In one of the school's landmark studies, for example, it found the concentration of schizophrenia to be highest in inner-city neighborhoods characterized by transience and social isolation and lowest in affluent suburban districts, while the reverse pattern was found for manic depression (Faris and Dunham 1939). Both Durkheim and the Chicago school conducted **ecologic studies** in that they compared the rates of disorder across societies or communities with different characteristics (see part VIII). Their intention was to study these societal or community characteristics, rather than to elucidate individual-level risk factors for the outcomes they were evaluating. These profound works still serve as cornerstones for research on the societal determinants of mental disorders. Moreover, they are increasingly recognized as the antecedents of the burgeoning field of social epidemiology.

The Development of Community Surveys

In the period after World War II, a distinct discipline of psychiatric epidemiology emerged. Some investigators continued to explore the social determinants of suicide and schizophrenia. But the studies in this period focused more on individual-level social risk factors, and accordingly, they were generally conducted *within* rather than *across* societies or communities. Notably, studies of suicide made innovative forays into risk factor research using case-control designs (e.g., MacMahon and Pugh 1965; Kreitman 1977), and studies of schizophrenia focused on the association between social class and disease (e.g., Hollingshead and Redlich 1958).

A predominant thrust of psychiatric epidemiology in the United States in the aftermath of World War II, however, pertained to psychological symptoms and impairments rather than to psychiatric disorders per se. Experience during World War II with psychological testing of incoming military recruits suggested that psychological impairments were far more common than had been previously suspected. This stimulated intriguing questions about the overall frequency of symptoms in the community and their relationship to social experiences.

To investigate these questions, psychiatric epidemiologists turned to the community survey, a method under development in sociology at the time. As used in psychiatric epidemiology, community surveys incorporated sophisticated sampling techniques to draw a representative sample and borrowed from the advances in psychological measurement made by U.S. Army psychologists during the war (Nunnally 1967). They generally measured the **point prevalence** of symptoms, that is, the proportion of persons with symptoms at the time of the survey (other measures of prevalence are defined in chapter 8).

Some of the most influential community surveys were designed and conducted by teams of psychiatrists, sociologists, and psychologists, setting a precedent for interdisciplinary work in psychiatric epidemiology that continues to this day. For example, the psychiatrist Thomas Rennie and sociologist Leo Srole designed the Midtown Manhattan Study in the early 1950s, in which approximately 1600 adults were interviewed with a detailed symptom inventory (Srole et al. 1962). This study captured the popular imagination—and provoked much criticism—by reporting that impairment due to psychological symptoms was surprisingly common in what was perceived as the most advanced locale on the globe. Eighty percent of respondents had current affective or psychophysiological symptoms, and 20 percent were judged by psychiatrists to be severely impaired. The correlates of psychological impairment included being female, having lower socioeconomic status, and experiencing greater social adversity.

Another landmark community survey took place in a rural county of Nova Scotia at about the same time (Leighton 1959). In this study, too, psychological impairment was found to be common, and was correlated with gender and social factors. The Nova Scotia study was led by Alexander Leighton, a professor of psychiatry, sociology, and anthropology. He was especially interested in comparing the mental health of communities with different sociocultural characteristics (Leighton 1959; Hughes et al. 1960; Leighton et al. 1963), and later went on to study mental disorders in the very different sociocultural setting of Nigeria (Leighton 1963). The Midtown and Nova Scotia samples were also reinterviewed many years later (e.g., Srole and Fischer 1980; Murphy et al. 2004).

Short screening scales were derived from each of these studies: the 22-Item Scale from the Midtown study and the Health Opinion Survey from the Nova Scotia study. These scales were subsequently used in many community surveys examining the relationship of stress to symptomatology. Looking for such associations can be seen as a first step toward understanding causes (Schwab and Schwab 1978). However, the results for psychological symptoms could not be directly related to specific mental disorders.

The field developed somewhat differently in Europe during this period. Commentaries and textbooks tended to emphasize the commonalities between the application of epidemiology to psychiatric disorders and application to other diseases (Lin and Standley 1962; Susser 1968; Cooper and Morgan 1973). Although excellent community surveys were conducted (Essen-Möller et al. 1956; Goodman and Tizard 1962; Rutter et al. 1970; Graham and Rutter 1973), more attention was given to studying disorders, as well as symptoms;

incidence, as well as prevalence; genetic, as well as social environmental, causes; and psychiatric registry patients, as well as community populations. In addition, the study of mental disorders in primary care was launched in England, with the pioneering work of Michael Shepherd and colleagues (Shepherd 1985) showing that mental disorders were common in general medical practice and that it was sometimes difficult to demarcate clear boundaries between mental and physical disorders. The importance of these European contributions to building a foundation for causal research will be evident, as we take up these themes in later chapters.

Diagnosing Mental Disorders in Community Surveys

By the 1980s, psychiatric epidemiologists in the United States had shifted their focus from symptoms to diagnosable disorders (Weissman and Klerman 1978). The design of the community survey was adapted to measure the frequency of psychiatric diagnoses rather than psychological symptoms. Three watershed events set the stage for this development.

First, a series of studies produced evidence that psychiatric disorders in adults could be reliably diagnosed. This was achieved by using clinician-administered standardized assessments with systematic diagnostic criteria: for example, the Renard Diagnostic Interview with Feighner criteria (Robins et al. 1981), and the Schedule for Affective Disorders and Schizophrenia with Research Diagnostic Criteria (Rice et al. 1989). The usefulness of the approach was demonstrated in the U.S.-U.K. project that showed that a previously observed striking difference between the two countries—a higher frequency of schizophrenia in U.S. psychiatric patients and a higher frequency of depression in U.K. psychiatric patients—disappeared when comparable diagnostic criteria and systematic interviewing techniques were used (Cooper et al. 1972). Also influential was WHO's cross-national program of research on schizophrenia (WHO 1974), which verified that a core set of criteria and a standard assessment instrument, the Present State Examination (Wing et al. 1974; Wing and Nixon 1975), could be applied reliably in diverse cultures around the globe.

Second, studies demonstrated that it was feasible to administer these diagnostic assessments to adults in community settings. In New Haven (Weissman and Myers 1980) and in the Three Mile Island area after the nuclear power plant accident (Bromet et al. 1982), the Schedule for Affective Disorders and Schizophrenia was employed in follow-ups of community samples. In the WHO Ten Country Study, the Present State Examination was adopted to determine the incidence and early manifestations of schizophrenia in defined communities across the globe (Jablensky et al. 1992). Meanwhile, the Isle of Wight study developed and employed standardized methods to assess psychiatric and behavioral, as well as other, disorders among children in a community sample (Rutter et al. 1970).

Third, in 1980 the American Psychiatric Association published the third edition of the *Diagnostic and Statistical Manual of Mental Disorders* (*DSM-III*). This was the first official nosology to include operational criteria for all major diagnoses. The criteria were chosen to facilitate reliable diagnoses and derived in part from previous research studies (Feighner et al. 1972; Spitzer et al. 1978). Successive editions of the *DSM* and the *ICD* (*International Classification of Diseases*, published by WHO) nosologies have continued and refined this approach (Mezzich et al. 1994).

Shortly after these watershed events, community surveys in the United States incorporated the *DSM-III* criteria and thereby took a quantum leap (Klerman 1990; Robins 1990). The Epidemiologic Catchment Area study launched by the National Institute of Mental Health (NIMH) determined the frequency of psychiatric diagnoses in approximately 20,000 adults living in selected neighborhoods of five U.S. communities (Regier et al. 1984; Robins and Regier 1991). The Diagnostic Interview Schedule (DIS), a fully structured interview designed to yield *DSM-III* diagnoses, was administered by lay (non–clinically trained) interviewers, which reduced the cost of such a large-scale undertaking. The training of the interviewers was standardized, and the diagnostic algorithm was computer scored. The subsequent 1990–1992 and 2001–2002 National Comorbidity Surveys (Kessler et al. 1994; Kessler et al. 2003) took the process still another step, assessing mental disorders in a national probability sample in the United States, with a modified version of the Composite International Diagnostic Interview (CIDI), also administered by lay interviewers.

Taken together, these studies suggested that in the United States approximately 15–25 percent of adults age 18–64 currently suffer from one or more mental disorders (Regier et al. 1988; Robins and Regier 1991; Kessler et al. 1994; Satcher 2000; Narrow et al. 2002). Moreover, they demonstrated that mental disorders are highly comorbid with one another and that for a great many disorders of adulthood the onset of symptoms occurs in childhood or adolescence. Though fewer studies have been conducted with children and the elderly, the evidence suggests the prevalence is at least as high in these age groups (NIMH 1999; Tsuang and Tohen 2002). Thus, the high prevalence of psychological symptoms and impairment reported by the early community surveys, dismissed by many as implausible, was replicated in studies of psychiatric diagnoses. Moreover, several correlates of psychological symptoms identified in the earlier surveys, such as gender, social class, family dysfunction, and environmental adversity, were shown to be associated with specific diagnosable disorders.

Global Burden of Disease

The DIS and the CIDI have now been used in numerous surveys of adults in communities across the globe (Wittchen et al. 1994; Weissman et al. 1996; Kessler 1999; Patel 2001). Most recently, a revised version of the CIDI (Kessler and Üstün 2004) was used in more than 30 countries as part of the World Mental Health initiative (Üstün 1999). As expected from previous surveys, the preliminary results indicate a consistently high overall prevalence of mental disorder, but they also suggest important variations in specific mental disorders across these countries (Demyttenaere et al. 2004).

High as the prevalence figures may be, they do not capture the full magnitude of the impact of psychiatric disorders. This requires considering not only the frequency of these disorders, but also their impact on individual quality of life and on societal development. By conceptualizing the burden of diseases in terms of the years of disability they cause (Murray and Lopez 1996; Mathers et al. 2000; Olesen and Leonardi 2003), one sees the true centrality of mental disorders in human societies. From this broader perspective, WHO has projected that depression will be the second leading cause of disability across the globe by the year 2020 (cardiovascular disease is first; Murray and Lopez 1996; Üstün et al. 2004).

To place mental disorders within this broader perspective required other kinds of studies in addition to the community surveys. First, epidemiologists quantified the impact of mental disorders on outcomes such as days absent from work and use of health care services (Ormel et al. 1994; Goldberg and Lecrubier 1995; Alonso et al. 2004; Simon et al. 2004). Second, they traced the long-term course of severe mental disorders, which are difficult to diagnose in community surveys (Anthony et al. 1985; Kendler et al. 1996) and are relatively rare, but which may cause decades or even a lifetime of disability in an affected individual, as well as call upon the resources of family members and health care systems over a long period (Jarbrink et al. 2003). Third, they explored the consequences of mental disorders across different cultural and socioeconomic contexts (Desjarlais et al. 1996). All this work together provided the foundation to comprehend the global burden of mental illness.

Limitations of Community Surveys

Successful in establishing the frequency and correlates of mental disorders in communities, surveys proved to have limited utility in establishing causes and prognosis. As we explain in later chapters, this is in part because prevalence reflects two distinct components: **incidence** and **duration** (see chapter 8). Studies that separate these components are more informative about causes and about prognosis.

Though often overshadowed, the search for causes continued alongside the community surveys throughout this time. There were studies that compared mental disorders across different kinds of societies (Murphy 1976). A prime example is the WHO Ten-Country Study that was used to compare the incidence and prognosis of schizophrenia and other psychotic disorders in developing and developed country sites (Jablensky et al. 1992; Susser and Wanderling 1994). There were also numerous studies using risk factor designs, such as cohort and case-control studies. In the next chapters, we turn to the development of risk factor studies and the potential for building upon them.

Conclusion

Over a 50-year period, psychiatric morbidity surveys have brought remarkable advances in knowledge. Ultimately, these studies helped to fulfill an overarching mission of psychiatric epidemiology: to bring about the recognition of mental disorders in public health. With this achievement behind us, we and others believe that the time has come to shift the balance from examining prevalence to finding the causes of these conditions (Mann 1997; Anthony and Van Etten 1998; Eaton and Merikangas 2000; Wyatt and Susser 2000; McGrath 2003).

References

Alonso J, Angermeyer MC, and Lepine JP (2004). The European Study of the Epidemiology of Mental Disorders (ESEMeD) Project: an Epidemiological Basis for Informing Mental Health Policies in Europe. *Acta Psychiatr. Scand. Suppl.* 420:5–7.

Anthony JC, Folstein M, Romanoski AJ, et al. (1985). Comparison of the Lay Diagnostic Interview Schedule and a Standardized Psychiatric Diagnosis. Experience in Eastern Baltimore. *Arch. Gen. Psychiatry* 42:667–675.

Anthony JC and Van Etten ML (1998). Epidemiology and Its Rubrics. In Bellack and Hersen, eds., *Comprehensive Clinical Psychology*, 355–390. Amsterdam: Pergamon Press.

Bromet E, Schulberg HC, and Dunn L (1982). Reactions of Psychiatric Patients to the Three Mile Island Nuclear Accident. *Arch. Gen. Psychiatry* 39:725–730.

Cooper B and Morgan HG (1973). *Epidemiological Psychiatry*. Springfield, Ill.: Thomas.

Cooper JE, Kendell RE, Gurland BJ, Sharpe L, and Copeland JRM (1972). *Psychiatric Diagnosis in New York and London: A Comparative Study of Mental Hospital Admissions*. London: Oxford University Press.

Demyttenaere K, Bruffaerts R, Posada-Villa J, et al. (2004). Prevalence, Severity, and Unmet Need for Treatment of Mental Disorders in the World Health Organization World Mental Health Surveys. *JAMA* 291:2581–2590.

Desjarlais R, Eisenberg L, Good B, and Kleinman A, eds. (1996). *World Mental Health: Problems and Priorities in Low-Income Countries*. New York: Oxford University Press.

Durkheim E (1987/1897). *Le Suicide*. New York: Free Press.

Eaton W (2001). *The Sociology of Mental Disorders*, 3rd ed. Westport Conn.: Praeger.

Eaton WW and Merikangas KR (2000). Psychiatric Epidemiology: Progress and Prospects in the Year 2000. *Epidemiol. Rev.* 22:29–34.

Essen-Möller E, Larsson H, Uddenberg CE, and White G (1956). Individual Traits and Morbidity in a Swedish Rural Population. *Acta Psychiatr. Neurol. Scand.* (*Suppl.* 100):1–160.

Faris R and Dunham H (1939). *Mental Disorders in Urban Areas: an Ecological Study of Schizophrenia and Other Psychoses*. New York: Hafner Publishing.

Feighner JP, Robins E, Guze SB, Woodruff RA, Jr., Winokur G, and Munoz R (1972). Diagnostic Criteria for Use in Psychiatric Research. *Arch. Gen. Psychiatry* 26:57–63.

Goldberg D and Lecrubier Y (1995). Form and Frequency of Mental Disorders Across Centres. In Üstün TB and Sartorius N, eds. *Mental Illness in General Health Care: An International Study*. Chichester, U.K.: Wiley.

Goodman N and Tizard J (1962). Prevalence of Imbecility and Idiocy among Children. *BMJ* 5273:216–219.

Graham P and Rutter M (1973). Psychiatric Disorder in the Young Adolescent: a Follow-up Study. *Proc. R. Soc. Med.* 66:1226–1229.

Hollingshead A and Redlich F (1958). *Social Class and Mental Illness*. New York: Wiley.

Hughes CC, Tremblay MA, Rapoport RN, and Leighton AH (1960). *People of Cove and Woodlot: Communities from the Viewpoint of Social Psychiatry*. Vol. 2, *Stirling County Study of Psychiatric Disorder and Sociocultural Environment*. New York: Basic Books.

Jablensky A, Sartorius N, Ernberg G, Anker M, Korten A, Cooper JE, Day R, and Bertelsen A (1992). Schizophrenia: Manifestations, Incidence and Course in Different Cultures. A World Health Organization Ten-Country Study. *Psychol. Med. Monogr. Suppl.* 20:1–97.

Jarbrink K, Fombonne E, and Knapp M (2003). Measuring the Parental, Service and Cost Impacts of Children with Autistic Spectrum Disorder: A Pilot Study. *J. Autism Dev. Disord.* 33:395–402.

Kandel ER (1998). A New Intellectual Framework for Psychiatry. *Am. J. Psychiatry* 155:457–469.

Kendler KS, Gallagher TJ, Abelson JM, and Kessler RC (1996). Lifetime Prevalence, Demographic Risk Factors, and Diagnostic Validity of Nonaffective Psychosis as Assessed in a U.S. Community Sample. The National Comorbidity Survey. *Arch. Gen. Psychiatry* 53:1022–1031.

Kessler RC (1999). The World Health Organization International Consortium in Psychiatric Epidemiology (ICPE): Initial Work and Future Directions—the NAPE Lecture 1998. Nordic Association for Psychiatric Epidemiology. *Acta Psychiatr. Scand.* 99:2–9.

Kessler RC, Berglund P, Demler O, Jin R, Koretz D, Merikangas KR, Rush AJ, Walters EE, and Wang PS (2003). The Epidemiology of Major Depressive Disorder: Results from the National Comorbidity Survey Replication (NCS-R). *JAMA* 289: 3095–3105.

Kessler RC, McGonagle KA, Zhao S, Nelson CB, Hughes M, Eshleman S, Wittchen HU, and Kendler KS (1994). Lifetime and 12-Month Prevalence of *DSM-III-R* Psychiatric Disorders in the United States. Results from the National Comorbidity Survey. *Arch. Gen. Psychiatry* 51:8–19.

Kessler RC and Üstün TB (2004). The World Mental Health (WMH) Survey Initiative Version of the World Health Organization (WHO) Composite International Diagnostic Interview (CIDI). *Int. J. Methods Psychiatr. Res.* 13:93–121.

Klerman GL (1990). Paradigm Shifts in USA Psychiatric Epidemiology since World War II. *Soc. Psychiatry Psychiatr. Epidemiol.* 25:27–32.

Kreitman N (1977). *Parasuicide.* London: Wiley.

Leighton AH (1959). *My Name Is Legion: Foundations for a Theory of Man in Relation to Culture.* Vol 1, *The Stirling County Study of Psychiatric Disorder and Sociocultural Environment.* New York: Basic Books.

Leighton AH (1963). *Psychiatric Disorder among the Yoruba: A Report from the Cornell-Aro Mental Health Research Project in the Western Region, Nigeria.* Ithaca, N.Y.: Cornell University Press.

Leighton DC, Harding JS, Macklin DB, MacMillan AM, and Leighton AH (1963). *The Character of Danger: Psychiatric Symptoms in Selected Communities.* Vol. 3, *Stirling County Study of Psychiatric Disorder and Sociocultural Environment.* New York: Basic Books.

Lin T and Standley C (1962). *The Scope of Epidemiology in Psychiatry.* Geneva, Switzerland: World Health Organization.

MacMahon B and Pugh T (1965). Suicide in the Widowed. *Am. J. Epidemiol.* 81:23–31.

Mann A (1997). The Evolving Face of Psychiatric Epidemiology. *Br. J. Psychiatry* 171:314–318.

Mathers CD, Stein C, and Fath DM (2000). *Global Burden of Disease 2000: Discussion Paper No. 50.* Geneva, Switzerland: World Health Organization.

McGrath JJ (2003). Invited Commentary: Gaining Traction on the Epidemiologic Landscape of Schizophrenia. *Am. J. Epidemiol.* 158:301–304.

Mezzich JE, Jorge MR, and Salloum IM (1994). *Psychiatric Epidemiology: Assessment of Concepts and Methods.* Baltimore: Johns Hopkins University Press.

Murphy JM (1976). Psychiatric Labeling in Cross-Cultural Perspective. *Science* 191:1019–1028.

Murphy JM, Horton NJ, Laird NM, Monson RR, Sobol AM, and Leighton AH (2004). Anxiety and Depression: A 40-Year Perspective on Relationships Regarding Prevalence, Distribution, and Comorbidity. *Acta Psychiatr. Scand.* 109:355–375.

Murray CJL and Lopez AD (1996). *The Global Burden of Disease: a Comprehensive Assessment of Mortality and Disability from Diseases, Injuries, and Risk Factors in 1990 and Projected to 2020.* Cambridge, Mass.: Harvard University Press.

Narrow WE, Rae DS, Robins LN, and Regier DA (2002). Revised Prevalence Estimates of Mental Disorders in the United States: Using a Clinical Significance Criterion to Reconcile 2 Surveys' Estimates. *Arch. Gen. Psychiatry* 59:115–123.

National Institute of Mental Health (2001). *Mental Health: Culture, Race, and Ethnicity. A Supplement to Mental Health: A Reports of the Surgeon General.* Rockville, Md.: National Institute of Mental Health.

Nunnally JC (1967). *Psychometric Theory.* London: McGraw-Hill.

Olesen J and Leonardi M (2003). The Burden of Brain Diseases in Europe. *Eur. J. Neurol.* 10:471–477.

Ormel J, VonKorff M, Ustun TB, Pini S, Korten A, and Oldehinkel T (1994). Common Mental Disorders and Disability across Cultures. Results from the WHO Collaborative Study on Psychological Problems in General Health Care. *JAMA* 272:1741–1748.

Patel V (2001). Poverty, Inequality, and Mental Health in Developing Countries. In Leon DA and Walt G, eds., *Poverty, Inequality, and Health*, pp. 247–262. Oxford, U.K.: Oxford University Press.

Regier DA, Boyd JH, Burke JD, Jr., et al. (1988). One-Month Prevalence of Mental Disorders in the United States. Based on Five Epidemiologic Catchment Area Sites. *Arch. Gen. Psychiatry* 45:977–986.

Regier DA, Myers JK, Kramer M, Robins LN, Blazer DG, Hough RL, Eaton WW, and Locke BZ (1984). The NIMH Epidemiologic Catchment Area Program. Historical Context, Major Objectives, and Study Population Characteristics. *Arch. Gen. Psychiatry* 41:934–941.

Rice J, Andreasen NC, Coryell W, et al. (1989). NIMH Collaborative Program on the Psychobiology of Depression: Clinical. *Genet. Epidemiol.* 6:179–182.

Robins LN (1990). Psychiatric Epidemiology—a Historic Review. *Soc. Psychiatry Psychiatr. Epidemiol.* 25:16–26.

Robins LN, Helzer JE, Croughan J, and Ratcliff KS (1981). National Institute of Mental Health Diagnostic Interview Schedule. Its History, Characteristics, and Validity. *Arch. Gen. Psychiatry* 38:381–389.

Robins LN and Regier DA, eds. (1991). *Psychiatric Disorders in America: The Epidemiological Catchment Area Study.* New York: Free Press.

Rutter M, Tizard J, and Whitmore K (1970). *Education, Health and Behaviour.* Harlow, U.K.: Longman.

Satcher D (2000). Mental Health: A Report of the Surgeon General. *Prof. Psychol. Res. Prac.* 31:5–13.

Schwab J and Schwab ME (1978). *Sociocultural Roots of Mental Illness: An Epidemiologic Survey.* New York: Plenum Medical Book Co.

Shepherd M (1985). Psychiatric Epidemiology and Epidemiological Psychiatry. *Am. J. Public Health* 75:275–276.

Simon GE, Fleck M, Lucas R, and Bushnell DM (2004). Prevalence and Predictors of Depression Treatment in an International Primary Care Study. *Am. J. Psychiatry* 161:1626–1634.

Spitzer RL, Endicott J, and Robins E (1978). Research Diagnostic Criteria: Rationale and Reliability. *Arch. Gen. Psychiatry* 35:773–782.

Srole L and Fischer AK (1980). The Midtown Manhattan Longitudinal Study vs. "the Mental Paradise Lost" Doctrine. A Controversy Joined. *Arch. Gen. Psychiatry* 37:209–221.

Srole L, Langer TS, Michael ST, Kirkpatrick P, Opler M, and Rennie TA (1962). *Mental Health in the Metropolis.* New York: Harper & Row.

Susser E and Wanderling J (1994). Epidemiology of Nonaffective Acute Remitting Psychosis vs. Schizophrenia. Sex and Sociocultural Setting. *Arch. Gen. Psychiatry* 51:294–301.

Susser M (1968). *Community Psychiatry: Epidemiology and Social Themes.* New York: Random House.

Tsuang M and Tohen M, eds. (2002). *Textbook In Psychiatric Epidemiology*, 2nd ed. New York: Wiley.

Üstün TB (1999). The Global Burden of Mental Disorders. *Am. J. Public Health* 89:1315–1318.

Üstün TB, Ayuso-Mateos JL, Chatterji S, Mathers C, and Murray CJ (2004). Global Burden of Depressive Disorders in the Year 2000. *Br. J. Psychiatry* 184:386–392.

U.S. Department of Health and Human Services, (1999). *Mental Health: A Report of the Surgeon General*. Rockville, Md.: U.S. Department of Health and Human Services.

Weissman MM, Bland RC, Canino GJ, et al. (1996). Cross-National Epidemiology of Major Depression and Bipolar Disorder. *JAMA* 276:293–299.

Weissman MM and Klerman GL (1978). Epidemiology of Mental Disorders: Emerging Trends in the United States. *Arch. Gen. Psychiatry* 35:705–712.

Weissman MM and Myers JK (1980). Psychiatric Disorders in a U.S. Community. The Application of Research Diagnostic Criteria to a Resurveyed Community Sample. *Acta Psychiatr. Scand.* 62:99–111.

Wing J and Nixon J (1975). Discriminating Symptoms in Schizophrenia. A Report from the International Pilot Study of Schizophrenia. *Arch. Gen. Psychiatry* 32:853–859.

Wing JK, Cooper JE, and Sartorius N (1974). *The Measurement and Classification of Psychiatric Symptoms*. New York: Cambridge University Press.

Wittchen HU, Zhao S, Kessler RC, and Eaton WW (1994). *DSM-III-R* Generalized Anxiety Disorder in the National Comorbidity Survey. *Arch. Gen. Psychiatry* 51:355–364.

World Health Organization (1974). The International Pilot Study of Schizophrenia. *Schizophr. Bull.* 1:21–34.

World Health Organization (2001). *The World Health Report: 2001; Mental Health: New Understanding, New Hope*. Geneva, Switzerland: World Health Organization.

Wyatt RJ and Susser E (2000). U.S. Birth Cohort Studies of Schizophrenia: A Sea Change. *Schizophr. Bull.* 26:255–256.

The Arc of Epidemiology

2

Ezra Susser and Alfredo Morabia

It is useful to view epidemiology through a lens that connects the underlying assumptions about causes of disease with the methods used to find them (Schwartz et al. 1999). Here we offer a historical overview along these lines, necessarily brief and selective. We trace the evolution of causal concepts up to the present time, and within this evolution locate findings about mental disorders, findings that serve as important precedents for our endeavor.

From this vantage point, the past evolution of epidemiology comprised three broad eras spanning the period from the beginning of the 19th to the close of the 20th century (Susser and Susser 1996). Each era lasted about 50–75 years and introduced a distinctive way of thinking about the causes of disease. The transition from one era to the next brought a powerful new strategy for finding causes and improving public health, but also led to the neglect of approaches developed in the previous eras, so that the field took "three steps forward and one step back."

A fourth era is emerging, although its shape is not yet clear. In the next chapter, we outline how we hope to see it evolve. In retrospect, each of the three previous eras—sanitary, infectious disease, and risk factor epidemiology—can be seen as focusing on causes at a particular level: the societal, cellular, and individual level, respectively. Our conceptual schema seeks to integrate the causal concepts that were dominant in each of these eras, in order to illuminate the causes and prevention of disease at multiple levels. Therefore, we also identify within each of the past eras epidemiologists who embraced an integrated approach along the lines that we and others now espouse.

Sanitary Era (Approximately 1840–1890)

The crucible for the birth of public health was 19th century Europe amid the throes of the Industrial Revolution (Susser 1973; Hamlin 1998; Porter 1999). In England, which set the precedent for many other countries, the earliest practitioners of public health were social reformers concerned with all aspects of society, not only health but also demographic, social, political, and economic conditions.[1] A movement specifically concerned with public health reform emerged around midcentury. Public health reformers collecting and analyzing empirical data acquired the appellation of "epidemiologists."

The leaders of public health reform harbored the belief that overcrowding in urban areas was toxic to the physical and mental health of the population. Poor sanitary conditions were often seen as the chief culprit. Hence, they were labeled "sanitarians." With some success, they advocated for urban sewage systems and cleaner water supplies, which remain basic goals of public health that are still not met in large parts of the world. The sanitarians were reformers, not revolutionaries; sometimes sanitary reforms were even advocated as a means to stave off the threat of revolution (Hamlin 1998).

The sanitarians rightly perceived that the societal transformation of the Industrial Revolution was the engine driving the population's ill health. Rapid urbanization and stark social inequalities were indeed producing overcrowding and poor sanitation, among other harmful effects. Most of them also believed, however, that these factors contributed to the proliferation of disease by generating "miasma," a noxious vapor that arose from decaying organic matter such as sewage. So strongly did some of the sanitary era's leaders believe in miasma, that they fought hard and long, even until the century's end, against the competing idea that germs transmitted diseases.

The miasma theory was dominant but by no means unchallenged. An especially significant challenge came from John Snow, who established that cholera was transmitted by the water supply, well before the discovery of the vibrio cholera bacterium. Snow entertained ideas about causes at many levels: societal change created a favorable context for epidemic spread of cholera, the privately owned and profitable water supply was the primary mode of transmission within this context, household and individual habits also influenced disease transmission, and a microorganism was likely to be discovered as the primary source (Davey Smith 2002; Vinten-Johansen et al. 2003).

Although mistaken about miasma, 19th century public health reformers were correct in recognizing that toxic environmental exposures could have adverse health effects (Lilienfeld 2000; Vandenbroucke 2000). At least some were aware that specific environmental toxins could produce mental disorders. Mercury exposure, for example, was understood to be a cause of psychosis (Chapin 1863; Baldi et al. 1953). Mercury was extensively used in the hat-making trade, and Lewis Carroll referred to the Hatter in Alice in Wonderland as "mad." The commonly used phrase, "mad as a hatter," referred to the hallucinations, delusions, and mania seen in aging workers in the hat industry who had high-level exposure to mercury.[2] Lead is another example

---

[1] Some countries, most notably France, developed public health in parallel along broadly similar lines. The French Revolution and Napoleonic wars were important influences in France even before industrialization. Pinel in France (and also Leuret) preceded William Farr in collecting quantitative data on mental patients (Coleman 1982; Morens D, personal communication, April 2004).

[2] Although the connection between mercury-soaked materials handled by hat makers and their tremors, confused speech, and other symptoms was commonly accepted, in fact the phrase "mad as a hatter" may have had other origins (Ward 1980).

of a toxic exposure long suspected to have adverse effects on the mind (Hernberg 2000). In the subsequent era, the evidence for these connections was sometimes overlooked, in part because powerful industrialists sought to suppress it (Markowitz and Rosner 2002).

William Farr, one of epidemiology's founders, reconstructed and analyzed the national registry of vital statistics. Notably, he was among the first epidemiologists to concern himself with the study of mental illness. In an early intimation of what we now call clinical epidemiology, Farr investigated mortality among inmates of English asylums in the 1830s (Farr 1841; Susser and Adelstein 1975). The findings were grim. Annual patient death rates in these institutions ranged from 11 to 27 percent; 27 percent was "as high as the rate of mortality experienced by the British troops on the western coast of Africa and by the population of London when the plague rendered its habitations desolate" (Susser and Adelstein 1975, p. 429).

During the sanitary era, many argued that there was an epidemic of insanity, and some attributed it to the stresses of urban life. John Snow was among those who turned their attention to this debate. He argued that the apparent increase in insanity was more likely due to an increase in detection and detention of the mentally ill than to incidence (Westminster Medical Society 1841). This question is still unresolved and continues to intrigue researchers today (Bresnahan et al. 2003).

Infectious Disease Era (Approximately 1890–1950)

At the turn of the century, epidemiology underwent a dramatic transition spurred by the new science of microbiology—fostered by Henle, Pasteur, Koch, and others—which had produced definitive evidence that germs were causes of human disease (Winslow 1943). Instead of focusing on societal-level causes, epidemiologists now focused on a different kind of cause—a germ— and as a result they also changed their methods for identifying causes. In this period, epidemiology came to be defined as the study of infectious diseases.

The infectious agents were identified by analysis of biological specimens. Furthermore, these infectious causes were viewed as specific and unique to the disease; that is, a cause was related to one disorder and a disorder was related to one cause (Susser 1973; Evans 1993). The goal was to detect the **"necessary"** and preferably **"sufficient" cause** of a disease. These concepts were embodied in the famous Henle-Koch postulates—still used by some microbiologists today—for establishing an infectious agent as a cause of disease. The postulates require, among other things, that the causative agent be present in all individuals with the disease and absent in individuals without the disease.

The identification of infectious agents led to powerful new insights about the etiology of many diseases. In some exceptional instances, it also led quite rapidly to therapeutic interventions. General paresis, a late consequence of syphilis, was one of the main causes of insanity and of mental hospital admissions. The discovery of the spirochete causing syphilis was followed by the development of Salvarsan 606, the first therapeutic drug chemically designed to counter an infectious agent and so named because it took 606 experiments to find the compound that worked (Ehrlich 1911; Himmelweit and Dale 1956). The drug was partially effective and no doubt prevented many cases of syphilis from progressing to insanity.

Learning how to apply these insights to improve public health was a long process, however, and the resulting changes were gradual and difficult to gauge. The early microbiologists did not fully understand that whether an individual reaches the point of disease depends upon many other factors within the individual. This delayed the recognition that an individual can harbor a silent infection without manifesting the disease and transmit this infection to others (Winslow 1943). It also led some epidemiologists to focus narrowly on interrupting transmission of specific germs and pay little attention to sanitary improvements and other general public health measures.

Germs were studied by microscopic examination at the cellular level. A bacterium is a cell, and it produces disease by attacking the cells of the afflicted person. To understand the onset of disease in an individual, however, requires studying a higher level of organization than the cell. For disease to occur, the cumulative damage must be enough to disrupt the functioning of a system of cells such as the neural system and, ultimately, the individual human being. To understand the emergence of an epidemic in a human population requires studying a still higher level of organization, the social relationships among individuals in the population (see part VIII).

In the first large-scale attempt to apply microbiology to public health practice (Markel 1997; Hammonds 1999; Winkelstein 2000), microscopic examination was brought into play in the response to epidemics of cholera, typhoid, and diphtheria in New York City. Shortly thereafter, in both the United States and Europe the colonial expansion stimulated investment in conquering "tropical" diseases such as yellow fever and malaria (Stepan 1978; Farley 1991). In the course of these efforts, the importance of also studying the host and the population (and sometimes the vector) became evident. Ultimately, infectious disease epidemiologists broadened their perspective, adopting the notion of a system comprising the infectious agent, the host, and the environment.

Despite the preoccupation with infectious diseases, some epidemiologists pursued other lines of investigation (Hardy 2004). An especially important discovery of this era was that a nutritional deficiency causes pellagra (Terris 1964; Barrett-Connor 1967; Etheridge 1972; Kraut 2003). Pellagra was recognized as epidemic in the south of the United States in the early twentieth century and was often attributed to an infectious agent. Public Health Service physician Joseph Goldberger disputed this view and examined nutritional causes in what became a multifaceted research program. In experimental studies, mainly in institutions, he showed that giving better food prevented pellagra. In observational studies of South Carolina mill villages (done with economist and statistician Edgar Sydenstricker (Kasius 1974), he showed that diets deficient in fresh meat and milk products were associated with pellagra. Laboratory research was initiated to identify the lacking micronutrient.[3]

---

[3] Ultimately, in 1937 Conrad Elvehjem, an agricultural chemist, pinpointed that niacin (vitamin B-3) cured "black tongue," a condition analogous to pellagra in dogs (Elvehjem et al. 2002).

Campaigns were launched for improved economic and social conditions as required for better nutrition. Thus was pioneered a multilevel research program to elucidate a cause of disease and then prevent it.

This program of research was stimulated in part by startling outbreaks of pellagra mortality among patients in "insane asylums." Goldberger's nutritional hypothesis derived in large part from observations that the disease affected the inmates but not the staff of these asylums, a pattern that seemed incompatible with an infectious cause. A puzzle was that asylum staff allegedly ate the same meals as patients. By actually observing the interactions among patients and staff, Goldberger solved the puzzle. The staff kept the meat and milk mainly for themselves and supplemented their diet with outside food.

There was also another connection between pellagra and mental illness. Pellagra often had psychiatric manifestations and was recognized as an important cause of mental illness in the south. Thus, it could be a cause as well as a consequence of being in an insane asylum. It is not surprising, then, that psychiatrists played a leading role in the study of pellagra before and then with Goldberger. Psychiatric patients were often the subjects of Goldberger's experiments. An experiment typically involved giving one group of patients nutritious food while keeping the others on the usual deficient diet. Although these groundbreaking studies were ethical by the standards of the time, some of this work was clearly unethical by today's standards. One study even included the experimental induction of pellagra by giving a deficient diet to prisoner volunteers.

Risk Factor Era (Approximately 1950–2010)

In the period after World War II, epidemiology once again changed radically. In the developed countries, infectious diseases were declining while the so-called diseases of civilization—notably cardiovascular disease, cancer, and peptic ulcer—were increasing at an alarming rate. In this context, leading epidemiologists turned away from the search for infectious agents and took up the challenge of discovering the causes of the new, apparently noninfectious, disease epidemics (Ryle 1948; Morris 1957; Lilienfeld 1976).

As interest shifted away from infectious diseases, the singular notion of necessary and sufficient causes was replaced by the concept of risk factors, that is, a combination of factors causes the disease, and each of them increases the probability of disease in an individual. Thus, we no longer think of *the* cause of a disease, but rather assume that diseases are produced by multiple interacting causes and that the same disease may be caused through different pathways. In the following chapters we will describe this causal paradigm in some detail.

In parallel, step by step, the methods for identifying risk factors, such as cohort and case-control designs, were developed, articulated, and refined (Susser 1985; Morabia 2004). The approach was labeled chronic disease epidemiology. Although the label stuck, it was a misnomer, because the approach is relevant to any kind of disease, indeed, any health outcome. Therefore, we prefer the term **risk factor epidemiology**.

In later chapters, using a current formulation of risk factor designs, we give logical preeminence to the cohort over the case-control design. But historically the case-control study came first (Paneth et al. 2004). The most dramatic early breakthrough for risk factor epidemiology came from research on cigarette smoking and lung cancer. Case-control studies of cigarette smoking and lung cancer were undertaken as early as the 1940s.[4] Although these studies detected a strong association, the inference of a causal connection was not widely accepted. Faced with the challenge of finding more definitive evidence, Doll and Hill devised an alternative approach, establishing a cohort of British doctors within which they demonstrated that cigarette smoking increased the subsequent risk of lung cancer (Doll 2004).[5] By the 1960s, as summarized in the surgeon general's report (U.S. Department of Health, Education, and Welfare 1964), epidemiologic research had proved that cigarette smoking was a cause of lung cancer, and it was clear that an increase in cigarette smoking had contributed to the epidemic of lung cancer (as well as cardiovascular disease) in the 20th century. Although these investigations are not considered to be in the realm of psychiatric epidemiology, it is worth noting that nicotine dependence is a psychiatric diagnosis and clearly part of the causal chain.

A more recent success of risk factor epidemiology pertains to neurodevelopmental disorders (see chapter 6). Prenatal folate supplementation was shown to prevent neural tube defects, one of the most common birth defects in developed countries (MRC Vitamin Study Research Group 1991). The work on folate was in one sense more successful than that on cigarette smoking. It led quickly to effective public health actions, such as fortifying bread with folate and encouraging the use of prenatal supplements that reduced the occurrence of neural tube defects (Erickson et al. 2002; Williams et al. 2002).

As in previous eras, other approaches coexisted with the dominant one. Consider peptic ulcer, once thought the exemplar "disease of civilization," surely related to the mental stress of modern life (see chapter 36). While most searched for risk factors, a scientist using the Henle-Koch postulates discovered that an infectious agent, the *Helicobacter pylori*, plays a key role in causing peptic ulcer (Marshall et al. 1985).

As already noted, the public health applications of infectious disease epidemiology often lagged far behind the discovered microbal causes. Accordingly, some of the most important applications of infectious disease epidemiology to public health occurred in this era, among them the elimination of small pox (Fenner 1988). Similarly, in the 21st century, smoking, diet, and exercise, major risk factors identified in the 1950s, are still the foci of large public health campaigns.

Multilevel thinkers were in evidence, too, during this period. The inspiring and imaginative book by Jeremy Morris, *The Uses of Epidemiology* (Morris 1957), was among the first to articulate an epidemiology for noncommunicable diseases. However, Morris took a very broad view of the matter and did not intend to limit epidemiology to any particular kind of causal hypothesis

---

[4] Recently, it has come to light that studies in Nazi Germany in the 1930s indicated a causal connection between smoking and lung cancer (see Proctor 1999).

[5] For other studies that played a key role in developing the cohort design, such as the Framingham Heart Study, see Susser (1985).

(Davey Smith 2001). He has criticized the subsequent narrowing of the focus to risk factors.

Risk Factor Studies of Mental Disorders

At the dawn of risk factor epidemiology, mental disorders were counted among the chronic diseases important to investigate. As early as the 1930s, just as epidemiologists were taking their first halting steps to extend to cancer and heart disease, there were calls for an "epidemiology of mental disease" (Elkind 1938). Not infrequently, leading epidemiologists emphasized the significance of mental disorders (see Morris 1964, pp. 218–223; Winslow 1999/1926, p. 1646).

Soon, there were also applications that attested to the usefulness of risk factor methods in this domain (Susser 1968; Cooper and Morgan 1973). Some of these studies are used for illustration later in this book. One of the earliest and most influential was Lee Robins's investigation of the relationship between childhood behavior problems and adult antisocial behavior (Robins 1966). Using the records of a child guidance clinic in St. Louis, Robins retrospectively identified children with well-described psychiatric problems and then selected age- and sex-matched children without such problems from the same school as the psychiatric cohort. The two groups were followed up 30 years later to determine whether they differed as adults with respect to psychiatric disorders. Not only were the rates of disorder significantly different, but the study found that specific childhood anti-social behaviors were risk factors for adult "sociopathic personality." This finding had a profound influence on subsequent diagnostic criteria created by the American Psychiatric Association for antisocial personality disorder (American Psychiatric Association 1980), as well as on our understanding of the antecedents of adult antisocial behavior.

Despite these promising beginnings, as represented by Robins and other examples throughout this book, the enormous potential of risk factor methods for revealing the causes of mental disorders remained largely untapped. Until recently, while risk factor studies proliferated in other domains of epidemiology, there were relatively few cohort and fewer case-control studies of mental disorders. Psychiatric epidemiologists, especially in the United States, gave more attention to community surveys than to studying risk factors (see chapter 1).

Conclusion

Using different approaches across successive eras, epidemiologists have sought to understand the nature and the causes of "mental" and "physical" diseases. Among the landmark events, a bacterium was found to cause syphilis, and a nutritional deficiency was found to cause pellagra. Both these diseases were leading causes of insanity that now can be prevented, as well as cured.

We believe that in the present era epidemiologists are exceptionally well positioned to search for causes of mental disorders. These disorders can now be reliably diagnosed, and their pathophysiology is increasingly accessible, bringing their causes within reach of our investigations. To find these causes, psychiatric epidemiologists will need to much more fully exploit the risk factor designs for this purpose.

Our call, though, is not only for the wider adoption of risk factor studies in psychiatry. Risk factor methods also have limitations. We propose in the next chapter an integrative approach in which causes can be studied at multiple levels and across the life course. This integrative approach is nascent in epidemiology and still in need of development. Psychiatric epidemiologists have much to contribute to it. We bring a unique history of interdisciplinary work. Drawing from sociology, psychiatric epidemiologists have developed ecologic designs to examine societal-level factors, a method vital to a multilevel strategy. Drawing from psychology, we have developed sophisticated approaches to measurement. Psychiatric epidemiologists have the opportunity to be partners, and sometimes leaders, in shaping the wider field of epidemiology in the coming era.

References

American Psychiatric Association (1980). *Diagnostic and Statistical Manual of Mental Disorders*, 3rd ed. Washington, D.C.: American Psychiatric Association.

Baldi G, Vigliani EC, and Zurlo N (1953). Mercury Poisoning in Hat Industry. *Med. Lav.* 44:161–198.

Barrett-Connor E (1967). The Etiology of Pellagra and Its Significance for Modern Medicine. *Am. J. Med.* 42:859–867.

Bresnahan M, Boydell J, Murray R, and Susser E (2003). Temporal Variation in the Incidence, Course and Outcome of Schizophrenia. In Murray RM, Jones PB, Susser E, van Os J, and Cannon M, eds., *The Epidemiology of Schizophrenia*, 34–48. Cambridge: Cambridge University Press.

Chapin JB (1863). Insanity Following Exposure to Fumes of Mercury. *Am. J. Insan.* 20:335–338.

Coleman W (1982). *Death Is a Social Disease: Public Health and Political Economy in Early Industrial France*. Madison: University of Wisconsin Press.

Cooper B and Morgan HG (1973). *Epidemiological Psychiatry*. Springfield, Ill.: Thomas.

Davey Smith G (2001). The Uses of "Uses of Epidemiology." *Int. J. Epidemiol.* 30:1146–1155.

Davey Smith G (2002). Commentary: Behind the Broad Street Pump: Aetiology, Epidemiology and Prevention of Cholera in Mid-19th Century Britain. *Int. J. Epidemiol.* 31:920–932.

Doll R (2004). Cohort Studies: History of the Method. In Morabia A, ed., *History of Epidemiologic Methods and Concepts*, 243–274. Boston: Birkhauser.

Ehrlich P (1911). *The Experimental Chemotherapy of Spirilloses: (Syphilis, Relapsing Fever, Spirillosis of Fowls, Framboesia)*. New York: Rebman.

Elkind HB (1938). Is There an Epidemiology of Mental Disease? *Am. J. Public Health* 28:245–250.

Elvehjem CA, Madden RJ, Strong FM, and Wolley DW (2002). The Isolation and Identification of the Anti–Black Tongue Factor, 1937. *J. Biol. Chem.* 277(34):e22.

Erickson JD, Mulinare J, Yang Q, Johnson CL, Pfeiffer C, Gunter EW, Giles WH, and Bowman BA (2002). Folate Status in Women of Childbearing Age, by Race/Ethnicity—United States, 1999–2000. *Morb. Mortal. Wkly. Rep.* 51:808–810.

Etheridge EW (1972). *The Butterfly Caste: A Social History of Pellagra in the South*. Westport, Conn.: Greenwood.

Evans A (1993). *Causation and Disease: A Chronological Journey.* New York: Plenum Medical Book Co.

Farley J (1991). *Bilharzia: A History of Imperial Tropical Medicine.* Cambridge: Cambridge University Press.

Farr W (1841). Report upon the Mortality of Lunatics. *J. Stat. Soc. Lond.* 4:17–33.

Fenner F (1988). *Smallpox and Its Eradication.* Geneva, Switzerland: World Health Organization.

Hamlin C (1998). *Public Health and Social Justice in the Age of Chadwick: Britain, 1800–1854.* Cambridge: Cambridge University Press.

Hammonds EM (1999). *Childhood's Deadly Scourge: The Campaign to Control Diptheria in New York City, 1880–1930.* Baltimore: Johns Hopkins University Press.

Hardy A (2004). Methods of Outbreak Investigation in the "Era of Bacteriology" 1880–1920. In Morabia A, ed., *History of Epidemiologic Methods and Concepts*, 199–206. Boston: Birkhauser.

Hernberg S (2000). Lead Poisoning in a Historical Perspective. *Am. J. Ind. Med.* 38:244–254.

Himmelweit F and Dale H, eds. (1956). *Collected Papers of Paul Ehrlich.* New York: Pergamon Press.

Kasius RV, ed. (1974). *The Challenge of Facts: Selected Public Health Papers of Edgar Sydenstricker.* New York: Prodist.

Kraut AM (2003). *Goldberger's War: The Life and Work of a Public Health Crusader.* New York: Hill & Wang.

Lilienfeld A (1976). *Foundations of Epidemiology.* New York: Oxford University Press.

Lilienfeld DE (2000). John Snow: The First Hired Gun? *Am. J. Epidemiol.* 152:4–9.

Markel H (1997). *Quarantine! East European Jewish Immigrants and the New York City Epidemics of 1892.* Baltimore: Johns Hopkins University Press.

Markowitz GE and Rosner D (2002). *Deceit and Denial: The Deadly Politics of Industrial Pollution.* Berkeley: University of California Press.

Marshall BJ, Armstrong JA, McGechie DB, and Glancy RJ (1985). Attempt to Fulfill Koch's Postulates for Pyloric Campylobacter. *Med. J. Aust.* 142:436–439.

Morabia A, ed. (2004). *History of Epidemiologic Methods and Concepts.* Boston: Birkhauser.

Morris JN (1957). *Uses of Epidemiology.* Edinburgh, Scotland: Livingstone.

Morris JN (1964). *Uses of Epidemiology*, 2nd ed. Edinburgh, Scotland: Livingstone.

MRC Vitamin Study Research Group (1991). Prevention of Neural Tube Defects: Results of the Medical Research Council Vitamin Study. *Lancet* 338:131–137.

Paneth N, Susser E, and Susser M (2004). Origins and Early Development of the Case-Control Study. In Morabia A, ed., *History of Epidemiologic Methods and Concepts*, 291–311. Boston: Birkhauser.

Porter D (1999). *Health, Civilization and the State: A History of Public Health from Ancient to Modern Times.* New York: Routledge.

Proctor R (1999). *The Nazi War on Cancer.* Princeton, N.J.: Princeton University Press.

Robins LN (1966). *Deviant Children Grow Up.* Baltimore: Williams & Wilkins.

Ryle JA (1948). *Changing Disciplines: Lectures on the History, Method, and Motives of Social Pathology.* London: Oxford University Press.

Schwartz S, Susser E, and Susser M (1999). A Future for Epidemiology? *Annu. Rev. Public Health* 20:15–33.

Stepan N (1978). The Interplay Between Socio-Economic Factors and Medical Science: Yellow Fever Research, Cuba and the United States. *Soc. Stud. Sci.* 8:397–423.

Susser M (1968). *Community Psychiatry: Epidemiology and Social Themes.* New York: Random House.

Susser M (1973). *Causal Thinking in the Health Sciences: Concepts and Strategies of Epidemiology.* New York: Oxford University Press.

Susser M (1985). Epidemiology in the United States after World War II: The Evolution of Technique. *Epidemiol. Rev.* 7:147–177.

Susser M and Adelstein A, eds. (1975). *Vital Statistics: A Memorial Volume of Selections from the Reports and Writings of William Farr.* Metuchen, N.J.: Scarecrow Press.

Susser M and Susser E (1996). Choosing a Future for Epidemiology: I. Eras and Paradigms. *Am. J. Public Health* 86:668–673.

Terris M, ed. (1964). *Goldberger on Pellagra.* Baton Rouge: Louisiana State University Press.

U.S. Department of Health, Education, and Welfare, Public Health Service (1964). *Smoking and Health: Report of the Advisory Committee to the Surgeon General of the Public Health Service.* Washington, D.C.: U.S. Government Printing Office.

Vandenbroucke JP (2000). Invited Commentary: The Testimony of Dr. Snow. *Am. J. Epidemiol.* 152:10–12.

Vinten-Johansen P, Brody H, Paneth N, Rachman S, and Rip MR (2003). *Cholera, Chloroform and the Science of Medicine: A Life of John Snow.* New York: Oxford University Press.

Ward P (1980). *A Dictionary of Common Fallacies,* 2nd ed. Cambridge: Oleander Press.

Westminster Medical Society Discussion of Nov. 27 on Hereditary Insanity (1841). *Lancet* 1:341–342.

Williams LJ, Mai CT, Edmonds LD, et al. (2002). Prevalence of Spina Bifida and Anencephaly During the Transition to Mandatory Folic Acid Fortification in the United States. *Teratology* 66:33–39.

Winkelstein W, Jr. (2000). Interface of Epidemiology and History: A Commentary on Past, Present, and Future. *Epidemiol. Rev.* 22:2–6.

Winslow CE (1999). Public Health at the Crossroads. 1926. *Am. J. Public Health* 89:1645–1648.

Winslow CEA (1943). *The Conquest of Epidemic Disease.* Princeton, N.J.: Princeton University Press.

Searching for the Causes of Mental Disorders

3

Ezra Susser, Sharon Schwartz, Alfredo Morabia, and Evelyn J. Bromet

A new way of thinking is emerging in epidemiology (Krieger 1994; Susser and Susser 1996; McMichael 1999). The causes of health outcomes are being conceptualized at multiple levels: at macro levels, as in the distribution of wealth in a society; at the individual level, as in the forms of personal behavior; and at micro levels, as in the cellular and molecular processes that generate disease. With hindsight, we can see that each of the successive eras of epidemiology focused on causes at one level to the relative exclusion of other levels. Thus, in the sanitary era epidemiologists focused on the societal level; in the infectious disease era, at least initially, they focused on the cellular level; and in the risk factor era they focused on the individual level (chapter 2).

One can locate epidemiologists within each era who were thinking about causes at many levels. However, this perspective was never the dominant one and was never fully articulated. What was lacking was an explicit conceptual framework that tied these causes together. In addition, the field was constrained by the tools available for research in the past. With the scientific and statistical advances of the past 50 years, we believe it is now possible to build upon the insights of those exceptional epidemiologists and develop an integrated approach to the study of causes.

Indeed, the pursuit of public health demands that we bring together these levels of investigation. Consider the epic challenge of the HIV/AIDS epidemic devastating the countries of sub-Saharan Africa (UNAIDS 2003). To gain the upper hand on HIV/AIDS, we need to answer questions on all these levels. We need to understand the societal causes that produce patterns of sexual relationships facilitating its spread (Myer et al. 2003), the sexual and other behaviors of individuals that increase their risk of infection with HIV, and the way in which the virus produces the disease in individuals who are infected. Furthermore, we need to develop vaccines and treatments for HIV/AIDS and grasp the dynamic relationships among causes, treatments, and the spread of the epidemic.

To illustrate how this conception of multilevel causation applies to a psychiatric disorder, we use the example of anorexia nervosa, a disorder that occurs mainly in young women and carries some risk of mortality. The biological underpinnings of anorexia are strong (Hoek et al. 1998); it is associated with fundamental changes in metabolism and with the disruption of basic bodily functions such as appetite and menstruation. The societal roots of anorexia are also compelling; it is rarely seen in the sociocultural environment of low-income countries.

How then do we think about the causes of anorexia nervosa? To encompass the different etiologies, we need to think of causes at different levels. At a global level, the high-income countries are evolving differently from the low-income countries, and the sociocultural environment of the high-income countries is somehow fostering the occurrence of this severe psychiatric disorder. We do not really know the reason, but the emergence of anorexia is thought to be related to both the sufficiency of food and the dominant attitudes about female body size and shape in these societies.

Within a given society, anorexia may affect the constituent social groups in different ways. In a study of anorexia in the former Dutch colony of Curaçao (Hoek et al. 2005), among the minority white and mixed-race population the incidence was similar to that of the Netherlands and the United States. By contrast, among the majority black population, descended from the slaves of the old plantation system, no cases of anorexia were found. Apparently, one segment of the population is economically better off and has adopted many of the values and practices of high-income countries, and anorexia occurs within that segment. The coexistence side by side of social groups with contrasting health profiles is also found in other societies (Susser et al. 1985, p. 13).

There are reasons that some young women acquire anorexia and others do not, even though they live in the same social milieu. The variation in risk across individuals may be explained by environmental exposures or by genetic factors that influence biological differences and the individual's response to them. All of these may be considered risk factors.

Finally, within the individual, the pathophysiology may be understood at various levels. We may consider the neural system, the neurons that comprise that system, or even the molecular constituents of the neurons. With the progress of neuroscience, the cellular processes underlying mental disorders are becoming accessible to investigation.

Thus, capturing the causes of a psychiatric disorder such as anorexia and grasping the full potential for intervention require the ability to differentiate and study causes at multiple levels.

The Context of Time

Just as we need to consider how causes operate across levels of causation, we also need to consider how causes operate over time. Within an individual, the previous life course represents the context of time. As we age, we carry with us the effects of our previous biological and social experience. In other words, our past is embodied in our present biology and behavior (Krieger and Davey Smith 2004). In addition, as an individual develops through the stages of the life course, the individual provides a different context for exposure and disease. The effect of an exposure depends upon this developmental context. So does the expression of disease.

Again consider anorexia nervosa. Suppose an intrauterine exposure could increase the risk of developing anorexia. The exposure may have this effect only if it occurs at a critical point in fetal development of the neuroendocrine system. Furthermore, the resulting abnormality would not be expressed as anorexia until puberty. The vulnerability of young women to anorexia seems to be related to the hormonal milieu of the adolescent female body, indicating the importance of developmental context for the expression of disease.

At the societal level, too, it can be illuminating to consider the context of time. As we explain in a later chapter (chapter 36), current secular trends in disease reflect long past, as well as contemporary, societal change. Therefore, to understand changing patterns of disease, we are compelled to consider the historical context.

The Task of Integration

Epidemiologists increasingly investigate causes beyond the individual level and incorporate the context of time (Susser 2004). Social epidemiologists are moving "upstream" from risk factors to the social processes that create the patterns of exposure to them. Some are attempting to understand the means by which social inequality produces health inequality within a given society (Link and Phelan 1995; Marmot and Wilkinson 1999; Shaw et al. 1999; Berkman and Kawachi 2000). Others are tracing the connections between the global economy, the stark inequalities between societies, and the ill health of large segments of the world population (Desjarlais et al. 1996; Beaglehole and Bonita 1998; Howson et al. 1998; Leon and Walt 2001). Such investigations pick up a thread developed early in the risk factor era (e.g., Morris 1957; Susser and Watson 1962), though later overshadowed.

Molecular and genetic epidemiologists are moving "downstream" from risk factors to study the biological processes that translate them into diseases. The spectacular advances of molecular and genetic research have created a drive to investigate causes at the cellular and even molecular level. Like the epidemiologists of a previous era, who were captivated by stunning discoveries in microbiology and who turned their attention to the ways in which germs cause disease, many today are drawn to investigate the ways in which new-found molecular pathways cause disease.

Life course epidemiologists are examining the trajectory of exposure and disease across the life cycle. Life course epidemiology has taken a quantum leap in the past decade. This is in part because exposure and disease can now be examined within cohorts established at or before birth and traced through midlife. The study of these cohorts has opened new windows on causes and, in particular, on the antecedents and evolution of psychiatric disorder over the life course.

It is therefore timely to bring together our thinking about causes across multiple levels and across time into a single rubric. One such rubric termed **eco-epidemiology** is described in part VIII. It seeks to incorporate different levels of causation, individual development over the life cycle, and historical change. We also advocate a common framework for examining different kinds of causes and health outcomes (physical and mental, genetic and nongenetic, infectious and noninfectious). Implicit in our approach is this notion: if epidemiologists are sharply divided into specialties examining but one level or one route of the causal pathway, the collective endeavor will be weakened.

An integrated approach does not imply that a given study should necessarily encompass causes at more than one level. Rather, it means considering the whole picture and strategically selecting the level or levels of causation to investigate. Sometimes it means looking at the interaction between causes at different levels. Similarly, it does not imply that a given study should necessarily encompass many points in the life cycle. We can achieve an integrated understanding through a series of studies with a much more limited purview. The goal is always to make the design as simple as possible —but not too simple—to answer a specific question, without losing sight of the larger context.

Thus, epidemiologists can now envision an integrative causal schema and use it to help frame hypotheses, design studies, interpret results, and extract implications for public health. However, the process of integration is still at an embryonic stage. We have yet to complement risk factor strategies with similarly rigorous designs for investigating both the upstream antecedents and the downstream biological consequences of risk factors. We are still learning how best to incorporate the context of time, in order to analyze the trajectory of health and illness over the life course, and the relation between historical change and societal patterns of disease. We also have yet to breach the divisions between epidemiologists who focus on different kinds of causes and outcomes. Completing the project is the collective endeavour of many epidemiologists and already underway (e.g., Diez Roux 1998; Khoury 1998; Koopman and Lynch 1999; Perera and Weinstein 2000; Krieger and Davey Smith 2004; Kuh and Ben-Schlomo 2004).

The maturation of such an integrated approach in psychiatric research will require at least four preliminary steps. First, psychiatric epidemiologists need to adopt risk factor designs more fully to integrate epidemiology across the key domains of mental and physical health. To do so will require that we take into account certain issues that pertain especially to mental disorders, such as the complexities of defining and measuring them (Helzer and Hudziak 2002), their underlying continuity yet variable expression over the life course (Costello and Angold 1991; Rapoport 2000; Susser and Factor-Litvak 2004), and the comorbidity patterns among them (Boyd et al. 1984; Kessler 1995).

Second, the connections between epidemiology and biological research in psychiatry need to be strengthened. In contrast to exposures such as life events, biological factors tend to be proximal to the disease process and pertain closely to its pathophysiology. Epidemiologic principles are nevertheless adaptable to biological research in psychiatry and can advance it substantially.

Third, consideration of genetic designs from an epidemiologic perspective is necessary for developing a unified framework for investigating genetic and nongenetic causes. Epidemiologic designs can be adapted to incorporate gene biology, and epidemiologic principles can help clarify some key genetic designs. Such an approach may help resolve apparent discrepant inferences from epidemiologic and genetic studies of the same question.

Fourth, we need to develop a broader conception of causes that includes a central but not exclusive role for risk factors at the individual level. A key tenet is that emergent phenomena arise at each level of organization; in other words, the whole signifies more than the sum of its constituent parts. Another tenet is that what happened before always provides part of the context for what happens now. Thus, we need to reinvigorate the insights of early psychiatric epidemiologists who thought about causes on multiple levels and across the life course (e.g., Leighton 1959) to approach the subsequent refinements of methods in epidemiology.

Conclusion

Building upon its past achievements, psychiatric epidemiology is well positioned for a concentrated search for the causes of mental disorders. We propose that risk factor methods be fully exploited in this endeavor. We also advocate the adoption of a broad conceptual framework, an integrative approach suitable for studying biological, genetic, psychological and societal causes of mental (and other) disorders. The framework is still embryonic, and in this book we hope to make a modest contribution to its development and use in psychiatric epidemiology.

References

Beaglehole R and Bonita R (1998). Public Health at the Crossroads: Which Way Forward? *Lancet* 351:590–592.

Berkman L and Kawachi I, eds. (2000). *Social Epidemiology*. New York: Oxford University Press.

Boyd JH, Burke JD, Jr., Gruenberg E, et al. (1984). Exclusion Criteria of *DSM-III*. A Study of Co-occurrence of Hierarchy-Free Syndromes. *Arch. Gen. Psychiatry* 41:983–989.

Costello EJ and Angold A (1991). Developmental Epidemiology. In Cicchetti D and Toth S, eds., *Rochester Symposium on Developmental Psychopathology*, 23–56. Hillsdale, N.J.: Erlbaum.

Desjarlais R, Eisenberg L, Good B, and Kleinman A, eds. (1996). *World Mental Health: Problems and Priorities in Low-Income Countries*. New York: Oxford University Press.

Diez Roux AV (1998). On Genes, Individuals, Society, and Epidemiology. *Am. J. Epidemiol.* 148:1027–1032.

Helzer JE and Hudziak JJ, eds. (2002). *Defining Psychopathology in the 21st Century: DSM-V and Beyond*. Washington D.C.: American Psychiatric Publishing.

Hoek HW, Treasure JL, and Katzman MA, eds. (1998). *Neurobiology in the Treatment of Eating Disorders*. Chichester, England: Wiley.

Hoek HW, van Harten PN, Hermans KM, Katzman MA, Matroos GE, and Susser E (2005). The Incidence of Anorexia Nervosa on Curaçao. *Am. J. Psychiatry* 162:748–752.

Howson CP, Fineberg HV, and Bloom BR (1998). The Pursuit of Global Health: The Relevance of Engagement for Developed Countries. *Lancet* 351:586–590.

Kessler R (1995). Epidemiology of Psychiatric Comorbidity. In Tsuang MT, Tohen M, and Zahner GEP, eds., *Textbook in Psychiatric Epidemiology*, pp. 179–197. New York: Wiley.

Khoury MJ (1998). Genetic Epidemiology. In Rothman KJ and Greenland S, eds. *Modern Epidemiology*, 2nd ed., 609–622. Philadelphia: Lippincott-Raven.

Koopman JS and Lynch JW (1999). Individual Causal Models and Population System Models in Epidemiology. *Am. J. Public Health* 89:1170–1174.

Krieger N (1994). Epidemiology and the Web of Causation: Has Anyone Seen the Spider? *Soc. Sci. Med.* 39:887–903.

Krieger N and Davey Smith G (2004). "Bodies Count," and Body Counts: Social Epidemiology and Embodying Inequality. *Epidemiol. Rev.* 26:92–103.

Kuh D and Ben-Schlomo Y (2004). *A Life Course Approach to Chronic Disease Epidemiology.* New York: Oxford University Press.

Leighton AH (1959). *My Name Is Legion: Foundations for a Theory of Man in Relation to Culture.* Vol. 1, *The Stirling County Study of Psychiatric Disorder and Sociocultural Environment.* New York: Basic Books.

Leon DA and Walt G (2001). *Poverty, Inequality and Health: An International Perspective.* Oxford: Oxford University Press.

Link BG and Phelan J (1995). Social Conditions as Fundamental Causes of Disease. *J. Health Soc. Behav.* (Extra Issue):80–94.

Marmot M and Wilkinson R, eds. (1999). *Social Determinants of Health.* Oxford: Oxford University Press.

McMichael AJ (1999). Prisoners of the Proximate: Loosening the Constraints on Epidemiology in an Age of Change. *Am. J. Epidemiol.* 149:887–897.

Morris JN (1957). *Uses of Epidemiology.* Edinburgh, Scotland: Livingstone.

Myer L, Morroni C, and Susser ES (2003). Commentary: The Social Pathology of the HIV/AIDS Pandemic. *Int. J. Epidemiol.* 32:189–192.

Perera FP and Weinstein IB (2000). Molecular Epidemiology: Recent Advances and Future Directions. *Carcinogenesis* 21:517–524.

Rapoport JL (2000). *Childhood Onset of "Adult" Psychopathology: Clinical and Research Advances.* Washington, D.C.: American Psychiatric Press.

Shaw M, Dorling D, Gorden D, and Davey Smith G (1999). *The Widening Gap: Health Inequalities and Policy in Britain.* Bristol, U.K.: Policy Press.

Susser E (2004). Eco-Epidemiology: Thinking Outside the Black Box. *Epidemiology* 15:519–520.

Susser E and Factor-Litvak P (2004). A Life Course Approach to Neuropsychiatric Disorders. In Kuh D and Ben-Shlomo Y, eds., *A Life Course Approach to Chronic Disease Epidemiology*, 2nd ed., pp. 324–342. New York: Oxford University Press.

Susser M and Susser E (1996). Choosing a Future for Epidemiology: II. From Black Box to Chinese Boxes and Eco-Epidemiology. *Am. J. Public Health* 86:674–677.

Susser MW and Watson W (1962). *Sociology in Medicine.* London: Oxford University Press.

Susser MW, Watson W, and Hopper K (1985). *Sociology in Medicine,* 3rd ed. New York: Oxford University Press.

UNAIDS (2003). *AIDS Epidemic Update 2003: Follow-up to the 2001 United Nations General Assembly Special Session on HIV/AIDS.* Geneva, Switzerland: World Health Organization.

RISK FACTORS AS CAUSES OF MENTAL DISORDERS

What Is a Cause?

4

Sharon Schwartz and Ezra Susser

Risk factor designs are still the most fully developed methods for the investigation of causes. Although new approaches are emerging in the current era, these approaches retain the risk factor paradigm as the basis for epidemiologic investigation in some very important contexts (see part VIII). We begin with the underlying principles that have guided the era of risk factor epidemiology.

The Concept of a Risk Factor

In the aftermath of World War II, as the uses of epidemiology were redefined (Morris 1957), so were the concepts of causation (Susser 1973). During the preceding era of infectious disease epidemiology, a cause was related to one disorder and a disorder was related to one cause (Evans 1993). The chronic diseases that were epidemic after World War II, however, were not easily attributable to single etiologic agents. The notion of specific necessary and sufficient causes lost its utility. What emerged in its place was the notion that multiple risk factors cause or prevent disorders.

In one of the first textbooks to focus on the epidemiology of chronic diseases, MacMahon et al. (1960) proposed the metaphor of a "web of causation" for thinking about multiple causes of a disease. The web is made of many strands. For exposition, the authors separated out the strands of the web, and pictured them along the lines of figure 4.1.[1] In the hypothetical scenario of figure 4.1, one strand that leads to schizophrenia includes genetic vulnerability, prenatal exposure to a virus, and adolescent cannabis use, as well as some other unknown causes. None of these causes is necessary for the development of schizophrenia. Other strands involving other combinations of factors can also lead to schizophrenia. In addition, none of these causes is sufficient for the development of schizophrenia. Rather, the combination of them is thought

---

[1] MacMahon et al. (1960) called them "chains" not "strands"; we avoid calling them "chains" so as not to confuse them with the chains of causation discussed later in the book.

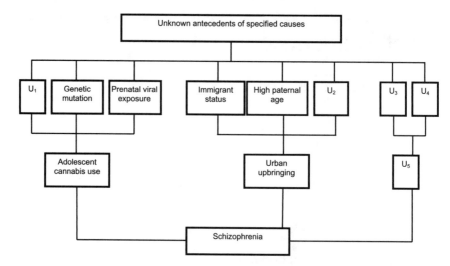

Figure 4.1 Strands of causation for schizophrenia: hypothetical example. U = unknown causes. (The links among the exposures do not indicate mediational relationships.)

to be responsible for the development of the disorder. Finally, the specified causes themselves have unspecified or unknown antecedents. Based on this and other attempts to conceptualize multiple causes (Hill 1965; Susser 1973; Lilienfeld 1976; Lilienfeld and Stolley 1994), and to distill the interpretation of epidemiologic data (Oppenheimer in press), the concept of a risk factor gradually emerged. The term came to mean a factor that contributes to the risk of a disease, but may be neither necessary nor sufficient to produce it.

Searching for Risk Factors

With this concept of a cause, epidemiologists began to see their task as identifying risk factors. In order to evaluate whether an exposure (e.g., smoking cigarettes) was a risk factor for a disease (e.g., lung cancer), the effects of the exposure had to be isolated, and the conditions of observation had to be simplified. Accordingly, researchers focused on separating risk factors out of the web of causation, rather than on understanding the workings of the web as a whole.

Identifying risk factors, even without understanding all the conditions under which they cause disease, has great significance for public health action. Removing a risk factor from a population breaks a particular strand in the web of causation and thereby prevents some cases of the disease. Also, in the long term, identifying the risk factors for a disease helps researchers piece together the causal process.

In the example of schizophrenia, we might attempt to identify prenatal viral infection as a risk factor, without necessarily understanding how it combines with genetic vulnerability and adolescent cannabis use, and without understanding all the other pathways that can lead to schizophrenia. By identifying and eliminating this risk factor we could reduce the incidence of schizophrenia, even without understanding how the virus affects the brain of a developing fetus. Moreover, the knowledge that this exposure plays a role in causing the disease would help direct research into causal mechanisms.

Nonetheless, epidemiologists using this approach continued to dispute precisely what constitutes a cause and how to determine when one has found a cause. Some attempted to avoid the fray by proposing that epidemiologists identify risk factors that elevate or decrease the chances of having an illness, regardless of whether they are actually causes. But such avoidance hinders the articulation of our purposes and methods. We do indeed want to identify causes. In what follows, we more closely examine the meaning of a cause in risk factor epidemiology and introduce the **counterfactual** approach that has gained broad if not universal acceptance.

Separating Cause from Coincidence

The potential of science for locating causes occupies a central place in the philosophy of science (Klee 1997). One definition of a cause that is being productively used in epidemiology and other scientific disciplines is rooted in the way we think about causes in our everyday lives. The main problem is distinguishing coincidence (i.e., noncausal sequence of events), from sequences that are causal. For example, suppose your phone rings and then the teakettle whistles. You would probably label the sequential events of the phone ringing and the teakettle whistling a coincidence. However, if a stranger approaches your house and the dog barks, you might assume a causal connection between these two events. What distinguishes these two event sequences?

Typically, although not consciously, we use a type of thought experiment to infer the causal sequence (Mackie 1974). We think about what the outcome would have been if the prior event had not occurred. In the first case, we think that if the phone had not rung, the teakettle would have whistled anyway, so we label this sequence a coincidence. In the second case, however, we assume that if the stranger had not approached the house, the dog would not have barked. We label this sequence causal, because without the prior event (the approach of the stranger) the outcome (the barking) would not have occurred. This type of thought experiment has been termed counterfactual because we imagine a situation counter to the actual facts.

Two qualifications should be noted about the way we infer causes in such thought experiments. First, we do not require that this causal sequence be the only one that can produce the outcome. In our example, any number of other causal sequences could also have resulted in the dog's barking. In other words, we did not infer that this cause (e.g., the approach of the stranger) is necessary to produce the outcome (e.g., the dog's barking) in all other instances.

Second, we remove only the one prior event that we are considering a cause. In our example, we assumed that all remained constant in the world except for the stranger's approaching. The dog maintained his temperament, the physical layout of the house did not change, no household member acted differently, and the laws of nature still applied. In other words, we did not infer that this cause was sufficient to produce the outcome in any other set of circumstances.

Thus, this application of the counterfactual leads us away from the notion of single causes that are necessary and sufficient. It leads us to ask instead whether the removal of one component of the constellation of circumstances (the stranger's approaching) would have prevented the outcome (dog's barking) from occurring in this particular instance. We think about a cause as something that contributes to the outcome in a certain context but which may be neither necessary nor sufficient to produce the outcome.

Revisiting the Concept of a Risk Factor

The counterfactual has been adopted as a central tenet by many, though not all, epidemiologists (Kaufman and Poole 2000; Maldonado and Greenland 2002). The following definition of a cause consistent with a counterfactual approach is offered in a current textbook, *Modern Epidemiology*: "We can define a cause of a specific disease event as an antecedent event, condition, or characteristic that was necessary for the occurrence of the disease at the moment it occurred, given that other conditions are fixed" (Rothman and Greenland 1998, p. 8).

An early attempt to explicitly formulate the concept of a cause based on the counterfactual was developed by the philosopher Mackie in the 1970s (Mackie 1974) and refined by Meehl (1977), a psychologist who applied it to mental disorders. Mackie (1974) referred to risk factor causes as *insufficient but necessary components of unnecessary but sufficient causes* (sometimes called, for short, **INUS causes**).[2] This phrase embodies the central characteristics of such causes. In our scenario in figure 4.1, in order for schizophrenia to have resulted from a prenatal viral exposure, the individual also had to have a genetic vulnerability and exposure to cannabis in adolescence. The prenatal viral exposure was an *insufficient* (since it alone would not have caused the disease) but *necessary* (since without it, the disease would not have occurred in this individual) component of an *unnecessary* (this was not the only combination of events that could produce the disease) but *sufficient* (this combination of events was enough for the disease to occur) cause. The concept of an INUS cause may be seen as extending and formalizing the earlier approaches to defining risk factors. Logically grounded in the counterfactual, it provided a more solid foundation on which to build.

Such causes can be portrayed in pictures of "causal pies," a device originally developed by Rothman (1976). The same risk factors pictured as strands in figure 4.1 are pictured as causal pies in figure 4.2. Each "pie" can be thought of as a set of causal partners that leads to disease occurrence. Thus, the pie represents a sufficient cause. Each slice in the pie represents a risk factor (or component cause, in Rothman's terminology). All the slices in the pie are necessary for the disease to occur from that pie.

---

[2] Note that the "n" in Mackie's (1974) formulation stands for *nonredundant*. We use the term *necessary*, because we have found it a simpler way to convey the idea of nonredundancy.

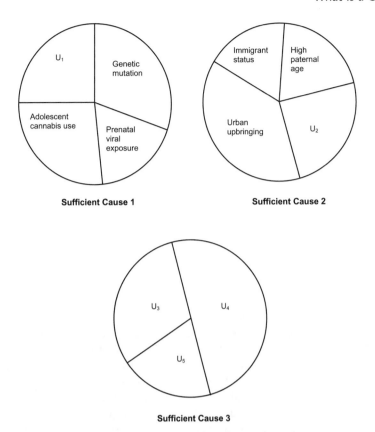

Figure 4.2 Causal pies for schizophrenia: hypothetical example. U = unknown causes.

A risk factor may be part of several different sufficient causes for the disease and therefore lead to the disease in conjunction with different causal partners. Any risk factor that is a causal partner in all the sufficient causes for a disease is deemed a **necessary cause**: the disease will not occur without it under any circumstances. In figure 4.2, if we learned that one of the unknown causes was another genetic mutation, and this mutation included in sufficient causes 1, 2, and 3, then it would be a necessary cause.

Note that in figure 4.2 a risk factor such as prenatal viral exposure is an INUS cause. Thus, the causal pie provides a way to picture INUS causes and helps clarify the implications of this concept of causation for epidemiologic research. Also note that the unspecified or unknown antecedents of figure 4.1 no longer have a place in figure 4.2; this point becomes important in the later critique of risk factor epidemiology (see part VIII).

As these and other authors developed similar ideas, they also generated different terminology for risk factor causes. For example, while Mackie referred to *INUS causes*, Rothman used the term *component causes*. Throughout this book, to avoid confusion, we will adhere to the term *risk factor*. When two or more risk factors are involved in a causal pathway, we will refer to them as **causal partners**. When a variable is being investigated to determine whether it is a risk factor, we will refer to it as an **exposure**.

Implications of the Counterfactual Approach

Although initially more difficult to understand, the counterfactual offers important advantages over earlier approaches. Most crucially, it provides a sound logical basis for the risk factor designs. Under this concept of causation, an exposure is a cause if some of the exposed people who incurred the disease would not have incurred it without the exposure. In a population, this is reflected in a disease risk that is higher than it would be in the absence of the exposure.[3] Accordingly, our risk factor designs can be understood as methods for determining whether the disease risk is higher in the presence of the exposure than it "would have been" in the absence of the exposure. This will be the topic of the next chapter.

By formalizing the logic of causation, the counterfactual helps clarify the implications of risk factors. Three of the more far-reaching implications are explained next.

Causal Relationships as Context-Dependent

The first implication derives directly from our definition of a risk factor. A risk factor leads to disease only in the presence of its causal partners. In the formal counterfactual definition already cited, this notion is represented in the phrase, "given that other conditions are fixed." This qualification means that the strength of a risk factor for a disease in a given population depends on the prevalence of its causal partners in the population.

This point can be illustrated in our hypothetical scenario for schizophrenia (see figure 4.2). In this scenario, prenatal viral exposure leads to disease only if, in addition, the individual has a genetic vulnerability to schizophrenia and uses cannabis in adolescence. In a given population, the number of people who would incur schizophrenia as a result of the prenatal viral exposure would depend on how many people have its causal partners, genetic vulnerability and cannabis exposure.

Let us examine more specifically how the prevalence of the causal partners can determine the strength of the risk factor. Suppose that a risk factor for autism is a specific genetic abnormality and its causal partner is a specific prenatal insult.[4] If the prenatal insult is rare, then the genetic abnormality will rarely result in autism. The gene will display "reduced **penetrance**." If, on the other hand, the prenatal insult is ubiquitous, then the genetic abnormality will always result in autism. The gene will now display "full penetrance."

More generally, if the causal partners of the risk factor are rare, the people exposed to the risk factor will rarely develop the disease. It will be a weak risk factor. If, on the other hand, the causal partners are common, the people exposed to the risk factor will often develop the disease. It will be a strong

---

[3] It should be noted, however, that the population risk is the average of the disease experience of individuals in the population. Therefore, a risk factor could cause disease in some individuals without its influence being reflected in an increased population risk. This can happen if there is a balancing of preventive and causal effects of the same risk factor. This point is fully addressed in part VIII.

[4] A genetic abnormality can be considered a risk factor (see part VII).

risk factor (Rothman 1976; Rothman and Greenland 1998). Therefore, depending on the characteristics of the population, risk factors may be strong or weak, as will be illustrated.

The underlying causal process that accounts for these relationships is **synergy**. One cause (e.g., genetic abnormality) combines with another cause (e.g., prenatal insult) to produce the outcome (e.g., autism). As we shall see later, in part VI and part VIII, this is the process that epidemiologists term **interaction** and that they try to capture when they use statistical measures of interaction. (However, not all statistical measures of interaction are suited to this purpose; see part VIII.)

Neural tube defects (NTDs) such as spina bifida and anencephaly provide a good example of a putative interaction. It has been hypothesized that many cases of NTDs are caused by a combination of genetic and dietary causes. A simple version of this interaction may be as follows.[5] A maternal genetic defect increases the need for folate. When the maternal intake of folate is insufficient to meet the increased need, the development of the fetus is affected. The offspring has an increased risk of being born with a NTD.

Consider what happens under different scenarios that involve different frequencies of the hypothesized genetic and dietary causes of NTDs. In a population where the genetic cause is ubiquitous (every mother has the defect), but the dietary cause is rare (few pregnant women have a low folate intake), the dietary cause will be a strong risk factor. Every fetus exposed to the dietary cause will also be exposed to the genetic cause that allows the dietary cause to act. In this scenario, the genetic defect will not even be detectable as a risk factor, because being exposed to the genetic defect does not distinguish fetuses with and without NTDs.

Now consider a second scenario of a population where the converse applies. In this population, the genetic cause is rare but the dietary cause is ubiquitous (every pregnant woman has low folate intake). Now the genetic cause will be a strong risk factor, whereas the dietary cause will not be detectable as a risk factor (maternal folate intake will not distinguish fetuses with and without NTDs).

These contrasting scenarios put a different slant on the issue of generalizability. It should not be automatically assumed that the relationship between any particular risk factor and a disease outcome should be consistent across populations. Since the frequency of risk factors differs between populations, so will the strength of these causes.

Thinking about consistency across populations leads us beyond identifying risk factors, into the realm of explaining causal processes. Inconsistent relationships across populations may provide clues about the causal partners of a risk factor. For example, some studies might find a risk ratio for the relationship between stressful life events and depression that indicates a large effect. Other studies may show no effect at all. Although these inconsistencies may be due to methodological artifacts, they may also result from differences in

---

[5] The hypothesized causal relationships are simplified for exposition. We assume a single genetic cause that is in the mother's genotype and that leads to disease only in combination with the environmental cause. Current theories about the causes of NTDs suggest synergy but do not impose these restrictions.

the conditions under which life events do and do not lead to depression. For example, contexts that lack sufficient social support may be necessary for life events to cause depression. These inconsistencies may serve as clues to the identification of the causal partners of life events and thereby enhance our understanding of the etiology of depression. Differences in the strength of a risk factor across persons, places, and times (Shadish et al. 2002) are therefore of great importance in explicating disease processes.

The Summed Contributions of Different Causes: More Than 100 Percent

A second implication derives from the relationship of each of the risk factors in a sufficient cause to its causal partners: they are equally necessary. This means that the elimination of any one of them will prevent all the disease due to the entire sufficient cause.

This point can be illustrated in our hypothetical scenario for schizophrenia. Suppose that 50 percent of the people with schizophrenia in a population developed the disease from the same sufficient cause (a combination of genetic vulnerability, viral exposure, and adolescent cannabis use). Then removing any one of the three causal partners will prevent all of the cases due to this sufficient cause; it will prevent 50 percent of the cases in the population. This quantity is referred to as the **attributable proportion** for the risk factor.

It makes no sense to add up the attributable proportions for different risk factors in a sufficient cause as though they were supposed to sum to 100 percent. In this example, if we were to add up the proportion of cases of schizophrenia that are attributable to the three risk factors, the result would be 150 pecent (i.e., 50 percent from genetic vulnerability, 50 percent from viral exposure, and 50 percent from adolescent cannabis use). But only 50 percent of all the cases of schizophrenia in the population were related to the sufficient cause comprising the three factors in the first place. After removal of one of the three factors, the removal of the other two is redundant and makes no further impact.

Like the concept that the strength of a cause depends upon the prevalence of its causal partners, the concept that all of the disease attributable to a sufficient cause is attributable to any one of the risk factors in the set is counterintuitive. Perhaps for that reason, authors of journal articles sometimes add up the attributable proportions of risk factors, even when these risk factors are considered to be part of the same sufficient cause. As will be discussed in more detail in part VII, the same misunderstanding underlies a common misinterpretation of heritability estimates.

Although we may try to parcel out effects of different causes from each other, when causes participate in the same sufficient cause—that is, when they "interact"—their effects are not separable. In our schizophrenia example, we cannot ask what proportion of the disease was due to genetic vulnerability as opposed to adolescent cannabis use as opposed to prenatal viral exposure. Fifty percent of cases of the disease were caused by a combination of all three. When all three were present, each had a role in causing the disease. When any one of them was absent, none had a role in the disease, at least within this sufficient cause.

Clearly, we cannot attribute unique proportions of disease occurrence to any specific cause. Nonetheless, we *can* estimate the proportion of disease that would have been prevented through the elimination of a specific cause within a designated context. This estimate, of the attributable proportion or attributable fraction (see chapter 8), has important public health applications.

The Definition of the Causal Field as Value Judgment

A third implication derives from the fact that the search for risk factors requires restriction of focus to only a small part of the causal field. This means that there is a potential for some factors to be considered "fixed" (i.e., outside the causal field of interest). The designation of what is fixed involves a value judgment.

By necessity, we make our search for causes manageable by looking for risk factors within a limited causal field. Factors that fall outside this causal field are accepted as the background for causal actions as expressed in phrases such as, "given that other conditions are fixed," "all other things being equal," or "ceteris paribus." For example, when we conduct a study within a given population, characteristics shared by all members of that population become fixed exposures: they do not vary. These characteristics become part of the unexamined causal field (Mackie 1974).

Some aspects of our causal field are temporary, with various factors defined as fixed in any particular study simply to allow for the examination of a limited number of exposures at a time. In our schizophrenia example, for a particular study we may want to examine the effects of adolescent cannabis use and treat genetic vulnerability as outside the causal field. As we explain later (chapter 11), if we do not measure genetic vulnerability in our study, we will observe the "average" effect of cannabis use, across individuals with and without the genetic vulnerability. In other studies, we may want to examine genetic vulnerability and treat adolescent cannabis use as outside the causal field. Again, this focus means we will observe the "average" effect.

Other aspects may be defined as permanently outside the causal field of interest. Researchers may consistently treat some factors as in the background. Most typically, factors considered to be immutable or dangerous to change are taken to be permanently part of the background context in which all causal action takes place. Phenomena thought to be mutable are more frequently placed within the field of investigation. Some factors may be universally accepted as part of the background context. Thus, we may consider the human genome as outside the causal field and only examine specific genetic variation within the genome. For many factors, however, our values determine what is considered immutable and outside the causal field. In this, as in other endeavors, sometimes "one person's meat is another person's poison." For example, some epidemiologists investigate social inequality as a cause of disorders such as anxiety and depression, whereas others consider it as part of the immutable background.

We cannot avoid the fact that our values necessarily play an important role in defining the causal field of interest for our studies. However, we can try to recognize the ways in which our values direct our research, so that we explicitly justify our approaches and modify them as needed. A prevailing paradigm often serves to define what is considered within and outside the causal field of interest. Debate about the boundaries of the legitimate causal field is generating some of the turbulence about the risk factor paradigm in epidemiology, as we shall see in part VIII.

Conclusion

The investigation of diseases that became epidemic after World War II, such as cardiovascular disease, lung cancer, and peptic ulcer, generated a new concept of the cause of a disease. The search for an infectious agent that caused a disease gave way to the search for the more elusive risk factors for a disease. Since a risk factor may be neither necessary nor sufficient to cause a disease, its effect depends on the presence of its causal partners. Therefore, the unique contribution of a risk factor to disease causation is inextricable from that of its causal partners, and its detection is context-dependent. To see the effect, we have to select the right context for the search. Methods suitable for finding these new types of causes had to be developed. From epidemiologists grappling with this task emerged the randomized trial, the cohort study, and the case control study. In the next chapter, we examine these strategies for the detection of risk factor causes.

References

Evans A (1993). *Causation and Disease: A Chronological Journey.* New York: Plenum Press.

Hill AB (1965). The Environment and Disease: Association or Causation? *Proc. R. Soc. Med.* 58:295–300.

Kaufman JS and Poole C (2000). Looking Back on "Causal Thinking in the Health Sciences." *Annu. Rev. Public Health* 21:101–119.

Klee R (1997). *Introduction to the Philosophy of Science: Cutting Nature at Its Seams.* New York: Oxford University Press.

Lilienfeld A (1976). *Foundations of Epidemiology.* New York: Oxford University Press.

Lilienfeld D and Stolley P (1994). *Foundations of Epidemiology.* New York: Oxford University Press.

Mackie JL (1974). The Cement of the Universe: A Study of Causation. New York: Oxford University Press.

MacMahon B, Pugh T, and Ipsen J (1960). *Epidemiologic Methods.* Boston: Little, Brown.

Maldonado G and Greenland S (2002). Estimating Causal Effects. *Int. J. Epidemiol.* 31:422–429.

Meehl P (1977). Specific Etiology and Other Forms of Strong Influence: Some Quantitative Meanings. *J. Med. Philos.* 2:33–53.

Morris JN (1957). *Uses of Epidemiology.* Edinburgh, Scotland: Livingstone.

Oppenheimer G (in press). The Emergence of Coronary Heart Disease Epidemiology in the U.S., 1947–1970. *Int. J. Epidemiol.*

Rothman KJ (1976). Causes. *Am. J. Epidemiol.* 104:587–592.

Rothman KJ and Greenland S (1998). *Modern Epidemiology,* 2nd ed. Philadelphia: Lippincott-Raven.

Shadish WR, Cook TD, and Campbell DT (2002). Experimental and Quasi-experimental Designs for Generalized Causal Inference. Boston: Houghton Mifflin.

Susser M (1973). *Causal Thinking in the Health Sciences: Concepts and Strategies of Epidemiology.* New York: Oxford University Press.

Detecting Causes

5

Sharon Schwartz and Ezra Susser

We can now proceed from the general concept of a cause to the ways in which causes can be detected. In this chapter, we provide the foundation for understanding how studies are designed for this purpose. The framework we present derives from two sources: psychology and epidemiology. Our starting point is a schema widely adopted in psychological research (Cook and Campbell 1979; Shadish et al. 2002) and influential in many other fields, including social sciences and epidemiology. Drawing upon the work of epidemiologists such as Susser (1973) and Rothman and Greenland (1998), we tailor this schema for use in epidemiology.[1] By distilling key ideas from these sources, we hope to provide readers with a clear, consistent, and broadly applicable conceptual foundation.

The identification of causes is problematic because it depends on an intangible. As described in the previous chapter, an exposure is a cause of a given outcome if, within the circumstances, the outcome would not have occurred had the exposure been absent. Since the exposure is present, this alternate "counterfactual" world is not visible. How then do we find causes? Although causes cannot be seen, they leave "footprints" or markers that aid in their identification. Epidemiologic studies are designed to help ascertain the presence or absence of these telltale signs and thus identify causes.

The Footprints That Causes Leave Behind

Just as our conceptualization of a cause in the counterfactual mirrors the way we approach causal questions in daily life, so does the way in which we examine causal hypotheses in epidemiology mirror more familiar processes. Imagine, for example, that we found some chickens mangled in the henhouse and hypothesized that a fox had gotten into it. We might go into the woods behind the henhouse to see if there were any indications that a fox had been there. We might find in the ground some evidence of a disturbance that looks

---

[1] See Appendix 1 for a full discussion of and justification for our adaptations.

like a footprint. We would try to recall if this footprint were new or had been there the previous day. Then we would carefully examine the footprint, noting its shape, depth, contours, and similarity to a fox's paw. If we could determine that the footprint were new and eliminate all other plausible explanations for the presence of the footprint, we would infer that, as hypothesized, the fox had been there. Similarly, we look at the "footprints" that risk factors leave behind in the real world to help us to identify them.

The footprint metaphor is apt. Identifying an animal by the footprints left behind is a difficult and uncertain task. Footprints can be washed away by rain, be made indistinct by wind, be too faint if the surface in which they are imprinted is hard, and be smudged if the surface is soft. Two different animals may leave footprints that are virtually indistinguishable. Nonetheless, if we search for footprints in a systematic way and attempt to eliminate as many alternative explanations as possible, we can often gain clues as to whether a particular animal has been there. Similarly, the search for causes is uncertain and our results can be indeterminate, but by following a systematic approach we can often arrive at a valid inference.

When an exposure is a cause of a disease, certain kinds of exposure-disease relationships will usually pertain in populations. To identify causes, we examine our data for indications of these relationships. Above all, we try to discern whether the exposure and disease are associated with one another, whether the exposure was temporally prior to the disease, and whether the exposure is the sole plausible explanation for the association (Mill 1843; Susser 1991; Shadish et al. 2002). **Association** is the co-occurrence of the exposure and disease; the disease is more common when the exposure is present than when the exposure is absent. Since it is not assumed that causes are necessary or sufficient, there is neither a requirement that the exposure be present in everyone who has the disease, nor that the disease be present in everyone who has the exposure.[2] **Temporal priority** exists when the exposure is present before the disease. Associations between the exposure and the disease can occur not only because the exposure leads to the disease, but also because the disease leads to the exposure. For example, stressful life events may be associated with depression either because stressful life events cause depression, or because depression causes stressful life events. To establish a cause, therefore, we must rule out reverse causation as the full explanation for the association.

Sole plausible explanation means that, after one considers all the alternative explanations for the observed association between the exposure and the disease, the only plausible explanation is that the exposure has caused the disease. It is possible for an exposure to be associated with a disease and be prior to the disease and still not be a cause of the disease. Rather, the association between the exposure and the disease may be explained by a **third variable**, that is, some variable, or set of variables, other than the exposure and

---

[2] Indeed, since this association is the average of the causal and protective effects of the exposure, the rate will be higher only if there are more people in the population for whom the exposure is causal than people for whom the exposure is protective.

disease (Susser 1973; Shadish et al. 2002). For example, infants born after obstetric complications may appear to be more likely to develop schizophrenia than infants born with no complications (Cannon et al. 2002). The obstetric complications will always occur temporally prior to the onset of schizophrenia. Yet the obstetric complications are not necessarily a causal factor in the development of schizophrenia. Rather, the association may be due to some other factor (e.g., maternal infection) that causes both the exposure (obstetric complications) and the outcome (schizophrenia).

The primary challenge for epidemiologic research is to establish the presence of all three signs (association, temporal priority, and sole plausible explanation) in order to infer that a variable is a true cause. Indeed, the difficulties of discerning these signs are the main source of indeterminacy in our studies, as explained next.

Exposure-Disease Association

In a multilayered dynamic world, exposure-disease associations are observed through a cloud of extraneous factors. Whether we can see the associations will depend on their size and our observational acuity. Our study designs and analytic approaches are the means by which we sharpen our vision.

To reveal associations, we begin by conceptualizing the exposure and the disease that we want to measure. We need to formulate a clear conception of the exposure we hypothesize to be causally relevant. The specification of the disease poses a similar challenge. We then need not only good measures of both of them, but also a study design in which they are both present in sufficient numbers; that is, we need **statistical power** (see part VI).

We will focus here on the exposure measure. This focus will illustrate the role of extraneous factors in our measures and how to minimize them. (We will discuss the disease measures in chapter 9.) Suppose we conduct a study of life events as a risk factor for depression. To begin, we develop a concept or construct of what we mean by exposure to life events. We think about the differences between various kinds of life events, consider the different meanings that the same life event may have in different contexts and for different people, try to relate the social concept of life events to the physiological concept of stress, and ultimately specify the kind of life events that are potentially causes of depression. This is by no means a small step. In the example of life events, investigators have vigorously debated the proper meaning and measurement of stressful life events for over thirty years (e.g., Brown and Harris 1989; Dohrenwend and Raphael 1993).

Suppose we determine that the construct we want to investigate is "adverse, stressful life events." We attempt to develop measures that tap into this construct in a meaningful way. Unless our measure differentiates life events that are "adverse and stressful" from those that are not, it will reflect many extraneous life events, as well as the actual hypothesized exposure.

We might try to measure "adverse, stressful life events" by asking about every possible stressful life event over the past year, giving a point to each one, and then summing the points for a "stressful life events" score. Under this procedure, for a given individual, the death of a grandmother and the loss of a job might each contribute one point to the score. Whether these life events are "adverse and stressful" for this individual depends, however, on their meaning in the specific social context. The death of a grandmother in some contexts could mean the loss of the most vital support from kin, but in other contexts could mean relief from the stress and burden of caring for someone with severe dementia. Similarly, losing a job in some contexts could be devastating, but in other contexts could create the opportunity to find more satisfying employment. Consequently, life events that are not truly "adverse and stressful" could enter the life events score.

In addition, random measurement error enters the picture even with the most carefully developed measures. We would probably find that if we repeated this life events measure on 3 successive days, we would get a slightly different score each day. Instruments are inexact, and people tend to have imperfect recall and change in their characterization of events. They might report eight life events on the first day, six on the second, and seven on the third day. Similarly, when we measure blood pressure, three readings taken on the same occasion will be slightly different from one another. This kind of variability can be attributed to random measurement error.

Systematic errors may also arise in our measure of life events. By systematic we mean that there is a pattern in the errors: it is not just random. For example, very embarrassing life events may never be reported by people who did not experience them but may sometimes be forgotten by people who did. In this circumstance, everyone without an event would be correctly classified, but some people with an event would be misclassified. This type of systematic error could also obscure our observation of an exposure-disease association.

The same logical sequence can be applied to the measurement of almost any exposure that is being investigated as a risk factor. It can also be applied to the measurement of the disease (see chapter 9). By giving thought to every step in the sequence, we can minimize the irrelevancies that ultimately enter into our measure of association. Thus, we sharpen our vision and enhance the determinacy of our study.

Temporal Order

Temporal order is the second marker of a cause. There are many examples in which clinicians and researchers evaded the question of temporal order over a long period. One example pertains to alcohol dependence and seizures. A long-held belief in medicine was that alcohol withdrawal caused seizures. In emergency rooms, seizures were frequently observed along with alcohol withdrawal symptoms, and the association was taken for a causal relationship (Ng et al. 1988). When the temporal order was finally investigated, it appeared that the seizures often preceded and were coincidental to the alcohol withdrawal. The high frequency of emergency room seizures among these patients could be better explained by a combination of antecedent heavy alcohol intake and medications given in the emergency rooms.

Temporal order is often difficult to discern because exposures and diseases overlap in time, with an exposure beginning before disease onset and continuing after onset. We may lack a clear sense of when an exposure begins or when it has continued long enough to have impact. For example, "chronic strain," which implies a persistently high background level of stressful life experiences rather than one or a few discrete insults, is an exposure of interest in many psychiatric studies. Strain seldom has a demarcated onset, and it is often not clear how long the strain must exist before it becomes chronic and of etiologic significance.

We may find it difficult to separate disease onset from prodromal symptoms. The problem is exacerbated in psychiatric research by the frequent **comorbidity** of diagnoses. Chronic dysthymia may precede the first onset of a depressive episode, and the coexistence of dysthymia and depression has been called "double depression." For some research questions, we may want to define the disease onset as the time that depression became "diagnosable" in the sense that the symptoms met currently prevailing criteria for a depressive episode. On the other hand, for other research questions, we may want to define the disease onset as the time that the dysthymic syndrome developed, on the grounds that the dysthymia was a manifestation of an underlying mood disorder from the start.

This problem is also exacerbated when prevalent rather than incident cases are studied, as is commonly done in psychiatric research. **Prevalence** is a measure of extant disease, regardless of onset recency or presence of past episodes (chapter 8). **Incidence** is a measure of new onsets of disease—for example, first episode of depression. Temporality is more difficult to establish when the disease is not the first episode or is not of recent onset. To make matters still more complicated, causes can become consequences and consequences can become causes, creating a dynamic relationship among exposures and diseases. In our example, chronic strain could contribute to depression, while depression contributes to chronic strain. This process may already be ongoing before the times we designate as representing the start of the exposure and the disease—that is, before strain is chronic and before depressive symptoms are diagnosable as depression.

There is no way to dodge the complexity of these relationships by applying some standard algorithm or statistical technique. In any particular study, the possible relationships must be delineated, a careful measure must be created, and a design must be selected that establishes the temporal order insofar as doing so is possible.

Sole Plausibility

To ascertain sole plausibility, we attempt to eliminate any remaining plausible explanations for the exposure-disease association other than the causal effect of the exposure. This is the most difficult marker to determine and is at the heart of epidemiologic methods.

The history of the AIDS pandemic provides an instructive example (Morabia 1995). Early on, in the 1980s, the use of "poppers" (amyl nitrite) was found to be associated with AIDS, and inferred by some to be a cause of it. Later, it became evident that the use of poppers was merely correlated with the disease. The observed association was entirely due to a third variable, unprotected anal sex. Some gay men both had unprotected anal sex and used poppers, and unprotected anal sex was a risk factor for AIDS. If this alternative explanation for the AIDS-popper association had not been quickly realized, the observed association could have led to preventive measures such as reducing the use of poppers, which would have been entirely ineffective. Associations that have other plausible explanations are produced by **confounding**, which will be further explained, or by phenomena that are closely related to it.

To determine whether there are other plausible explanations for an exposure-disease relationship, risk factor studies attempt to isolate the effects of the exposure on the disease from the effects of other factors. We will rely upon the concept of **full comparability** to explain the challenges of isolating the effects of a risk factor and thereby evaluating it in terms of sole plausibility.[3]

Full Comparability

As we emphasized in the previous chapter, the causal effect of an exposure depends not only on its biological actions, but also on the constellation of other risk factors in the population. Therefore, an exposure that is a cause of a disease in one population and historical context may not be a cause in another population or another historical context. For example, a genetic vulnerability may be a cause of anorexia nervosa in societies in which food is abundant and slimness is seen as an ideal female characteristic, but may not lead to anorexia nervosa in societies in which food is scarce and different norms about female beauty prevail.

What, then, do we mean when we say a risk factor is a cause of a disease? In line with the approach introduced in the last chapter, we mean that the removal of the risk factor would make a difference to the disease risk in the population we have in mind. "Make a difference" means that in these circumstances at least some people with the risk factor who incurred the disease would not have incurred it without the risk factor. Such causes are universal in the sense that, given the same circumstances, this risk factor would always be a cause of disease.

The preceding paragraphs are full of conditional statements: "would not have," "would be," "would make a difference." The problem is that causation is not directly observable; it can only be inferred. We can surmise that removal of an exposure "would" change the disease risk, but we can never actually observe whether it does, for the following reason: we can observe an exposed group of people and determine the proportion that develops the disease, but we cannot know what would have happened to the same group

---

[3] The concept of *full comparability* is an extension of the concept of *exchangeability* proposed by Greenland and Robins (1986). However, their concept of exchangeability applies only to true risk factors for the disease. We extend the notion to include factors that influence disease detection, as well. To avoid confusion, we use a different term for this more general notion.

of people if they had not been exposed. Getting the information we need would mean going back in time and then observing history again under different conditions.

The situation we face is directly parallel to the one we faced when we had to determine whether there was a causal relationship between a stranger's approaching the house and the dog's barking (see chapter 4). Conducting a thought experiment, we inferred that the dog would not have barked if the stranger had not approached. We concluded that the relationship was causal rather than merely coincidental. The difference here is that we collect data to test the counterfactual rather than depend exclusively on the thought experiment.

Suppose we make a clinical observation that mothers giving birth to babies with neural tube defects (NTDs) did not use folate supplements during the prenatal period. We can design a study that helps us judge whether our clinical observation is a clue to a causal connection between low folate intake and risk of NTDs. We begin by defining babies as exposed to low folate if their mothers did not take prenatal folate supplements. We collect a sample of exposed babies and observe the proportion that have NTDs to be 0.2 percent. How do we then gauge the impact of the exposure?

Imagine that we can go back in time, remove the exposure, and observe the same babies in the unexposed condition, that is, having mothers who took prenatal folate supplements. We now see that only 0.1 percent of these babies are born with NTDs. The difference between these two proportions is 0.1 percent. We conclude that removal of the exposure reduced the NTD risk in these babies by 50 percent. This is the true measure of the causal effect that we would like to observe.

Of course, we cannot travel backwards in time. We therefore look for an observable substitute. We look for a group of people whose disease experience can be used as a proxy for what would have happened if we had traveled back in time, removed the exposure, and observed the exposed people under the unexposed condition. A surrogate group that serves as an accurate stand-in for this counterfactual scenario is fully comparable to the exposed group. In other words, an unexposed group is fully comparable to the exposed group if it represents what would have happened to the exposed group under the unexposed condition.

In our example of NTDs, using this reasoning, who would we look for as our unexposed group? We would want to find an unexposed group of babies who are identical to the exposed babies in terms of all factors influencing the development of the disease (and its ascertainment, as will be discussed), except for the exposure to low folate. If we succeed in selecting an unexposed group of babies who are fully comparable to the exposed babies, then the unexposed group will truly represent the counterfactual scenario. We will observe that 0.1 percent of them have NTDs, as in the counterfactual scenario. Using this information, we will correctly infer that in the exposed group the removal of the low folate exposure would have reduced NTD risk from 0.2 percent to 0.1 percent.

In this scenario, the exposed and the unexposed do not differ on any factors that influence the disease other than the exposure. In this context, it is safe to infer that the exposure is the sole plausible explanation for any difference in disease risk between the two groups. On the other hand, if we select a group of unexposed babies who are not fully comparable to the exposed babies, we can be misled. Suppose we select a group of unexposed babies from a population with a lower risk of NTDs: only 0.05 percent are born with NTDs, rather than 0.1 percent. A comparison of the exposed and unexposed babies would suggest that removing the exposure to low folate would reduce NTD risk from 0.2 percent to 0.05 percent (a risk ratio of $0.2 \div 0.05 = 4$), when in fact it would reduce NTD risk only from 0.2 percent to 0.1 percent (a risk ratio $0.2 \div 0.1 = 2$). The overestimate of the effect of the exposure arises from noncomparability between the exposed and unexposed groups (see figure 5.1). The observed risk ratio reflects the effect of other causes of NTDS, in addition to the causal effect of folate. Noncomparability can also hide true associations. In our example, if 0.2 percent of the unexposed babies had developed NTDs, the risk ratio would have been 1, indicating no effect. We would wrongly conclude that removing the exposure would not make a difference.

Finally, it should be noted that we have been discussing causal effects in terms of increasing disease risk. Exposures can also have causal effects by reducing disease risk. In fact, our example of taking folate supplements could be easily reframed in this way. We could think of the folate supplement as an exposure that prevents NTDs. We would then classify women taking folate supplements as the exposed and other women as unexposed, rather than

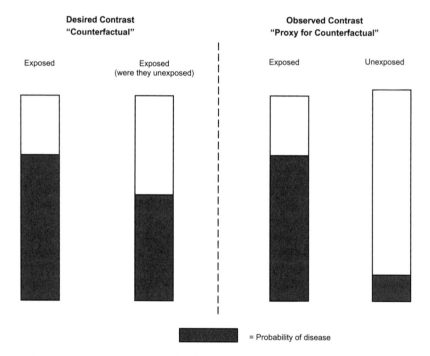

Figure 5.1 Noncomparability of proxy for the counterfactual: hypothetical example of folate as factor in neural tube defects.

vice-versa. The risk ratio would be less than 1, indicating that the exposure reduced the risk of the outcome.

Sources of Noncomparability

Noncomparability means that the probability of disease in the unexposed does not equal the probability of disease that the exposed would have shown if they had not been exposed. In the example we used, this noncomparability occurred because the exposed and unexposed differed on one or more third variables that are risk factors for the disease. This is what epidemiologists mean by confounding (Greenland and Robins 1986).

There are other ways, however, in which the groups may not be comparable. The disease frequencies that we assess in our studies are not the true disease proportions. Rather, they are the disease frequencies as refracted through our observations and measurements. Thus, we need to broaden our view and consider not only whether the exposed and unexposed groups differ on true causes of disease, but also whether they differ on factors related to the detection and labeling of the disease.

For example, suppose that in our NTD study, we recruit and assess 1000 exposed (low-folate) and 1000 unexposed women very early in pregnancy. At the start of the study, the exposed and unexposed are equal on all other risk factors for NTDs. We collect further information in a 6-month follow-up assessment and determine the NTD outcomes in a one-year follow-up assessment. However, one half of the unexposed women drop out of the study between the 6-month and the one-year follow-up. At the end of the study, we compute the proportions of the exposed and unexposed women who gave birth to babies with NTDs. Suppose that for each exposure group we use the number of women reporting NTDs at one-year follow-up as the numerator, and 1000 as the denominator. Using this procedure, we would underestimate the proportion of NTDs in the unexposed group, because we would miss the NTDs among the study dropouts. The difference in follow-up time between the exposed and unexposed would be a source of noncomparability that created an association between the exposure and the disease. In other words, follow-up time would be an alternative explanation for the observed exposure-disease relationship.

In a similar way, noncomparability may arise when the exposed and unexposed are differentially labeled as diseased. For example, researchers who are convinced that low folate is related to NTDs may be more vigilant in assigning the diagnosis of NTDs to the exposed (low-folate) babies. This differential misclassification can also create an exposure-disease association.

With this broader perspective, we can distinguish three sources of noncomparability that are central to evaluating sole plausibility in epidemiologic studies. The exposed and unexposed may differ on other risk factors for the disease, observation time, and disease labeling errors. We refer to these as **confounding**, **unequal attrition**, and **differential misclassification**, respectively. All three provide an alternative explanation for the relationship between the exposure and the disease. We elaborate on these different sources of noncomparability in chapter 11.

Conclusion

Given the complexity of the web of causation and the infinite number of potential causes that could be investigated, the discoveries of risk factor epidemiology are truly remarkable. Pioneering epidemiologists were able to distill the infinite complexity into a few relationships of central interest, study these relationships, and produce results with lasting impact on population health. How did they do it? At the heart of their approach were two elements. One was a well-formulated initial hypothesis that focused on one or a few exposures. The other was a study design that isolated the effects of these from all other factors. In the next chapter we will describe the major epidemiologic study designs and how they utilize full comparability to accomplish this goal.

References

Brown GW and Harris T (1989). *Life Events and Illness.* New York: Guilford Press.

Cannon M, Jones PB, and Murray RM (2002). Obstetric Complications and Schizophrenia: Historical and Meta-Analytic Review. *Am. J. Psychiatry* 159:1080–1092.

Cook TD and Campbell DT (1979). *Quasi-experimentation: Design and Analysis Issues for Field Settings.* Boston: Houghton Mifflin.

Dohrenwend BP and Raphael KG (1993). The Structured Event Probe and Narrative Rating Method for Measuring Stressful Life Events. In Goldberger L and Breznitz S, eds. *Handbook of Stress: Theoretical and Clinical Aspects.* New York: Free Press.

Greenland S and Robins JM (1986). Identifiability, Exchangeability, and Epidemiological Confounding. *Int. J. Epidemiol.* 15:413–419.

Mill JS (1843). *A System of Logic.* London: Parker.

Morabia A (1995). Poppers, Kaposi's Sarcoma, and HIV Infection: Empirical Example of a Strong Confounding Effect? *Prev. Med.* 24:90–95.

Ng SK, Hauser WA, Brust JC, and Susser M (1988). Alcohol Consumption and Withdrawal in New-Onset Seizures. *N. Engl. J. Med.* 319:666–673.

Rothman KJ and Greenland S (1998). *Modern Epidemiology,* 2nd ed. Philadelphia: Lippincott-Raven.

Shadish WR, Cook TD, and Campbell DT (2002). *Experimental and Quasi-experimental Designs for Generalized Causal Inference.* Boston: Houghton Mifflin.

Susser M (1973). *Causal Thinking in the Health Sciences: Concepts and Strategies of Epidemiology.* New York: Oxford University Press.

Susser M (1991). What Is a Cause and How Do We Know One? A Grammar for Pragmatic Epidemiology. *Am. J. Epidemiol.* 133:635–648.

Study Designs

6

Sharon Schwartz and Ezra Susser

As ideal types, risk factor study designs can be ordered in terms of how effectively they can simulate conditions of full comparability between the exposed and unexposed groups.[1] By this standard, the strongest design is a preventive intervention trial and in particular the randomized controlled trial. Next is the cohort design, which includes the natural experiment, as well as the ordinary cohort study. The case-control study is further from this ideal. A final study design, the cross-sectional study, poses the most difficulty for the identification of causes and is used more for nonetiologic research, such as studies to establish the prevalence of psychiatric disorders in the population.

We use the caveat "as ideal types" because in practice the validity of results from these designs does not follow any rigid hierarchy. It depends very much upon the conditions and quality of the particular study (Miettinen and Cook 1981; Susser 1995; Shapiro 2000). In addition, the designs fall into a different order on other dimensions, such as their breadth of application. Nonetheless, ordering them by the standard of full comparability is a logical and useful approach.

To see the relation of these designs to each other, we describe each of them in turn, with reference to the standard of full comparability. We then illustrate how each was actually used to investigate the causal effect of low prenatal folate intake on neural tube defects (NTDs).

Preventive Intervention Trials

The defining feature of a preventive intervention trial is that the researcher decides which people are assigned to which condition (Lilienfeld 1982). The hypothesized exposure is purposely removed from one group (unexposed) but not from the other group (exposed). Thus, the exposed are the no-intervention (or placebo intervention) group and the unexposed are the intervention group.

---

[1] Here we consider epidemiologic study designs with only individuals as the units of analytic interest. Study designs that deal with other levels of organization are discussed in part VIII.

The two groups are then observed for a period of time to ascertain the proportion in each group who develop the study outcome. Similar principles apply to treatment trials (although in treatment trials, the exposed are the intervention group and the unexposed are the no-intervention group).

Preventive intervention trials have produced some of the most important findings on the causes of neuropsychiatric disorders. In a famous historical example, Goldberger and Sydenstricker (Goldberger et al. 1915, 1920; for collected papers, see Terris M 1964) used preventive intervention trials to establish a nutritional etiology for pellagra. Pellagra was an important cause of psychosis at that time (see chapter 2).

We will discuss only one kind of preventive intervention trial, the *double-blind randomized controlled trial* (for a comprehensive discussion of intervention trials, see Friedman et al. 1996). **Randomized controlled** means that we randomly assign people to the exposed or the unexposed group. **Double-blind** means that neither the field research team nor the participants know which participants are in which group. This design is a gold standard for approximating full comparability of the exposed and unexposed, and serves as a useful referent when one considers the other risk factor designs.

The random assignment ensures that the groups do not differ due to systematic factors at the start of the trial. All of the ways in which exposures cluster because of individual choices and societal pressures are eliminated through random assignment. There can, however, be differences between the two groups caused by random processes at the start of the trial.

After the start of a trial, sources of noncomparability can be introduced and lead to bias. A classic scenario is when one group has a more burdensome regimen than the other group, leading to follow-up rates that are different for the two groups. This creates the potential for bias due to unequal attrition.

Another classic scenario is when the research team, the participants, or both have a strong belief in the intervention, leading them to look more carefully for disease among the exposed (no-intervention) than the unexposed (intervention) group. The double blind provides a partial safeguard against this practice but may not eliminate it. To produce a complete double blind requires that the no-intervention group receive a placebo that is indistinguishable from the intervention. When this is only partly realized, the field research team and the participants may be able to guess the assigned group correctly. This creates the potential for bias due to differential misclassification.

The double-blind randomized controlled trial has been used on several occasions to investigate whether prenatal folate supplements reduce the risk of NTDs. In the first such trial (MRC Vitamin Study Research Group 1991), women planning a pregnancy were randomly assigned to receive one of four supplements—folic acid, other vitamins, both, or neither. Offspring exposed to low folate (mother received no vitamins or other vitamins alone) had a nearly fourfold higher risk of NTDs than offspring unexposed to low folate (mother received folic acid with or without other vitamins).This trial and later ones produced definitive evidence that prenatal folate was related to the risk of NTDs. More precisely, these trials demonstrated that removing exposure to low prenatal folate (by providing vitamin supplements) reduced the risk of

NTDs. The randomized controlled trial results will be compared with the results from other designs as we progress through the chapter.

Natural Experiments

The cohort study is second to the preventive intervention trial in terms of simulating full comparability. A cohort study begins with exposed and unexposed people who are free of the outcome of interest. The **natural experiment** is a kind of cohort study, but not the most common kind. It bears special consideration because it represents a particularly effective strategy for controlling sources of noncomparability. Just as the randomized controlled trial sets the standard among preventive intervention trials, the natural experiment sets the standard among cohort studies.

Natural experiments are sometimes founded on historical events that "assign" individuals to exposed and unexposed groups (other kinds of natural experiments are described in chapter 10). One group is affected by an event (exposed), whereas a second otherwise similar group is not (unexposed). The design is termed a natural experiment because, unlike an ordinary experiment, the investigator does not assign individuals to exposed and unexposed groups. In a well-designed natural experiment, the selection of the populations exposed and unexposed is largely by chance or, at the very least, largely outside the control of the people affected. Natural experiments based on historical events tend to approximate these conditions best when they are based on catastrophic events, such as famines, floods, hurricanes, earthquakes, and wars. Typically, the population of one area is afflicted by a sudden and unexpected disaster (exposed), while the population of a neighboring area is not (unexposed).

The Dutch Famine Study was a natural experiment that provided an early clue that prenatal diet was related to NTDs (Stein et al. 1975). A Nazi blockade of western Holland toward the end of World War II precipitated a severe famine that was tightly circumscribed in both time and place. In the famine cities, the birth cohort in gestation during the famine period was exposed to prenatal nutritional deficiency. Birth cohorts in the same cities born before or conceived after the famine were unexposed to prenatal nutritional deficiency. Birth cohorts in other areas of Holland during the famine period were also unexposed.

The Dutch Famine Study compared the exposed with the unexposed birth cohorts. The strength of the design rested on the overall similarity between the exposed and unexposed cohorts, except for the dramatic difference in prenatal nutrition. The authors noted that the birth cohort exposed in early gestation had a higher frequency of congenital anomalies of the central nervous system, including NTDs (Stein et al. 1975), a finding that helped stimulate much of the later epidemiologic research on prenatal folate and NTDs. The Dutch Famine Study illustrates a rigorous natural experiment, but also how the natural experiment is more vulnerable than the randomized controlled trial to sources of noncomparability. Exposure status was determined primarily by chance, in the sense of being conceived in a particular time and place. The exposure was pervasive in the famine cities. Yet the mothers of the exposed birth cohort did have some ability to mitigate the exposure by obtaining black market and other supplementary food supplies, so the wealthy were less affected than the poor. Further complicating matters, starvation suppresses fertility, so that the wealthy were more likely than the poor to conceive a baby at the height of the famine. The complex social class differences between the exposed and unexposed birth cohorts continue to generate debate about the findings even today. We will return to discuss these aspects of the study in the context of adult schizophrenia outcomes in chapter 10.

Ordinary Cohort Studies

An ordinary **cohort study** is one further step removed from simulating full comparability. As in the natural experiment, the investigator does not control the assignment of the participants to the exposed and unexposed groups. Unlike the natural experiment, we cannot assume that selection into exposure was largely beyond the control of the participants.

Exposures are not distributed independently of one another, but rather tend to cluster together. Socioeconomic status, individual personality, gender, age, and ethnicity are among the many forces that shape life experience such that exposures tend to co-occur. People who live in extreme poverty may suffer unemployment, homelessness, assault, hunger, and a profound sense of social exclusion. People who are health conscious may eat green leaf vegetables, exercise regularly, take vitamin supplements, and avoid cigarette smoke. When risk factors cluster together in this way, the exposed and unexposed will differ on many exposures, not just the one under investigation.

For these and other reasons, in a cohort study the exposed and unexposed groups tend to differ in regard to a large number of third variables. (As noted in chapter 5, third variables are all the factors other than exposure and disease). If any of these third variables are risk factors for the disease, they will be a potent source of noncomparability between the exposed and unexposed. These third variables will provide an alternative explanation for the observed association between the exposure and disease; in other words, there will be confounding.

Researchers have used the ordinary cohort design to examine the relation of prenatal folate to NTDs. In one such study, the authors identified women at prenatal screening and determined whether or not they had been taking folate supplements (Milunsky et al. 1989). They then compared the frequency of NTDs in the exposed (mother did not take folate supplements) and unexposed (mother took folate supplements) babies. The risk of NTDs was 3.7 times higher among the exposed. This study well illustrates the problems that arise because of clustering of risk factors. The women who took folate supplements generally also took other vitamins (often in the same pill). Therefore, the exposed and unexposed babies also differed on a third variable, other vitamins. The authors could not be entirely sure that the difference in NTD risk between the exposed and unexposed babies was not due to these other vitamins rather than to folate. A further source of concern was that a major case-control study, published at the same time, found no relation of prenatal folate to NTDs. The question could not be resolved until the randomized controlled trials were completed.

Case-Control Study

Case-control studies play a central role in epidemiology. They are not prominent, however, in the specialty of psychiatric epidemiology. One of our goals in this book is to increase the understanding and proper use of this design in psychiatric epidemiology; another related goal is to show how it can be used in biological psychiatry.

Under certain circumstances, a case-control study can arrive at the same result as a cohort study, using a fraction of the sample size, in less time and at less expense. Thus, it is a far more efficient design. However, it is also a less secure design in terms of simulating full comparability.

Many people find it difficult to draw the connection to full comparability for the case-control design. Full comparability has to do with differences between the exposed and the unexposed, whereas in a case-control study we are comparing cases and controls. One way to bring this connection to light is to look at a case-control study as though it were being done in the same population as a cohort study. Taking this perspective, we can begin to see the efficiency as well as the logic of the design. We will use an imaginary scenario to illustrate this point, which will be discussed in detail in part IV.

Suppose we conducted the cohort study exhibited in table 6.1, examining the relation of prenatal viral exposure to schizophrenia. After completing the study at great effort and expense, we display the results in a fourfold table where the cells represent the number of people with the four possible combinations of exposure-disease experience. The odds ratio is 5.21 which suggests that the exposed have a fivefold greater risk of schizophrenia than the unexposed (in chapter 8, we will explain how to compute and interpret odds ratios). Inspecting this fourfold table, we mull over a striking feature: the disproportionate sizes of the cells. Those without the disease far outnumber those with the disease. We followed 20,000 people over a long time to identify 600 people with the disease and 19,400 without the disease. We wonder whether there might be a better way. It would certainly be more efficient if

Table 6.1 Relation of Prenatal Viral Exposure to Schizophrenia in a Hypothetical Cohort Study

	Disease		No Disease		
	Schizophrenia	+	Schizophrenia	−	Total
Exposed	500		9,500		10,000
Unexposed	100		9,900		10,000

Note: Odds ratio = 5.21.

we could get the same result by using only a sample of the nondiseased, instead of having to follow and assess all 19,400. A great deal of time and expense would be saved if the study could be done with only 20 percent, 10 percent, or perhaps one percent, or even 0.1 percent of the nondiseased people.

Case-control studies do just that. Consider what would have happened in this imaginary study of prenatal viral exposure and schizophrenia if, instead of doing a cohort study using the whole cohort, we had done a case-control study using only 10 percent (i.e., 1,940) of the nondiseased. Suppose that we could select this 10 percent so as to keep the proportion exposed the same as among all the nondiseased. Under this condition, as shown in table 6.2, we would get the same result as in the cohort study: the odds ratio is 5.21.

Currently, epidemiologists conceptualize the case-control study in just this way. It is seen as an abbreviated form of the cohort study, the efficiency of which derives from using a sample of the noncases instead of all of them. In part IV we will explain in detail how this is done. For now, we ask the reader to accept this formulation and consider the implications.

Epidemiologists, following the pioneering work of Cornfield (1951), have reframed the case-control study as a design that samples from an underlying cohort to arrive at the same result that we would have obtained by studying the entire cohort. Hence, everything that pertains to the validity of the cohort result also pertains to the validity of the case-control result. In particular, the exposed and unexposed groups of the underlying cohort must be fully comparable, whether we are studying the whole cohort (cohort design) or a sample of it (case-control design).

Once we adopt this perspective, it becomes obvious that the same sources of noncomparability that threaten the cohort study also threaten the case-control study. In the case-control study, however, we cannot visualize them easily. What we have at hand are only the cases and controls. Although we may understand the controls to represent a sample of the noncases in some underlying cohort, we may not be able to delineate that underlying cohort. To discern how the exposed and unexposed groups might be different without having the whole cohort at hand is a real intellectual challenge.

Furthermore, the case-control study presumes that we can take a representative sample of the noncases in a sometimes intangible underlying cohort. Otherwise, we will arrive at a different result. In part IV, we will describe what we mean by representative in this context and how best to select controls

Table 6.2 Relation of Prenatal Viral Exposure to Schizophrenia in a Hypothetical Case Control Study

| | Cases | | Controls | | |
	Schizophrenia	+	Schizophrenia	−	Total
Exposed	500		950		1,450
Unexposed	100		990		1,090

Note: Odds ratio = 5.21.

to represent the noncases in the underlying cohort. For now, it is sufficient to appreciate that the case-control study brings a remarkable gain in efficiency but, at the same time, adds another level of complexity to the comparison of exposed and unexposed.

In addition to the efficiency afforded by requiring a smaller sample size, the case-control study can be done in a shorter time frame. The cohort study begins before disease onset and follows the cohort over time to measure the disease risk. By contrast, the case-control study is done after the disease has developed. The time frame is therefore compressed. But this efficiency also comes with a cost—temporal order is more difficult to discern with surety. We try to limit this problem by using incident cases and by measuring only the exposures that were antecedent to the disease. Even for incident cases, however, the measurement of the exposure is often colored by the disease experience, especially when the measurement depends upon recall (see chapter 16).

Researchers have applied the case-control design to investigate the relation of prenatal folate to the risk of NTDs. In one influential study (Mills et al. 1989), mothers with and without offspring with NTDs were asked to recall their use of vitamin supplements around the time of conception. The authors found no relation between prenatal folate supplementation and NTDs. It was a well-designed investigation and for that reason cast considerable doubt on the hypothesis until the matter was resolved by the randomized controlled trials already described. This discrepancy is not typical, because in general case-control studies do yield similar results to cohort studies and randomized controlled trials. But it is instructive to keep this example in mind as a caution; they sometimes do not.

Cross-sectional Studies

Cross-sectional studies generally take a random sample of a population at a specific moment in time. Most often, community surveys to estimate prevalences of mental disorders are cross-sectional studies. Thus, the design has been a mainstay of psychiatric epidemiology. Cross-sectional studies are sometimes also used to identify causes of psychiatric disorders. Here we consider their application for this purpose.

The hallmark of a cross-sectional study is that individuals in a defined population are cross-classified on their exposure and disease experience as it is extant during a specified time period. In contrast to a cohort or case-control study, cases in a cross-sectional study are, by definition, prevalent cases (see chapter 8). They represent the proportion of people in a population who have a disease during a specified time period, regardless of time of onset.

Similar to the case-control study, the cases and noncases can be understood to be derived from an underlying cohort. Problems regarding comparability can be difficult to discern because the study is compressed in time. Instead of our following the underlying cohort through time, a snap shot is taken of the cohort at a particular moment. From the original underlying cohort, the cross-sectional study brings into view only the exposed and unexposed who survived to the time at which the cross-sectional study is done. All the sources of noncomparability in a cohort study (confounding, unequal attrition, and differential misclassification) can exist in the cross-sectional study, but may be difficult to see.

In addition, the use of prevalent cases makes cross-sectional studies more problematic for causal inference than case-control studies. With prevalent cases, it is often difficult to assess temporal order. Researchers try to overcome this problem through attempts to date the onset of the exposure and the disease. Prevalent cases also tend to underrepresent individuals who either recover or die after a short duration of illness. Thus, an exposure that is a cause of a long duration of illness may be misidentified as a cause of the disease itself.

It should be noted, however, that in some instances these problems do not arise. When considering exposures that are present from conception (e.g., maternal age) and outcomes that are long-lasting (e.g., Down's syndrome), the cross-sectional study may not be more problematic for the identification of causes than case-control studies. It still presumes, however, that the exposure is not related to the survival of the cases (e.g., maternal age does not influence survival of children with Down's syndrome).

Cross-sectional studies are not often suited to the investigation of specific risk factors for rare diseases. It is difficult to justify the cost of establishing exposure in large numbers of nondiseased individuals for a design that offers less rigorous causal inference. Cross-sectional studies relating folate intake and NTDs were not undertaken. Nevertheless cross-sectional studies of social class and NTDs provided indirect evidence supporting nutritional hypotheses. Elwood and Nevin (1973) surveyed still and live births in Belfast (1964–1968), and found rates of NTDs were lowest in the highest social classes (Elwood and Nevin 1973). These and other similar findings drew attention to dietary factors as a possible explanation of the social class distribution, and as potential risk factors for NTDs.

Conclusion

Study designs can be viewed as techniques for organizing our observations in ways that can reveal the causes of disease. The risk factor study designs attempt to do this by mimicking the counterfactual, which is the true test of causal effects. When the mimicry is successful, our studies isolate the effects of the exposure on the disease.

In regard to this mimicry, the randomized controlled trial is the simplest and most direct, but practical for only a small number of exposures. The cohort study is much more widely applicable, but selection into exposure is not random. The case-control study is more complex and indirect but often the most useful. Although the specific techniques differ among designs, the underlying strategy is the same—the examination of fully comparable groups of exposed and unexposed individuals to isolate the effects of specific risk factors. Whatever design is chosen, the validity of the study depends upon the degree to which we achieve this goal.

References

Cornfield JA (1951). A Method of Estimating Comparative Rates from Clinical Data. *J. Natl. Cancer Inst.* 11:1269–1275.

Elwood JH and Nevin NC (1973). Factors Associated with Anencephalus and Spina Bifida in Belfast. *Br. J. Prev. Soc. Med.* 27:73–80.

Friedman LM, Furberg CD, and Demets DL, eds. (1996). *Fundamentals of Clinical Trials*, 3rd ed. Littleton, Mass.: PSG Publishing.

Goldberger J, Waring CH, and Willets DG (1915). The Prevention of Pellagra: a Test of Diet Among Institutional inmates. *Public Health Rep.* 30:3117–3131.

Goldberger J, Wheeler GA, and Sydenstricker E (1920). A Study of the Relation of Diet to Pellagra Incidence in Seven Textile-Mill Communities of South Carolina in 1916. *Public Health Rep.* 35:648–713.

Lilienfeld AM (1982). The Fielding H. Garrison Lecture: *CeterisPparibus:* The Evolution of the Clinical Trial. *Bul. Hist. Med.* 56:1–18.

Miettinen OS and Cook EF (1981). Confounding: Essence and Detection. *Am. J Epidemiol.* 114:593–603.

Mills JL, Rhoads GG, Simpson JL, Cunningham GC, Conley MR, Lassman MR, Walden ME, Depp OR, and Hoffman HJ (1989). The Absence of a Relation between the Periconceptional Use of Vitamins and Neural-Tube Defects. National Institute of Child Health and Human Development Neural Tube Defects Study Group. *N. Engl. J. Med.* 321:430–435.

Milunsky A, Jick H, Jick SS, Bruell CL, MacLaughlin DS, Rothman KJ, and Willett W (1989). Multivitamin/Folic Acid Supplementation in Early Pregnancy Reduces the Prevalence of Neural Tube Defects. *JAMA* 262:2847–2852.

MRC Vitamin Study Research Group (1991). Prevention of Neural Tube Defects: Results of the Medical Research Council Vitamin Study. *Lancet* 338:131–137.

Shapiro S (2000). Bias in the Evaluation of Low-Magnitude Associations: An Empirical Perspective. *Am. J. Epidemiol.* 151:939–945.

Stein ZA, Susser M, and Saenger G, Marolla F (1975). *Famine and Human Development: The Dutch Hunger Winter of 1944–1945.* New York: Oxford University Press.

Susser M (1995). The Tribulations of Trials—Intervention in Communities. *Am. J. Public Health* 85:156–158.

Terris M, ed. (1964). *Goldberger on Pellagra.* Baton Rouge: Louisiana State University Press.

7 Relationships among Causes

Sharon Schwartz and Ezra Susser

Over the past 50 years, epidemiologists have refined the methods for isolating risk factors and put them to extremely good use. By examining one risk factor at a time, however, we cannot fully understand the etiology of a disease. Causes interact with one another and change one another in a dynamic process.

In this chapter, we present and illustrate an elementary framework for translating our ideas about disease causation into a set of predicted relationships among several variables in the web of causation, rather than merely into a predicted relationship between the exposure and the disease. Having such a framework represents a first step toward using our study designs for understanding the role of a risk factor in the web of causation, that is, for **causal explanation** (Shadish et al. 2002). In part VIII, we build upon and extend this framework.

Elaborating and Testing Causal Ideas

In what follows, we refer to ideas or theories about the causation of a disease as causal ideas. Causal ideas generate hypotheses, and hypotheses in turn are operationalized as predictions about the relationships among variables, such as an association between exposure and disease. The process of hypothesis testing can be thought of as a series of studies in which we collect and analyze the data needed to evaluate these predictions (Platt 1964; Shadish et al. 2002).

An apparently simple hypothesis—that a certain exposure is a risk factor for a disease—may already embody some key assumptions that predict relationships among variables. It assumes the potential for other causal pathways; not all persons with the disease have necessarily had this exposure. It also assumes that the exposure works in tandem with other causes, that the disease would not follow inevitably from this exposure alone. In other words, by specifying that the exposure is a risk factor, we predict that it will be associated with the disease but neither necessary nor sufficient to produce the disease.

To elaborate other predictions, we can think about roles that other variables may play in relationship to our (hypothesized) risk factor of central interest. Of paramount concern are relationships that could pose alternative explanations for an association between the exposure and the disease. By considering these relationships in advance of our study, we can refine our predictions to take them into account and arm ourselves with the data necessary to do so (Maclure 1985).

The process is exemplified in the investigations of social causation of schizophrenia. Social causation posits that social disadvantage can play a role in the development of this disease. In accordance with this causal idea, it was hypothesized that low social class is a risk factor for schizophrenia. This hypothesis predicts that low social class should—like any risk factor—be associated with schizophrenia, be temporally antecedent to it, and be the sole plausible explanation for at least part of the association (chapter 5). An association between low social class and schizophrenia was readily established (Eaton 1985; Dohrenwend et al. 1992). In fact, early evidence for this association helped stimulate the idea of social causation.

It was far more difficult, however, to discern the temporal order. Reverse causation was a potent possibility. On the one hand, as predicted by the theory of social causation, low social class might increase the risk for the disease. On the other hand, as predicted by a competing theory of social selection, early manifestations of schizophrenia might cause individuals to attain a lower than expected social class (Dohrenwend et al. 1992). In a classic study, Goldberg and Morrison (1963) devised a means to determine the temporal order. They reasoned that under social causation but not social selection the low socioeconomic status of the family of origin—as well as that of the afflicted individual—would be associated with schizophrenia. They found that low socioeconomic status of the family of origin was *not* associated with schizophrenia. They concluded that social causation did not match the data. Later, studies in Israel and elsewhere, using varying approaches, came to similar conclusions (Dohrenwend et al. 1992; Hafner and an der Heiden 1997; Mulvany et al. 2001; Lawlor et al. 2003).

Thus, investigators over a period of time generated a causal idea, formulated a hypothesis, elaborated a set of predictions from this hypothesis, designed studies to test the predictions in empirical data, and ultimately rejected the idea, at least in its original form. Foreseeing and specifying the competing explanations for the exposure-disease association was a crucial part of this process. This enabled investigators to design studies that afforded a rigorous test of the causal idea.

Causal Explanation

Causal explanation involves consideration of the variables that produce, mediate, and modify the hypothesized exposure-disease relationship. The goal of causal explanation is to go beyond the identification of the causes of the disease to an understanding of the interplay among causes.

Attempting causal explanation has value for several reasons. One is that we decrease the number of plausible alternative explanations for the observed exposure-disease association. Suppose we postulate a causal explanation; spell out its predictions for the relationships among the exposure, the disease, and other variables; and observe these relationships in our data. Then any viable alternative would also have to explain not only the exposure-disease association, but also this set of relationships among the exposure, the disease, and other variables. Another reason is that, as we will show later, it suggests alternative loci for public health interventions.

As the research proceeds, even the most elementary causal idea can usually be elaborated to generate hypotheses pertaining to causal explanation. We may do this, for example, by considering the characteristics of persons, places, and time periods that provide the conditions necessary for the cause to have an effect—that is, the causal partners as defined in chapter 4. In what follows we discuss how we can elaborate our causal ideas to postulate causal explanations. This requires consideration of the relationships among the variables in the web of causation. In an elementary framework, we describe five kinds of relationships. The first two relationships are part of causal identification described in earlier chapters. We include them here for completeness of the schema. The last three relate to causal explanation.

An Elementary Framework

From the vantage point of a particular exposure, we can specify five roles that other variables can play in relation to it (Susser 1973; Shadish et al. 2002). These relationships—independent risk factors, confounders, antecedents, mediators, and causal partners—are depicted in figure 7.1. We first describe and illustrate each role and then provide an example to show how this schema can be applied.

Independent Risk Factors

Independent risk factors cause disease through causal pathways other than the exposure of interest (i.e., through different sufficient causes). In addition, they are not associated with the exposure of interest (figure 7.1). In chapter 4, we offered an imaginary scenario in which three different sufficient causes led to schizophrenia (see figure 4.2). In this scenario, the exposure of interest was prenatal viral exposure, which was a partner in one sufficient cause comprising prenatal viral exposure, genetic mutation, adolescent cannabis use, and other unknown causes (sufficient cause 1 in figure 4.2). Immigrant status was a risk factor belonging to a different sufficient cause (sufficient cause 2 in figure 4.2). Immigrant status would then be an independent risk factor, provided that immigrants and nonimmigrants had the same frequency of prenatal viral exposure.

Ultimately, our explanation of disease etiology will be incomplete without consideration of these independent risk factors. In terms of identifying and explaining the causal effect of our exposure of interest, however, they can be ignored, because they do not influence or explain the association between the exposure of interest and the disease.

A. Independent Risk Factors

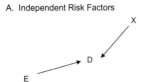

B. Confounders (Alternatives to Sole Plausibility)

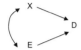

C. Antecedents

X ⟶ E ⟶ D

D. Mediators

E ⟶ X ⟶ D

E. Causal Partners

X

+ ⟶ D

E

Figure 7.1 Relationship among variables. E = exposure of interest; X = other variables (third variable); D = disease of interest.

Confounders

Like independent risk factors, confounders are risk factors that cause disease through different causal pathways than the exposure of interest. However, in contrast to independent risk factors, they are associated with the exposure of interest (figure 7.1). Confounders represent competing explanations for an exposure-disease association. For example, in the consideration of negative, stressful life events as a cause of depression, low self-esteem is a potential confounder. Negative events and depression may be associated not only through a causal effect of this exposure on the disease, but also because low self-esteem causes both negative events and depression. Thus confounding by low self-esteem provides a competing explanation for at least part of the association between life events and depression. By specifying confounders, we elaborate our causal idea and can make more specific predictions. In our example, we would elaborate our idea by specifying that negative events are a cause of depression regardless of self-esteem. This elaborated causal idea makes the more specific prediction that life events are associated with depression even among people with similar levels of self-esteem.

The alternative explanations of most theoretical interest are **natural confounders**. These confounders co-occur with the exposure of interest due to characteristics of individuals' and the environments in which they reside. The relationship between the exposure and the third variable exists in naturally occurring populations. However, **artifactual confounders** need to be considered, as well. These are confounders associated with the exposure of interest only (or more strongly) within the context of the study, as a result of selective recruitment or other methodological artifacts. We will revisit this distinction in chapter 11 and discuss its implications in part VIII.

Antecedents

An **antecedent** is a cause of the exposure of interest (figure 7.1). The identification of antecedents embeds the exposure of interest within a causal chain leading to disease. Such "upstream" causes may provide promising loci for intervention.

For example, suppose we find that a mother's smoking cigarettes at home (the exposure of interest) increases the risk of tobacco use dependence in her adolescent daughter. An antecedent of the mother's smoking cigarettes at home may be her own tobacco use dependence. Reducing tobacco use dependence in mothers may be an important intervention in preventing tobacco use dependence in their adolescent daughters.

An antecedent is not necessarily detectable within the population of interest (Rose 1992), because everyone in the population may have been exposed to it. To be detectable as a cause within a population, a factor must show variation within the population. In the smoking example, if we look further upstream, we may suspect that the unrestricted marketing of cigarettes is an important antecedent of mothers' tobacco use dependence. But this antecedent will not be detectable if everyone in the population has been exposed to the unrestricted marketing.

Antecedents shared by everyone within a population may, however, vary across populations. Restrictions on cigarette marketing may vary when legal restrictions are imposed in some but not other nations. Therefore, the hypothesis that unrestricted cigarette marketing is an antecedent of mothers' tobacco use dependence could be tested in cross-population studies as described in part VIII.

Mediators

A **mediator** (also referred to as an intervening or intermediate variable) is a risk factor that links the exposure of interest to the disease (figure 7.1). As with confounding variables, mediators are causes of the disease and are associated with the exposure of interest. Unlike confounders, however, mediators do not provide an alternative explanation for an exposure-disease association. Rather, they are situated in the causal chain of interest between the exposure and the outcome, and therefore are part of the explanation of how the exposure causes disease.

In the smoking example, suppose the mother's smoking is the exposure of interest. The mother's smoking at home may be causally relevant only insofar as it leads to the daughter's seeing the mother's smoking. The daughter's *seeing* her mother's smoking is then a mediator. A mediator can be thought of as the "active ingredient" of a more broadly measured exposure. Following the same hypothetical example, the active ingredient of the exposure of interest (mother's smoking at home) is the daughter's seeing the mother's smoking. Mother's smoking at home when the daughter is out has no effect.

Causal Partners

Causal partners are risk factors that work together (or in "synergy") with the exposure of interest to cause the disease (figure 7.1). As noted earlier, the causal partners are the characteristics of persons, places, and times that provide the context in which the exposure has an effect. In the terms introduced in chapter 4, they are causal partners in the same sufficient cause. In the imaginary scenario of figure 4.2, for example, genetic mutation, and adolescent cannabis use were causal partners of prenatal viral exposure in a sufficient cause of schizophrenia.

The process of specifying causal partners can be illustrated with the example of social causation of schizophrenia. After studies refuting the prediction that low social class was antecedent to schizophrenia, this theory was at a low ebb, despite some useful refinements (Link et al. 1986). This position was reconsidered, however, when a series of studies suggested that second generation Afro-Caribbean immigrants to the United Kingdom had a markedly increased risk of schizophrenia (reviewed in Boydell and Murray 2003). Shortly thereafter, studies in other European countries produced striking results along the same lines. Social causation—for example, unemployment and discrimination—is considered by many to be the most plausible explanation for these findings. The causal idea now has been reformulated, however, to explain why the combination of immigrant parents, low socioeconomic status and discrimination, but not socioeconomic status alone, might increase the risk of schizophrenia. Thus, the original idea was refuted by the data, but subsequently new data led to its appearance in a new context. The reformulated idea suggests specific hypotheses about causal partners needed for low socioeconomic status to have an effect. This represents a first step toward causal explanation (Murray and Hutchinson 1999; Susser and Mojtabai 1999; Cooper 2005).

To understand the context in which an exposure has an effect, we need a well-developed theory and a large data set in which to examine the synergistic effects of causal partners predicted by the theory. Perhaps because these preconditions are often lacking, the methods used to study causal partners (or synergy) are often inadequate. Synergy is typically examined with use of tests of statistical interaction or effect modification, but different statistical methods can lead to different conclusions. To avoid contributing to further misunderstanding, we defer a full consideration of synergy, effect modification, and interaction to part VIII.

Risk Factor Epidemiology and Causal Explanation

Contemporary critiques of risk factor epidemiology have focused on its relative neglect of some of these relationships and in particular of antecedents and mediators. Without specifying the antecedents, such as the marketing of cigarettes in the earlier example, we may not appreciate the implications for public health action (e.g., Lawlor et al. 2003). Without specification of the mediators, the exposure and disease are connected only by a "black box" (Susser and Susser 1996; Weed 2000).

In this regard, the progress of risk factor epidemiology described in chapter 4, may be seen as "three steps forward but one step back." Moving from strands of causation (see figure 4.1) to causal pies (see figure 4.2) brought the discipline to a concept of cause that could be grounded in the logic of the counterfactual. This enhanced the development of methods for causal identification and clarified the role of causal partners. At the same time, however, this approach drew our attention away from other aspects of causal explanation. As we explain in Part VIII, this approach does not easily accommodate antecedents and mediators.

Illustration: Elaborating Our Causal Ideas

Suppose we develop a causal idea about fetal origins of schizophrenia, and it leads us to hypothesize that prenatal exposure to the influenza virus is a risk factor for schizophrenia. This hypothesis predicts that the risk of schizophrenia is higher among those with prenatal influenza exposure than among those who have not been exposed (Brown et al. 2004). However, we would want to generate more precise predictions and provide the beginning of a causal explanation.

Our framework can provide some guidance. First, we could look for confounders that provide alternative explanations for the same pattern of results. Older paternal age is a risk factor for schizophrenia (Malaspina et al. 2001) and could be a confounder as follows. Older women may be more likely to develop prenatal influenza infections. Since older women tend to have children with older men, the risk factor of older paternal age may occur more frequently among the exposed. The risk factor hypothesis, then, also predicts that the association between prenatal influenza exposure and schizophrenia be independent of paternal age. Next, we could look for antecedents and mediators. Crowded housing conditions may be hypothesized to be an antecedent of prenatal influenza exposure. Disturbances in the production of cytokines (which are part of the biological response to infections and also play a role in neurodevelopment) may be a hypothesized mediator. Finally, we may specify one of the conditions under which prenatal influenza exposure may produce schizophrenia—for example, the presence of a genetic mutation. That is, we could posit that genetic mutation and prenatal influenza exposure are causal partners in a sufficient cause leading to schizophrenia. The postulated causal explanation would now be as follows: Prenatal influenza exposure, generated in part by crowded housing conditions, causes schizophrenia through the disruption of cytokines when the child has a genetic predisposition to schizophrenia. This relationship between prenatal influenza exposure and schizophrenia is independent of paternal age.

This is a very simple example using only one variable in each role: confounder, antecedent, mediator, and causal partner. The causal explanation can be specified further to take into consideration multiple variables in one or more of these roles. In addition, the same variable can play multiple roles as a mediator-confounder, antecedent-confounder, or causal partner–confounder.

The patterns brought into view by our studies can be compared with the predictions generated by our causal explanation. To concisely state these predictions, we often frame them in terms of the effects of "adjusting" for variables (for detailed explanation of this terminology, see chapter 12). Having specified the potential confounders, antecedents, mediators, and causal partners, as well as the exposure being investigated as a risk factor, we make the following predictions: there should be an association between the exposure and the disease, this association should persist after adjustment for potential confounding exposures, adjusting for the exposure of interest should decrease the relationship between the antecedent and the disease, the exposure's relationship with the disease should be decreased after adjustment for the potential mediator, and the exposure's effect should be more pronounced in the presence of its causal partners.

When variables play multiple roles, however, the assessment becomes quite complicated. The designs and statistical procedures for assessing these relationships are elaborated later in this book.

Drawing Conclusions from Our Data

A good fit between our study data and our predictions gives us more confidence in the hypotheses and the underlying theory. Note, however, that this confidence does not confirm the theory. Since all observations are fallible, and alternative explanations are always possible, our conclusions are almost always tentative.

In addition, any conclusion deriving from a good fit between our hypothesis and our data is predicated on the assumption that our data faithfully represent the pattern of facts in the "real" world. As discussed in previous sections and reiterated throughout, data reflect the facts, but imperfectly. Our vision is "blurred" by measurement errors and chance distortions, as well as by conceptual lapses.

How then do we know that our data are trustworthy? How do we know if we can believe what they tell us? Two approaches, null hypothesis testing and the application of **causal criteria** are often used as decision rules to answer these questions. Although neither method was developed to be used in this way, our desire for certainty sometimes leads to over reliance on them. We will consider each approach and its appropriate and inappropriate application, and some available alternatives.

Null Hypothesis Testing and Alternative Procedures

In null hypothesis testing, commonly used in psychiatric research, data associations are juxtaposed with a hypothesis of no association. Statistical tests are applied to assess the probability of the data, or more extreme values, when one assumes the null to be true. If this probability dips below a cut-point, traditionally 5 percent (i.e., "p-value" less than 0.05), the null hypothesis is rejected.

A null hypothesis test may be useful but is not nearly sufficient for assessing whether an observed association is due to chance (and is not helpful at all for assessing whether it is due to bias). Researchers often conclude from a null hypothesis test with a p-value less than 0.05 that they are 95 percent confident that the data are true. Unfortunately, as has been discussed extensively in the literature (Cohen 1994), this conclusion demands more of the statistical test than it can deliver. The p-value does not tell us the probability that the data are true, which is what we really want to know. It tells us only the probability of these or more extreme values if the null is true, assuming no bias or misclassification error.

To illustrate this point, suppose we test 10,000 hypothesized associations, of which 100 (one percent) are true associations. We conduct each test with a statistical power of 80 percent, which means that in the presence of a true association there is an 80 percent chance that the null hypothesis will be rejected. In this scenario, we expect that in 80 (80 percent) of the 100 studies testing true associations, the null hypothesis will be rejected, but also that in 495 (5 percent) of the 9,900 other studies the null hypothesis will be rejected. Thus, among the studies in which the null hypothesis will be rejected, only a small fraction (80 of 575) would have detected a true association. In the vast majority (495 of 575), the observed association would be due to chance.

To improve the proportion of tests that reveal true associations, we seek to improve the prior probability that a hypothesized association will be true. In this scenario, suppose the prior probability had been 25 percent rather than one percent, or in other words, 2,500 rather than 100 of the 10,000 associations we tested were true associations. Then the vast majority of tests that rejected the null hypothesis would reveal true associations (80 percent of 2500 = 2000, versus 5 percent of 7500 = 375). We improve the prior probability by testing associations for which we have previous findings and good theories. Thus, to properly interpret the result of a null hypothesis test, we must consider not only the p-value but also the prior probability as indicated by the weight of prior evidence and supporting theory.

Notwithstanding its limitations, this approach is the one most often used in psychiatric research, and in fact in all medical research at the present time. Therefore, even though few epidemiologists would endorse this approach, it is vital to be familiar with it. In part VI we describe the approach, and steer readers toward the more appropriate uses and interpretations.

Causal "Criteria"

Epidemiologists often use guidelines or causal "criteria" to help them draw conclusions from their study results. The best known are the guidelines developed by Austin Bradford Hill (1965), which suggest that exposure-disease associations are more likely to be causal if they exhibit (1) strength (a large effect size), (2) consistency (the relationship has been observed in different times, places, and persons), (3) specificity (the exposure is related to a narrow outcome, and the outcome is related to a narrow set of causes), (4) temporality (the exposure is prior to the outcome), (5) biologic gradient (the association evidences a dose-response curve), (6) plausibility (there is a biologically plausible explanation for the relationship), (7) coherence (with respect to the negative side of plausibility, the association does not violate known aspects of the pathophysiology of the disease), (8) experiment (there is evidence from experimental manipulations for the relationship), and (9) analogy (the exposure-disease relationship is analogous to other types of relationships).

Although researchers often use these or similar guidelines as causal criteria against which to evaluate their results at the end of a particular study (Weed and Gorelic 1996; Weed 1997), the guidelines were not intended to be used in this way and their application for this purpose can be problematic. As many people, including Hill (1965), have noted, the extent to which the criteria apply to a particular study depends on the theory under investigation. For example, when biological phenomena create threshold effects, the characteristic of a biologic gradient is not applicable. Similarly, there are many potent causes, such as smoking or socioeconomic status, which do not evidence specificity; they are causally related to many outcomes.

Our own view is that causal criteria are of limited value for drawing conclusions from our study results. Although it is perfectly legitimate to synthesize all the available evidence after the study is completed, this practice does not substitute for the process of specifying what conclusions can be drawn from the results of our particular study. The causal criteria do not offer a systematic approach to assessing how much the study data have shifted the balance of evidence for a causal hypothesis.

On the other hand, these causal criteria offer extremely valuable guidelines in the planning stages of a study (Maclure 1985). Before beginning a study, we need to consider the strength and consistency of the current evidence, and postulate explanations for inconsistencies between previous studies. How well tested are the hypothesized causal effects? How consistent are past results? Are the inconsistencies between studies due to differences in methods? How large are the effects found in previous studies? Do the effect sizes differ and, if so, are they within the range of sampling variations, or do they represent real effect modification due to true differences in the contexts under which the exposure has an effect? We also need to develop reasonable theories about disease causation. For this purpose, we consider coherence, biological plausibility, and analogy. Finally, to devise tests of our theories, we specify the mediators and causal partners implied by these theories, and identify patterns of results that would discriminate among competing theories. Reference to the guidelines helps to systematize our thinking throughout this process.

Bayesian Approaches

Generally, in epidemiologic research we do not aim to reach a final decision on a causal relationship in a single study. The goal of a particular study is to increase or decrease our confidence in a hypothesized causal relationship, and to help us to refine or reformulate our causal idea. To reach that goal, we want each study to be as strong as possible (Platt 1964).

In this context, what do we mean by a strong study? Ideally, before we do a study we assess our confidence in the hypothesized causal relationship. A strong study should be able to shift the balance of evidence toward or away from a particular hypothesis about disease causation. In other words, strong studies are those that adequately confront and challenge our hypotheses and are therefore capable of changing our confidence in them (Platt 1964).

Methodologies for quantifying the changes in our beliefs due to our study results are at the heart of Baysean approaches to decision making (for a full discussion, see Howson and Urbach 1993). Although formal Bayesian approaches are not yet common in epidemiology, this way of thinking corresponds well with how epidemiologists think about their results and draw their conclusions (Rothman and Greenland 1998; Schwartz and Susser, in press).

Sensitivity Analysis

Although there is no litmus test for the validity of a result, **sensitivity analyses** can be used to probe our data for this characteristic. Sensitivity analyses examine the robustness of our data patterns to errors related to bias or chance (Weinstein 1980; Rothman and Greenland 1998). We examine our data, making different assumptions about the amount of measurement error, unmeasured confounding, and other methodological artifacts. Trustworthy data will show the same basic pattern of results over a broad range of assumptions. For example, if we suspect that part of the association between our exposure and disease is due to recall bias, we can reanalyze the data to see how large this bias would have to be to appreciably change the association. If the results change only under unreasonable scenarios, we have more confidence in our data patterns. We provide an example of the use of this approach in part III.

Epidemiologists increasingly employ sensitivity analyses, and epidemiology journals encourage reporting such analyses to help readers assess the validity of the main results. Sensitivity analyses have also begun to appear in the analysis and interpretation of results in medical journals. If in the future sensitivity analysis were to become a routine part of data analysis, it would be a welcome development.

Conclusion

Epidemiologists aim not only to identify causes, but also to explain the causal processes that lead to disease. Causal explanation requires us to elaborate our causal ideas through the specification and examination of alternative explanations, antecedents, mediators, and causal partners. This process helps to create strong studies.

The elucidation of causal pathways also helps to locate points for public health intervention. It is important to note, however, that confidence in our theories of disease causation does not automatically translate into a solid basis for public health action. This basis may require assessment, in addition, of the consequences of acting or not acting to remove an exposure from a particular context. Because of the dynamic interplay among risk factors, the removal of a single exposure can have reverberations that lead to unintended consequences for both the disease of interest and other outcomes.

For purposes of exposition, we have presented an idealized version of the relationship between causal ideas and the conduct of studies. In the real world, data spark theories even as they are testing them, and everything is sprinkled with a layer of serendipity. However, by starting with a well-formulated, theory-driven plan, we will make the most progress.

References

Boydell J and Murray R (2003). Urbanization, Migration, and Risk of Schizophrenia. In Murray RM, Jones PB, Susser E, van Os J, and Cannon M, eds., *The Epidemiology of Schizophrenia*. New York: Cambridge University Press.

Brown AS, Begg MD, Gravenstein S, Schaefer CA, Wyatt RJ, Bresnahan M, Babulas VP, and Susser E (2004). Serologic Evidence of Prenatal Influenza in the Etiology of Schizophrenia. *Arch. Gen. Psychiatry* 61:774–780.

Cohen J (1994). The Earth Is Round ($p < .05$). *Am. Psychol.* 49:997–1003.

Cooper B (2005). Immigration and Schizophrenia: The Social Causation Hypothesis Revisited. *Br. J. Psychiatry* 186:361–363.

Dohrenwend BP, Levav I, Shrout PE, Schwartz S, Naveh G, Link BG, Skodol AE, and Stueve A (1992). Socioeconomic Status and Psychiatric Disorders: The Causation-Selection Issue. *Science* 255:946–952.

Eaton WW (1985). Epidemiology of Schizophrenia. *Epidemiol. Rev.* 7:105–126.

Goldberg EM and Morrison SL (1963). Schizophrenia and Social Class. *Br. J. Psychiatry* 109:785–802.

Hafner H and an der Heiden W (1997). Epidemiology of Schizophrenia. *Can. J. Psychiatry* 42:139–151.

Hill AB (1965). The Environment and Disease: Association or Causation? *Proc. R. Soc. Med.* 58:295–300.

Howson C and Urbach P (1993). *Scientific Reasoning: The Bayesian Approach*, 2nd ed. Chicago: Open Court.

Lawlor DA, Frankel S, Shaw M, Ebrahim S, and Davey Smith G (2003). Smoking and Ill Health: Does Lay Epidemiology Explain the Failure of Smoking Cessation Programs among Deprived Populations? *Am. J. Public Health* 93:266–270.

Link B, Dohrenwend BP, and Skodol AE (1986). Socio-Economic Status and Schizophrenia: Noisome Occupational Characteristics as a Risk Factor. *Am. Sociol. Rev.* 51: 242–258.

Maclure M (1985). Popperian Refutation in Epidemiology. *Am. J. Epidemiol.* 121: 343–350.

Malaspina D, Harlap S, Fennig S, Heiman D, Nahon D, Feldman D, and Susser E (2001). Advancing Paternal Age and the Risk of Schizophrenia. *Arch. Gen. Psychiatry* 58:361–367.

Mulvany F, O'Callaghan E, Takei N, Byrne M, Fearon P, and Larkin C (2001). Effect of Social Class at Birth on Risk and Presentation of Schizophrenia: Case-Control Study. *BMJ* 323:1398–1401.

Murray RM and Hutchinson G (1999). Psychosis in Migrants: The Striking Example of Afro-Caribbeans Resident in England. In Gattaz WF and Hafner H, eds., *Search for the Causes of Schizophrenia: Balance of the Century*. Vol. 4. New York: Springer.

Platt J (1964). Strong Inference. *Science* 146:347–353.

Rose G (1992). *The Strategy of Preventive Medicine*. New York: Oxford University Press.

Rothman KJ and Greenland S (1998). *Modern Epidemiology*, 2nd ed. Philadelphia: Lippincott-Raven.

Schwartz S and Susser E. (in press). What Can Epidemiology Accomplish? *Int. J. Epidemiol.*

Shadish WR, Cook TD, and Campbell DT (2002). *Experimental and Quasi-experimental Designs for Generalized Causal Inference.* Boston: Houghton Mifflin Co.

Susser E and Mojtabai R (1999). Epidemiology in Schizophrenia Research: The Untapped Potential. In Gattaz WF and Hafner H, eds., *Search for the Causes of Schizophrenia: Balance of the Century.* Vol. 4. New York: Springer.

Susser M (1973). *Causal Thinking in the Health Sciences: Concepts and Strategies of Epidemiology.* New York: Oxford University Press.

Susser M and Susser E (1996). Choosing a Future for Epidemiology: II. From Black Box to Chinese Boxes and Eco-Epidemiology. *Am. J. Public Health* 86:674–677.

Weed DL (1997). On the Use of Causal Criteria. *Int. J. Epidemiol.* 26:1137–1141.

Weed DL (2000). Beyond Black Box Epidemiology. *Am. J. of Public Health* 88:12–14.

Weed DL and Gorelic LS (1996). The Practice of Causal Inference in Cancer Epidemiology. *Cancer Epidemiol. Biomarkers Prev.* 5:303–311.

Weinstein MC (1980). *Clinical Decision Analysis.* Philadelphia: W.B. Saunders.

Measures of Association

8

Ezra Susser and Sharon Schwartz

We usually begin the investigation of an exposure-disease relationship by looking for an association between the exposure and the disease. We evaluate this association by generating some simple quantitative measure that describes the strength of their association as fairly and accurately as possible. This chapter introduces the measures of association used for this purpose and some of the impediments to obtaining good measures. In part VI, we will show how to gauge the precision of these measures and how to "adjust" them to remove the contributions of confounding variables as required to examine sole plausibility.

Cohort and Case Control Studies

Cohort and case-control studies often examine the association between a dichotomous exposure (exposed or unexposed) and a dichotomous outcome (diseased or nondiseased). We focus primarily on this simplest scenario, in which the data can be displayed in a 2×2 or fourfold table. We also briefly discuss nondichotomous exposures and examine the implications of time for measures of association.

The Fourfold Table

The data from a cohort or case-control study may be summarized in a fourfold table such as table 8.1. Each of the cells (a, b, c, d) in the fourfold table gives the count of the number of individuals with a given combination of exposure and disease. For example, a represents the number of subjects who are exposed and diseased, and d represents the number of subjects who are unexposed and nondiseased. The row totals (m_1, m_2) are the numbers of exposed and unexposed, the column totals (n_1, n_2) are the numbers of diseased and nondiseased, and the total number of study subjects is t.

To assess the association between a dichotomous exposure and a dichotomous outcome, we rely on three types of probabilities (joint, marginal, and conditional) that can be derived from the fourfold table. The four **joint**

75

Table 8.1 Fourfold Table in Cohort and Case-Control Studies

	Diseased	Nondiseased	Row Totals
Exposed	a	b	m_1
Unexposed	c	d	m_2
Column totals	n_1	n_2	t

probabilities (a/t, b/t, c/t, and d/t) refer to the probability of two conditions occurring at once. For example, a/t is the probability that a subject is both exposed and diseased. The sum of the four joint probabilities is one. The four **marginal probabilities** (m_1/t, m_2/t, n_1/t, n_2/t) refer to the presence or absence of only one condition. For example, m_1/t is the probability of exposure among the study subjects. The eight **conditional probabilities** refer to the probability of one condition, given another specified condition. For instance, a/m_1 is the probability of disease, given that an individual is exposed.

Although the data from both cohort and case-control studies can be displayed in a fourfold table, the interpretation of the data depends on the study design. When the data are generated from a population cohort such as a birth cohort (see chapter 9), all of the joint, conditional, and marginal probabilities can be given meaningful interpretations. The cohort can be considered as a sample of some larger population of interest, and the probabilities can be interpreted as estimates of the true probabilities in that population.

But a cohort study can also be built around a specific exposed population where the numbers of exposed and unexposed are specified beforehand. For instance, in a study of posttraumatic stress disorder among rescue workers at the World Trade Center on September 11, 2001, one might compare 1000 rescue workers with 1000 unexposed workers. The equal numbers of exposed and unexposed are an artifact of design and do not represent the frequency of exposure in any population. Therefore, we cannot give a meaningful interpretation to any of the joint or marginal probabilities. We can, however, interpret two of the conditional probabilities: disease given the presence of exposure, and disease given the absence of exposure.

Now consider the case-control study. The number of subjects with and without disease is an artifact of design. Therefore, we cannot interpret the joint or marginal probabilities. We also cannot interpret the conditional probabilities of disease given exposure status. We can nonetheless interpret two other conditional probabilities: exposure, given presence of disease, and exposure, given absence of disease.

Measures of Association

The probabilities of greatest interest in the assessment of association are the two conditional probabilities of disease given exposure status: $Pr(\text{disease}|\text{exposed}) = a/m_1$ and $Pr(\text{disease}|\text{unexposed}) = c/m_2$. These two probabilities are referred to in epidemiology as the risk of disease in the exposed and in the unexposed, respectively. The **risk** is more precisely the probability of developing the disease over a time period specified by the study.

The comparison between these two key probabilities represents our effort to compare the disease experienced by the exposed with the disease experience they would have had were they not exposed. To make this comparison, we calculate summary values. Three popular choices are the **risk difference**, the **risk ratio** (or **relative risk**), and the **disease odds ratio**. In a cohort study, the two key probabilities (a/m_1, c/m_2), derived directly from the fourfold table, are used to compute a risk difference and risk ratio. The risk difference is simply the difference between the risks in the exposed and the unexposed ($a/m_1 - c/m_2$). The risk ratio is the ratio of the risk in the exposed to the risk in the unexposed (a/m_1 divided by c/m_2). In a case-control study, since the two component probabilities are uninterpretable, we cannot compute a valid risk difference or risk ratio. We can, however, use the fourfold table from a case-control study to compute a valid odds ratio. This is, in large part, why the odds ratio is so frequently reported in epidemiologic studies. Later we will explain why this is possible.

The disease odds ratio is the odds of disease in the exposed divided by the odds of disease in the unexposed. The **odds** are the probability of disease divided by its complement. Thus, the disease odds ratio is given by (a/m_1) / ($1 - a/m_1$) divided by (c/m_2) / ($1 - c/m_2$). This can be rewritten as (a/m_1) / (b/m_1) divided by (c/m_2) / (d/m_2). After cancellation of terms, this becomes simply a/b divided by c/d. The last expression is often rewritten as ad/bc.

The disease odds ratio, based on the risk of disease in the exposed and unexposed, can be obtained directly from a cohort but not from a case-control study. However, the disease odds ratio is identical to the exposure odds ratio (defined below). The terms in the exposure odds ratio can be derived from a case-control study. Thus, we compute the exposure odds ratio and automatically also obtain the disease odds ratio.

The equality of the disease odds ratio and the exposure odds ratio can be demonstrated by simple algebra. We have showed that the disease odds ratio can be rewritten as ad/bc. Likewise, the *exposure odds ratio* = odds of exposure in diseased divided by odds of exposure in nondiseased = (a/n_1) /($1 - a/n_1$) divided by (b/n_2) / ($1 - b/n_2$) = (a/n_1) / (c/n_1) divided by (b/n_2) / (d/n_2) = a/c divided by $b/d = ad/bc$. (For further discussion, see part IV.)

The odds ratio has another very useful property. When the probability of disease is low, the $[1 - Pr(disease)]$ term in the denominator of the odds is close to one. For a rare disease, therefore, the odds approximates its numerator, the $Pr(disease)$, that is, the risk; and the odds ratio approximates the risk ratio. Generally, the odds ratio will provide a close approximation of the risk ratios for a disease that affects less than one percent of the population, and a reasonable approximation for a disease that affects less than 10 percent in both the exposed and the unexposed groups.

There is more than one way of deriving an odds ratio. Unless otherwise specified, in this book the term **odds ratio** refers to the odds ratio just described. On occasion, we will refer to this odds ratio as the **traditional odds ratio**, in order to clearly distinguish it from other forms of the odds ratio described later (see chapter 18).

Properties of the Measures

When one compares the three measures of association (risk difference, risk ratio, and odds ratio), it is important to bear in mind that the three measures are not expressed in the same scale. For example, suppose that the probability of disease among the exposed is 20 percent and that among the unexposed it is 5 percent. The risk difference is 15 percent, or 0.15. The risk ratio is 4, indicating that the risk of disease is 4 times greater among exposed subjects than among unexposed people. Finally, the odds ratio is 4.75, revealing that the odds of disease are 4.75 times higher among exposed subjects than among unexposed people.

In addition, the range of the measures is different. The range of the risk difference is −1 to +1. The range of the risk ratio and odds ratio is zero to positive infinity. When exposure decreases disease risk, in other words, when it has a preventive effect, the risk difference is negative, and the risk ratio and odds ratio are less than one. Under the no-association scenario, the risk difference will be approximately zero, and the odds ratio and risk ratio are approximately one.

Nondichotomous Exposures

The form of the exposure variable influences the choice of measure of association. Exposure variables may be dichotomous as already described, multilevel categorical, or continuous. A multilevel exposure can take on one of a limited number (say, three, four, or more) of possible values. A continuous exposure, strictly defined, can take on any one of an infinite number of values in a given range. In practice, however, the number of possible values of a continuous variable is limited by the accuracy of the measuring instrument and by the number of digits available for recording it.

Many exposure variables can be expressed in more than one of these forms. We then choose for a specific analysis the form that is appropriate for the question being addressed. Consider the exposure maternal body mass index in the Prenatal Determinants of Schizophrenia Example (PDSE) study, which will be described in chapter 10. The PDSE examines maternal body mass index as a risk factor for schizophrenia spectrum disorder in a birth cohort study (for a summary, see chapter 10, Figure 10.1 and tables 10.6 and 10.7). The outcome is dichotomous: presence or absence of schizophrenia spectrum disorder. On the original scale, the exposure is continuous (kilograms per meter squared). For purposes of analysis, however, body mass index could be converted into a five-level categorical exposure (*very low, low, average, high, very high*); or could be converted into a dichotomous exposure (*very low/low/average* and *high/very high*). In the PDSE, maternal body mass index was converted into a dichotomous exposure, in accordance with the hypothesis that maternal overweight was a risk factor for offspring schizophrenia spectrum disorder.

Note that multilevel categorical variables can be subdivided into two types: nominal and ordinal. Nominal variables have no ordering to their categories (an example is race/ethnicity defined as *white, black, Latino, Asian*, or *other*).

In contrast, ordinal variables have an inherent ordering (the categorized version of maternal body mass index is an example). Methods for describing nominal variables can always be applied to ordinal variables, but methods for ordinal variables may or may not apply to nominal variables.

Multilevel Categorical Exposures. The concepts presented for the evaluation of association between a dichotomous exposure and disease can be easily extended to multilevel categorical exposures. Instead of summarizing the data by means of a 2×2 table, we construct a $k \times 2$ table, where k is the number of distinct levels of the categorical exposure variable, as shown in table 8.2.

In this table, we can compare any pair of exposure categories by temporarily "ignoring" the other rows in the table. By focusing on only two rows of the table, we can proceed as though we are analyzing a 2×2 table and generate any of the three measures of association already described: the risk difference, risk ratio, or odds ratio. If level 1 of the exposure variable represents a "comparison" or "unexposed" group, then it becomes the natural choice for comparison with subsequent categories. In this case, we refer to level 1 as the referent category with respect to exposure.

As in the case of the 2×2 table, only certain measures of association can be estimated from the $k \times 2$ table, depending on the design of the study. If the data come from a cohort study, we can estimate any of the three measures of association introduced previously (risk difference, risk ratio, and odds ratio). If the data come from a case-control study, only odds ratios can be computed.

Continuous Exposures. When the exposure of interest is a continuous variable, the 2×2 and the $k \times 2$ tables are inapplicable. To estimate the effect of an increase in exposure on the risk or the odds of disease, we have to resort to statistical modeling. Without statistical modeling, however, we can make some useful comparisons in the preliminary examination of the data. In a cohort study, we might categorize the exposure variable, as already described for the example of body mass index in the PDSE, and compare the disease risk in the exposure groups. In a case-control study, we might compare the

Table 8.2 A $k \times 2$ Table for Multilevel Exposures

	Diseased	Nondiseased	Row Totals
Exposure level 1	r_1	s_1	m_1
Exposure level 2	r_2	s_2	m_2
Exposure level 3	r_3	s_3	m_3
.	.	.	.
.	.	.	.
.	.	.	.
Exposure level k	r_k	s_k	m_k
Column totals	n_1	n_2	t

mean or median exposure of the diseased and nondiseased respondents. Methods for analyzing continuous exposure data are introduced in part VI.

The Element of Time

In the preceding discussion of the fourfold table, we used the terms *probability* and *risk* of disease as though they were synonymous. A disease risk, however, is not simply a probability. It is the probability of developing the disease *over a specified time period*.

Suppose we follow 1000 individuals over a 5-year period. Ten of them develop the disease. Then the disease risk is one percent or 0.01 *over five years*. The risk would not be the same for a one-year period, or for a 10-year period. By extension, the measures of association already described also pertain to a specified time period. An easy way to see this is to consider the outcome of mortality. Over a limited time period, the exposed might have a higher mortality than the unexposed. Over a period of 300 years, however, everyone will die in both the exposed and unexposed groups. The risk ratio and odds ratio will necessarily equal one, and the risk difference will be zero.

In the cohort study, the element of time is quite apparent in the process of collecting the data. We explicitly measure the risk (also known as the **cumulative incidence**) of disease in the exposed and unexposed groups over a specified time period (or **risk period**; see chapter 9) by counting the number of new or incident cases that develop in each group. We can then display these results in a fourfold table and estimate the risk ratio in the population as described.

In the case-control study, the time period may also be explicit. The recommended practice for case-control studies is to restrict attention to *incident cases collected over some specified time period*. In the simplest scenario, we include all new cases occurring in a defined population over a specified time period. But, in some case-control studies, the time period is only implicit or is unspecified. We defer further discussion of this point to part IV.

The element of time requires us to consider two further aspects of measures of association in the cohort study: the incidence rate and cohort attrition. These also have implications for the case-control study.

Incidence Rate.   Introducing the element of time enables us to consider another approach to comparing the occurrence of disease in the exposed and unexposed groups. As an alternative to comparing their disease risks, we can compare their disease rates.

An **incidence rate**, or simply *rate*, is defined in terms of number of new cases per observed person-time. Suppose we follow 1003 persons over a period of one year. Assume the rate is constant over the year of the study. Six individuals develop the disease at the midpoint of the year. Therefore, the numerator of the rate is 6 cases. The denominator is the total amount of observed person-time. This is computed by assuming that each individual contributes observed person-time until he or she either develops the disease, reaches the end of the study, or is lost to observation. In this instance, we will assume that no one is lost to observation. Then the denominator is 1000

Table 8.3 Person-Time and Rate Ratio

	Exposed	Unexposed	Total
Cases	a	b	m_1
Person-time	n_1	n_2	t

Note: Here a and b represent the number of new cases occurring over the study period among exposed and unexposed people; m_1 equals the total number of cases $(a + b)$; n_1 and n_2 represent the total person-time of exposed and unexposed people (i.e., the total amount of time the exposed and unexposed were observed while they were at risk for the disease); t equals the total amount of time all subjects were observed $(n_1 + n_2)$. The rate in exposed $= a/n_1$; in unexposed, b/n_2. The rate ratio $= [a/n_1] / [b/n_2]$.

person-years: 997 person-years (for the 997 who were disease-free for the entire year) plus 3 person-years (for the 6 who were disease-free for one half of a year). The rate is 6/1000 person-years. This could also be expressed as 6 cases/12,000 person-months, or as 6 cases/52,000 person-weeks.

To display the data, we use a different kind of fourfold table (see table 8.3). To compare the exposed and unexposed groups, we compute an **incidence rate ratio** (or *rate ratio*): rate in exposed over rate in unexposed. Although it is less often done, we could also compute an incidence rate difference (or rate difference): rate in exposed minus rate in unexposed. In later chapters, we will discuss the concept of person-time, the subtleties of the rate, and the relationship of the rate ratio to the risk ratio and the odds ratio.

Table 8.4 draws on a different example to illustrate the relationship among the different ratio measures of association for dichotomous variables. In this example, the period of observation is 17 years (6,209 days). In general, when calculated over the same time period, the risk ratio is the smallest, followed by the rate ratio. The odds ratio is larger than both. When the disease rate is low, the values of all three ratio measures converge.

Population Attributable Proportion. In etiologic research, the ratio measures we have described are most commonly employed. For some public health purposes, however, the **population attributable proportion** is more useful. It represents the proportion of cases in a population that can be "attributed" to a specific exposure. From the fourfold table, it is calculated as the risk in the population $(a + c)/t$ minus the risk in the unexposed (c/m_2), over the risk in the population $(a + c)/t$. Then we multiply by 100 to obtain a percentage. The population attributable proportion of exposure for disease, computed from the data in table 8.4, is 11 percent: the risk in the population (50/6,800) minus the risk in the unexposed (40/6,096), over the risk in the population (50/6,800), multiplied by 100 (see table 8.5).

The attributable proportion is an important statistic but needs to be interpreted with caution. First, the same proportion of disease that is attributed to a risk factor can also be attributed to the causal partners with which the risk factor interacts in causing the disease (see chapter 4). For this reason, we prefer to think of the attributable proportion as describing the proportion of disease that could be eliminated in this population through the removal of the risk factor. Second, the attributable proportion is dependent not only on the size of the ratio measures, but also on the proportion of the population

Table 8.4 Risk, Rate, and Odds

	Cases (50)	Noncases (6,750)	Total Subjects (6,800)	Person-days[a]	Risk[b]	Rate[c]	Odds[d]
Exposed	10	694	704	4,347,098	.01420455	2.300385×10^{-6}	.01440922
Unexposed	40	6,056	6,096	37,714,032	.00656168	1.060613×10^{-6}	.00660502
Measures of effect: (ratios)					2.165	2.169	2.182

[a] Sum across persons (days observed at risk for disease).
[b] The number of cases ÷ total subjects.
[c] The number of cases ÷ the number person-days.
[d] The number of cases ÷ the number of non-cases.

82

Table 8.5 Attributable Proportion

	Cases	Noncases	Total
Exposed	10	694	704
Unexposed	40	6,056	6,096
	50	1,350	6,800

$$\text{Attributable proportion} = \frac{(a+c)/t-(c/m_2)}{(a+c)/t} = \frac{50/6800-(40/6096)}{50/6800} = .11, \text{ or } 11\%.$$

that is exposed. A risk factor that has a modest influence on the disease as measured by a ratio measure could have a very large public health impact if it is very common. In the example in table 8.5, if the prevalence of exposure in the population increased from approximately 10 percent to 50 percent, the attributable proportion would more than triple even if the risk ratio remained the same.

Cross-sectional Studies

In a cross-sectional study, as opposed to a cohort or case-control study, we do not examine the association between exposure and disease risk. Instead, we examine the association between exposure and disease prevalence. The **point prevalence** (or prevalence proportion) is the proportion of people who have the disease at the time of the study; the **period prevalence** is the proportion who have had the disease over some past time interval, such as the past three years; and the **lifetime prevalence** is the proportion who have ever had the disease.

The disease prevalence is numerically different from the disease risk and has a different meaning. A cross-sectional study does not specify a time period over which incident cases are identified. In fact, it does not restrict attention to incident cases.

Although the joint, marginal, and conditional probabilities in the fourfold table can be computed, they should be interpreted in terms of prevalence, not risk. The most appropriate terms for the results of a cross-sectional study are prevalence difference, prevalence ratio, and prevalence odds ratio. Investigators nonetheless sometimes use the terms *risk difference, risk ratio* (or *relative risk*), and *odds ratio* for the results of a cross-sectional study. When this terminology is used, it is important to keep in mind the distinctly different meaning of these measures in the context of cross-sectional studies. Consider the risk ratio. In the cohort study, the risk ratio estimates only the effect of the exposure on the risk of the disease. In the cross-sectional study, on the other hand, the "risk ratio" estimates a mixture of three effects: the effect of the exposure on the risk of the disease, the effect of the exposure on the duration of the disease, and the effect of the disease on the exposure. Because the contributions of these three effects cannot be disentangled, we cannot estimate any one of them alone with the "risk ratio" from a cross-sectional study.

Although the prevalence should not be confused with the risk or rate of disease, there is a relationship between them. This is expressed in the following formula: prevalence odds = prevalence / (1 − prevalence) = rate × average duration. (This formula holds under the assumption that both the incidence rate and the disease duration are stable.) Thus, an increase (or decrease) in the prevalence of a disease can be due to either a change in its incidence or a change in its duration.

Impediments to Finding Associations

Obtaining good estimates of the association between our exposure and disease can be challenging. As described in chapter 5, the relationship between the exposure and disease is always viewed through a cloud of irrelevancies. Two important sources of irrelevancies that can obscure our vision are sampling variation and measurement errors.

Sampling Variation

The measures we obtain in our studies are used to make inferences about the true values of these measures in a population of interest. Our study measures are variable in nature. That is, if we repeated the same study by drawing a second sample from the same population, the results obtained would differ somewhat from those we obtained in the first study. The amount of sampling error in an estimate reflects its **precision**; the less sampling error, the more precise the estimate. All else being equal, larger samples yield more precise estimates. Methods for gauging the precision of each sample estimator are described in part VI.

The population of interest may sometimes be explicitly defined by the investigator. If we were to randomly sample all pregnant mothers in California in 2003, we could state explicitly that our results pertain to that population. More often, the population of interest is only implicit and somewhat ambiguous. If we were to study all pregnant women attending one prenatal clinic in California in 2003, we might think of the population of interest more broadly than as the users of this particular clinic in this particular year, without specifying precisely the boundaries of reasonable generalization. Notwithstanding these ambiguities, the interpretation of the sample values depends upon the assumption that the sample is drawn from some larger population of interest (see part VI).

The standard notation for sample estimates is $\hat{\theta}$, indicating that these are sample estimates, not true population parameters. For simplicity we will not use this notation, except in part VI, where we explain how to gauge the precision of the sample value. However, it is important to keep in mind the distinction between study sample estimates and true population parameters.

Measurement Error

A second source of difficulty in viewing associations is measurement error. For dichotomous variables, measurement errors are referred to as **misclassi-**

fication. Each individual in a study is classified as belonging in one particular cell of the fourfold table (table 8.1). If there is error in the measurement of the exposure or the disease, then the person will be misclassified and put in the wrong cell.

There are two major types of misclassification, nondifferential and differential. Nondifferential misclassification means that the misclassification of exposure status is independent of disease status and the misclassification of disease status is independent of exposure status. For example, if 20 percent of those without a disease were misclassified as diseased in both the exposed and unexposed groups, this error would be nondifferential. Similarly, if 20 percent of those without an exposure were misclassified as exposed in both the diseased and the nondiseased groups, this error, too, would be nondifferential.

Differential misclassification pertains when the misclassification of the disease depends on the exposure status (more common in cohort studies) or misclassification of the exposure depends on disease status (more common in case control studies).[1] For example, if in a cohort study, among the exposed, 20 percent of the nondiseased were misclassified as diseased, but among the unexposed only 5 percent of the nondiseased were misclassified as diseased, the error would be differential. Similarly, if in a case-control study, among the diseased (cases), 20 percent of the exposed were misclassified as unexposed, but among the nondiseased (controls) only 5 percent of the exposed were misclassified as unexposed, the error would again be differential.

This distinction is important. In general, nondifferential misclassification of dichotomous variables makes the observed association between exposure and disease smaller than the true association. Differential misclassification, on the other hand, can either strengthen or weaken the apparent association between exposure and disease. Because of this characteristic, differential misclassification can also pose an alternative explanation for an observed exposure-disease association. Here we will discuss only nondifferential misclassification, which is a threat to our observing an association. We defer a discussion of the consequences of differential misclassification to chapters 14 and 16.

Nondifferential Misclassification.   The measures in our study are numerical representations of some concept, or construct, that we have in mind. We can think of the construct as the true variable, as opposed to the variable that we measure.

There is always some difference between the construct we want to measure and the measure that we use. In the example of stressful life events used in chapter 5, people were asked to report their events. Some people did not recall

---

[1] Differential misclassification occurs when errors in exposure classification are associated with the true disease status, or errors in disease classification are associated with the true exposure status (or both). However, the same type of consequences can result from linkages among the misclassification errors, as well. We refer to this as **dependent nondifferential misclassification** in this book. We discuss dependent nondifferential misclassification with differential misclassification in chapter 14.

their events, others did not think they were worth reporting, and still others did not feel comfortable enough to report them. These phenomena created a gap between the true classification of the construct we had in mind and the measure of that construct.

Some measurement error is random; there is no discernable pattern to the error. Some exposed are classified as unexposed, and some unexposed are classified as exposed. For example, if in an unpredictable way people forget life events or remember having events that did not happen, such error would be random error. Similarly, our measures of disease also reflect random error. All random error is nondifferential. Since random error has no pattern, the misclassification of exposure cannot be linked with the disease, and misclassification of disease cannot be linked with the exposure.

Random measurement error undermines the reliability of the measure. **Reliability** refers to the replicability of our measures, our ability to obtain the same answer across different tests, testers, and time periods (for a full discussion of reliability, see Carmines and Zeller 1979; Crocker and Algina 1986). Devising a reliable measure is an important part of devising a valid measure, because an unreliable measure will be to some extent invalid, in the sense that it will reflect measurement error, as well as the true value.

Other errors are systematic; they have a pattern. Suppose that in a given study some individuals forget their events, but no individuals report events they did not have. In this study, some of the exposed will be misclassified as unexposed, but none of the unexposed will be misclassified as exposed. A systematic error of this kind will be nondifferential if the errors are independent of disease status. (It can also be differential. For example, in a case-control study of depression, one may find that the cases are more likely than the controls to forget their life events.)

Systematic errors do not necessarily undermine the reliability of a measure. In fact, systematic errors can be very reliable. The same errors may occur across tests, testers, or time periods. However, systematic errors make the measure invalid. For example, a thermometer that is constantly 2 degrees too low, can provide a consistent, reliable measure that is invalid.

Sensitivity and Specificity. It is useful to quantify measurement errors to see their effects and to understand what types of errors can cause problems and how. When one uses dichotomous variables, measurement error is often assessed through sensitivity and specificity. **Sensitivity** refers to the proportion of people who have a trait who are correctly classified as having a trait. **Specificity** refers to the proportion of people who do not have the trait who are correctly classified as not having the trait. Frequently, sensitivity and specificity are used to compare a less than perfect but more practical measure against a gold standard measure. More generally, we can think about sensitivity and specificity as relating an individual's measured classification to his or her true classification.

In table 8.6 we have arrayed the individuals from table 8.4 according to their true exposure classification (the columns) and according to their measured exposure classification (the rows). For illustrative purposes, we have assumed the numbers in table 8.4 are the true values. The sensitivity of the

Table 8.6 Sensitivity and Specificity of Exposure Measure

Measured Classification	True Classification		
	Exposed	Unexposed	
Exposed	634	610	**1,244**
Unexposed	70	5,486	**5,556**
	704	**6,096**	**6,800**

$$\text{Sensitivity} = \frac{634}{704} = 0.90. \quad \text{Specificity} = \frac{5486}{6096} = 0.90.$$

Table 8.7 Effect of Nondifferential Misclassification of Exposure Status on the Risk Ratio

	True 2 × 2		As Measured				Study 2 × 2	
			Correctly Classified on Exposure		Incorrectly Classified on Exposure			
	Disease +	Disease −	Disease +	Disease −	Disease +	Disease −	Disease +	Disease −
Exposed	10	694	9	625	4	606	13	1,231
Unexposed	40	6,056	36	5,450	1	69	37	5,519
	50	**6,750**	**45**	**6,075**	**5**	**675**	**50**	**6,750**
RR	2.165						1.569	

Note: RR = risk ratio.

exposure measure in this example is 90 percent; of the 704 people who were exposed, 634 were correctly classified. The specificity is also 90 percent; of the 6096 individuals who were not exposed, 5,486 were correctly classified.

What would be the consequences of nondifferential misclassification of this magnitude on our measures of association? In the first two columns of table 8.7, we display the relationship between exposure and disease from table 8.4. The risk ratio, assuming the measures are the true values, is 2.165. The last two columns presents the data as they would appear in a study with this type of measurement error. The risk ratio calculated from this study would be 1.569.

The columns in between reveal how we would arrive at this discrepant result. We would assume perfect classification of disease, and 90 percent sensitivity and specificity for the measure of the exposure. Since the misclassification of the exposure is nondifferential, the sensitivity and specificity of the exposure measure is 90 percent for those with and without the disease. The third and fourth columns show the numbers of diseased and nondiseased among the 90 percent who were correctly classified as exposed (sensitivity) or as unexposed (specificity) in our study. The fifth and sixth columns show the numbers of diseased and nondiseased among the 10 percent who were incorrectly classified on exposure. By simply adding the numbers from the middle columns, we obtain the 2×2 table in the last columns. For example, 9 are correctly and 4 are incorrectly classified as exposed among the diseased, yielding 13 classified as exposed among the diseased in our study.

This numeric example illustrates the profound effect that nondifferential misclassification of exposure can have on an exposure-disease association. A sensitivity and specificity of 90 percent would represent a good measure. Nonetheless, the risk ratio is considerably underestimated. The same pertains to nondifferential misclassification of disease.

In one circumstance, however, the risk ratio (but not the risk difference) can be unbiased in the presence of nondifferential misclassification. This will occur when there is nondifferential misclassification of disease caused by a uniform underestimation of the disease risk; that is, the disease is measured with perfect specificity but imperfect sensitivity.

Conclusion

Measuring the association between exposure and disease is usually the first step in the investigation of a cause. Our measures of association compare the disease outcome of the exposed and unexposed groups. This comparison can be expressed in terms of risks, rates, or odds, and in terms of ratio or difference measures. Regardless of the measures used, sampling error, combined with misclassification, either random or systematic, can obscure our view of exposure-disease associations. Having a sufficiently large sample size and measures that are as reliable and accurate as possible will help to thwart these threats to finding associations.

Difficult as it is to obtain a valid measure of the exposure-disease association, it is not usually as problematic as determining that the exposure was antecedent to the disease, and that the effect of the exposure on the disease is the sole plausible explanation for their association. In the next part, we discuss different study designs and how they are used for this purpose.

References

Carmines EG and Zeller RA (1979). *Reliability and Validity Assessment*. Beverly Hills, Calif.: Sage Publications.

Crocker LM and Algina J (1986). *Introduction to Classical and Modern Test Theory*. New York: Holt, Rinehart, and Winston.

COHORT DESIGNS IN PSYCHIATRIC EPIDEMIOLOGY

Prototypical Cohort Study

9

Ezra Susser and Sharon Schwartz

The cohort design emerged from an intellectual revolution in epidemiology after World War II (see chapter 2). By the 1950s, epidemiologists had articulated the concept of a risk factor, developed the cohort study as a method for identifying risk factors, and demonstrated the potency of this method in early applications to cancer and cardiovascular disease (MacMahon et al. 1960; Hill 1965; Susser 1985; Morabia 2004; Doll 2004; Oppenheimer in press). The design has withstood the test of time over the ensuing half century. In fact, the scope and flexibility of the cohort study have been vastly extended. Numerous variants have been devised and analytic techniques have been continually refined (Rothman and Greenland 1998; Samet and Munoz 1998; Szklo and Nieto 2000; Greenland and Brumback 2002).

In a cohort study, we compare individuals exposed and unexposed to a hypothesized risk factor, and the respective proportions who develop the disease over a specified period of time. Since this strategy requires the exposure status to be determined before the onset of the disease, it minimizes uncertainty about the temporal order of exposure and disease. It does not, however, ensure the equivalence of the exposed and unexposed groups on all factors other than the exposure. Thus, the exposure groups may not be fully comparable (as defined in chapter 5), which poses problems for causal inference.

The key innovation of the cohort design was to start with disease-free individuals as the base for a study of disease. Ideally, all individuals in the cohort are followed until they develop the disease, succumb to another condition (e.g., death) that precludes the disease, or reach the predetermined endpoint of the study. In other words, the investigator attempts to observe the entire disease experience of the cohort members for the duration of the study.

The word *cohort* originates from the Latin *cohors*, which referred to a unit of soldiers in a Roman army. It implies a group bound together and remaining together whatever happens. Likewise, once an individual enters an epidemiologic cohort, there is no exit from it. The individual is bound to the cohort under any and all circumstances. As we shall see in a later chapter, all the members of the cohort have to be taken into account in the analysis of the study results, whether or not they remain under the investigator's observation for the duration of the study.

In this chapter, we introduce the main elements of the design. To facilitate exposition, we describe as a prototype a prospective **population cohort** study. A diverse array of studies falls under the rubric of the cohort design, however, and the subsequent chapter takes up some of these variants. Chapters 11–14 discuss the principles of causal inference that pertain to such studies.

Throughout, we use examples from psychiatric epidemiology that were chosen to convey the great variety of applications, and include some of the studies that influenced the evolution of the field. In addition, we pay special attention to the salient challenges that mental disorders pose for cohort studies. Many of these challenges derive from the intrinsic complexity of disorders defined by thoughts, behaviors, and feelings. With few exceptions, the relationships between the underlying pathophysiology of the brain and these outward manifestations have yet to be well delineated.

A Prospective Population Cohort Study

Although a prospective population cohort study is but one of many kinds of cohort studies, it serves well as a prototype, both because it is most easily described and because other kinds of cohort studies can be derived by varying one or more elements of it (see chapter 10). By **prospective**, we mean that both the exposure and the outcome data are collected in the course of the investigation, rather than being culled from previously existing records.[1] A prospective cohort study may begin at any phase of the life cycle: before or at birth (table 9.1), in childhood (table 9.2), or in adulthood (table 9.3).

By population cohort (also called *general population cohort*; Rothman and Greenland 1998, p. 91), we mean that it is assembled from a naturally occurring population. Thus, the exposed and unexposed individuals are identified within the same population. Examples are persons living in a given community, or children attending a given school. Any naturally occurring population will have many kinds of exposures, so the consequences of multiple exposures can be examined within the same cohort.

Six successive steps characterize a prospective population cohort study: (1) articulating the questions, (2) defining the source population, (3) measuring the exposures, (4) following the cohort, (5) classifying the outcomes, and (6) analyzing the data. (We defer discussion of the last step to later chapters.) In a real study, where circumstance and serendipity always play a role, a researcher might not actually follow these steps in sequence. Nonetheless, the sequence is useful for introducing the main elements of the design and the points at which bias can be introduced.

---

[1] All cohort studies are prospective in the sense that they proceed from the exposure to the study outcome. By convention, however, the term prospective cohort usually refers to a cohort in which the data are collected as described here.

Table 9.1 Prospective Population Cohort Studies: Examples of Cohorts Assembled from Pregnancy/Birth

Sources	Study Description and Selected Findings
Buka et al. (1993) *See also*: Buka et al. (2001) Broman (1984)	*Study*: National Collaborative Perinatal Project (NCPP)–Providence Center *Cohort (N = 4,140)*: Pregnancies enrolled in NCPP 1959–1966. Offspring followed in childhood ages 4 and 8 months, and ages 1,3,5, and 7. Selected for follow-up in adulthood (ages 18–27) were offspring exposed to pregnancy and delivery complications, and matched unexposed offspring (total N = 1,068). *Finding*: Exposed and unexposed did not differ overall on psychiatric disorders. Findings for some specific disorders were suggestive, for example, of a relation of chronic fetal hypoxia to psychotic disorders.
Caspi et al. (2002) *See also*: Cannon et al. (2002) Silva and Stanton (1997)	*Study*: Dunedin Multi-disciplinary Child Development Study *Cohort (N = 1,037)*: All births at Queen Mary Maternity Hospital in Dunedin, New Zealand, from April 1, 1972, through March 31, 1973, alive at age 3 and residing in the health district; 91% of eligible sample enrolled in the study (N = 1,037). Follow-up in childhood and adolescence ages 3, 5, 7, 9, 11, 13, 15, and 18; in adulthood, ages 21 and 26; and ongoing. *Finding*: Maltreatment in childhood increased risk of conduct disorder and other indicators of antisocial behavior in adolescence among males with low *MAOA* activity genotype, and not among males with high *MAOA* activity genotype. This analysis was based on a subset of 442 males with complete data.

Table 9.2 Prospective Population Cohort Studies: Examples of Cohorts Assembled from Children

Sources	Study Description and Selected Findings
Johnson et al. (2002) *See also*: Cohen and Cohen (1996)	*Study*: Children in the Community Study *Cohort (N = 976 families)*: Children age 1–10 years from a random sample of 976 families from two counties in northern New York recruited in 1975. Includes 659 families with information on key variables from 1975, 1985–1986, and 1991–1993 interviews. *Finding*: Children exposed to maladaptive parenting or abuse had increased risk of attempting suicide in late adolescence or early adulthood. This effect was mediated by interpersonal difficulties during adolescence.
Ensminger et al. (2002) *See also*: Kellam et al. (1983)	*Study*: Woodlawn Study *Cohort (N = 1,242)*: First-grade children in 12 schools in the Woodlawn district of Chicago academic year 1966–67. Followed up as teenagers in 1975–1976 (N = 705), and as adults in 1992–1993 (N = 952). *Finding*: Boys exhibiting both shy and aggressive behavior in childhood were at increased risk of substance use in teenage years and in adulthood. This relationship was not evident in girls.

Table 9.3 Prospective Population Cohort Studies: Examples of Cohorts Assembled from Adults

Sources	Study Description and Selected Findings
van Os et al. (2002)	*Study*: The Netherlands Mental Health Survey and Incidence Study (NEMESIS)
See also: Bijl et al. (1998a) Bijl et al. (1998b)	*Cohort (N = 7,076)*: A multistage, stratified random sample of the Netherlands population (age 18–64) enrolled at baseline in 1996. Follow-up interviews in 1997 and 1999.
	Finding: Individuals reporting cannabis use at baseline had increased risk of psychotic symptoms at 3 years follow-up. This analysis was restricted to those with no history of psychotic symptoms at baseline, and with follow-up assessments in 1999 (N = 4,045).
Weitoft et al. (2000)	*Study*: Swedish Mothers Study
See also: Weitoft et al. (2002)	*Cohort (N = 712,479)*: Women age 29–54 years in the Swedish Population and Housing Census of 1990 who had children under 15 years old. Follow-up in Death Registry 1991–1995.
	Finding: Mothers living alone (1985, 1990, or both) compared to mothers with partners (1985 and 1990) had increased risk of overall mortality and suicide.

Articulating the Questions

A cohort study is meant to answer a particular kind of question: is there a causal relationship between an exposure and a subsequent health outcome? This kind of question was posed by the researchers in a cohort study of children in New York State (table 9.2; Johnson et al. 2002). The authors asked whether an adverse childhood family environment was a risk factor for suicide attempts in adolescence and young adulthood. The assembled cohort provided the basis to answer this question. In childhood, the family environment was directly measured; at later time points, information on suicide attempts was systematically collected. The analysis compared children exposed and unexposed to maladaptive parenting behaviors such as harsh punishment, verbal abuse, and the like. Such parenting, the data suggested, did indeed relate to subsequent suicide attempts.

In this instance, the authors also examined the pathways linking the risk factor to the outcome. The hypothesis that interpersonal difficulties during middle adolescence mediated the effect of these childhood experiences on suicide attempts could be tested in the data collected at several time points from childhood to young adulthood. The results were compatible with the hypothesized pathway. The pathway, thus elucidated, added strength and coherence to the results and pointed the way toward preventive interventions.

Some important etiologic questions in psychiatric epidemiology, however, are not suited to the cohort design (see part VIII). A cohort study would not serve to examine the impact of historical change on the incidence of depression (Weissman and Klerman 1992) or schizophrenia (Bresnahan et al. 2003) (see chapter 10). Nor would it serve to model the pattern of epidemic spread of drug use in a community (Anthony 1992).

Other questions, seemingly appropriate to the design in theory, may not be amenable in practice. Thus, a cohort study will yield little when only minor variation in the exposure of interest is to be found in the study population. Likewise, a cohort study of a very rare disease presents the difficulty of accumulating a sufficient number of cases, unless it is an extremely large cohort. The prospective cohort study also encounters difficulty when the interval between the postulated exposure and the outcome spans many decades.

Despite these restrictions, the design has proved to be a powerful strategy for detecting causes. It is being applied in an increasingly wide range of circumstances. Some of the first cohorts of individual births, established a half century ago, are being followed into late life; in these special cohorts, investigators can examine risk factors over the full life course up to the present. Thus, recorded fetal exposures can be related to late-life outcomes. With the advent of very large cohorts of several hundred thousand individuals (Riboli 1992), rare exposures can also be investigated. The design is also being extended to new domains, such as genetic risk factors (see part VII).

Defining the Source Population

With the research questions articulated, the next task in designing a cohort study is to identify a population or setting in which these questions can be answered. The population may be defined in terms of personal characteristics, place, and time. It must be a population in which the exposure can be determined at the outset and in which it is feasible to determine the outcomes upon follow-up. Populations appropriate to the questions asked can be of all sorts and may be found in a school, a community, a nation, or some other setting.

Once a population or setting is chosen, we define the **source population** for the study. The source population is comprised of the people we would like to have in our study. Hence, the investigator stipulates the inclusion and exclusion criteria for selection and entry to the study. People who already have the study outcome are excluded. Other inclusion and exclusion criteria may vary from study to study, although a crucial requirement is that they be precisely specified.

The **study population** comprises only the people who actually enter our study, which will rarely be the entire source population. Some of the individuals in the source population (i.e., those eligible for the study) may not be located. Some of those located may refuse to participate in the study.

In psychiatric epidemiology, an increasingly popular strategy is to follow up the subjects of a community survey along the lines of a prospective population cohort study. Thus, the community survey becomes a resource for causal research. In this design, the chosen population is one step removed from a naturally occurring population in the sense that the participants in the survey are already a selected subgroup from the community. We define the source population for our cohort study only among these survey participants. As always, the members of the source population who actually enter our cohort study become the study population.

The Netherlands Mental Health Survey and Incidence Study (NEMESIS) cohort study followed up a community survey of mental disorders in Holland (table 9.3; Bijl et al. 1998a; Bijl et al. 1998b). The sample for the community survey was restricted to people between age 18 and 64. It was selected with a multistage, stratified random sampling procedure: selecting 90 Dutch municipalities, selecting households within each municipality, and choosing persons to interview within each household. The investigators were able to locate and assess 70 percent of the individuals chosen for the community survey. The remaining 30 percent could not be included in the source population defined for any subsequent cohort study.

All of the individuals assessed in the community survey were designated for follow-up in the NEMESIS study. The follow-up assessment covered a wide range of mental disorders and any of them can be examined as an outcome in a cohort study. When analyzing a particular outcome, however, one must exclude from the source population individuals who had the outcome at the start. A cohort study of depression in NEMESIS, for example, would exclude people diagnosed with depression in the community survey from the source population. Similarly, as in the example in table 9.3, a cohort study of psychotic symptoms would exclude from the source population people reporting these symptoms in the community survey. Thus, the survey serves as a repository within which many source populations for cohort studies can be defined. Each source population is defined by the inclusion or exclusion criteria specific to the question under investigation.

Measuring the Exposures

The exposures are measured at or before the start of the follow-up period. Exposures may be measured in a number of ways, from questionnaire responses, biological indicators, or current medical records. Reliable and valid measures of the exposure improve the power of a study to detect true associations.

In the simplest version of the cohort study, each individual is assigned to a fixed category according to exposure to the factor under investigation. The classification as exposed or unexposed holds for the duration of the study. When more than two exposure categories are used, individuals are classified into one of several exposure groups. Exposures may also be finely categorized, virtually on a continuum, although the data analysis will then depend upon statistical models such as logistic regression.

In practice, the exposure status of the cohort members may change during the course of the study. The Swedish Mothers Study (table 9.3) investigated whether living without a partner had adverse effects on the health of single mothers (Weitoft et al. 2000). A report from this study focused on mortality during 1991–1995. The source population was defined from 1990 census data, exposure to living without a partner was defined from 1985 and 1990 census data, and mortality was determined from the national death index for 1991–1995. Mothers living without a partner in both 1985 and 1990 had an increased risk of suicide during 1991–1995. The authors recognized, however, that, unknown to them, the gain or loss of partners during the follow-up period of 1991–1995 could have modified the degree, as well as the nature, of the exposure.

In some circumstances, current statistical methods can take changes in exposure status into account during the analysis of the data, provided that the changes are documented (Rothman and Greenland 1998; Kalbfleisch and Prentice 2002). In other circumstances, one may confront more complexity, perhaps even a dynamic, ever-changing exposure status. The available analytic approaches for changes in exposure status may then be inadequate (see part VIII).

An additional complexity is that cohort studies sometimes introduce new exposure measures as the cohort is followed over time. A birth cohort in Dunedin, New Zealand, provides an example. The cohort was assembled from births at a maternity hospital in 1972–1973 and assessed at 10 time points between ages 3 and 26 (Silva and Stanton 1997). A potentially important finding from this study concerned a gene-environment interaction in which the environmental exposure was maltreatment in childhood (table 9.1; Caspi et al. 2002). The exposure to maltreatment was defined as a composite both of measures built into the original design and of measures added later. Some of these additions were made even in adulthood, after the outcomes had been determined (the adults were asked to recall their childhood experiences). Thus, the study departed from the standard procedures of the cohort design, to capture needed exposure information not collected when the cohort was initiated.

In a prospective study of this kind, one can purposefully build in some potential for unanticipated future uses. This may mean collecting a fairly wide range of exposure data. It is increasingly common to collect and archive biological specimens that serve this purpose.

Following the Cohort

As noted earlier, we attempt to follow all the individuals in the cohort until they develop the disease, succumb to another condition (e.g., death) that precludes the disease, or reach the end of the study. An individual who is lost to observation while still at risk of disease introduces a potential for bias. In practice, despite our best efforts, cohort members will be lost to observation, sometimes in substantial numbers.

The Woodlawn Study (table 9.2; Kellam et al. 1983) illustrates the uncertainties introduced by heavy loss to follow-up. This was one of a number of early cohort studies designed from a developmental life course perspective. The investigators sought to trace the pathways linking childhood experiences to teenage psychiatric symptoms and substance use. They began with a survey and other studies of schoolchildren in an African American inner city community on the south side of Chicago. The first-grade schoolchildren of 1966–1967 were then selected for follow-up in their teenage years. At the 10-year follow-up, however, many of the families could not be located, and among those located some of the teenagers were unwilling to be assessed. All together, 43 percent of the children could not be reassessed.

Among the 57 percent reassessed, the first-grade boys judged to be both shy and aggressive were more likely to use substances in their teenage years. In any interpretation of this finding, however, the potential bias due to loss to follow-up had to be considered. For this purpose, the authors compared the 43 percent lost to observation with the 57 percent reassessed. The groups were substantially similar at baseline. Subsequently, in a much more successful follow-up at age 32 (Ensminger et al. 2002), the results were consonant in suggesting that the shy-aggressive first-grade boys were also more likely to be adult drug users. The coherence of these results from teenage and adult follow-ups suggests that there was not substantial bias due to the loss to follow-up and lends credence to the results.

Specifying the Risk Period

The risk period is the time period during which cases of disease are identified in a cohort. The risk period may begin later than the follow-up period. Suppose we are using a birth cohort to investigate whether low birthweight is a risk factor for postpubertal depression. Then the follow-up would begin at the time of birth, whereas the risk period would begin at puberty.

There may also be practical reasons for defining the start of the risk period after the start of follow-up. A common reason is that systematic outcome data are not available until a certain time point. Any cases that happen to be identified before that time point might reflect an idiosyncratic process of ascertainment. For example, they may have come to attention because of some unusual characteristic. If one suspects that the inclusion of these earlier identified cases could introduce bias, the risk period might be defined as starting at the time that systematic outcome data became available.

The risk period may be defined so that the cohort members are followed over the same historical period. In the Dutch NEMESIS study, various cohort studies drew their source populations from the participants in a survey of the Dutch population age 18–64 in 1996. The survey participants were followed up to 1999 (table 9.3; Bijl et al. 1998a; Bijl et al. 1998b). As a result, in each of these studies the cohort members were followed over the same historical period, 1996–1999, but over different age spans. Over the 3-year follow-up, the youngest members of the cohort were age 18–21, while the oldest were age 64–67. We then have to take age effects into account in the analysis and interpretation of the data.

Alternatively, the risk period may be defined so that cohort members are followed over the same phase of the life cycle. In some instances, this will result in different cohort members being followed over different historical periods. A simple scenario would be a birth cohort, assembled from births at a given hospital over a 25-year period, in which the investigator defines the date of birth as the start of the risk period and age 21 as the end of it. This ensures that the members of the cohort are followed over the same phase of the life cycle, birth to age 21. But it also means that they are followed over different historical periods. The oldest cohort members will reach age 21 before the youngest cohort members are born. We then have to take the effects of the historical period into account in the analysis and interpretation of the data.

In certain circumstances, a further differentiation becomes important. We may need to disentangle the effects of age, current historical period, and past historical experience. An approach referred to as age-period-cohort analysis is used for this purpose. When applicable, this kind of analysis can illuminate causes that are not otherwise evident. An age-period-cohort analysis is not usually applicable, however, in the data of an ordinary cohort study, and we therefore defer further discussion to part VIII, where we demonstrate its usefulness for the analysis of secular trends in disease rates.

The Timing of Follow-Up Assessments

Once the risk period has been defined, we choose the timing of the follow-up assessments. Several different approaches may be used, with different implications for potential bias. Here we describe three approaches that are commonly used in psychiatric epidemiology. In later chapters, we will discuss their implications for bias.

The simplest approach is an **end-of-study case ascertainment**. We attempt to identify all the cases that occurred at any time during the risk period by means of a single assessment at the end of the risk period. Although this is a common method and sometimes considered the prototype, it is often problematic for psychiatric disorders. For example, the diagnosis of a mental disorder may depend upon the temporal sequence and co-occurrence of signs and symptoms, and individuals may find it difficult to recall their past mental states with any precision.

In general, periodic assessments over a given time interval allow for more valid psychiatric diagnoses than a single assessment at the end of the interval. Therefore, unless the risk period is very short, it may be preferable to evaluate the cohort at several time points during the risk period. This was done in the Dunedin cohort described earlier, which was assessed 10 times between ages 3 and 26. We shall refer to this approach as **periodic case ascertainment**.

Still another approach is to continually monitor the treatment experience of the cohort during the risk period by means of a case registry. A case registry accumulates the history of an individual's treatment contacts with a defined set of health services in a defined population (Laska et al. 1983; Ten Horn 1983; Ten Horn 1986). As we will explain in later chapters, this approach may confer important advantages in minimizing bias due to attrition. On the other hand, it restricts the study to treated cases, and for some mental disorders only a minority of people with the disorder are treated. We shall refer to this approach as **ongoing case registry ascertainment**.

Classifying the Outcomes

The cohort design presumes that the outcome data we have collected will enable us to classify the cohort members as "cases" or "noncases." But what is a "case"? The question is profound and in psychiatric epidemiology has a contentious history (Gruenberg 1950; Wing et al. 1981; Helzer and Hudziak 2002).

In practice, investigators most often define a case as someone who meets the *DSM* diagnostic criteria of the American Psychiatric Association or the *ICD* criteria from the World Health Organization for the disorder under investigation. These criteria may at least ensure that the measurement of case status is reasonably reliable and comparable across studies. They do not necessarily represent the most valid or appropriate definition of a case for any particular study. Next we discuss in turn the reliability and validity of classification.

Choosing Reliable Measures

The reliable measurement of disorder is an area in which psychiatric research has made great strides. In its broadest sense, reliability means that diagnoses are replicable across raters, studies, settings, and time. Otherwise, one researcher does not know the meaning of a diagnosis assigned by another; studies cannot be replicated and results cannot be meaningfully compared.

Reliable diagnosis requires a commonly agreed upon nosology that can be operationalized to allow different observers to make the same diagnosis when presented with the same information. Until the 1980s, psychiatric nosology had not met this standard (Frances et al. 2002). The Rubella Birth Defects Evaluation Project (Chess et al. 1971) provides a good illustration of the barriers this shortcoming posed for cohort studies of psychiatric disorders. Stella Chess—famed for her work on childhood temperament—followed a cohort of 243 children who had been exposed to rubella in utero to determine if such exposure was a risk factor for childhood disorders, including autism. This original and careful study lacked two safeguards that today are considered mandatory: namely, an unexposed comparison group and an assessment that was blind to the antecedent history of the exposure.[2] Nonetheless, in its time, the study was groundbreaking. Based on intensive clinical evaluations at several time points, a surprisingly large number of cases of autism were diagnosed in the cohort, suggesting that their risk of autism far exceeded the risk in other populations. The study preceded the development of standardized approaches to eliciting and rating information for making diagnoses of psychiatric disorders among children. Thus, although the diagnoses were more systematic than other contemporary studies, we cannot know whether other clinicians would have diagnosed autism in these cases. The important finding of increased autism in this cohort is still questioned on these grounds.

---

[2] Because it lacks an explicit unexposed group, we did not include this study in the tables of cohort studies. The results for the exposed group can be compared only with "what would be expected" in the general population.

The publication of the *DSM-III* in 1980 was a landmark event because it was the first official nosology to adopt systematic and explicit criteria that facilitated diagnostic reliability. Currently, either *DSM* or *ICD* diagnostic criteria can help clinicians reach the same diagnosis when they are observing the same clinical phenomena. To take full advantage, cohort studies may employ standardized assessments, intensive interviewer training, and formal diagnostic protocols.

In cohort studies that rely upon direct assessments to collect outcome data, investigators typically use structured instruments administered by lay interviewers. This approach makes it possible to obtain reliable diagnoses without incurring prohibitive costs (see chapter 1). In one of the earlier large-scale uses of this approach, part of a birth cohort in Providence, Rhode Island, was traced at ages 18–27 and assessed with the Diagnostic Interview Schedule (table 9.1; Buka et al. 1993). The follow-up of this cohort was subsequently extended and produced a number of intriguing results (Kremen et al. 1998; Zornberg et al. 2000; Buka et al. 2001).

Cohort studies with ongoing case ascertainment from a case registry may be limited to routine clinical diagnoses, the reliability of which is sometimes suspect. However, national registry diagnoses tend to be more reliable in countries with uniform training in psychiatry, such as Holland or Denmark. Case registries meeting these standards provided the basis for some remarkable cohort studies, encompassing all hospitalized cases in an entire nation over a long period of time. Since these were usually historical cohort studies, we provide examples in the next chapter.

In an extension of this approach, registry diagnoses may be verified by direct and reliable assessments of the identified cases (Hoek et al. 1998). In a still further extension, the researchers may cast a broad net of registry diagnoses and use them only to screen for potential cases. The potential cases are then administered full diagnostic assessments with established reliability. This was done in the Prenatal Determinants of Schizophrenia study, which we will describe in detail in the next chapter.

As we discuss below, the case definition in a particular study may not necessarily follow the convention of the official *DSM* or *ICD* nosology. It may be tailored to the research question. It is then all the more important to demonstrate that the study outcome can be measured reliably. When the investigator is departing from official nosology and standardized methods of assessment, the definition of a case for the study should be specified with explicit criteria, and the measurement protocol should be pretested in a field study of the same type of population.

Choosing Valid Measures

For some psychiatric disorders, the *DSM* and *ICD* diagnoses can be shown to be valid in the sense that they correspond reasonably well with an underlying pathophysiology. A diagnosis of Alzheimer's disease based on repeated neuropsychologic testing and other evaluations strongly predicts that the brain pathology of Alzheimer's disease—plaques and neurofibrillary tangles—will be seen on postmortem examination (Hogervorst et al. 2003).

Although the correspondence is impressive, it is not one to one; the postmortem will sometimes reveal a different pathology and refute the Alzheimer's diagnosis (e.g., the patient may have Lewy-body dementia).

More typically for psychiatric diagnoses, the pathophysiology is not so well understood. A classic article by Robins and Guze (1970) sets out an alternative approach for establishing the validity of a psychiatric diagnosis, centered on familial aggregation, response to treatment, and phenomenology. These dimensions do not always lead to concordant results, however, and the sought-after "valid" diagnosis may be elusive. In addition, official diagnostic criteria change over time, and the *DSM* and *ICD* nosologies differ in some important respects.

Ultimately, neither medicine nor public health can offer any universally applicable definition of what comprises a disease or disorder in any health domain. Defining a disease is an iterative process. A diagnosis usually begins as a label for a pattern of signs and symptoms observed in a clinical setting (Scadding 1996). As causes are elucidated, the disease may be redefined on the basis of one or more of these causes. In a historical example, many cases of insanity were reclassified as syphilitic disease after the discovery of an infectious agent, a diagnostic test, and a treatment for it (see chapter 2). In a recent example, some patterns of anxiety and depressive symptoms were reclassified in the *DSM-III* as constituting posttraumatic stress disorder, following the recognition that they can be produced by traumatic experiences (Kutchins and Kirk 1997). In this genomic era, we may anticipate that some mental disorders will be redefined to correspond more closely with specified genetic causes (Insel and Collins 2003).

Although these problems of case definition pertain to some degree in all cohort studies, they are especially salient for cohort studies of mental disorders. The dilemmas are exacerbated by the limited knowledge of the pathophysiology of mental disorders (Wakefield 1992), the comorbidity among mental disorders (Boyd and Hauenstein 1997), and the difficulties of measuring them (Dohrenwend and Dohrenwend 1982; Bromet et al. 1986). Social and political controversies are also woven into the disputes about mental disorders (Bayer 1981; Caplan 1995; Kutchins and Kirk 1997).

In the context of such uncertainty about how best to define a case, rigid adherence to official nosology may not always be appropriate. In some instances, diagnostic criteria are slightly refined for a particular study. Current nosologies often set a threshold for diagnosis—such as having a minimum number of symptoms or a minimum duration of illness—and the threshold may be disputed. If research findings have outpaced the official nosology, or if a specific theory warrants it, an alternative threshold may be justified (Regier et al. 1998; Mojtabai et al. 2000; Kessler et al. 2003).

In other instances, the tailoring may be more fundamental. Genetic epidemiologists may define the outcome as an **endophenotype** instead of a diagnosable disorder (see part VII). Endophenotypes are postulated to be intermediate outcomes that are on the pathway between the genetic determinant and the disease. They are usually measured by neuropsychological or physiological testing. The rationale for their use is that different genes may be determinants of different endophenotypes, the confluence of which emerges as a diagnosable psychiatric disorder.

In a still further departure from standard practice, we may study a disease-related functional disability or social handicap (Susser 1990). Health researchers increasingly acknowledge the importance of studying such outcomes. The World Health Organization now publishes a separate *ICD* classification system for them (World Health Organization 2001). Mental disorders are among the most prominent causes of disability (see chapter 1), and the use of these outcomes may be compelling for some purposes in psychiatric epidemiology.

At times the outcome of a cohort study may even be measured on a continuum. We may study outcomes such as birthweight, blood pressure, and IQ that are continuously distributed in the population and not readily categorized into health and disorder (Swales 1985; Rose 1992; Wilcox 2001; Wasserman et al. 2003). Some investigators have argued persuasively that certain kinds of psychiatric symptoms are—like birthweight, blood pressure, and IQ—continuously distributed in the population (Anderson et al. 1993; van Os et al. 2000; Mirowsky and Ross 2002).

In order to apply the prototypical cohort design to a continuously distributed outcome, it may still be reasonable to invoke the notion of a case for scores above or below some threshold. This is often done for low birthweight, high blood pressure, and low IQ and is similarly applicable for psychiatric symptom scores. A cohort study may then define a case by a score above a threshold on a symptom inventory such as the Center for Epidemiologic Studies of Depression scale (Weissman et al. 1977) or the Child Behavior Checklist (Achenbach and Edelbrock 1983).

A report from the Dutch NEMESIS study offers an intriguing illustration of how an outcome that is conceptualized as a continuous variable may nonetheless be used to define a "case" in a cohort study (table 9.3). This report examined cannabis use as a risk factor for the onset of psychosis-like symptoms such as delusional ideation (table 9.3; van Os et al 2002). The authors conceptualized psychosis-like symptoms as a continuous phenomenon, which could be related to the risk of clinical psychotic disorders, analogous to the relation between increases in blood pressure and the risk of cardiovascular disease. To protect the validity of causal inference, however, they excluded from their main analyses all individuals who reported any psychotic ideation in the baseline community survey. Thus, they defined a cohort that was free of psychotic ideation at the start of the risk period. They then defined the outcome as the new onset of any psychotic ideation during the 3-year follow-up, as would be done for new onset of "cases" of disorder. In these data, cannabis use at baselines was associated with onset of psychosis outcome at follow-up, although the finding was based on small numbers.

It may be legitimately argued that, in some instances, we could take an entirely different perspective. We might instead group together otherwise heterogeneous disorders that share a common psychosocial cause that is known to be readily modifiable. In theory at least, this approach to classification of the study outcome could provide the most useful guide to preventive intervention (Cassel 1964).

An important caveat to all these options is that any departure from the official psychiatric nosology should be fully justified and undertaken with appropriate caution. An excessive proliferation of outcomes will impede comparison of results and the collective progress of research. Even when using alternative definitions, studies should be designed so that the implications of the results for official nosologic categories can be discerned.

Misclassification

Despite the progress, many problems remain for attaining reliable and valid psychiatric diagnoses in cohort studies (Kendler 1999). Standardized diagnostic assessments by lay interviewers confer reliability, but not necessarily validity. Individuals with mental disorders may have a limited awareness of their condition, or may be unable to provide an accurate history in response to rigidly prespecified questions. A systematized clinician-administered interview should improve validity but is not a panacea. A full clinical history may require integration of multiple and sometimes conflicting sources of information, including family members and clinicians, as well as the individual affected. The process is not easily standardized (Buchan et al. 2002), and different researchers may elicit somewhat different clinical pictures for the same person. In studies of children, to standardize the process of integrating information, most studies require at least two (mother and child) and sometimes three (teacher) informants, and the diagnosis is based on a positive report by any one of them (Jensen et al. 1999).

Inevitably, under any approach some cases will be misclassified as noncases, and vice-versa. Most crucially, the misclassification should not be influenced by exposure status, or the comparison of exposed with unexposed will be biased. Careful investigators will go to some lengths to minimize any possible influence of exposure on the ascertainment of the outcome (see chapter 14). The most important safeguard is that those who conduct the outcome assessments be blind to the exposure status.

Conclusion

By way of introduction, we have described a prospective population cohort study as a prototype of the cohort study. In real applications, however, we may choose any one of a wide array of cohort study designs. We also must consider all the plausible alternative explanations for an observed association between exposure and disease. These complexities will unfold in the following chapters.

References

Achenbach TM and Edelbrock CS (1983). *Manual for the Child Behavior Checklist and Child Behavior Profile*. Burlington: University of Vermont.

Anderson J, Huppert F, and Rose G (1993). Normality, Deviance and Minor Psychiatric Morbidity in the Community. A Population-Based Approach to General Health Questionnaire Data in the Health and Lifestyle Survey. *Psychol. Med.* 23:475–485.

Anthony JC (1992). Epidemiological Research on Cocaine Use in the USA. *Ciba Found. Symp.* 166:20–33.

Bayer R (1981). *Homosexuality and American Psychiatry: The Politics of Diagnosis.* New York: Basic Books.

Bijl RV, Ravelli A, and van Zessen G (1998a). Prevalence of Psychiatric Disorder in the General Population: Results of the Netherlands Mental Health Survey and Incidence Study (NEMESIS). *Soc. Psychiatry Psychiatr. Epidemiol.* 33:587–595.

Bijl RV, van Zessen G, Ravelli A, de Rijk C, and Langendoen Y (1998b). The Netherlands Mental Health Survey and Incidence Study (NEMESIS): Objectives and Design. *Soc. Psychiatry Psychiatr. Epidemiol.* 33:581–586.

Boyd MR and Hauenstein EJ (1997). Psychiatric Assessment and Confirmation of Dual Disorders in Rural Substance Abusing Women. *Arch. Psychiatr. Nurs.* 11:74–81.

Bresnahan M, Boydell J, Murray R, and Susser E (2003). Temporal Variation in the Incidence, Course and Outcome of Schizophrenia. In Murray RM, Jones PB, Susser E, van Os J, and Cannon M, eds., *The Epidemiology of Schizophrenia*, 34–48. Cambridge: Cambridge University Press.

Broman, SH (1984). The Collaborative Perinatal Project: An Overview. In Mednick SA, Harway M, and Finello KM, eds., *Handbook of Longitudinal Research*, 185–227. Vol. 1. New York: Praeger.

Bromet EJ, Dunn LO, Connell MM, Dew MA, and Schulberg HC (1986). Long-Term Reliability of Diagnosing Lifetime Major Depression in a Community Sample. *Arch. Gen. Psychiatry* 43:435–440.

Buchan BJ, Dennis ML, Tims FM, and Diamond GS (2002). Cannabis Use Consistency and Validity of Self-Report, On-site Urine Testing and Laboratory Testing. *Addiction* 97 (Suppl.) 98–108.

Buka SL, Tsuang MT, and Lipsitt LP (1993). Pregnancy/Delivery Complications and Psychiatric Diagnosis. A Prospective Study. *Arch. Gen. Psychiatry* 50:151–156.

Buka SL, Tsuang MT, Torrey EF, Klebanoff MA, Bernstein D, and Yolken RH (2001). Maternal Infections and Subsequent Psychosis among Offspring. *Arch. Gen. Psychiatry* 58:1032–1037.

Cannon M, Caspi A, Moffitt TE, Harrington H, Taylor A, Murray RM, and Poulton R (2002). Evidence for Early-Childhood, Pan-Developmental Impairment Specific to Schizophreniform Disorder: Results from a Longitudinal Birth Cohort. *Arch. Gen. Psychiatry* 59:449–456.

Caplan P (1995). *They Say You're Crazy: How the World's Most Powerful Psychiatrists Decide Who's Normal.* Reading, Mass. Addison-Wesley.

Caspi A, McClay J, Moffitt TE, Mill J, Martin J, Craig IW, Taylor A, and Poulton R (2002). Role of Genotype in the Cycle of Violence in Maltreated Children. *Science* 297:851–854.

Cassel J (1964). Social Science Theory as a Source of Hypotheses in Epidemiological Research. *Am. J. Public Health Nations Health* 54:1482–1488.

Chess S, Korn S, and Fernandez P (1971). *Psychiatric Disorders of Children with Congenital Rubella.* New York: Brunner/Mazel.

Cohen P and Cohen J (1996). *Life Values and Adolescent Mental Health.* Mahwah, N.J.: Erlbaum.

Dohrenwend BP and Dohrenwend BS (1982). Perspectives on the Past and Future of Psychiatric Epidemiology. The 1981 Rema Lapouse Lecture. *Am. J. Public Health* 72:1271–1279.

Doll R (2004). Cohort Studies: History of the Method. In Morabia A, ed., *History of Epidemiologic Methods and Concepts*, 243–274. Boston: Birkhauser.

Ensminger ME, Juon HS, and Fothergill KE (2002). Childhood and Adolescent Antecedents of Substance Use in Adulthood. *Addiction* 97:833–844.

Frances A, Mack AH, First MB, Widiger T, Ford S, Vetterello N, and Ross R (2002). *DSM-IV* and Psychiatric Epidemiology. In Tsuang MT and Tohen M, eds., *Textbook in Psychiatric Epidemiology*, 273–279. New York: Wiley.

Greenland S and Brumback B (2002). An Overview of Relations among Causal Modelling Methods. *Int. J. Epidemiol.* 31:1030–1037.

Gruenberg, EM (1950). Review of Available Material on Patterns of Occurrence of Mental Disorders: Major Disorders. New York: Milbank Memorial Fund.

Helzer JE and Hudziak JJ, eds. (2002). *Defining Psychopathology in the 21st Century: DSM-V and Beyond.* Arlington, Vir.: American Psychiatric Publishing.

Hill AB (1965). The Environment and Disease: Association or Causation? *Proc. R. Soc. Med.* 58:295–300.

Hoek HW, Brown AS, and Susser E (1998). The Dutch Famine and Schizophrenia Spectrum Disorders. *Soc. Psychiatry Psychiatr. Epidemiol.* 33:373–379.

Hogervorst E, Bandelow S, Combrinck M, Irani S, and Smith AD (2003). The Validity and Reliability of Six Sets of Clinical Criteria to Classify Alzheimer's Disease and Vascular Dementia in Cases Confirmed Post-Mortem: Added Value of a Decision Tree Approach. *Dement. Geriatr. Cogn. Disord.* 16:170–180.

Insel TR and Collins FS (2003). Psychiatry in the Genomics Era. *Am. J. Psychiatry* 160:616–620.

Jensen PS, Rubio-Stipec M, Canino G, Bird HR, Dulcan MK, Schwab-Stone ME, Lahey BB (1999) Parent and Child Contributions to Diagnosis of Mental Disorder: Are Both Information Always Necessary? *J. Am. Acad. Child Adolesc. Psychiatry* 38:1569–1579.

Johnson JG, Cohen P, Gould MS, Kasen S, Brown J, and Brook JS (2002). Childhood Adversities, Interpersonal Difficulties, and Risk for Suicide Attempts during Late Adolescence and Early Adulthood. *Arch. Gen. Psychiatry* 59:741–749.

Kalbfleisch JD and Prentice RL (2002). *The Statistical Analysis of Failure Time Data,* 2nd ed. New York: Wiley.

Kellam, SG, Brown CH, Rubin BR, and Ensminger ME (1983). Paths Leading to Teenage Psychiatric Symptoms and Substance Use: Developmental Epidemiologic Studies in Woodlawn. In Guze SB, Earls FJ, and Barret JE, eds., *Childhood Psychopathology and Development,* 17–51. New York: Raven Press.

Kendler KS (1999). Setting Boundaries for Psychiatric Disorders. *Am. J. Psychiatry* 156:1845–1848.

Kessler RC, Merikangas KR, Berglund P, Eaton WW, Koretz DS, and Walters EE (2003). Mild Disorders Should Not Be Eliminated from the *DSM-V. Arch. Gen. Psychiatry* 60:1117–1122.

Kremen WS, Buka SL, Seidman LJ, Goldstein JM, Koren D, and Tsuang MT (1998). IQ Decline during Childhood and Adult Psychotic Symptoms in a Community Sample: A 19-Year Longitudinal Study. *Am. J. Psychiatry* 155:672–677.

Kutchins H and Kirk S (1997). *Making Us Crazy: DSM—The Psychiatric Bible and the Creation of Mental Disorders.* New York: Free Press.

Laska EM, Gulbinat WH, and Regier DA (1983). *Information Support to Mental Health Programs: An International Perspective.* New York: Human Sciences Press.

MacMahon B, Pugh T, and Ipsen J (1960). *Epidemiologic Methods.* Boston: Little, Brown.

Mirowsky J and Ross CE (2002). Measurement for a Human Science. *J. Health Soc. Behav.* 43:152–170.

Mojtabai R, Bromet EJ, Harvey PD, Carlson GA, Craig TJ, and Fennig S (2000). Neuropsychological Differences between First-Admission Schizophrenia and Psychotic Affective Disorders. *Am. J. Psychiatry* 157:1453–1460.

Morabia A, ed. (2004). *History of Epidemiologic Methods and Concepts.* Boston: Birkhauser.

Oppenheimer G (in press). The Emergence of Coronary Heart Disease Epidemiology in the U.S., 1947–1970. *Int. J. Epidemiol.*

Regier DA, Kaelber CT, Rae DS, Farmer ME, Knauper B, Kessler RC, and Norquist GS (1998). Limitations of Diagnostic Criteria and Assessment Instruments for Mental Disorders. Implications for Research and Policy. *Arch. Gen. Psychiatry* 55:109–115.

Riboli E (1992). Nutrition and Cancer: Background and Rationale of the European Prospective Investigation into Cancer and Nutrition (EPIC). *Ann. Oncol.* 3:783–791.

Robins E and Guze SB (1970). Establishment of Diagnostic Validity in Psychiatric Illness: Its Application to Schizophrenia. *Am. J. Psychiatry* 126:983–987.

Rose G (1992). *The Strategy of Preventive Medicine.* New York: Oxford University Press.

Rothman KJ and Greenland S (1998). *Modern Epidemiology,* 2nd ed. Philadelphia: Lippincott-Raven.

Samet JM and Munoz A (1998). Cohort Studies. *Epidemiol. Rev.* 20:135–136.

Scadding JG (1996). Essentialism and Nominalism in Medicine: Logic of Diagnosis in Disease Terminology. *Lancet* 348:594–596.

Silva PA and Stanton WR (1997). *From Child to Adult: The Dunedin Multidisciplinary Health and Development Study.* New York: Oxford University Press.

Susser M (1985). Epidemiology in the United States after World War II: The Evolution of Technique. *Epidemiol. Rev.* 7:147–177.

Susser M (1990). Disease, Illness, Sickness; Impairment, Disability and Handicap. *Psychol. Med.* 20:471–473.

Swales JD (1985). *Platt versus Pickering: An Episode in Recent Medical History.* London: Cambridge University Press.

Szklo M and Nieto FJ (2000). *Epidemiology: Beyond the Basics.* Gaithersburg, Md.: Aspen Publishing.

Ten Horn GHMM (1983). Psychiatric Case Registries, Report on a Working Group. Geneva, Switzerland: World Health Organization.

Ten Horn GHMM (1986). A Classification of Different Types of Psychiatric Case Registers. In Ten Horn GHMM et al., eds., *Psychiatric Case Registers in Public Health: A Worldwide Inventory 1960–1985.* Amsterdam: Elsevier.

van Os J, Bak M, Hanssen M, Bijl RV, de Graaf R, and Verdoux H (2002). Cannabis Use and Psychosis: a Longitudinal Population-Based Study. *Am. J. Epidemiol.* 156:319–327.

van Os J, Hanssen M, Bijl RV, and Ravelli A (2000). Strauss (1969) Revisited: A Psychosis Continuum in the General Population? *Schizophr. Res.* 45:11–20.

Wakefield JC (1992). The Concept of Mental Disorder. On the Boundary between Biological Facts and Social Values. *Am. Psychol.* 47:373–388.

Wasserman GA, Factor-Litvak P, Liu X, Todd AC, Kline JK, Slavkovich V, Popovac D, and Graziano JH (2003). The Relationship between Blood Lead, Bone Lead and Child Intelligence. *Neuropsychol. Dev. Cogn. Sect. C. Child Neuropsychol.* 9:22–34.

Weissman MM and Klerman GL (1992). Depression: Current Understanding and Changing Trends. *Annu. Rev. Public Health* 13:319–339.

Weissman MM, Sholomskas D, Pottenger M, Prusoff BA, and Locke BZ (1977). Assessing Depressive Symptoms in Five Psychiatric Populations: A Validation Study. *Am. J. Epidemiol.* 106:203–214.

Weitoft GR, Haglund B, Hjern A, and Rosen M (2002). Mortality, Severe Morbidity and Injury among Long-Term Lone Mothers in Sweden. *Int. J. Epidemiol.* 31:573–580.

Weitoft GR, Haglund B, and Rosen M (2000). Mortality among Lone Mothers in Sweden: A Population Study. *Lancet* 355:1215–1219.

Wilcox AJ (2001). On the Importance—and the Unimportance—of Birthweight. *Int. J. Epidemiol.* 30:1233–1241.

Wing JK, Bebbington PE, and Robins LN (1981). *What Is a Case? The Problem of Definition in Community Surveys.* London: Grant McIntyre Medical & Scientific.

World Health Organization (2001). *International Statistical Classification of Functioning, Disability and Health.* Geneva Switzerland: Author.

Zornberg GL, Buka SL, and Tsuang MT (2000). Hypoxic-Ischemia-Related Fetal/Neonatal Complications and Risk of Schizophrenia and Other Nonaffective Psychoses: A 19-Year Longitudinal Study. *Am. J. Psychiatry* 157:196–202.

10 Diversity of Cohort Studies

Ezra Susser and Sharon Schwartz

The versatility of the cohort design is evident in its many forms and wide range of application. In the previous chapter, we described a prospective population cohort study as a prototype. By modifying one or another element of this prototype, we construct natural experiments, **historical cohorts**, and **special exposure cohorts**. To these three major variants we here add a fourth, the **clinical cohort**, the purpose of which is to discover the determinants of the course and outcome of a disorder. This variant, close kin to the etiologic cohort, has been prominent in psychiatric epidemiology. Furthermore, an ongoing cohort study can assume different forms over time. Once we have described these four major forms of the cohort design, we give an account of a cohort study that has evolved over a period of more than 50 years. Finally, we introduce a data set, the Prenatal Determinants of Schizophrenia Example (PDSE) study, for illustration in this and other parts of the book.

Natural Experiments

In a natural experiment, people are selected into the exposed or unexposed group by some event that is largely or entirely outside their own control. As in an ordinary experiment, the event is imposed upon some but not others. Unlike an ordinary experiment, the event is a natural one in the sense that it is not created by the investigator.

People have significant scope to shape their own environmental exposures, although always constrained by their particular social and physical circumstances. Health-conscious people with adequate resources and time might eat more nutritious foods than the rest of the population, and at the same time they might be more likely to take vitamin supplements, abstain from smoking, exercise vigorously, and attend yoga classes. Also, well-off people can afford to live in safer and less polluted neighborhoods when the poor cannot. For these and other reasons, those exposed and unexposed to a factor under study are likely to differ on many other factors that influence the outcome. To isolate the effects of a single exposure from all the others is often difficult.

108

In a natural experiment, however, individuals have little or no leeway to select themselves into the exposed or unexposed group. Thus, the design confers a major advantage for causal inference. It removes one of the most important reasons that exposed and unexposed people differ on other causes of the disease. In other words, it removes a major source of confounding in a cohort study.

In devising natural experiments to study environmental exposures, we often exploit the occurrence of a circumscribed historical event in a known population (Susser 1991). We may compare psychiatric outcomes in people exposed and unexposed to an unpredictable or at least unanticipated disaster, such as the Chernobyl nuclear accident of 1986, the World Trade Center terrorist attack of September 11, 2001, on the Asian tsunami of 2004. A natural experiment can also be built around a beneficial event. If the event is entirely unanticipated, a cohort study cannot be planned in advance. Instead it takes the form of a historical cohort study (described later), which is constructed after the event has already occurred. The Dutch Famine Study described in chapter 6, for example, was both a natural experiment and a historical cohort study.

Occasionally, however, an unanticipated event befalls a prospective cohort already established for other purposes. The Great Smoky Mountains Study of Youth is an ongoing prospective population cohort study of childhood psychiatric disorders in rural North Carolina (Costello et al. 1996). Serendipity provided the basis for a natural experiment (table 10.1; Costello et al. 2003;

Table 10.1 Examples of Natural Experiments

Sources	Study Description and Selected Findings
Costello et al. (2003) See also: Costello et al. (1996)	*Study*: The Great Smoky Mountains Study
	Cohort (N = 1,420): A representative sample of rural children followed annually from 1993–2000. Includes 350 children from Cherokee Indian families. Beginning in 1996, tribal members began to receive revenues from a casino, and a significant number of families moved out of poverty.
	Finding: Psychiatric symptoms were reduced in children in families who moved out of poverty; there was no change in children in families who remained poor, or in children in families who were never poor.
Heston (1966)	*Study*: Oregon Study of Schizophrenia in Foster Home Children
	Cohort (N = 116): Exposed were offspring of mothers with schizophrenia who were separated from their mothers upon birth and put in care of foundling homes or relatives. Unexposed were from the same foundling homes but were offspring of mothers without schizophrenia. Births were from 1915 to 1945 and follow-up assessments started in 1964.
	Finding: Children of mothers with schizophrenia were at increased risk of schizophrenia. Among offspring of mothers with schizophrenia, 5 of 47 were diagnosed with schizophrenia at follow-up; among offspring of mothers without schizophrenia, none were diagnosed with schizophrenia at follow-up.

Rutter 2003). In this instance, the unanticipated event was beneficial: the introduction of a lucrative casino into a Native American Indian community whose children comprised 25 percent of the cohort. Once the casino began operation, families received extra income from profits distributed to all members of the Indian community. Before the casino, the majority of families in this community lived in poverty, that is, below the official federal poverty line. Afterward, a significant number moved out of poverty, although many did not.

These historical circumstances prepared the ground for the researchers to pose an important question: did the alleviation of family poverty reduce child psychopathology? In the families who moved out of poverty, the children did exhibit a reduction in psychopathology, more pronounced for behavioral than for emotional symptoms. This effect appeared to be mediated by improved parental supervision of the children. On the other hand, as with many well-designed studies, some of the results pose further questions. In families who remained below the poverty line, and in families who were never below it, the event had no effect on child psychopathology. It is not readily apparent why the same extra income should not have also had a beneficial effect in these families.

Natural Experiments to Study Genetic Causes

Natural experiments of a somewhat different ilk have been developed to study genetic causes. Since individuals cannot choose their genes, any cohort study that examines the association between a specific gene and a disease includes a defining feature of a natural experiment (see chapter 29). Of more interest for the present discussion, however, are natural experiments specially crafted to isolate genetic causes, such as studies of adoptees, of twins (chapter 31), and of familial clusters of cases (chapter 30).

A classic example is an **adoption study** devised to isolate the effects of genes from the effects of environment. This type of adoption study conforms to the natural experiment because adoptees choose neither their biological parents, who contribute their genes, nor their adoptive parents, who contribute the environment in which they are reared. At the same time, adoptions are predictable, so studies can be planned around them.

A natural experiment of this kind produced some of the earliest evidence for a genetic contribution to the familial transmission of schizophrenia (table 10.1; Heston 1966). The offspring of women with a diagnosis of schizophrenia in an Oregon psychiatric hospital comprised the exposed group. All had been separated from their biological mothers at birth and placed in the care of foundling homes or relatives. The offspring of women without schizophrenia, who had also been separated at birth from their biological mothers and had been placed in the same foundling homes, comprised the unexposed group. Thus, the exposed and unexposed offspring had a similar rearing environment but different genetic exposures. In adulthood, schizophrenia was diagnosed in a substantial proportion (5/47) of the offspring of biological mothers with schizophrenia, but in none of the offspring whose biological mothers were unaffected by schizophrenia.

A genetic study of a family with multiple cases of a disorder across several generations also conforms to a natural experiment (see chapter 33). Such familial clusters are sometimes (but not always) produced by the transmission of a genetic allele with a strong effect on the disorder. The individuals within a pedigree do not choose their genes. Equally important, it is likely that the cases within a single pedigree are all related to the same genetic allele. Hence, the design isolates this particular genetic allele from the many others that may be related to the disorder in the population as a whole.

Potential for Bias

We have emphasized that the natural experiment is a particularly strong cohort design because it mitigates a major source of confounding. On the other hand, it is important not to underestimate the potential for confounding (and other bias).

Suppose we compare the individuals in a community that was in the path of a hurricane (exposed) with the individuals in a community that was not (unexposed). If there were advance warning, people in the exposed community would be able to influence their exposure status. To the extent that this occurs, the design of a natural experiment is undermined. When Hurricane Katrina struck New Orleans in 2005, most of the population had evacuated the city; those remaining were a large but highly selected group.

With no advance warning, people could not influence whether they were exposed or unexposed. Nonetheless, there would be potential for confounding. The exposed community could provide a healthier living environment than the unexposed community, for example, better recreational facilities, better garbage pick-up, and better access to health care. To adjust our results for the potential bias, we would need to obtain data on the characteristics of the two communities (see part VIII). Also, since the two communities differ, the exposed individuals may tend to have higher incomes than the unexposed individuals within our cohort study. To adjust for this potential bias, we would need to obtain data on the incomes of the individuals in our study (see chapter 12).

This caveat also pertains to natural experiments in genetic epidemiology. It is perhaps most obvious in cohort studies examining the association between a genetic allele and a disease. The individuals in the study do not choose their genes. But they may differ in their ancestry, belonging to groups that have different kinship patterns, dietary habits, and disease risks. For this and other reasons, these studies can pose difficult problems for causal inference (see chapter 29).

Historical Cohorts

The historical (or retrospective) cohort study departs from our prototype in that the researcher makes use of existing data that yield the necessary measures of exposure and outcome. An investigation of early prenatal exposure to famine as a risk factor for schizophrenia provides a clear example of a historical cohort study (table 10.2; Susser et al. 1996). The study drew on the birth cohorts assembled for the Dutch Famine Study, a natural experiment described in chapter 6 (Stein et al. 1975). In the 1990s, when the schizophrenia study was undertaken, the Dutch Hunger Winter of 1944–1945 was long past. Historical records were used to determine how many individuals met the entry criterion: birth in a city of western Holland during the years 1944–1946. The date of birth determined the assignment to famine exposure according to the stage of gestation during the peak of the Hunger Winter. It was hypothesized that the birth cohorts exposed in early gestation, who had shown an increased risk of congenital anomalies of the central nervous system in the original Dutch Famine Study, would also have an increased risk of schizophrenia. Those who developed schizophrenia were identified from the Dutch national psychiatric registry for 1970–1992. The risk of schizophrenia was about twice as high in the exposed as in the unexposed. Subsequently this result was replicated in a study based on the Chinese famine of 1959–1961 (St. Clair et al. 2005).

A great many cohort studies in psychiatric epidemiology have been historical cohort studies. This type follows from the frequently long interval between the time of exposure and the onset of diagnosable disorder. Mental disorders diagnosed in adulthood are often viewed as having origins in fetal and child development (Costello and Angold 1991). To define a cohort of births or children in the present and then follow the cohort until enough cases have been diagnosed in adulthood may require an inordinate lapse of time. To

Table 10.2 Examples of Historical Cohort Studies

Sources	Study Description and Selected Findings
Susser et al. (1996)	*Study*: Dutch Famine Study
See also: Stein et al. (1975) Susser et al. (1998)	*Cohort (N = 146,347)*: All births in major cities of Holland conceived during 1944–1946, who were still alive at age 19. Exposed were children born between Nov. 15, 1945, and Dec. 31, 1945, conceived at the height of the famine; less exposed were children born between Aug. 1, 1945 and Nov. 14, 1945, conceived in the early months of the famine; unexposed were children born between Jan. 1, 1944 and July 31, 1945, and between Jan. 1, 1946 and Dec. 31, 1946. National psychiatric registry follow-up was ongoing, 1970–1992.
	Finding: Offspring conceived at the height of the famine were at increased risk of schizophrenia.
Mortensen et al. (2003)	*Study*: Bipolar Affective Disorders in Denmark
	Cohort (N = 2,100,000): Individuals with known maternal identity born in Denmark between Jan. 1, 1950 and Dec. 31, 1983. National psychiatric registry follow-up from April 1, 1970, or from their 15th birthday, whichever came later, to Dec. 31, 1998.
	Finding: Loss of mother before fifth birthday increased risk of bipolar affective disorder in adulthood.

Note: Historical cohort studies are also called *retrospective cohort studies*.

follow the cohort of the Dutch Famine Study from the Hunger Winter of 1944–1945 up to 1992 would have required a study lasting nearly 50 years.

Like the Dutch Famine Study, most other large-scale, long-term historical cohort studies of mental disorders have relied on the use of national psychiatric registry data to determine the outcomes. In several countries, excellent national registries have been developed and maintained for long periods of time—for example, in Denmark (Munk-Jorgensen and Mortensen 1997; Mortensen et al. 1999) and Israel (Davidson et al. 1999; Malaspina et al. 2001). National or regional registries are often kept anonymous to preserve confidentiality. Under controlled conditions and with proper safeguards, however, they may still allow linkage to birth, death, and other registries (Rabinowitz 1998). The Danish registry has probably been used more extensively than any other. A study of bipolar disorder in this registry illustrates the power that can be derived from a long-standing national registry (Mortensen et al. 2003). This study found that individuals who lost their mother in childhood had an increased risk of bipolar disorder (table 10.2). Since both the exposure and the outcome are rare, the relationship could be effectively examined only in a very large national database.

To preserve the full advantages of the cohort design when using a historical cohort study, the investigator sometimes has to take extra precautions. Suppose that, to reflect current science, one decides to make new ratings of exposure status, using the raw data initially collected at the time of exposure. To avoid biased judgment, the new raters must be kept blind to any knowledge of outcomes already observed. In some historical birth cohort studies, for example, the observations recorded during labor and delivery have provided the opportunity to apply new rating scales for obstetric complications that accord with current convention. The people applying the new obstetric ratings to the previously recorded obstetric data must be kept blind to the study outcomes.

The problems associated with data collected in the past are reduced in a variant that is sometimes referred to as a **historical cohort with concurrent follow-up** (Lilienfeld and Lilienfeld 1980). In this type of study, the entry criteria and the exposure assessment are based on historical data. The study outcomes, by contrast, are determined by a follow-up assessment. Earlier in the chapter, we described a study that compared offspring of women with and without schizophrenia, who had been separated at birth from their biological mothers (table 10.1; Heston 1966). Although the exposed and unexposed groups in this study were retrospectively assembled in accordance with historical data, a concurrent follow-up was used to assess the outcomes in the offspring.

Special Exposure Cohort Studies

Cohort studies of another type can be built around a population subgroup that has suffered an unusual adverse exposure. These special exposure cohort designs begin with the identification of an exposed group and select an

Table 10.3 Example of a Special Exposure Cohort

Sources	Study Description and Selected Findings
Quinton et al. (1984)	*Study*: Institutional Rearing and Adult Adjustment
	Cohort (N = 145): Exposed were girls being reared in children's homes in 1964. Unexposed were a random sample of same-age girls living with their families from the same London area. Adult follow-up assessment at age 21–27 in 1978.
	Finding: The girls raised in children's homes had more parenting difficulties as adult women. Factors promoting resilience were also identified, for example, the presence of a supportive male partner.

Note: Special exposure cohorts are built around a single exposure. A subset of special exposure cohorts is sometimes referred to as *cohorts with external comparison groups*. In genetic epidemiology, when the exposed group is offspring of parents with the disorder, it may be referred to as a *high-risk study*.

unexposed group to serve for comparison.[1] A special exposure cohort study can also be built around a population subgroup with a beneficial exposure.

This design is exemplified by a study built around a sample of girls who had been exposed to institutional care "because their parents could not cope with child rearing rather than because of . . . the children themselves" (table 10.3; Quinton et al. 1984, p. 109). The exposed girls had been identified and assessed in a previous study of children's homes. The comparison was to girls raised by their own families who had been part of a different previous study. Strictly speaking, the two groups of girls were not drawn from the same population, but they had been assessed at about the same age and with similar measures, and originated from the same general area of inner London.

In the cohort study, the authors followed up and compared the "ex-care" (exposed) and "family reared" (unexposed) groups as young women with respect to parenting of their own children (outcome). On average, the ex-care women exhibited far more parenting difficulties than the family-reared women. One-third of the ex-care women but none of the family-reared women had a child placed in the care of someone else for 6 months or more. Clearly, parenting difficulties had been transmitted across the two generations by childhood experiences and possibly by genetic factors.

The study also searched for factors that might interrupt the transmission. Many of the ex-care women, despite adverse childhood experience, showed good parenting skills, and among them some pathways to resilience were identified. For instance, a supportive male partner made a vital difference; in such instances, parenting skills were similar to those of family-reared women.

In special exposure studies, bias is a particular concern when the exposed and unexposed samples are drawn from quite distinct populations. In

---

[1] There are several different terms in use for this type of cohort study. When the unexposed group has to be selected from a different population, this type of study may be referred to as a cohort study with an external comparison group (Kelsey et al. 1986). In genetic epidemiology, when the exposed groups are offspring of parents with the disorder, it may be referred to as a high-risk study.

addition, ratings of outcome made blind to the exposure status of the participants are then more important but also more difficult to achieve (see chapter 14).

Clinical Cohorts

A clinical cohort study (or natural history study) departs from our prototype in that it examines the determinants of disorder outcome rather than of onset (Liddell 1988). The study may examine both negative outcomes (such as relapse, mortality, and homelessness) and positive outcomes (such as recovery, a supportive partner, and a stable job). The course of the disorder, too, may be followed in its many aspects: whether it is continuous or intermittent; whether the trend is toward improvement or deterioration; and the frequency, severity, and duration of episodes of illness and disability (see, e.g., Jablensky et al. 1992; Susser et al. 2000a).

Clinical cohort studies have a long and rich tradition in psychiatric epidemiology. For developing valid diagnoses, the course and outcome have been considered a crucial dimension of phenomenology (Robins and Guze 1970; see also chapter 9). Also, psychiatric disorders often lead to intermittent or ongoing manifestations over a long period, and prognosis cannot be captured in simple measures such as mortality.

A famous example is Manfred Bleuler's long-term follow-up of his clinic patients with schizophrenia (Bleuler 1978). Bleuler assembled a cohort of patients in the 1940s and personally followed them for 20 years. He examined many potential determinants of outcome. For example, he compared the outcomes of patients with and without childhood experiences of institutional care. But his most important and enduring finding was simply that the majority of patients improved, and a significant minority recovered. This result refuted the prevailing belief that schizophrenia almost always had a very poor long-term outcome. Initially greeted with skepticism, Bleuler's finding was later confirmed by numerous long-term follow-up studies.

In the assembly of a clinical cohort, it is important to recruit persons at some defined time point in their illness. Studying a heterogeneous mix of persons at various stages of illness can render results uninterpretable. Often the most informative studies begin at the first episode of illness (or a proxy for it, such as the time of first treatment for the illness). A current example is an ongoing follow-up of first-admission patients with psychosis identified in psychiatric hospitals in Suffolk County, New York (table 10.4; Bromet et al. 1996). The study has examined determinants of outcome at 6-month, 2-year, 4-year, and 10-year follow-ups. Comparison groups are internal to the study and depend upon the question being addressed. For example, one report compared patients with varying durations of untreated psychosis before hospitalization with respect to their outcome after 2 years. Data were analyzed separately for patients with diagnoses of schizophrenia, bipolar disorder, and depression (Craig et al. 2000). In contrast to some previous studies, duration of untreated psychosis was not related to outcome within any diagnostic group.

Table 10.4 Examples of Clinical Cohorts*

Sources	Study Description and Selected Findings
Craig et al. (2000) *See also*: Bromet and Fennig (1999)	*Study*: Suffolk County Mental Health Project *Cohort (N = 696)*: First-admission patients age 15–60 with evidence of psychosis recruited at inpatient facilities in Suffolk County (1989–1995). Follow-up interviews at 6 months, and at 2, 4, and 10 years.
Mojtabai et al. (2000)	*Finding*: Duration of untreated psychosis was not associated with illness course or clinical outcomes at 24-month follow-up within any diagnostic group. This analysis was based on a subset of 349 subjects.
Graham and Rutter (1973) *See also*: Rutter et al. (1970)	*Study*: Isle of Wight *Cohort (N = 126)*: Total population of children age 10 and 11 living on the Isle of Wight were surveyed in 1965. Derivative clinical cohort was the 126 children with significant psychiatric disorders. This cohort followed up at age 14–15.
	Finding: An appreciable minority of children with conduct disorder at age 10–11 developed emotional disorder by age 14–15.
Vaillant (1996) *See also*: Vaillant et al. (1991)	*Study*: The Harvard Grant Cohort *Cohort (N = 268)*: Harvard sophomores recruited 1938–1942. At age 47 follow-up interview, 249 remained under study; 52 had *DSM-III* alcohol abuse or dependence. Follow-up to age 70 with biennial questionnaires and every 5 years with physical exam.
	Selected finding: Those who developed alcohol abuse or dependence by age 47 had two times higher mortality compared to nonabusers by age 70.

* Also called natural history studies.

Thorough diagnosis is often essential to the interpretation of a clinical cohort study. In the Suffolk County study, information was collected from several sources, including diagnostic interviews with patients, hospital discharge summaries, and reports from clinicians and significant others. Diagnosticians met to review the information from all sources to arrive at consensus ratings. In fact, clinical cohort studies with thorough diagnostic information are often used to refine the diagnoses themselves. This is one of the important uses of epidemiology (Morris 1957) and, as already noted, especially of psychiatric epidemiology. For example, the Suffolk County study was used (Mojtabai et al. 2003), along with other studies (Susser and Wanderling 1994; Mojtabai et al. 2001), to generate a proposed refinement in the classification of acute and transient psychoses.

Ideally, to capture the full range of course and outcome, a clinical cohort should include untreated, as well as treated, cases. In practice, it is not often feasible to recruit a cohort outside of a clinical setting, but some studies have achieved it (Graham and Rutter 1973; Hasin et al. 1990). A clinical cohort derived from the Isle of Wight study provides an example (table 10.4). The original study sought to identify psychiatric disorders among all 10- to 11-

year-old children on the island (Rutter et al. 1970). The derivative clinical cohort comprised all those identified as having psychiatric disorders, which were classified as emotional, conduct, or mixed emotional/conduct disorders (Graham and Rutter 1973). Only about 10 percent of the 10 to 11-year-old children with disorders were attending a psychiatric clinic. A cohort based on these treated cases alone would have excluded 90 percent of the cases. The derivative cohort was followed up at age 14–15 (Graham and Rutter 1973; Rutter et al. 1976). Among children with conduct disorders at age 10–11, an appreciable minority had also developed emotional disturbances by age 14–15. Because the cohort included all cases, rather than only the 10 percent treated in psychiatric clinics, this result was informative about the developmental course of psychopathology in children.

A clinical cohort may also be constructed within a prospective population cohort study. In the Dunedin birth cohort study (see Table 9.1), psychiatric disorders were identified in the entire cohort at each of the 10 follow-up assessments from age 3 to 26. The investigators sought to shed light on the evolution of untreated, as well as treated, psychiatric disorders over the course of development. The cohort data enabled them to determine whether specific childhood disorders subsequently led to particular adult disorders (McGee et al. 1991). Analyzing the study from another perspective, they also examined whether specific adult disorders were preceded by particular kinds of childhood psychiatric disorders (Kim-Cohen et al. 2003).

To follow the effects of a disorder on later health and mental health, a clinical cohort study will sometimes include a control comparison group without a psychiatric disorder. The approach has been used, for example, to compare the long-term outcomes of psychiatric and surgical patients (Tsuang and Winokur 1975), of depressed and nondepressed children (Weissman et al. 1999), and of alcohol abusers and nonalcohol abusers (Vaillant 1996). In the latter study, Harvard undergraduates, all men, were followed from college up to age 70 (table 10.4). Mortality was about twofold higher in the men who developed alcoholism than in those who did not.

In still another variation, a clinical cohort is sometimes used as a natural experiment in which to examine the effects of changing patterns of treatment. This use can be traced as far back as a study of psychiatric patients in mid-19th century England, to which we referred in chapter 2. William Farr sought to determine the impact of reforms that were being implemented in some "insane asylums." For this purpose, he devised a comparison of mortality rates for patients living in the reformed Hanwell asylum and in other unreformed asylums (Susser and Adelstein 1975).[2] The mortality rate was lower in the reformed than the unreformed asylums, but in all asylums the mortality rate far exceeded that of the general population. Furthermore, being admitted as a pauper appeared to have a greater effect on mortality than the asylum to which one was admitted.

---

[2] Since Farr's evaluation of reformed care was conceived after its introduction by others, we consider this study a natural experiment. It might also be legitimate to consider this study a quasi-experiment, because the asylum reform was a planned intervention, if not by the researcher himself (Shadish et al. 2002).

Other Variations

We have construed the natural experiment, historical cohort, and special exposure cohort as variants that modify one of the key elements of a prospective population cohort study. However, we can also modify more than one element at the same time. As we have noted, for example, the Dutch Famine Study is both a natural experiment and an historical cohort. Thus, many other variations are possible. A cohort study may, simultaneously, encompass a natural experiment, a historical cohort, and a special exposure cohort. A clinical cohort may even be built into the same study.

Some epidemiology textbooks have also described "open" cohorts in which cohort members may enter or leave the population after the start of follow-up. These are dynamic populations, well exemplified by the population of any city: every day there are births and deaths, and immigration and emigration, so the populations are constantly in flux. Strictly speaking, such studies of dynamic populations are not cohort studies, and we do not include them here.

Evolution of a Cohort Study

A cohort study may evolve over several decades and generations of researchers. Long after the original questions have been addressed, researchers return to examine other questions in the data. In addition, as we have seen, investigators may initiate further follow-ups or derivative studies of the same cohort.

The National Survey of Health and Development offers an extraordinary example (Wadsworth 1991; Wadsworth et al. 2003). It began as a study of all births in England, Scotland, and Wales during March 3–9, 1946. One of its purposes was to shed light on the declining birth rate, a purpose that soon became irrelevant because of the post–World War II baby boom. Another purpose was to aid in planning the new National Health Service.

Shortly thereafter, this cross-sectional maternity study started to evolve into a cohort study. A subsample of 5,362 births was selected for another assessment at age 2. The subsample comprised one-quarter of the offspring of manual workers (who were the great majority) and all offspring of non-manual and agricultural workers. Twin and illegitimate births were excluded. With another follow-up of this subsample at age 4, it had become an ongoing cohort study. By age 60 (2006), the cohort will have been followed up 23 times (MRC National Survey of Health and Development 2004). Though each follow-up has a somewhat distinct focus, some information pertaining to cognitive ability and mental health is usually included.

The results of this cohort study—which we refer to as the 1946 British birth cohort (see table 10.5)—have been informative for mental disorders at every stage of the life cycle. For example, reports have suggested that death of a parent and parental separation or divorce are risk factors for childhood enuresis (Douglas 1973); that among adolescent school leavers frequent job changes predict (but may not be a cause of) later psychiatric problems (Cherry 1976);

Table 10.5 Studies of Mental Disorders over the Life Course in the National Survey of Health and Development (the 1946 British Birth Cohort; $N = 5,362$)

Sources	Study Description and Selected Findings
Douglas (1973)	*Study*: Parental loss and enuresis in childhood
	Cohort subset (N = 3,393): Subset of the cohort with information on life events in the first 6 years, and on enuresis at ages 6, 8, 9, 11, and 15.
	Finding: Children whose mother died or whose parents divorced or separated before age 6 were more than twice as likely to have enuresis at later ages (6, 8, 9, 11, 15 years) than children from intact homes.
Cherry (1976)	*Study*: The association between persistent job changing and personal problems.
	Cohort subset (N = 4,330): Subset of the cohort that left school at age 15,[a] and completed a questionnaire at age 26. Persistent job changing defined as 4 or more job changes prior to 18 years; personal problems defined as illegitimate births, broken marriages, psychiatric problems, and unemployment after age 18.
	Finding: Those with a history of persistent job changing before age 18 were at higher risk for subsequent personal problems, including nervous troubles, in comparison to those with stable employment. The association remained among men after controlling for earlier poor adjustment.
Rodgers (1978)	*Study*: The association between bottle feeding in infancy and cognitive ability and achievement in childhood and adolescence.
	Cohort subset (N = 2,424): Subset of cohort known to be exclusively bottle fed or exclusively breastfed in infancy. Cognitive and achievement tests available at age 8 (picture intelligence, word reading) and age 15 (nonverbal ability, mathematical achievement, sentence completion). Main analyses restricted to those of birthweight $> = 6$ lbs. with complete information on family background variables, and relevant test scores at age 8 (N = 1,464) and age 15 (N = 1,398).
	Finding: Children who were bottle fed had significantly lower scores on four of five tests of cognitive ability and achievement. These associations remained after controlling for family background.
Jones et al. (1994)	*Study*: The association between early developmental delay and risk of schizophrenia in adulthood.
	Cohort subset (N = 4,746): A subset of those with childhood data and outcomes assessed at age 43. Early milestones were reported at age 2; physical development measured at birth, 6, 7, 11, and 15; educational achievement measured at 8, 11, and 15 years; social and behavioral characteristics measured at 4, 6, and 13. Cases of schizophrenia ascertained between 16 and 43 years.
	Finding: Children with developmental delays were at higher risk of schizophrenia in adulthood.

continued

Table 10.5 continued

Sources	Study Description and Selected Findings
Richards et al. (2004)	*Study*: The association between cognitive ability in childhood and cognitive decline in midlife (ages 43–53).
	Cohort subset (N = 2,058): A subset consisting of those followed at age 53 for whom there was complete information on cognitive ability at age 15, memory and search speed at ages 43 and 53, reading test scores at age 53, and adult educational attainment and social class.
	Finding: Childhood cognitive ability was inversely associated with rate of memory decline in midlife.
Richards et al. (2003)	*Study*: The association between smoking and cognitive decline in middle age.
	Cohort subset (N = 1,941): A subset consisting of those followed at age 53, for whom there was complete information on smoking at ages 36, 43, and 53; measures of verbal memory, speed and concentration at ages 43 and 53; cognitive ability at age 15; and adult measures of education and occupational social class.
	Finding: Heavy smoking at age 43 was associated with more rapid decline in memory from ages 43 to 53.

Note: The National Survey of Health and Development included all live births in England, Scotland, and Wales during the week March 3–9, 1946 (N = 13,687). The 1946 British birth cohort comprises a stratified random sample of the surveyed group selected for follow-up (N = 5,362; Wadsworth 1991). The cohort was followed 22 times from birth to age 53 years; an additional 8 annual postal questionnaires were sent to women during middle age. Follow-up is ongoing.
[a] Over three-quarters of the cohort left school at the earliest opportunity, either upon their 15th birthday or at the end of the school year after turning 15 years old.

that bottle feeding as opposed to breastfeeding is associated with lower cognitive and achievement scores in childhood and adolescence (Rodgers 1978); that childhood developmental delay is a risk factor for adult schizophrenia (Jones et al. 1994); and that childhood cognitive ability might protect against cognitive decline in midlife and beyond (Richards et al. 2004).

In the 1946 British birth cohort, with births from within a single week, the effects of age and of historical time are not separable. The cohort certainly bears the imprint of its historical time (for an in-depth account, see Wadsworth 1991). The cohort was born shortly after the election of a Labor government, which was committed to reducing social class inequalities and establishing a welfare state. The childhood of its members was spent in a period of relative prosperity in the 1950s and 1960s. Compared with their parents, they had better material conditions, social programs, and educational opportunities. They grew up, on average, taller and better educated. A question that cannot be answered in this design is the degree to which the causes of mental disorders over the life course of this cohort were shaped by the historical context.

The foremost recent publications from this cohort pertain to the links between early life experiences and adult health and mental health. But the cohort is also being used to answer questions that pertain exclusively to later stages of the lifespan. For instance, a recent report examined the relation of cigarette smoking to cognitive decline in mid-life (Richards et al. 2003).

Reflecting on the remarkable contributions of this and other highly evolved cohorts (e.g., Hardy et al. 1997), some have called for an investment of resources into "conception-to-death" cohorts that trace the trajectory of health and illness over the entire life course (Eaton 2002; Susser and Terry 2003).

The Prenatal Determinants of Schizophrenia Example (PDSE)

In any particular application, the basic elements of a cohort study are less straightforward than they may seem in the abstract. By examining one cohort study in more detail and presenting the data from it, we will follow the judgments that are made through a single study design and reveal some of the nuances. We will also use the data in subsequent chapters to illustrate potential sources of bias and how to deal with them, and to illustrate other points in later parts of the book.

We chose the PDSE study for this purpose (Susser et al. 2000b). The PDSE was a birth cohort study designed to examine whether prenatal exposures are causally related to schizophrenia spectrum disorder (see tables 10.6 and 10.7 and figure 10.1). A great wealth of prenatal data was available for this cohort,

Table 10.6 The Prenatal Determinants of Schizophrenia Study Example (PDSE)

Articulating the questions	Are prenatal exposures risk factors for schizophrenia spectrum disorders (SSD)? Specifically, does prenatal exposure to high maternal body mass index (BMI) increase risk for SSD?
Defining the source population	12,090 individuals who (a) were members of a birth cohort of 19,044 children born between 1959 and 1967 to mothers in the Kaiser Permanente Medical Care Plan in northern California, and (b) participated in Kaiser Permanente Medical Care Plan during the study period (Jan. 1, 1981 to Dec. 31, 1997). Of these, 9298 had data available for measurement of prepregnancy BMI.
Measuring the exposure	Prepregnancy height from prenatal visit records, and prepregnancy weight from maternal interview. High BMI $\geq 27 \, \mathrm{kg/m^2}$.
Following the cohort	The follow-up period was from birth to 1997; the risk period was 1981–1997. Computerized membership and psychiatric registries were used to monitor membership in the Kaiser Permanente Medical Care Plan and to identify potential cases of SSD.
Classifying the outcomes	Searched Kaiser Permanente Medical Care Plan registries to identify potential cases. Potential cases were diagnosed by face-to-face diagnostic assessment using the Diagnostic Instrument for Genetic Studies, by chart review, or both.

Table 10.7 Ages During the Study Period By Birth Year in the PSDE Cohort

Year of Birth	Age during Risk Period[a]	N in Birth Year	% of PDS Cohort	N Cases Birth Year
1959	21–38	129	1.4%	1
1960	20–37	945	10.2%	6
1961	19–36	825	8.9%	6
1962	18–35	1,737	18.7%	11
1963	17–34	1,680	18.1%	7
1964	16–33	1,560	16.8%	11
1965	15–32	1,128	12.1%	8
1966	14–31	1,085	11.7%	9
1967	13–30	209	2.2%	1
Total	13–38	9,298	100.0%	60

[a] Jan. 1, 1981 to Dec. 31, 1997.

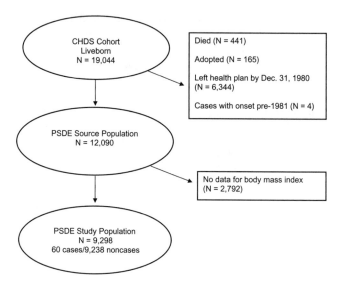

Figure 10.1 Derivation of the PDSE analytic cohort from the Child Health and Development Study (CHDS) cohort.

including archived serum samples collected from the mothers during pregnancy. Many findings have been published. For illustration, we chose one particular analysis that examined fetal exposure to high maternal body mass index as a risk factor for schizophrenia spectrum disorder (Schaefer et al. 2000). We have modified the analysis to simplify the presentation.[3] Therefore, in the text we always use the term *PDSE* in which "E" denotes *Example*.

---

[3] Any formal critique of the study should refer to the original publications (Schaefer et al. 2000; Susser et al. 2000b).

Articulating a Question

The analysis of maternal body mass index was motivated by evidence suggesting that fetal exposure to an adverse state of maternal nutrition might be related to the risk of schizophrenia spectrum disorder. The best-established summary measure of the overall state of maternal nutrition is the body mass index: weight in kilograms divided by height in meters squared (Willett 1998). Both the high and the low extremes of the body mass index represent adverse nutritional states related to morbidity and mortality in women and their offspring (Deckelbaum 1996; Hoek et al. 1998; Krebs and Jacobson 2003). Results from previous birth cohort studies had suggested that fetal exposure to either very high (Jones et al. 1998) or very low (Done et al. 1991; Susser et al. 1996; Wahlbeck et al. 2001) maternal body mass index might increase the risk of schizophrenia.

The PDSE was appropriate to address only one part of this hypothesis. In well-fed industrialized societies, the body mass index shows substantial variation above but not below the levels conducive to health. Therefore, a cohort study in such a society could readily detect effects of fetal exposure to high but not low maternal body mass index. Thus, the question posed in this analysis was whether exposure to a high maternal body mass index was a risk factor for schizophrenia spectrum disorder.

We noted in the previous chapter that cohort studies might be impractical when the disorder has a low incidence, and when there is a long interval between the exposure and the onset of disorder. In this instance, however, the cohort design was practical even though both these conditions pertained. As will be described, the PDSE was based on a large prospective cohort spanning the period from fetal exposure to adult life. Even so, the number of cases was limited and the statistical power was modest. It should be noted that this example was chosen to represent a typical rather than an extraordinary epidemiologic result. The association was of modest size and the causal inference was not definitive.

Defining the Source Population

The PDSE is derived from the Child Health and Development Study, a birth cohort study of 19,044 offspring. This prospective population cohort comprised births between 1959 and 1967 to mothers enrolled in the Kaiser Permanente Medical Care Plan (hereafter referred to as "health plan") in Alameda County, California (van den Berg 1984). Virtually all mothers giving birth participated in the study. The original follow-up study of the full cohort stopped in early childhood.

The PDSE follow-up of the cohort for schizophrenia spectrum disorder began in 1981, when the psychiatric registry of the health plan was computerized. To enter the source population for the PDSE, a cohort member had to meet two criteria: (1) be free of schizophrenia spectrum disorder until 1981, and (2) be a member of the health plan for some period after 1981. 12,090 offspring met these criteria (figure 10.1). Thus, the source population of the PDSE is a subset of the original birth cohort, subject to possible bias as a consequence, although the bias appears to be small (Susser et al. 2000b).

Measuring the Exposure

The assessment of the exposure required data on the mother's prepregnancy weight and height, to compute prepregnancy maternal body mass index. These data were available for the cohort members whose mothers completed a study assessment at a prenatal visit: 9,298 of the 12,090 in the PDSE cohort. Several legitimate but different approaches were available for categorizing the body mass index as "high." One option was to follow current guidelines, developed decades after the cohort was born (Health and Welfare Canada 1988; Institute of Medicine 1990; Flegal et al. 1998). Another was to use the distribution of body mass index within the PDSE, for example, defining the top 10th percentile as high. After examining these options, the research team chose a current definition (Najjar and Rowland 1987), with minor modifications, defining high body mass index as a score greater than or equal to 27. Under this definition, 9.8 percent of the individuals included in this analysis were exposed to high maternal body mass index.

Following the Cohort

The risk period in the PDSE was specified as 1981–1997. The start of the risk period was specified as January 1, 1981, for the practical reason that the computerized health plan registry used for the ascertainment of cases was begun at that time. A systematic ascertainment of cases before 1981 would have entailed searching through clinic cards in shoeboxes. Ascertainment was stopped in 1997, to allow for the analysis of the data. Thus, cohort members born in 1967 were followed from age 13 to 30, whereas those born in 1959 were followed from age 21 to 38 (see table 10.7).

There was ongoing case registry ascertainment in the health plan registry. The cohort members were under observation for as long as they were members of the health plan. The losses to follow-up over this period are displayed in Appendix B.

Classifying the Outcomes

Genetic studies indicate that a spectrum of schizophrenia-related diagnoses coaggregate in families. The results of the Dutch Famine Study suggested that exposure to prenatal famine also affected this broader spectrum (Hoek et al. 1996). Therefore, we chose to define the outcome as **schizophrenia spectrum disorder** (SSD), although results were also examined for schizophrenia alone. As defined in the PDSE, the spectrum includes schizophrenia, schizoaffective disorder, schizotypal personality disorder, delusional disorder, and psychotic disorder not otherwise specified. All diagnoses were based on *DSM-IV* criteria.

The health plan registries were searched for records of psychiatric treatments provided to cohort members during the period 1981–1997. These records, systematically abstracted and rated, yielded 183 potential cases of SSD. The 183 potential cases were further evaluated by face-to-face standardized clinical diagnostic assessments and chart reviews. The final yield was 67 individuals with a diagnosis of a SSD. Sixty of the 67 had the prenatal data required for computation of maternal body mass index.

Evolution of the Cohort Study

The PDSE combines elements of a prospective population cohort, a historical cohort, and a historical cohort with concurrent follow-up. Indeed, it illustrates how a cohort, once established, is often exploited anew with a concurrent follow-up to examine outcomes later in the life course. Further, as we will see in later chapters, the PDSE provided the basis for case-control studies nested within the cohort, studies in which the archived prenatal biological samples were used to devise new exposure measures.

Conclusion

We have described a diversity of cohort studies that fall within the rubric of the cohort design. The many variants differ somewhat in the foundation they provide for causal inference, the questions they can best address, and the practical problems they present for implementation. Nonetheless, they follow the same general theme of comparing an exposed group and an unexposed group with respect to the frequency of the study outcome over a specified period of time.

We have not yet considered how to evaluate alternative explanations for an association between exposure and disease. The cohort design is tailored to isolate this relationship and permit scrutiny of the evidence for a causal connection. In the following chapters, we offer a systematic approach to causal inference from a cohort study. Fortunately, we can distill a few general principles about the cohort design that are adaptable to a vast array of particular applications. To do so, however, we are compelled to develop a more sophisticated formulation of the cohort design. Readers will discover that it is a more subtle—and interesting—device than so far described.

References

Bleuler M (1978). *The Schizophrenic Disorders: Long-Term Patient and Family Studies.* New Haven: Yale University Press.

Bromet EJ and Fennig S (1999). Epidemiology and Natural History of Schizophrenia. *Biol. Psychiatry* 46:871–881.

Bromet EJ, Jandorf L, Fennig S, Lavelle J, Kovasznay B, Ram R, Tanenberg-Karant M, and Craig T (1996). The Suffolk County Mental Health Project: Demographic, Pre-Morbid and Clinical Correlates of 6-Month Outcome. *Psychol. Med.* 26:953–962.

Cherry N (1976). Persistent Job Changing: Is It a Problem? *J. Occup. Psychology* 49:203–221.

Costello EJ and Angold A (1991). Developmental Epidemiology. In Cicchetti D and Toth S, eds., *Rochester Symposium on Developmental Psychopathology,* 23–56. Hillsdale, N.J.: Erlbaum.

Costello EJ, Angold A, Burns BJ, Stangl DK, Tweed DL, Erkanli A, and Worthman CM (1996). The Great Smoky Mountains Study of Youth. Goals, Design, Methods, and the Prevalence of *DSM-III-R* Disorders. *Arch. Gen. Psychiatry* 53:1129–1136.

Costello EJ, Compton SN, Keeler G, and Angold A (2003). Relationships between Poverty and Psychopathology: A Natural Experiment. *JAMA* 290:2023–2029.

Craig TJ, Bromet EJ, Fennig S, Tanenberg-Karant M, Lavelle J, and Galambos N (2000). Is There an Association between Duration of Untreated Psychosis and 24-Month Clinical Outcome in a First-Admission Series? *Am. J. Psychiatry* 157:60–66.

Davidson M, Reichenberg A, Rabinowitz J, Weiser M, Kaplan Z, and Mark M (1999). Behavioral and Intellectual Markers for Schizophrenia in Apparently Healthy Male Adolescents. *Am. J. Psychiatry* 156:1328–1335.

Deckelbaum RJ (1996). Preventive Nutrition in Childhood: A Rationale. *Public Health Rev.* 24:105–111.

Done DJ, Johnstone EC, Frith CD, Golding J, Shepherd PM, and Crow TJ (1991). Complications of Pregnancy and Delivery in Relation to Psychosis in Adult Life: Data from the British Perinatal Mortality Survey Sample. *BMJ* 302:1576–1580.

Douglas J (1973). Early Disturbing Events and Later Enuresis. In Kolvin I, MacKeith Re, and Meadow SR, eds., *Bladder Control and Enuresis*, 109–117. London: Spastics International Medical Publications.

Eaton W (2002). The Logic for a Conception-to-Death Cohort Study. *Ann. Epidemiol.* 12:445–451.

Flegal KM, Carroll MD, Kuczmarski RJ, and Johnson CL (1998). Overweight and Obesity in the United States: Prevalence and Trends, 1960–1994. *Int. J. Obes. Relat. Metab. Disord.* 22:39–47.

Graham P and Rutter M (1973). Psychiatric Disorder in the Young Adolescent: A Follow-up Study. *Proc. R. Soc. Med.* 66:1226–1229.

Hardy JB, Shapiro S, Astone NM, Miller TL, Brooks-Gunn J, and Hilton SC (1997). Adolescent Childbearing Revisited: The Age of Inner-City Mothers at Delivery Is a Determinant of Their Children's Self-Sufficiency at Age 27 to 33. *Pediatrics* 100:802–809.

Hasin DS, Grant B, and Endicott J (1990). The Natural History of Alcohol Abuse: Implications for Definitions of Alcohol Use Disorders. *Am. J. Psychiatry* 147:1537–1541.

Health and Welfare Canada (1988). *Canadian Guidelines for Healthy Weights. Report of an Expert Group Convened by Health Promotion Directorate*. Ottawa: Author.

Heston LL (1966). Psychiatric Disorders in Foster Home Reared Children of Schizophrenic Mothers. *Br. J. Psychiatry* 112:819–825.

Hoek HW, Susser E, Buck KA, Lumey LH, Lin SP, and Gorman JM (1996). Schizoid Personality Disorder after Prenatal Exposure to Famine. *Am. J. Psychiatry* 153:1637–1639.

Hoek HW, Treasure JL, and Katzman MA, eds. (1998). *Neurobiology in the Treatment of Eating Disorders*. Chichester, U.K.: Wiley.

Institute of Medicine (1990). *Nutrition during Pregnancy: Weight Gain, Nutrient Supplements*. Washington, D.C.: National Academy Press.

Jablensky A, Sartorius N, Ernberg G, Anker M, Korten A, Cooper JE, Day R, and Bertelsen A (1992). Schizophrenia: Manifestations, Incidence and Course in Different Cultures. A World Health Organization Ten-Country Study. *Psychol. Med. Monogr. Suppl.* 20:1–97.

Jones P, Rodgers B, Murray R, and Marmot M (1994). Child Development Risk Factors for Adult Schizophrenia in the British 1946 Birth Cohort. *Lancet* 344:1398–1402.

Jones PB, Rantakallio P, Hartikainen AL, Isohanni M, and Sipila P (1998). Schizophrenia as a Long-Term Outcome of Pregnancy, Delivery, and Perinatal Complications: A 28-Year Follow-up of the 1966 North Finland General Population Birth Cohort. *Am. J. Psychiatry* 155:355–364.

Kelsey JL, Thompson WD, and Evans AS (1986). *Methods in Observational Epidemology*. New York: Oxford University Press.

Kim-Cohen J, Caspi A, Moffitt TE, Harrington H, Milne BJ, and Poulton R (2003). Prior Juvenile Diagnoses in Adults with Mental Disorder: Developmental Follow-Back of a Prospective-Longitudinal Cohort. *Arch. Gen. Psychiatry* 60:709–717.

Krebs NF and Jacobson MS (2003). Prevention of Pediatric Overweight and Obesity. *Pediatrics* 112:424–430.

Liddell FD (1988). The Development of Cohort Studies in Epidemiology: A Review. *J. Clin. Epidemiol.* 41:1217–1237.

Lilienfeld AM and Lilienfeld DE (1980). *Foundations of Epidemiology,* 2nd ed. New York: Oxford University Press.

Malaspina D, Harlap S, Fennig S, Heiman D, Nahon D, Feldman D, and Susser ES (2001). Advancing Paternal Age and the Risk of Schizophrenia. *Arch. Gen. Psychiatry* 58:361–367.

McGee R, Partridge F, Williams S, and Silva PA (1991). A Twelve-Year Follow-up of Preschool Hyperactive Children. *J. Am. Acad. Child Adolesc. Psychiatry* 30: 224–232.

Mojtabai R, Bromet EJ, Harvey PD, Carlson GA, Craig TJ, and Fennig S (2000). Neuropsychological Differences between First-Admission Schizophrenia and Psychotic Affective Disorders. *Am. J. Psychiatry* 157:1453–1460.

Mojtabai R, Susser ES, and Bromet EJ (2003). Clinical Characteristics, 4-Year Course, and *DSM-IV* Classification of Patients with Nonaffective Acute Remitting Psychosis. *Am. J. Psychiatry* 160:2108–2115.

Mojtabai R, Varma VK, Malhotra S, Mattoo SK, Misra AK, Wig NN, and Susser E (2001). Mortality and Long-Term Course in Schizophrenia with a Poor 2-Year Course: A Study in a Developing Country. *Br. J. Psychiatry* 178:71–75.

Morris JN (1957). *Uses of Epidemiology.* Edinburgh, Scotland: Livingstone.

Mortensen PB, Pedersen CB, Melbye M, Mors O, and Ewald H (2003). Individual and Familial Risk Factors for Bipolar Affective Disorders in Denmark. *Arch. Gen. Psychiatry* 60:1209–1215.

Mortensen PB, Pedersen CB, Westergaard T, Wohlfahrt J, Ewald H, Mors O, Andersen PK, and Melbye M (1999). Effects of Family History and Place and Season of Birth on the Risk of Schizophrenia. *N. Engl. J. Med.* 340:603–608.

MRC National Survey of Health and Development (2004). www.nshd.mrc.ac.uk. London: University College London.

Munk-Jorgensen P and Mortensen PB (1997). The Danish Psychiatric Central Register. *Dan. Med. Bull.* 44:82–84.

Najjar MF and Rowland M (1987). *Anthropometric Reference Data and Prevalence of Overweight, United States 1976–1980: Data From the National Health Survey.* Series 11. Washington, D.C.: National Center for Health Statistics, U.S. Public Health Service, U.S. Government Printing Office.

Quinton D, Rutter M, and Liddle C (1984). Institutional Rearing, Parenting Difficulties and Marital Support. *Psychol. Med.* 14:107–124.

Rabinowitz J (1998). A Method for Preserving Confidentiality when Linking Computerized Registries. *Am. J. Public Health* 88:836.

Richards M, Jarvis MJ, Thompson N, and Wadsworth ME (2003). Cigarette Smoking and Cognitive Decline in Midlife: Evidence from a Prospective Birth Cohort Study. *Am. J. Public Health* 93:994–998.

Richards M, Shipley B, Fuhrer R, and Wadsworth ME (2004). Cognitive Ability in Childhood and Cognitive Decline in Mid-Life: Longitudinal Birth Cohort Study. *BMJ* 328:552.

Robins E and Guze SB (1970). Establishment of Diagnostic Validity in Psychiatric Illness: Its Application to Schizophrenia. *Am. J. Psychiatry* 126:983–987.

Rodgers B (1978). Feeding in Infancy and Later Ability and Attainment: A Longitudinal Study. *Dev. Med. Child Neurol.* 20:421–426.

Rutter M (2003). Poverty and Child Mental Health: Natural Experiments and Social Causation. *JAMA* 290:2063–2064.

Rutter M, Tizard J, and Whitmore K (1970). *Education, Health and Behaviour.* Harlow, U.K.: Longman.

Rutter M, Tizard J, Yule W, Graham P, and Whitmore K (1976). Research Report: Isle of Wight Studies, 1964–1974. *Psychol. Med.* 6:313–332.

Schaefer CA, Brown AS, Wyatt RJ, Kline J, Begg MD, Bresnahan MA, and Susser ES (2000). Maternal Prepregnant Body Mass and Risk of Schizophrenia in Adult Offspring. *Schizophr. Bull.* 26:275–286.

Shadish WR, Cook TD, and Campbell DT (2002). *Experimental and Quasi-Experimental Design for Generalized Causal Inference.* Boston: Houghton Mifflin Co.

St. Clair D, Xu M, Wang P, Yu Y, Fang Y, Zhang F, Zheng X, Gu N, Feng G, Sham P, He (2005). Rates of Adult Schizophrenia Following Prenatal Exposure to the Chinese Famine of 1959–1961. *JAMA* 294:557–562.

Stein ZA, Susser M, Saenger G, and Marolla F (1975). *Famine and Human Development: The Dutch Hunger Winter of 1944–1945.* New York: Oxford University Press.

Susser E, Finnerty M, Mojtabai R, Yale S, Conover S, Goetz R, and Amador X (2000a). Reliability of the Life Chart Schedule for Assessment of the Long-Term Course of Schizophrenia. *Schizophr. Res.* 42:67–77.

Susser E, Hoek HW, and Brown A (1998). Neurodevelopmental Disorders after Prenatal Famine: The Story of the Dutch Famine Study. *Am. J. Epidemiol.* 147:213–216.

Susser E, Neugebauer R, Hoek HW, Brown AS, Lin S, Labovitz D, and Gorman JM (1996). Schizophrenia after Prenatal Famine. Further Evidence. *Arch. Gen. Psychiatry* 53:25–31.

Susser E, Schaefer CA, Brown AS, Begg MD, and Wyatt RJ (2000b). The Design of the Prenatal Determinants of Schizophrenia Study. *Schizophr. Bull.* 26:257–273.

Susser E and Terry MB (2003). A Conception-to-Death Cohort. *Lancet* 361:797–798.

Susser E and Wanderling J (1994). Epidemiology of Nonaffective Acute Remitting Psychosis vs. Schizophrenia. Sex and Sociocultural Setting. *Arch. Gen. Psychiatry* 51:294–301.

Susser M (1991). What Is a Cause and How Do We Know One? A Grammar for Pragmatic Epidemiology. *Am. J. Epidemiol.* 133:635–648.

Susser M and Adelstein A, eds. (1975). *Vital Statistics: A Memorial Volume of Selections from the Reports and Writings of William Farr.* Metuchen, N.J.: Scarecrow Press.

Tsuang MT and Winokur G (1975). The Iowa 500: Field Work in a 35-Year Follow-up of Depression, Mania, and Schizophrenia. *Can. Psychiatr. Assoc. J.* 20:359–365.

Vaillant GE (1996). A Long-Term Follow-up of Male Alcohol Abuse. *Arch. Gen. Psychiatry* 53:243–249.

Vaillant GE, Schnurr PP, Baron JA, and Gerber PD (1991). A Prospective Study of the Effects of Cigarette Smoking and Alcohol Abuse on Mortality. *J. Gen. Intern. Med.* 6:299–304.

van den Berg BJ (1984). The California Child Health and Development Studies. In Mednick SA, Harway M, and Finello K, eds., *Handbook of Longitudinal Research*, 166–179. New York: Praeger.

Wadsworth ME, Butterworth SL, Hardy RJ, Kuh DJ, Richards M, Langenberg C, Hilder WS, and Connor M (2003). The Life Course Prospective Design: An Example of Benefits and Problems Associated with Study Longevity. *Soc. Sci. Med.* 57: 2193–2205.

Wadsworth MEJ (1991). *The Imprint of Time: Childhood, History and Adult Life.* Oxford: Clarendon Press.

Wahlbeck K, Forsen T, Osmond C, Barker DJ, and Eriksson JG (2001). Association of Schizophrenia with Low Maternal Body Mass Index, Small Size at Birth, and Thinness during Childhood. *Arch. Gen. Psychiatry* 58:48–52.

Weissman MM, Wolk S, Goldstein RB, et al. (1999). Depressed Adolescents Grown Up. *JAMA* 281:1707–1713.

Willett W (1998). *Nutritional Epidemiology,* 2nd ed. Oxford: Oxford University Press.

Causal Inference: A Thought Experiment

11

Ezra Susser and Sharon Schwartz

We now take up the process of causal inference from cohort studies. We have proposed that the many forms of the cohort design represent variations on the same theme. This underlying unity makes it possible to distill a few principles that are adaptable to the diverse array of particular cohort studies and circumstances.

Within a given cohort study, causal inference is likely to be tentative rather than definitive. To reach firm conclusions, we generally require results from several cohort studies, as well as other designs. The root of the uncertainty is that the identification of risk factors depends on our ability to isolate the effects of the exposure from all other effects on the disease. This criterion can be met only when the exposure groups are fully comparable (as defined in chapter 5). Typically, however, they are not.

Consequently, a cohort study is always a kind of "thought experiment." We need to imagine what our result "would have been" if the exposed and the unexposed groups had in fact been fully comparable. This chapter sets up a framework for conducting this thought experiment in a systematic way.

The exposed and unexposed may differ on (1) other causes of the disease (confounding), (2) the length of time over which they are observed (unequal attrition), and (3) the accuracy with which cases are ascertained (differential misclassification). Each of these factors may account for part, or even all, of an apparent association between the exposure and the disease. These same factors can also suppress an association or reverse it.

The process of causal inference depends upon the identification and evaluation of these alternative explanations for our result. Below we show how confounding, unequal attrition, and differential misclassification can produce an association between exposure and disease. In the subsequent three chapters, using examples from cohort studies in psychiatric epidemiology, we will discuss each of these sources of bias in turn. As we seek to distill the complexity of these cohort studies, the framework presented here will serve as a vital referent.

Confounding

Confounding occurs when the exposed and unexposed groups differ on another cause of the disorder being investigated. Table 11.1 depicts a hypothetical scenario of confounding by gender. The cohort comprises 10,000 exposed and 10,000 unexposed individuals. In this cohort, gender is associated with the exposure: men are one half of the exposed (5,000 out of 10,000) but only one-quarter of the unexposed (2,500 out of 10,000). In addition, gender is a cause of the disease: men are four times as likely to get the disease as women within both the exposed (8 percent versus 2 percent) and the unexposed (1.6 percent versus 0.4 percent) groups. The risk ratios within each gender group are the same (5.0) and are correct. However, the risk ratio for the total cohort is 7.1. Thus, confounding by gender explains part of the association between exposure and disease in the total cohort.

Confounding occurs for two reasons. One reason resides in the naturally occurring population from which we select our source population. In a cohort study, we do not assign people to be exposed or unexposed, but instead accept their exposures as found "in nature." For a variety of reasons, including individual choices and social forces, the exposed and unexposed tend to differ on other causes of the disease. We refer to this as **natural confounding**. If in our example gender (the confounder) was associated with the exposure in the naturally occurring population, it would be a scenario of natural confounding.

Table 11.1 Hypothetical Scenario of a Confounder

TOTAL COHORT

	N	Cases N	Risk	Risk Ratio
Exposed	10,000	500	5.0%	7.1
Unexposed	10,000	70	0.7%	

MALES ONLY

	N	Cases N	Risk	Risk Ratio
Exposed	5,000	400	8.0%	5.0
Unexposed	2,500	40	1.6%	

FEMALES ONLY

	N	Cases N	Risk	Risk Ratio
Exposed	5,000	100	2.0%	5.0
Unexposed	7,500	30	0.4%	

Note: Gender is associated with exposure and is a cause of disease. The risk ratio for the total cohort is confounded by gender, while the risk ratios within each gender are correct.

Another reason for confounding derives from the selection of the people we study from the naturally occurring population. This selection may produce further differences between the exposed and unexposed groups on other risk factors for the disease. This kind of confounding is a methodological artifact and we refer to it as **artifactual confounding**. Artifactual confounding may be introduced into a population cohort study by selective recruitment of the source population from a naturally occurring population, as when the source population comprises the participants in a community survey; by selective recruitment of the study population from the source population, as when some members of the source population refuse to participate in the study; and in the selection of a subgroup of the cohort (e.g., people with adequate data on exposure and relevant confounders) for a particular analysis. In a special exposure cohort study, all artifactual confounding is a central concern; such a study is not based in a naturally occurring population.

Suppose that in our current example, gender were not associated with the exposure in the source population, but only in the study population. The association between gender and exposure in the cohort study in table 11.1 could have been produced by exposed women in the source population refusing participation in the study much more often than the three other subgroups, that is, much more often than unexposed women, exposed men, and unexposed men. This, then, would be a scenario of artifactual confounding.

We usually refer simply to *confounding* without differentiating natural and artifactual confounding. For certain purposes, however, the distinction becomes important. It can have implications for research design and for public health actions (Szklo and Nieto 2000; also see part VIII). Usually we have to consider not one but several variables as potential confounders, as well. In many studies, for example, gender, age, and socioeconomic status are all potential confounders. The observed association will reflect the net effect of all the confounders.

Although confounding is an ever-present danger in cohort studies, we have ways of counteracting it. We often use **matching** to reduce confounding in the study population and adjustment to compensate for it in the analysis of the data. Thus, we seek to infer what the association between exposure and disease would be if we could remove the contribution of confounders.

Unequal Attrition

Attrition that is unequal for the exposed and unexposed groups can also create the appearance of an association between exposure and disease. In this chapter, we assume that within each exposure group those who are lost and those who remain under observation have the same disease risk. Under this condition, the attrition may be unequal for the exposed and the unexposed, but it will not be differential. **Differential attrition** is an important and particularly damaging variant of unequal attrition, but because it is complex we defer discussion to chapter 13.

There are two main reasons for cohort attrition. One is **loss to follow-up**. Some members of the cohort may not be located or may not consent to a follow-up assessment. The other is **competing risk**. A competing risk is the risk of getting some other condition that precludes having the disease being studied. Suppose that in a study of suicide an individual dies from some other cause—a competing risk—before the end of the risk period. One does not know whether the individual would have committed suicide during the remainder of the risk period. So the outcome is unobserved, and the follow-up data are incomplete. Loss to follow-up is an artifact of the study, whereas competing risks generally arise from natural phenomena that have nothing to do with the conduct of the study.

The implications of unequal attrition are somewhat different under different approaches to follow-up of the cohort. To show how unequal attrition can alter the observed association, we restrict attention to a cohort study using a very simple though not uncommon approach. In chapter 13, we discuss the complexities of attrition under different approaches.

Suppose we have a national psychiatric registry to identify the cases as they arise, but lack data on deaths and emigration (i.e., attrition) for the population covered by the registry. In this type of study, we have to assume that anyone who is not ascertained by the registry does not have the disorder. In computation of the disease risk for the exposed (or unexposed) under this practice, the denominator is the number of exposed (or unexposed) at the start of the risk period, and the numerator is the number of cases observed in the exposed (or unexposed) over the entire risk period. Thus, the disease risks for the exposed and unexposed are computed for the entire risk period, as though there had been no attrition.

In the presence of attrition, the observed disease risk will underestimate the true disease risk. This occurs because our procedure assumes that all individuals were observed for the outcome over the entire risk period. In fact, the individuals who died or emigrated were observed for only part of the risk period. Over their shorter period of observation, these individuals had less chance to develop the disease. In the presence of unequal attrition, the underestimation will be different for the exposed and the unexposed groups. The unequal attrition will therefore increase (or decrease) the observed association between the exposure and the disease. It could even lead us to observe an association when there is no true association, or to observe no association when there is a true association.

Unequal attrition can arise not only from differences between exposure groups in the proportion of people lost to observation, but also from differences between exposure groups in the times at which people are lost. An extreme scenario is exhibited in table 11.2. One year into the study, before any cases occur, a war breaks out. Five thousand unexposed die or emigrate as refugees. Near the end of the study, after all the cases have occurred, war breaks out again. This time, five thousand exposed die or emigrate.

Under our approach to follow-up, because we lack information on deaths and emigration, we are unaware of this difference in the timing of attrition between the exposure groups. We simply count the number of cases detected in the exposed and the unexposed groups, regardless of attrition, as shown in

Table 11.2 Hypothetical Scenario of Unequal Timing of Attrition Between Exposure Groups

A. HYPOTHETICAL COHORT STUDY WITH 10-YEAR FOLLOW-UP: NO ATTRITION

	N	Cases N	Risk	Risk Ratio
Exposed	10,000	500	5.0%	5.0
Unexposed	10,000	100	1.0%	

B. UNEQUAL ATTRITION SCENARIO: HALF THE UNEXPOSED LOST EARLY IN FOLLOW-UP AND HALF THE EXPOSED LOST LATE IN FOLLOW-UP[a]

	N	Cases N	Risk	Risk Ratio
Exposed	10,000	500	5.0%	10.0
Unexposed	10,000	50	0.5%	

[a] War breaks out early in the study before any cases occur. Half the unexposed flee and are lost to follow-up. As a result, only half of the cases in the unexposed are observed. A second war breaks out near the end of the study. Half the exposed flee. Because all cases have occurred by this time, all cases among the exposed have been observed.

table 11.2. Since we lost half of the unexposed group before any cases arose, we find only half of the cases, and the observed risk in the unexposed is reduced by half (from 1 percent to 0.5 percent). The observed risk in the exposed is still 5 percent, because the loss of the exposed occurred after all the cases were counted. The observed relative risk is therefore increased from 5.0 to 10.0.

We can limit attrition by making use of various strategies to enhance the follow-up of the cohort. If the attrition is not differential, we can also reduce the bias in the analysis of the data, using methods such as restriction or survival analysis; the appropriate method depends upon the approach to follow-up.

Differential Misclassification

The exposed and the unexposed groups may also differ in the accuracy with which the cases are ascertained. As a result, they may differ in the proportion of cases misclassified as noncases, the proportion of noncases misclassified as cases, or both. When this happens, we have differential misclassification of the outcome; that is, the exposure is linked to misclassification of the disease.

Suppose the doctors of the exposed group suspect the exposure causes the disease and carefully scrutinize the exposed for signs of the disease, detecting all the cases. The doctors of the unexposed group, however, adhere to routine procedures and detect only half of the cases. As a result, we detect all the cases in the exposed, but only one-half the cases in the unexposed. This scenario is depicted in table 11.3. The observed risk remains 5 percent in the exposed, but is reduced from one percent to 0.5 percent in the unexposed. The observed relative risk is increased from 5.0 to 10.0.

Table 11.3 Hypothetical Scenario of Differential Misclassification of the Outcome

A. HYPOTHETICAL COHORT STUDY WITH 10-YEAR FOLLOW-UP: NO MISCLASSIFICATION

	N	Cases N	Risk	Risk Ratio
Exposed	10,000	500	5.0%	5.0
Unexposed	10,000	100	1.0%	

B. DIFFERENTIAL MISCLASSIFICATION SCENARIO: ALL EXPOSED CASES AND HALF OF UNEXPOSED CASES ASCERTAINED[a]

	N	Cases N	Risk	Risk Ratio
Exposed	10,000	500	5.0%	10.0
Unexposed	10,000	50	0.5%	

[a] Belief in the risk factor leads examiners to scrutinize the exposed more carefully than they do the unexposed, resulting in diagnosis of all cases in exposed, but only half of the cases in the unexposed.

Note that differential misclassification may also work the other way around. We may have differential misclassification of the exposure; that is, the disease may be linked to misclassification of the exposure. This kind of differential misclassification is more germane to the case-control than the cohort study, however, and is discussed in the chapters on the case-control design.

Nondifferential misclassification should also be considered in the design of the study, because it can prevent us from observing true associations (chapter 8). Except for one special case, however, nondifferential misclassification of dichotomous exposure and disease variables produces bias toward the null. Therefore, it does not represent a plausible alternative explanation for an observed association between exposure and disease. The special case is that of dependent nondifferential misclassification, which means that errors in the classification of the exposure are linked to errors in the classification of disease (see chapter 14).

We can build safeguards into a cohort study that reduce the possibilities for differential misclassification. For example, the outcome can be assessed blind to the exposure status. Prevention is especially important for this kind of bias, because we generally cannot adjust our results for it.

Steps of a Cohort Study

In chapter 9 we described implementation of a prototypical cohort study in terms of six steps: articulating the study questions, defining the source population, measuring the exposure, following the cohort, classifying the outcomes, and analyzing the data. As illustrated in figure 11.1, one can also consider the sources of bias in terms of these six steps.

We begin by articulating the study questions. Then we attempt to choose a population or setting in which the study questions can be answered and define a source population within that setting. In the source population—the people eligible for our study—we are likely to encounter natural confounding.

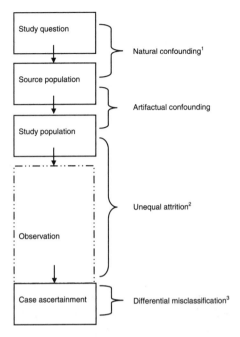

Sources of Noncomparability

Study question — Natural confounding[1]

Source population

Artifactual confounding

Study population

Observation — Unequal attrition[2]

Case ascertainment — Differential misclassification[3]

1. Also artifactual confounding if the source population is defined within a selected population.
2. Especially when it is differential attrition.
3. Also dependent non-differential misclassification.

Figure 11.1 Sources of noncomparability in a population cohort study.

If the source population is one step removed from a naturally occurring population, as in the examples of the Netherlands Mental Health Survey and Incidence Study (chapter 9) and the Prenatal Determinants of Schizophrenia Example (chapter 10), then we may also encounter some artifactual confounding in the source population. In the study population—the people who actually enter our study—nonresponse and other selection factors may produce artifactual confounding, in addition. Once the study population is assembled and the exposures are measured, we attempt to follow the cohort over the risk period. Now unequal attrition enters the stage. The exposed and unexposed may differ on loss to follow-up and competing risks. Furthermore, attrition may be related to disease risk within the exposure groups, leading to differential attrition. Then we classify the outcomes observed in the cohort. We are likely to classify some cases as noncases and classify some noncases as cases. If there is differential misclassification of the outcome—that is, if misclassification is linked to exposure status—it will introduce a bias.

Finally, we analyze the data. Suppose we find the disease risk to be different in the exposed and the unexposed. As shown in table 11.4, the (unadjusted) risk ratio that we observe reflects not only the causal effect of the exposure (what we want to isolate), but also the effects of other causes, attrition, and misclassification. In order to make a causal inference, we seek to rule out these alternative explanations for the observed result.

Table 11.4 Contributions to Noncomparability in a Cohort Study

	Observed Number of Cases	Contributions to Observed Number of Cases			
		Exposure	Effect of Other Causes	Attrition	Misclassification
E+ 100,000	30,000	20,000	10,000	0	0
E− 100,000	5,000	0	15,000	−5,000	−5,000

Note: The observed risk ratio is 6. However, the unbiased risk ratio is 3. The unbiased risk ratio is obtained as follows: (1) The risk in the exposed individuals = (30,000/100,000); (2) The "counterfactual" risk in these individuals had they not been exposed = (10,000/100,000); (3) The ratio of these two risks = 3. The difference between the observed risk ratio and the unbiased risk ratio arises from differences between the exposed and unexposed on other causes of disease (confounding), follow-up time (unequal attrition), and accuracy with which causes are observed (differential misclassification). While all three factors are a source of noncomparability, the methods for limiting their effects differ (see chapters 12–14).

Interaction

When the exposed and unexposed groups are fully comparable, the association between exposure and disease reflects the average effect of the exposure on the disease in the study population. Averages, while very informative, can sometimes be misleading, depending on the question under investigation. Many different underlying patterns across the subgroups of a cohort can produce the same average.

Suppose the risk ratio is one. This could mean that the exposure has no effect on anyone in the cohort. But it could also mean that the exposure is protective for one half of the cohort and harmful for the other half. Such a cohort is heterogeneous in important ways that influence the effect of the exposure. Although it is true that the exposure has no effect "on average," we would want to identify the subgroups in the cohort for whom the exposure is protective or harmful.

Gene environment interactions are abundant, and sometimes a gene has a strong effect within a subgroup with a specific environmental exposure, but a very small effect in the population as a whole. In this instance, again, the effect of the genetic exposure in a subgroup (people with the environmental exposure) may be more informative for some questions than the average effect. The Dunedin study described in chapter 9 reported that a polymorphism of the *MAOA* gene was associated with a high risk of antisocial behavior among boys with a history of childhood maltreatment (see table 9.1). Averaged over the total cohort, however, the association between the genetic allele and antisocial behavior was small and not readily interpretable.

We should expect some heterogeneity in a cohort, because the exposure will have an effect only in the presence of its causal partners. Since the frequency of the causal partners will vary somewhat across subgroups of the population, so will the effect of the exposure. This is what we mean by interaction.

Most of the time, however, population heterogeneity is not so extreme. Typically, the magnitude of the effect varies somewhat across subgroups, but the effect is in the same direction. In such circumstances, the average risk is meaningful. Nonetheless, by examining the variation in the effect across subgroups, we may better understand how and under what circumstances the exposure has an effect. For example, if the exposure doubles the risk for men but quadruples the risk for women, it is meaningful to say that, on average, the exposure triples the risk. This tells us that the exposure is a potent cause of disease in this population. However, it would also be useful to know that the effect differs in magnitude for men and women and to explore the reasons for this difference.

Although it is useful to identify interactions, it can be very difficult to do so in practice. Variation across subgroups can be produced by random fluctuation and methodological artifact, as well as population heterogeneity. In addition, epidemiologists have struggled to develop appropriate mathematical representations for interaction. The statistical methods currently used to assess and detect interactions are discussed in chapter 27. The conceptual meaning of interaction, the debate surrounding its detection, and recent methodological advances are discussed in part VIII.

Conclusion

In a cohort study in which we observe an association between exposure and disease, we cannot easily infer a causal connection between them. The next three chapters will guide the reader in approaching this task. Alternative explanations for the association can be found in whom we recruited into the cohort (confounding, chapter 12), what we observed of their subsequent experience (unequal attrition, chapter 13), and how we classified what we observed (differential misclassification, chapter 14). To make a causal inference, we have to rule out these other explanations. It can be a formidable challenge. In the words of Alice Stewart, a pioneer of epidemiology, "The epidemiologist is like a conductor—you must hear every note, you must be able to detect a false note anywhere" (Greene and Caldicott 1999, p. 216).

References

Greene G and Caldicott H (1999). *The Woman Who Knew Too Much—Alice Stewart and the Secrets of Radiation*. Ann Arbor: University of Michigan Press.

Szklo M and Nieto FJ (2000). *Epidemiology: Beyond the Basics*. Gaithersburg, Md.: Aspen Publishing.

12 Confounding: What It Is and What Can Be Done

Ezra Susser and Sharon Schwartz

Typically, the exposure groups differ on a baffling array of factors, but only a few factors are actually confounders. We must find a way to "sort the wheat from the chaff." The goal is to correctly identify and accurately measure the factors that might amplify or suppress the observed association between the exposure and the disease. We may then be able to safeguard our study from their confounding effects.

The first part of this chapter discusses the conditions under which a factor can confound the association between exposure and disease, and the conditions under which this cannot occur. We also differentiate confounders from antecedents or mediators. The next part discusses methods devised to neutralize the effects of confounders. Two standard methods are presented: matching to prevent confounding in the data by equalizing the exposed and the unexposed on a potential confounder, and statistical adjustment to compensate for confounding in the data by separating the effects of the exposure from the effects of the confounder.

What Is and What Is Not Confounding

A confounder is a third variable that contributes to the noncomparability of the exposed and unexposed on causes of disease. (The term third variable refers to any factor other than the exposure and disease under investigation; see chapter 5). Therefore, to be a confounder, a third variable must be a cause of the disease, and it must be associated with the exposure in the study. To identify potential confounders, we can start by restricting attention to the third variables that are thought to be risk factors for the disease. We can then assess their association with the exposure in the study.

An intriguing report from the Nun study of Alzheimer's disease examined whether lower linguistic ability in young adulthood was related to poor cognitive function and Alzheimer's disease in late life (table 12.1; Snowdon et al.

138

Table 12.1 Examples of Potential Confounding in Cohort Studies

Sources	Study Description and Potential Confounding
Cottler et al. (1987)	*Study*: St. Louis ECA
	Cohort (N = 3,004): A probability sample of adults in three St. Louis communities. Follow-up was one year later.
	Potential confounding: Examined number of contacts required to recruit participants with different characteristics. Increased number of contacts was required to recruit urban residents and alcohol abusers. The findings indicate the potential for selective recruitment and artifactual confounding in other studies.
Snowdon et al. (1996) *See also*: Snowdon et al. (1997)	*Study*: The Nun Study
	Cohort (N = 678): Notre Dame nuns, at least 75 years old, who agreed to annual assessment of cognitive and physical function and to donate their brains after death. A subset of 93 participants with an archived writing sample from youth was used for a cohort study of the relation between linguistic ability in youth and cognitive ability in old age, and Alzheimer's disease. Cognitive ability was assessed at follow-up in late life; Alzheimer's disease, following death. Low linguistic ability in youth was a strong predictor of poor cognitive function and Alzheimer's disease in late life.
	Potential confounding: Educational attainment could account in part for an association of linguistic ability in youth with cognitive ability and Alzheimer's disease in late life.

1996).[1] Ratings of linguistic ability were based on essays the nuns wrote at the time of entrance to their profession. Cognitive function was assessed in a follow-up study of the nuns in late life. For those who died (only a small number so far), postmortem brain pathology was used to diagnose Alzheimer's disease. The investigators found that in these nuns a low rating on linguistic ability in young adulthood was indeed associated with an increased risk of poor cognitive function and Alzheimer's in late life.

The authors were concerned, however, that part or all of the observed association might be due to the effects of confounders. One of these was low educational attainment. They were aware that low educational attainment is a purported risk factor for Alzheimer's disease (D'Arcy 1994; Stern et al. 1994). They examined whether it was also associated with low linguistic ability in their study.

Consider what would happen if they found no association between the nuns' linguistic ability and their educational attainment. In this instance, educational attainment would still be a presumed risk factor, but it would not

---

[1] This was actually a substudy within a cohort of nuns assembled for a follow-up study in late life. The analysis was restricted to the nuns in the cohort for whom the archival exposure data were available. Thus, the design used for this report is somewhat of a hybrid. For present purposes, we may think of it as a historical cohort study with concurrent follow-up (as defined in chapter 10).

be associated with the exposure being investigated. Therefore, educational attainment would not confound the association between linguistic ability and late life poor cognitive function or Alzheimer's disease in this study. In these nuns, however, low linguistic ability was associated with low educational attainment. Thus, low educational attainment was a presumed risk factor and associated with the exposure. Using procedures described later in the chapter, investigators adjusted the results for confounding by educational attainment.

Artifactual Confounding

In the previous chapter, we distinguished confounding present in the naturally occurring population (natural confounding) from confounding introduced by selective recruitment of the people we study (artifactual confounding). It is often difficult to gauge the degree to which selective recruitment has introduced artifactual confounding because of limited information on people who do not participate in a study. Useful insights can be gleaned, however, by comparing subjects who are recruited, with varying degrees of difficulty.

This gauging was done in an innovative report from the St. Louis site of the Epidemiologic Catchment Area (ECA) study (table 12.1; Cottler et al. 1987). The ECA was designed as a community survey with a longitudinal follow-up. The analysis of recruitment into the community survey in St. Louis was possible because the study made a large investment in recruiting respondents, continuing contact attempts beyond what is feasible in most studies. Fifty percent of the recruitments required more than four contact attempts; five percent required more than 14 (the maximum was 57). Two factors strongly associated with recruitment difficulty were urban residence and alcohol abuse. These findings illustrate the potential for artifactual confounding to be present in the source population in cohort studies designed as follow-ups of community surveys.[2]

It is useful to keep in mind the distinction between natural and artifactual confounding because it has implications for translating findings into public health actions. It does not have implications, however, for the topics addressed in the remainder of this chapter. Therefore we shall not make this distinction and defer further discussion of it to part VIII.

Mediators and Antecedents

There are two scenarios where, although a variable is associated with the exposure and is a cause of the disease, it is not a confounder. Mediators and

---

[2] Artifactual confounding is introduced only when recruitment depends upon both a risk factor for the disease and the exposure being investigated (see chapter 11). Suppose the ECA community survey provided the source population for a cohort study examining the relation of ethnicity to risk of depression. Alcohol abuse is a risk factor for depression. If the difficulty of recruiting alcohol abusers differed across ethnic groups, this would create (or magnify or suppress) an association between alcohol abuse and ethnic group within the study and thereby introduce artifactual confounding. If the difficulty of recruiting alcohol abusers did not differ across ethnic groups, it would not introduce artifactual confounding.

antecedents are part of a causal pathway that connects the exposure to the disease. We do not want to eliminate the effects of these variables from the effects of the exposure, but rather want to understand how they work together with the exposure to cause the disease.

In the scenario where a third variable acts as a mediator, the exposure causes the third variable, which in turn causes the disease. Suppose that in the Nun study already described low linguistic ability was actually a cause of low educational attainment among the nuns, as shown in figure 12.1A. This is plausible because low linguistic ability may pose a barrier to educational advancement. Suppose further that low linguistic ability led to a higher risk of Alzheimer's disease only because of this effect on educational attainment. Then, educational attainment would be a mediator of the effect of low linguistic ability, rather than a confounder.

In the other scenario, where a third variable acts as an antecedent, the third variable causes the exposure, which in turn causes the disease. Suppose now that among the nuns low educational attainment was a cause of low linguistic ability (figure 12.1B). This scenario is also plausible because education enhances linguistic skills. Suppose further that low educational attainment was a risk factor for Alzheimer's disease only because it lowered linguistic ability. Then, educational attainment would be an antecedent of low linguistic ability, rather than being a confounder.

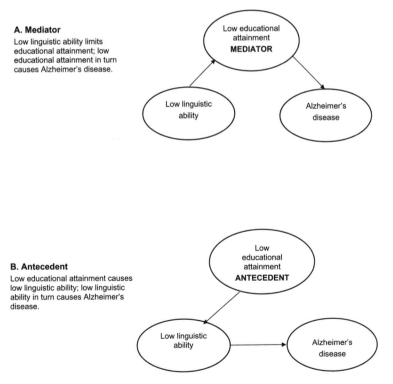

A. Mediator
Low linguistic ability limits educational attainment; low educational attainment in turn causes Alzheimer's disease.

B. Antecedent
Low educational attainment causes low linguistic ability; low linguistic ability in turn causes Alzheimer's disease.

Figure 12.1 Mediators and antecedents: low educational attainment as mediator and antecedent in the nun study.

We therefore require a further condition to be met before we consider a third variable to be acting as a confounder. The third variable must not be acting merely as a mediator or an antecedent of the exposure being studied. The word "merely" is included to acknowledge that these roles are not mutually exclusive. Because there may be several causal pathways that connect the exposure to the disease, a third variable may act as a mediator or antecedent in one pathway, and as a confounder of another pathway. In fact, in our example of the Nun study, low educational attainment could plausibly have been a confounder, a mediator, and an antecedent, all at the same time (see figure 12.2). Low educational attainment probably did play all of these roles to some degree in the Nun study. Thus, it would not be correct to simply state that a confounder cannot be a mediator or antecedent.

Magnitude of Confounding

Examples have been documented in which a single confounder could have produced a large spurious association between exposure and disease (Phillips

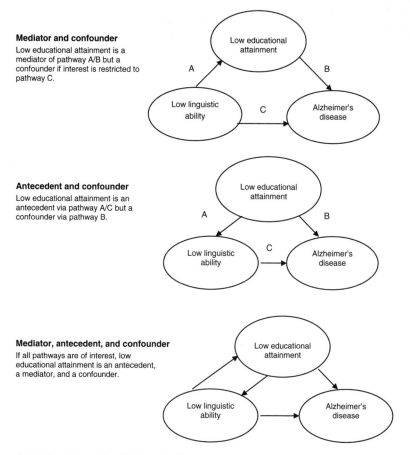

Figure 12.2 Variables with multiple roles: low educational attainment as confounder, mediator, and antecedent of the relationship between low linguistic ability and Alzheimer's disease in the Nun Study.

and Davey Smith 1993; Morabia 1995). A confounder needs to be very powerfully associated with both the exposure and the disease, however, to produce such an effect (Bross 1966). In most studies, a risk ratio of 2 or more is unlikely to be entirely explained by a single confounder.

The study of schizophrenia after early prenatal exposure to the Dutch Hunger Winter provides an example (Susser et al. 1996). As described in chapter 10, the authors reported a twofold increase in the risk of schizophrenia in the exposed cohort. A thoughtful letter to the editor posited that the association could have been due to social class confounding (van Os 1997). The letter noted correctly that during the famine higher social class women were somewhat better nourished than lower social class women and, therefore, more likely to conceive a child. Consequently, among the offspring, exposure to prenatal famine was associated with higher social class. In addition, the letter suggested that in Holland higher parental social class could be a risk factor for schizophrenia in offspring. If this were true, higher social class would indeed be a confounder in the Dutch Famine Study.

In their reply to the letter (Susser et al. 1997), the authors examined what might happen if in fact the relation between prenatal famine and schizophrenia were confounded by social class. Their numeric example assumed no causal relationship between prenatal famine and schizophrenia. Based on the empirical data of the Dutch Famine Study, it assumed a modest relationship between higher social class and prenatal famine (risk ratio = 1.47); and based on a report from Holland cited in the letter (Wiersma et al. 1983), it assumed a modest relationship between higher social class and schizophrenia (risk ratio = 2.0). The example showed that under these conditions, confounding by social class would create a spurious effect, but it would be very small in magnitude (risk ratio = 1.07). Social class confounding of this magnitude was not a plausible explanation for the twofold effect reported in the Dutch Famine Study.

On the other hand, very small risk ratios are readily produced by a single confounder. This fact makes it extremely difficult to rule out confounding as an explanation for a small risk ratio. Consider the reported association between being born in the winter-spring and later risk of schizophrenia. The association has been found in numerous cohort studies, but the risk ratios are small, usually in the range of 1.05 to 1.15 (Torrey et al. 1997). A confounder with only a modest influence on both the timing of conception and the risk of schizophrenia in offspring could produce a spurious risk ratio of this magnitude.

In addition, confounding can be cumulative, and often several confounders co-occur. Several confounders may each have a modest impact but, taken together, may account for an appreciable risk ratio. Cumulative confounding offers a plausible explanation for some causal inferences that later turned out to be wrong. For example, recent randomized control trials of hormone replacement therapy from the Women's Health Initiative indicated deleterious effects on dementia (Rapp et al. 2003; Shumaker et al. 2003). These results were surprising—and disconcerting—because several observational studies had reported substantial protective effects of hormone replacement therapy on dementia (Nelson et al. 2002). The results of the Women's Health

Initiative and prior observational studies were similarly discrepant for some other diseases. One of the explanations that has been put forward for these discrepancies is that the cumulative effects of several (unidentified or unmeasured) confounding variables might have distorted the results of the observational studies (Michels and Manson 2003).

Matching to Prevent Confounding

Matching is a means to prevent confounding. The protocol for recruitment of subjects is devised to equalize the exposed and unexposed groups on one or more confounders.

Individual matching is a stringent approach. For each exposed individual, we choose an unexposed individual who has the same value on the confounder. If gender is a confounder and we decide to match on it, then for each exposed man, we choose an unexposed man, and for each exposed woman, we choose an unexposed woman. We can match on more than one variable. Also, we can match more than one unexposed individual to each exposed individual. Though providing strict control of confounding, this approach is costly, and the matching requirement may limit the attainable sample size and statistical power, especially when more than three variables are involved (see part VI).

A less costly approach, frequency matching, is often sufficient. Under frequency matching, the unexposed are chosen so that their distribution across the categories of the confounders is similar to that of the exposed. For example, if one-third of the exposed are men, we ensure that one-third of the unexposed are men.

An early example of frequency matching is found in the study by Lee Robins described in chapter 2. She compared children with and without behavior problems (exposed and unexposed) with respect to adult psychiatric outcomes (table 12.2; Robins 1966). To match for age, the proportion of the children with behavior problems who were born in each calendar year was calculated, and the children without behavioral problems were selected so that the same proportion of them was born in each calendar year. Similarly, she matched on sex and census tract.

In some circumstances, however, individual matching may be the only effective way to rule out confounding. This may be necessary when a risk factor has many strata, or is too difficult to quantify so as to equalize its distribution in the exposed and unexposed groups. This problem arises in studies that relate birthweight to childhood IQ, where the social environment of the family is a potential confounder. No single measure is known to capture the entire effect of family environment on children's IQ. One solution is to individually match same-sex siblings who share the family environment.

This strategy was adopted to prevent confounding by family social environment in a study of birthweight and childhood IQ (table 12.2; Matte et al. 2001). Although the original cohort did not employ a matched design, the authors selected for their study only the same-sex sibling pairs in the cohort.

Table 12.2 Examples of Matching to Prevent Confounding in Cohort Studies

Sources	Study Description and Matching Procedures
Robins (1966)	*Study*: Deviant Children Grow Up
	Cohort (N = 624): Exposed were children seen for behavioral problems 1924–1929. Unexposed were children without behavior problems. Follow-up was in 1955–1960. Childhood behavior problems predicted adult behavior problems.
	Matching: Exposed and unexposed children were matched on year of birth, sex, and socioeconomic status (census tract).
Matte et al. (2001)	*Study*: Birthweight and Childhood IQ, National Collaborative Perinatal Project
	Cohort (N = 3,366): 1,683 same-sex sibling pairs of birthweight 1500–3999 g and gestation > =37 weeks, assessed at birth and age 7. IQ measured at age 7 follow-up exams. Within sibling pairs, lower birthweight was associated with lower IQ; the association was stronger in boys than in girls.
	Matching: Same-sex sibs were used as matched pairs; sibship matches on family environment.

Within sibling pairs, lower birthweight was associated with lower IQ; the association was stronger in boys than in girls.[3]

Closely related to matching is the strategy of **restriction**. This means limiting the study to persons in one category of the potential confounder. A study restricting both the exposed and unexposed groups to females would be an example.

Matching or restriction in a cohort study is highly effective in preventing confounding, but may exact a substantial cost. When several matching factors are used, it can be burdensome, as well as expensive, to find unexposed individuals who are the same as the exposed individuals on all these factors. In general, it is best that the matching factors be carefully selected and few in number. As a rule, a matching factor should be a variable that has a strong effect on the disease, or has so many strata that adjustment in the analysis is impractical.

Adjustment for Confounding

Adjustment for confounding helps us to compensate for the effects of confounding in the data. We use it to infer what the association between exposure and disease would be if the exposed and unexposed groups were identical on the potential confounder, or confounders. The resulting estimate is referred

---

[3] Individual matching generally refers to the recruitment of subjects into a cohort. As this example shows, however, the same end may sometimes be achieved by selecting only a subset of a very large cohort for a specific analysis. Then the individual matching reduces the sample size but incurs no additional expense.

to as the adjusted result. Here we explain the logic of adjustment; the corresponding statistical procedures are described in part VI.

The logic is most easily seen in the simplest scenario. Suppose we adjust for a single confounder having two strata (e.g., gender). An adjusted result is obtained in three steps. First, we divide the cohort into the two strata of the confounder (e.g., males and females). Since the individuals within each stratum have the same value for gender, there is no confounding within a stratum. Second, the association between exposure and disease is computed separately for each of the two strata (e.g., for males and for females). Third, the results for the two strata are averaged, using some weighting procedure. The exact same logic can be extended to confounders with many strata.

An especially useful procedure for stratified analysis is the Mantel-Haenszel procedure for adjusted odds ratios (Mantel and Haenszel 1959; Fleiss et al. 2003). Separate tables are constructed for each stratum, and an odds ratio is computed for each stratum with use of a weighting procedure that accounts for the number of subjects in each stratum. These are then averaged across the strata. This procedure can also be extended to more than one confounder.

Alternatively, statistical models (such as logistic regression) use the same logic but assume a specific data structure. Statistical models are most useful when adjustment is needed for several variables and when the effects of the confounders themselves are of interest. A further advantage is that potential confounders in statistical models can be included as continuous variables. The procedures of Mantel-Haenszel and logistic regression analysis will be described in part VI.

Underadjustment

In the data analysis, investigators will usually adjust for any identified major confounder. Consequently, in practice the confounders carrying the greatest threat to validity are those that are unidentified. Investigators posed this problem in a reanalysis of the data from a cohort study that showed cigarette smoking was associated with both the risk of suicide and the risk of being murdered (Davey Smith et al. 1992). These authors deemed a causal connection between smoking and these outcomes to be biologically implausible. Yet there was no other evident explanation for the observed associations. They concluded that the effect of smoking on these outcomes was probably entangled with the effects of other as yet unidentified factors.

Identified but unmeasured confounders also carry a great threat. To reduce this threat, one may want to attempt at least a proxy adjustment for any confounders that are suspected to be important but were not measured. Suppose we are doing a cohort study of life events and depression in which we suspect socioeconomic status to be a confounder but have not measured it. Since we cannot adjust for socioeconomic status, we may adjust instead for a proxy of social class that was measured in the study. If owning a house was measured, for example, it might be used as a proxy. A proxy adjustment will, of course, be only partially successful. To the extent that it does not fully capture the effect of the confounder, there will be residual confounding.

Poorly measured confounders are underadjusted even when they are included in the data analysis. Suppose that in our study of life events and depression we did measure socioeconomic status, but our measure was unreliable. Like use of a proxy, the adjustment will be partial, leaving residual confounding. The amount of residual confounding can be considerable, too. If the measurement of a confounder does not properly capture the construct it is intended to measure (i.e., has poor validity), or is unreliable, then an effect reported as being adjusted may be virtually unadjusted (Phillips and Davey Smith 1994).

Sometimes residual confounding goes unrecognized because we adjust for measures without fully articulating the relationship between these measures and the confounding we want to control. Suppose that in our example we did precisely measure and adjust for current socioeconomic status. This measure would still not adjust for confounding effects of socioeconomic status at earlier points in the life course (e.g., childhood, or adolescence), which can be distinct and equally important, and which we would want to control (see chapter 36). Results may be reported as adjusted for socioeconomic status, without recognizing that there will be residual confounding due to socioeconomic status earlier in the life course.

Similarly, we may measure and adjust for ethnicity, without having a clear conception of the confounding we want to control. In some studies, ethnicity is used only to represent the net effect of various unidentified and unmeasured confounders that differ across ethnic groups (see chapter 29). In this context, adjusting for ethnicity is equivalent to using a proxy for these multiple confounders. Again, results may be reported as adjusted for ethnicity, without recognizing that there will be residual confounding.

Overadjustment

Overadjustment is also to be avoided. The simultaneous adjustment for too many potential confounders can obscure the main results. Adjusting for four or more confounders precludes the most transparent methods of adjustment. For example, the Mantel-Haenszel procedure is straightforward when one is simultaneously adjusting for one or two, or occasionally three, confounding variables. Beyond that, it becomes cumbersome, and the computations cannot be displayed concisely.

More complex statistical models, such as logistic regression, can accommodate numerous confounders in a single analysis. But the results tend to be less transparent and more prone to undetected errors. In addition, the inclusion of many variables in a logistic regression model tends to increase the variance in the statistical estimates, thereby reducing their precision. Any reduction in precision will make it more difficult to detect a true association between exposure and disease.

Investigators sometimes assume that an analysis will be more valid if more variables are adjusted in a statistical model. However, simultaneous adjustment for a large number of variables does not reveal, and may in fact obscure, the causal relationships among these variables. Sound causal inferences in epidemiologic studies depend upon postulating causal pathways, examining the relationships among the variables in these pathways, and drawing the implications for the analysis of the question at hand. An analysis that indiscriminately incorporates many variables into a statistical model can be quite misleading.

Finally, a thorny problem is that the effects of confounders can depend on the presence or absence of other confounders. Ultimately, confounding is the overall difference between the exposed and unexposed on all other causes of disease. Sometimes, these other causes can balance each other out, as when the unexposed have an excess of some protective factors and some causal factors. Adjusting for one of the confounders can upset this balance. Since the complex relationships among variables cannot be captured in our ordinary statistical procedures, the process of adjustment may alter the apparent associations in unpredictable ways (for further discussion, see part VIII).

Thus, it is important to select potential confounders judiciously. Although we never want to overlook potentially powerful confounders, these are usually few in number. After a thorough review of previous studies and potential biological pathways, and a careful examination of the associations between the candidate confounders and the exposure within the data set, one can usually limit the main analysis to a small number of major confounders.

Differentiating among Confounders, Mediator, and Antecedents

It can be very difficult to distinguish between a confounder and a mediator. The distinction cannot be based on our data alone. Rather, it is based on logic and on our causal ideas.

As described, we try to eliminate the effect of a confounder by adjusting for it. If the adjustment diminishes the association between the exposure and the disease, we conclude that the true effect is smaller than we had originally assumed. Similarly, we can eliminate the effect of a mediator by adjusting for it. Again, the adjustment may diminish the association between the exposure and the disease. In this instance, however, this result may actually increase our confidence in the causal role of the exposure. Rather than posing an alternative explanation, the mediator helps to explain how the exposure works.

In the Nun study, as described above, the authors examined whether lower linguistic ability in young adulthood was related to a higher risk of poor cognitive function and Alzheimer's disease in late life (table 12.1). Educational attainment may have confounded the effect of linguistic ability; it may also have mediated the effect. In either case, adjusting for educational attainment would diminish the association between linguistic ability and late life dementia.

Thus, adjustment for a confounder or a mediator can have the same result (with caveats discussed in part VIII), but the interpretation of the result is different. Distinguishing between them depends on our causal idea, which indicates whether the third variable is in the causal pathway of interest leading from the exposure to the disease (mediator) or is in a different causal pathway (confounder).

Separating an antecedent from a confounder is not as difficult. Adjusting for the antecedent should have no influence on the exposure-disease relationship. If the antecedent also has an independent effect on the disease, however, then it is also a confounder, and adjustment will change the association between the exposure and disease, as with any other confounder. We will return to these points in the final part of the book.

Conclusion

Confounding is virtually ubiquitous in cohort studies. Methods have been developed, however, to minimize confounding by matching or by adjustment in data analysis. The effective use of these methods depends upon both correctly identifying and accurately measuring the confounders. Indiscriminate adjustment for a large number of variables in the analytic phase, a weak though widely employed strategy for ruling out confounding, can be avoided by thoughtful decisions about design and analysis at the outset.

The logic behind both matching and adjustment is to divide the subjects into strata in which everyone has the same value for the third variable. Then, one averages the results for the different strata. We will see in the next chapter that this same logic can be extended to understand adjustment for follow-up time, with use of survival analysis.

References

Bross ID (1966). Spurious Effects from an Extraneous Variable. *J. Chronic. Dis.* 19:637–647.

Cottler LB, Zipp JF, Robins LN, and Spitznagel EL (1987). Difficult-to-Recruit Respondents and Their Effect on Prevalence Estimates in an Epidemiologic Survey. *Am. J. Epidemiol.* 125:329–339.

D'Arcy C (1994). Education and Socio-Economic Status as Risk Factors for Dementia: Data from the Canadian Study of Health and Aging. *Neurobiol. Aging* 15:S40.

Davey Smith G, Phillips AN, and Neaton JD (1992). Smoking As "Independent" Risk Factor for Suicide: Illustration of an Artifact from Observational Epidemiology? *Lancet* 340:709–712.

Fleiss JL, Levin BA, and Paik MC (2003). *Statistical Methods for Rates and Proportions*, 3rd ed. Hoboken, N.J.: Wiley.

Mantel N and Haenszel W (1959). Statistical Aspects of the Analysis of Data from Retrospective Studies of Disease. *J. Natl. Cancer Inst.* 22:719–748.

Matte TD, Bresnahan M, Begg MD, and Susser E (2001). Influence of Variation in Birth Weight within Normal Range and within Sibships on IQ at Age 7 Years: Cohort Study. *BMJ* 323:310–314.

Michels KB and Manson JE (2003). Postmenopausal Hormone Therapy: A Reversal of Fortune. *Circulation* 107:1830–1833.

Morabia A (1995). Poppers, Kaposi's Sarcoma, and HIV Infection: Empirical Example of a Strong Confounding Effect? *Prev. Med.* 24:90–95.

Nelson HD, Humphrey LL, Nygren P, Teutsch SM, and Allan JD (2002). Postmenopausal Hormone Replacement Therapy: Scientific Review. *JAMA* 288:872–881.

Phillips AN and Davey Smith G (1993). Smoking and Human Papillomavirus Infection. Causal Link Not Proved. *BMJ* 306:1268–1269.

Phillips AN and Davey Smith G (1994). Risk-Factor Epidemiology. *Lancet* 343:603.

Rapp SR, Espeland MA, Shumaker SA, et al. (2003). Effect of Estrogen Plus Progestin on Global Cognitive Function in Postmenopausal Women: The Women's Health Initiative Memory Study: A Randomized Controlled Trial. *JAMA* 289:2663–2672.

Robins LN (1966). *Deviant Children Grow Up*. Baltimore: Williams & Wilkins.

Shumaker SA, Legault C, Rapp SR, et al. (2003). Estrogen Plus Progestin and the Incidence of Dementia and Mild Cognitive Impairment in Postmenopausal Women: the Women's Health Initiative Memory Study: A Randomized Controlled Trial. *JAMA* 289:2651–2662.

Snowdon DA, Greiner LH, Mortimer JA, Riley KP, Greiner PA, and Markesbery WR (1997). Brain Infarction and the Clinical Expression of Alzheimer Disease. The Nun Study. *JAMA* 277:813–817.

Snowdon DA, Kemper SJ, Mortimer JA, Greiner LH, Wekstein DR, and Markesbery WR (1996). Linguistic Ability in Early Life and Cognitive Function and Alzheimer's Disease in Late Life. Findings from the Nun Study. *JAMA* 275:528–532.

Stern Y, Gurland B, Tatemichi TK, Tang MX, Wilder D, and Mayeux R (1994). Influence of Education and Occupation on the Incidence of Alzheimer's Disease. *JAMA* 271:1004–1010.

Susser E, Neugebauer R, Hoek HW, Brown A, and Lin S (1997). In Reply: Schizophrenia after Prenatal Famine. *Arch. Gen. Psychiatry* 53:25–31.

Susser E, Neugebauer R, Hoek HW, Brown AS, Lin S, Labovitz D, and Gorman JM (1996). Schizophrenia after Prenatal Famine. Further Evidence. *Arch. Gen. Psychiatry* 53:25–31.

Torrey EF, Miller J, Rawlings R, and Yolken RH (1997). Seasonality of Births in Schizophrenia and Bipolar Disorder: A Review of the Literature. *Schizophr. Res.* 28:1–38.

van Os J (1997). Schizophrenia after Prenatal Famine. *Arch. Gen. Psychiatry* 54:577–578.

Wiersma D, Giel R, De Jong A, and Slooff CJ (1983). Social Class and Schizophrenia in a Dutch Cohort. *Psychol. Med.* 13:141–150.

Unequal Attrition under Different Types of Follow-Up

13

Ezra Susser and Sharon Schwartz

In any kind of cohort study, some degree of attrition of members is to be expected. Attrition tends to be larger when the design calls for subjects to be assessed in person in order to determine outcome. The degree of attrition can be influenced also by the characteristics of the subjects under study, such as age, sex, education, and occupation, by the local culture, and even by the prospect of some reward for participation.

Since cohort studies of mental disorders must often rely upon diagnostic interviews to assess outcomes, they are especially vulnerable to attrition. The Netherlands Mental Health Survey and Incidence Study (NEMESIS) (see chapter 9 table 9.3) followed up the people who participated in a 1996 survey of the Dutch population age 18–64. Outcomes were assessed by diagnostic interview. At the one-year follow-up, one in five (20.6 percent) could either not be found or simply refused to participate (de Graaf et al. 2000; Janssen et al. 2003).

In older age groups, attrition can be compounded by mortality and morbidity, which represent competing risks (see chapter 11). The Amsterdam Study of the Elderly (Geerlings et al. 1999), also in Holland, recruited subjects age 65–84 from general medicine practices for a study of dementia (see table 13.1). At the first follow-up, after on average 3 years, the 21.2 percent loss to follow-up was augmented by a further 21.4 percent who had died or were too ill to participate.

Cohort attrition can become a source of bias when it is unequal for the exposed and the unexposed groups. In what follows, we describe strategies for limiting the attrition, and procedures to take it into account in the data analysis. Then we explain the conditions under which attrition can be differential as well as unequal, and the use of sensitivity analysis to gauge the potential bias.

Limiting the Attrition

Strategies to limit attrition focus on reducing loss to follow-up because one cannot reduce competing risks. They involve both locating the subjects and

Table 13.1 Examples of Attrition in Cohort Studies

Sources	Study Description, Selected Findings, and Follow-Up Yield
Geerlings et al. (1999)	*Study*: Amsterdam Study of the Elderly (AMSTEL)
See also: Schoevers et al. (2003) Launer et al. (1993)	*Cohort (N = 3,778)*: Age-stratified, random sample of the nondemented elderly (65–84) selected from 30 general practices in Amsterdam. Two-stage follow-up assessment: stage-1 screening (Mini-Mental State Examination and memory scales); stage-2 diagnostic exams of screen positives. Follow-up on average was 3.2 years.
	Finding: Low level of education was related to increased risk of Alzheimer's disease.
	Follow-up yield: stage-1 screening: 21.4% either died or were too ill; 21.2% were lost or refused; 57.4% were interviewed. Among those interviewed, 20.0% screened positive and were targeted for stage-2 diagnostic interview. Stage-2 diagnostic exams: among those targeted, 24% either died in the interim or were too ill; 14% were lost or refused diagnostic exams; 62% were interviewed.
Hagnell et al. (1986a)	*Study*: The Lundby Study
Hagnell et al. (1986b)	*Cohort (N = 2,612)*: All individuals living in "Lundby," Sweden, in 1957. Follow-up diagnostic assessments in 1972. Often the same psychiatrist conducted exams in 1957 and 1972.
See also: Essen-Möller et al. (1956)	*Finding*: Personality traits measured in 1957 were associated with an increased risk of alcoholism at follow-up.
Hagnell et al. (1994)	*Follow-up yield*: 16% of cohort died and 1% was lost; 83% were personally interviewed.
Helgason (1964)	*Study*: Epidemiology of Mental Disorders in Iceland
	Cohort (N = 5,395): All live births in Iceland 1895–1897 and living there on December 1, 1910. Data on residence and mortality obtained from population registries. Psychiatric outcome data abstracted from institutional records (to 1957) and physician interviews.
	Finding: Urban residence in adolescence was associated with an increased risk of alcoholism in adulthood among men.
	Follow-up yield: Based on death certificates, court records, and National Register data: 28% of the cohort died, and 1% were lost mostly to emigration. All others remained under observation (i.e., by institutional records or physicians).
Ron et al. (1988a)	*Study*: Radiation Exposure and Neural Tumors
See also: Ron et al. (1988b) Modan (1987)	*Cohort (N = 27,060)*: Israeli immigrant children who received X-ray therapy for tinea capitis (1948–1960), and matched unexposed children from general population registry, and matched unexposed sibs. Neural tumors ascertained through cancer registry linkage supplemented by hospital pathology records (1950–1982).
	Finding: Radiation exposure was associated with an increased risk of neural tumors.
	Follow-up yield: Based on linkage to Central Population Registry: 2–3% died, and an estimated 4–6% emigrated (Ron et al. 1988b). All others remained under observation by registry.

garnering their participation (Wadsworth 1991; Ribisl et al. 1996; Cotter et al. 2002). In contemporary studies, those refusing participation often outnumber those not located. At the one-year follow-up of the Dutch NEMESIS study, for example, 219 individuals could not be located, while 923 refused participation (de Graaf et al. 2000).

To locate subjects, we usually depend in part on large scale organized information systems. Several European countries maintain population registries that detail every change in residence for the complete population. In countries lacking population registries, such as the United States, commercial identification services may be available to locate individuals who have moved. A great variety of other information systems may be useful in a particular study, such as those derived from drivers' licenses, school records, or general practice doctors. Supplemental tracing methods may be available to locate people who have entered an institution, such as a jail or a hospital. When possible, we also obtain information about their location directly from the cohort members by means of ongoing regular contacts. People who migrate to another country are difficult to locate in any other way because few tracing systems extend across national boundaries.

An individual's participation in a follow-up study is influenced by his or her sense of affiliation with the project. Good follow-up teams think about ways to foster affiliation, are at pains to avoid actions that undermine trust, and try to gain an understanding of the particular study cohort's sensitivities. Some procedures that may facilitate affiliation include retaining the same interviewers, sending birthday cards and other acknowledgments, and distributing newsletters about the study and its results.

Sometimes these standard methods are not applicable or not adequate. The completion of follow-up assessments can be especially challenging in certain hard-to-reach populations of interest to psychiatric epidemiologists (Esbensen et al. 1999; Boys et al. 2003; Vlahov 1994; Cottler et al. 1996; Conover et al. 1997). In a cohort comprised of homeless people, for example, the participants may lack official documents and other identifying information, and have no postal address or telephone number. It can be extremely difficult to locate the members of such a cohort for an assessment.

In these circumstances, researchers may choose to employ more intensive strategies to limit attrition. Two of these strategies are described below: personal continuity of follow-up, and the incorporation of ethnographic methods. In general, they should be applied equally to the exposure groups; otherwise, they may produce differences between the groups.

Personal Continuity of Follow-Up

A continuous personal relationship between researcher and study participants may effectively limit attrition. Personal continuity is exemplified by an investigation of mental disorders in a geographically defined area of southern Sweden called "Lundby" by the authors (table 13.1; Hagnell et al. 1986a, 1986b; Hagnell et al. 1994). Originally, Erik Essen-Möller and his colleagues personally interviewed 99 percent of the inhabitants who in 1947 were registered in the parishes of the area. Subsequently, Olle Hagnell, who had been a student of Erik Essen-Möller, recognized that such a well-described population with a personal connection to a research team provided an excellent basis for a longitudinal study. Accordingly, he interviewed the residents of Lundby in 1957 and again in 1972. At both time points, Hagnell himself conducted many of the interviews. Ernest Gruenberg, one of the progenitors of psychiatric epidemiology in the United States, accompanied Hagnell on some of his interviews and described them as follows: "I could understand a great deal of the emotional communication that was going on between Dr. Hagnell and his subjects; these were very real interviews with real interactions between two people, and if the person had anything to say he was obviously saying it" (Hagnell 1989, p. 62).

In some contexts, personal continuity is virtually a prerequisite for the study—for example, in low-income countries lacking information systems. An example is the clinical cohort study by Rangaswamy Thara, using her own patients in Madras, India. She rated the patients in detail every month for 10 years. The information collected was used to analyze the patterns of relapse in schizophrenia (Eaton et al. 1995). In a clinical cohort such as this one, the methodological tradeoff is that the assessments could be influenced by the clinicians' knowledge and expectations of their patients. Investigators who personally interview their own patients over time may gain depth in the assessments, but sacrifice the independence of a "blinded" interviewer (see chapter 14).

In still another variation on this theme, the investigator may tap into the information accumulated by treatment providers who have established personal relationships with the cohort members. A historical cohort study of mental disorders in Iceland by Tomas Helgason provides a remarkable example (table 13.1; Helgason 1964). National census data were used to define a cohort comprising individuals born in Iceland between 1895 and 1897, and still residing there at the starting point of follow-up on December 1, 1910. To conduct a follow-up assessment in 1957, Helgason relied on information he elicited from general practice doctors who had ongoing relationships with the persons in their practices. In this way, he could indirectly assess almost the entire population of Iceland (Helgason 1964).

Incorporation of Ethnographic Methods

In studies of hard-to-reach populations, the research team often includes designated "locators" who take the lead in continually tracking the participants. The locators use any available registries or other information systems, maintain ongoing contact with the cohort members, and ensure personal continuity of follow-up. Some of the most successful teams add a further element, integrating ethnographic methods into the locators' follow-up protocol.

Conover (Conover et al. 1997) has described one of these approaches. The locators collect ethnographic data on the participants' customary movements, and these data become the basis for tracing. In a follow-up of hard-to-reach homeless individuals, for example, a follow-up worker succeeded in tracing a participant by spending an entire day and night waiting at a bus station where the participant, according to previously collected ethnographic data, was known to appear at irregular times on most days. In another follow-up, of injection drug users in Harlem, the follow-up workers were former injection drug users who knew the customs of street life and the local hangouts; they constructed detailed maps, marking each block according to the kind of street activity that was found there. Visiting these hangouts was one way to locate people in the cohort. The collection of this kind of ethnographic data requires the locator to become familiar with the participants and their daily routines. The method not only makes for effective tracing, but also fosters affiliation. Indeed, in very marginal settings, the warmth, dignity, and respect offered by the follow-up team might be the most crucial ingredient of a successful follow-up.

Ethical Issues

The process of recruiting and following participants raises a host of ethical issues. For example, in using personal continuity in a clinical cohort, we have to ensure that the participants fully understand the distinction between the research study and their clinical care. In using ethnographic approaches to locate an individual, we have to be careful not to violate the person's privacy or reveal information about that individual to family, friends, or neighbors. Some of the protocols used in the past do not meet current ethical guidelines for research.

A discussion of ethical issues in longitudinal research is beyond the scope of this book (see Roberts and Roberts 1999; Fisher 2004). Nevertheless, we can draw attention to some general principles. Useful guidelines for any research on human subjects are laid out in the landmark 1979 *Belmont Report* (National Institutes of Health 1979). The cardinal principles are identified as respect for persons, beneficence, and justice. In short, this means that researchers are responsible for respecting and honoring the decisions of participants, ensuring that they understand the benefits and risks of participating, and treating subjects fairly and ethically (Coughlin and Beauchamp 1996; Schulte et al. 1997; Steinberg 2001).

An additional principle in longitudinal research is that an investigation implies an ongoing moral contract between researchers and study participants. We are, after all, partners in the pursuit of knowledge. This principle is captured in a recent National Institutes of Health (NIH) report describing informed consent as "an ongoing, meaningful, and educational process that is woven throughout the course of a research study" (NIH Director's Council of Public Representatives 2001).

Estimating "True" Disease Risk

In a cohort with no attrition, the risk is directly observable as the proportion of individuals who develop the disease during the specified risk period (chapter 8). This concept is intuitive, easy to grasp. In a cohort with attrition, however, the risk is not directly observable because part of the cohort is lost to follow-up or competing risks. We do not know whether or not these people would have developed the disease during the risk period. The true risk is the proportion that would have developed the disease over the study period, had there been no attrition. The true risk is an abstraction, neither observable nor intuitive.

To estimate the true risk in the exposed and unexposed groups, we extrapolate from known to unknown, from the realm of what has happened to the realm of what would have happened. As discussed later, an important assumption is necessary for this extrapolation to be valid: the attrition cannot be differential. The appropriate way to estimate the true risk depends upon the time that the cases are ascertained, which may be at the end of the study, ongoing, or periodic (see chapter 9).

In end-of-study case ascertainment, the study outcomes are determined in a single follow-up assessment at the end of the risk period. In this design, we can take account of attrition by a procedure similar to restriction. We restrict the analysis of the data to the individuals with complete follow-up. In other words, we exclude the individuals who did not complete the follow-up assessment from both the numerator and the denominator of the risk. Under this restriction procedure, the risk ratio and odds ratio will generally be unbiased.[1] However, end-of-study case ascertainment has many disadvantages. If we wait until the end of the study to identify the cases, we ascertain prevalent rather than incident cases, the information about the time and nature of onset is limited by retrospective recall, and as explained later in the chapter, we increase the potential for differential attrition. The longer the follow-up, the more prominent these issues may be.

In ongoing case registry ascertainment, we identify the cases as they arise in the cohort over the risk period. Being limited to treated cases, this method is mainly suitable for disorders such as schizophrenia which are usually treated. In this design, the restriction procedure we have described is not appropriate, as explained later. Instead, we turn to survival analysis.

In a study with periodic case ascertainment, the cases are identified at multiple time points over the risk period. The number of time points and the intervals between them vary a great deal across studies. A further issue is that some studies supplement the periodic case ascertainment with ongoing case ascertainment (e.g., referrals by treatment providers and a case registry). Therefore, these studies present a mixed picture and may use restriction, survival analysis, or both. The most appropriate procedure will depend upon the particulars of the study and the question being addressed. For questions that pertain only to the disease risk over a single follow-up interval, the restriction procedure may be appropriate. For the analysis of outcomes over

---

[1] As a caveat, we note that there is one circumstance in which restriction may not entirely remove the bias even when it is not differential. The attrition may differ by disease risk without being differential. This happens when the attrition is unequal for the cases and the noncases, but to the same degree in the exposed and the unexposed groups. In this circumstance, the risk ratio will be unbiased under the null, but otherwise biased. Unless the attrition is extensive, however, the bias in the risk ratio will be small. The odds ratio will be unbiased even in this situation.

numerous short follow-up intervals, it may be appropriate to use a survival analysis.

Survival Analysis

We present here the logical foundation of a survival analysis for the disease risk, and in chapter 26, the statistical procedures. A survival analysis can often be understood in terms of three basic steps: (1) divide the risk period into many small time intervals, (2) compute a result for each interval, and (3) combine the results across the intervals (Clayton and Hills 1995). We present a hypothetical example in terms of these three steps and then discuss the premise on which it rests.

Hypothetical Example.   We apply a survival analysis to the data of a hypothetical cohort study with ongoing case registry ascertainment shown in table 13.2 (following the Kaplan-Meier approach, see chapter 23). The total cohort comprises 10 exposed and 10 unexposed individuals enrolled in a health plan. The risk period is approximately 10 years (3,650 days). We assume that the health plan has both a case registry and a membership registry by calendar date (the need for a membership registry is explained below). The outcomes for the 20 cohort members are shown in table 13.2A.

In the exposed group, 3 develop disease during the risk period; 3 are lost to follow-up (drop out of the health plan); 2 are lost to competing risks (death); and 2 remain disease-free and in the health plan until the end of the risk period. To compute the disease risk for the exposed group, we proceed as follows:

Step 1: Divide the risk period into many small time intervals. We divide the 10-year risk period into 3,650 one-day intervals. We choose one-day intervals because the registry data are by calendar date. The exposed cohort under observation at the start of the study comprises 10 individuals. The number declines across the intervals because some people drop out of the health plan and others develop the disease (table 13.2B). On day 2007, for example, 6 individuals remain under observation.

Step 2: Compute a result for each interval. Within each one-day interval, we compute the disease risk and its complement, the survival probability: 1 − disease risk = survival probability. In practice, we need compute a result only for the three intervals where a case occurred. As shown in table 13.2B, the first case occurs on day 182; disease risk is 1/10 = .100, and survival probability is .900. The second case occurs on day 547; disease risk is 1/9 = .111, and survival probability is .889. The third case occurs on day 2007; disease risk is 1/6 = .167, and survival probability is .833. In the 3,647 intervals where no case occurred, the disease risk is zero, and the survival probability is one.

Step 3: Combine the results across the intervals. We multiply the survival probabilities for the intervals to obtain a cumulative survival probability for the entire risk period. Again, we need to consider the survival probabilities only for the three informative intervals where a case occurred. We can disregard the other 3,647 intervals as uninformative because an interval with a

Table 13.2 Hypothetical Cohort study with Attrition: 20 Members of a Health Plan Followed over 10 Years

A. OUTCOME DATA FROM HEALTH PLAN REGISTRIES

Exposed (N = 10)		Unexposed (N = 10)	
Person	Outcome	Person	Outcome
1	Disease day 182	1	Disease day 365
2	Disease day 547	2	Disease day 730
3	Died day 912	3	Died day 1,277
4	Lost day 1,094	4	Lost day 1,459
5	Disease day 2,007	5	Disease day 1,642
6	Died day 2,189	6	Died day 1,825
7	Lost day 2,371	7	Lost day 2,737
8	Lost day 2,554	8	No disease by day 3,650
9	No disease by day 3,650	9	No disease by day 3,650
10	No disease by day 3,650	10	No disease by day 3,650

B. SURVIVAL ANALYSIS OF THE EXPOSED GROUP[a]

Day	N Cohort[b]	N Cases	Conditional Probability[c]		Cumulative Probability of Survival
			of Disease	of Survival	
1	10	0	0	1	1
182	10	1	1/10 = .100	1 − 0.100 = .900	.900
547	09	1	1/09 = .111	1 − 0.111 = .889	.800
2,007	06	1	1/06 = .167	1 − 0.167 = .833	.666
3,650	02	0	0	1	.666

Disease risk in the exposed: 1 − 0.666 = 0.334

Using the same procedure:
Disease risk in the unexposed: 1 − 0.833 = 0.167

Risk ratio = 0.334/0.167 = 2.000
Risk difference = 0.334 − 0.167 = 0.167

[a] Calculations rounded to three decimal points
[b] Refers to N in cohort remaining disease-free and under observation. N of total cohort is always 10.
[c] These are conditional survival probabilities and conditional disease risks: conditional on having reached the given interval.

C. INCIDENCE RATES UNDER ASSUMPTION OF CONSTANT INCIDENCE

Incidence exposed	3 cases/19,156 person-days = 3 cases/52.446 person-years = 0.057 case per person-year
Incidence unexposed	1 case/20,985 person-days = 1 case/57.454 = 0.017 case per person-year
Incidence rate ratio	3.353
Incidence rate difference	0.040

survival probability of one can have no impact on the result of the multiplication. The resulting cumulative survival probability is $.900 \times .889 \times .833 = .666$. Finally, we convert this cumulative survival probability to its complement: the disease risk for the entire 10-year risk period is $1 - .666 = .334$.

The disease risk in the unexposed group, computed in the same way, is .167 (table 13.2B). The risk ratio is $.334/.167 = 2.000$. The risk difference is .167.

Premise.   This survival analysis rested on the premise that we could obtain a valid result for the disease risk within each one-day interval. Each informative one-day interval was considered as a mini-cohort study. The mini-cohort study had its own study population: the cohort under observation at the beginning of the interval. Given a valid result for the disease risk within each mini-cohort, we could combine their results to compute a valid result for the entire risk period.

How can we ensure that we obtain a valid result within each mini-cohort? We make the intervals small enough that within each interval in which a case occurs, neither loss to follow-up nor competing risks occurs. That is, within each mini-cohort, there is no attrition; the follow-up data are complete. In our hypothetical example, we used an interval of one day. No one was lost to follow-up or competing risks on the same day on which a case occurred.[2] Thus, the interval was small enough to ensure complete follow-up of each mini-cohort.

What happens when the time intervals are not small enough? There is potential for attrition to affect the observed risk in the mini-cohorts and, by extension, the overall result for the risk. In other words, the computation of the disease risk takes account of some, but not all, of the attrition in the cohort.

Comparison with Other Procedures.   It is instructive to compare the true disease risks obtained from the survival analysis in our hypothetical example (.334 and .167 in the exposed and unexposed groups, respectively) with what would be obtained with other approaches. One option would be the restriction procedure described earlier. Under this approach, we would obtain as follows: disease risk in the exposed = $3/5 = .600$; disease risk in the unexposed = $1/4$ = .250. Another option would be to disregard the attrition entirely. Under this approach, we would obtain as follows: disease risk in the exposed = $3/10$ = .300; disease risk in the unexposed = $1/10 = .100$.

Note that these two approaches bias the disease risks in opposite directions: the former upward and the latter downward. This occurs because the former deletes all the cohort members lost to observation from the denominator, as though they had never been in the study, whereas the latter includes them all in the denominator, as though they had remained under observation until the end of the study. In fact, the truth is in between because these cohort members were under observation for part of the study. This truth is what is reflected in the result from the survival analysis.

---

[2] If a case and a loss to follow-up occur in the same time interval, the Kaplan-Meier approach assumes that the loss to follow-up survives to the end of the interval.

The rational for the survival analysis can be distilled as follows. If we include people observed to develop disease by a certain time point, we must also include people observed to not develop disease by a certain time point.

Enumeration of the Cohort.   To divide the risk period into very small time intervals as required for a complete survival analysis, we have to complement ongoing case ascertainment with ongoing enumeration of the cohort under observation. This is required to determine the denominator for each mini-cohort.

In a given application, the exact information required to enumerate the cohort under observation depends on what it means to remain under observation in the particular study. In our hypothetical example, where a health plan case registry was used for ongoing case ascertainment, the cohort under observation at a given time comprised the individuals who were still members of the health plan. Therefore, a health plan membership registry was used for ongoing enumeration of the cohort under observation, on each day of a ten-year risk period.

If instead the cases are ascertained by a national disease registry, the cohort under observation at a given time comprises the individuals living in the nation. Then we aim to obtain a complete picture of emigration and deaths in the cohort. If the cases are ascertained by a local municipal registry for residents of a city or county, then we also need to know whether individuals continue to live in the city or county.

Periodic Case Ascertainment.   We have presented survival analysis applied to studies with ongoing case registry ascertainment. In these studies, it is often feasible to divide the study into very small time intervals, such as calendar days. As noted earlier, however, a form of survival analysis may also be applied in a study with periodic case ascertainment. The study may be divided into time intervals which correspond to the periods between the successive follow-up assessments. Generally these time intervals will be measured in months or years rather than days, and will not be small enough to ensure complete follow-up within each mini cohort. Nonetheless, the survival analysis may diminish, if not eliminate, potential bias due to unequal attrition.

Application to a Complex Data Set.   For clarity of presentation, we have applied survival analysis to a very simple hypothetical example. However, a complex data set can be analyzed much the same way. For readers who wish to see an application, Appendix B exhibits an application of survival analysis to the data of the Prenatal Determinants of Schizophrenia Example.

Linking Information Systems.   Conducting a cohort study with ongoing case registry ascertainment and ongoing enumeration of the cohort under observation often requires linking information systems. For instance, cases may be ascertained in separate outpatient and inpatient registries, the population data may be kept in a different registry, and exposure information such as birth records and school records may be kept in still other registries. Currently, some regions are building systems of linked registries that will provide unprecedented opportunities for cohort studies in coming decades. These linked registries permit ongoing ascertainment of cases of many disorders within fully enumerated population cohorts. In some instances, the diagnoses of cases ascertained by the registry are verified by further assessments. An example is the registry system of western Australia for studies of neurodevelopmental disabilities (Bower et al. 2000), which includes a birth register, death register, Birth Defects Register, Cerebral Palsy Register, and Autism Spectrum Disorder Register, and has the flexibility to link with service-sector information systems.

The Incidence Rate

The results of a cohort study are often analyzed in terms of the incidence rate rather than the risk. Since the incidence rate is the number of cases per unit of time (chapter 8), more meaningful estimates are obtained in studies that ascertain the cases as they arise in the cohort. The computation of the incidence rate naturally takes account of attrition by dividing the observation period for each cohort member into small time units. To illustrate this procedure, we consider the simplified scenario of a constant incidence rate.

We use the concept of **person-time** that was introduced in chapter 8. One can think of each cohort member as having a cohort clock. The clock is set at time zero at the start of the risk period. The clock stops when the individual is ascertained as a case of the disease, is lost to follow-up, succumbs to a competing risk, or reaches the study conclusion without the disease. The time on the cohort clock represents the time contributed by the individual to the cohort study. We refer to this as the observed person-time contributed by the individual. The observed person-time may be measured in any unit of time, such as person-years, person-weeks, or person-days. For example, an individual ascertained as a case one year into the risk period contributes one person-year, or 52 person-weeks, or on average 365.25 person-days. Often we simply refer to observed person-time as person-time, and we will do so below.

The total person-time of the exposed group is the sum of the person-time of all the individuals in the exposed group. Similarly, the total person-time of the unexposed group is the sum of the person-time of all the individuals in the unexposed group. In each of the exposure groups, the incidence rate is the number of cases divided by the total person-time. This can be illustrated for the hypothetical study in table 13.2. By adding up the person-time contributed by each of the 10 individuals in the exposed group, we obtain the total person-time of 19,156 days (table 13.2C). The incidence rate is 3 cases/19,156 person-days = 0.057 cases/person-year. Using the same procedure for the unexposed group, the incidence rate is 0.017 cases/person-year. The incidence rate ratio is 3.353.

Thus, rates take account of the follow-up time by quantifying the units of person-time in the denominator. We think of the exposed and unexposed groups as comprising units of person-time rather than people. We try to divide the follow-up time of each individual into many small units of person-time. If the intervals are not small enough, we cannot quantify the person-time precisely. To divide the follow-up time into small units, we depend on ongoing case ascertainment and ongoing enumeration of the cohort under observation.

Statistical Models

In the publication of results, we tend to rely on the statistical models described in chapter 26. A survival analysis models the time until onset of a disorder. A very widely used approach is **proportional hazards regression**, which yields a concise single result (point estimate with confidence limits) for the rate ratio adjusted for attrition and confounders.

Nonetheless, the interpretation of these results still depends on thinking through the potential bias due to unequal attrition in our study. This is especially important when, as often happens, survival analysis is the appropriate analytic procedure but the available data limit its application. As we scrutinize the data for potential bias, it is often helpful to make use of the relatively simple and transparent procedures we have described here, and essential to keep in mind the premises of a survival analysis.

Differential Attrition

The most damaging kind of unequal attrition is differential attrition. Differential attrition depends upon both exposure status and disease risk. In the simplest scenario, a different proportion of the cases and the noncases are lost to observation, and the magnitude of this difference is unequal for the exposed and the unexposed groups.

When there is an interval between the onset and ascertainment of a case, during which the disease has (or may have) an effect on attrition, we need to be concerned about differential attrition. However, this instance will not by itself result in differential attrition as defined here. The attrition may be unequal for the cases and the noncases, but to the same degree in the exposed and the unexposed groups. To produce differential attrition, the exposure and the disease must have a synergistic effect on attrition.

Although it is inherently difficult to document differential attrition, we can imagine plausible scenarios. Indeed, we are compelled to do so in interpreting our studies. Suppose we study exposure to child abuse before age 6 as a risk factor for developing depression by age 30. Children age 6 with a documented history of abuse are selected for the exposed group, and children age 6 from the same schools are selected for the unexposed group, with appropriate matching for factors such as sex, ethnicity, and social class. We use end-of-study case ascertainment. That is, we follow up the exposed and unexposed groups at age 30 to determine the study outcomes. At follow-up, the individuals who had developed depression might be more likely to be lost to follow-up than those who did not. In addition, the selective loss might pertain to a different degree in the exposed and unexposed groups because depression may well have a different effect on the social lives of individuals with and without a history of childhood abuse.

For several reasons, we are especially concerned about this kind of differential attrition in cohort studies of mental disorders. Mental disorders increase the risk of homelessness, imprisonment, and other social conditions that make an individual hard to locate (Susser et al. 1993; Torrey 1995; Teplin et al. 1996;

Herman et al. 1998). They disrupt thoughts, behaviors, and feelings, which may influence an individual's inclination or ability to participate in a follow-up assessment. Finally, mental disorders are related to mortality and other competing risks. All these effects of mental disorders might differ for the exposed and unexposed groups in a given study.

The nature of the problem suggests the solution. We attempt to shorten the interval between the onset of the disorder and the ascertainment of the case in the study. This will limit the effect of the disease on attrition in both the exposed and the unexposed. It will thereby limit the potential size of any inequality in this effect between the exposure groups.

Cohort studies with periodic or ongoing ascertainment are generally less susceptible to differential attrition than cohorts with end-of-study ascertainment. Periodic case ascertainment limits the period between onset and ascertainment to the interval between follow-up assessments. Ongoing ascertainment by a registry limits it to the interval between onset and treatment. However, these designs are by no means immune to differential attrition. There will always be an interval between the onset and ascertainment, and it is also possible that premorbid manifestations of the disease will have an effect on attrition.

Other Kinds of Differential Attrition

There are other kinds of differential attrition, though they tend to be less damaging. Attrition related to a confounder will generally be differential. For example, age may be a confounder in a study of head trauma as a risk factor for late life dementia. (Older age is associated with an increased risk of head trauma, as well as of dementia.) As noted earlier, older age tends to be associated with increased attrition because of higher mortality in older age groups. Since older age is related to both exposure and disease, the increased attrition it causes will also be related to both exposure and disease: in other words, it will be differential. The bias will be mitigated, however, by adjusting for age.[3]

Sensitivity Analysis

The underlying problem in differential attrition is that individuals who remain under observation at any given time are a selected subgroup of the original study population. Within this subgroup, the relationship between exposure and disease may not be the same as within the original study population. When it occurs, this problem is not remedied by the analytic procedures of either restriction or survival analysis.

Although we cannot remedy the bias due to differential attrition, we can gauge its potential magnitude. To do so, we examine the cohort attrition as fully as possible. An example is a report on attrition at the 15-year follow-up of the Baltimore Epidemiologic Catchment Area (ECA) sample (Badawi et al. 1999). Since the source population was originally assembled for a community survey, the follow-up included individuals who had mental disorders

---

[3] One can extend this argument to show that differential attrition can produce confounding. This happens in the same way that selective recruitment can produce confounding as described in chapter 11. Again, the bias is mitigated by adjustment for the (artifactual) confounder.

diagnosed at baseline. This made it possible for the authors to examine the effect of psychopathology at baseline on attrition during follow-up. They found that psychopathology at baseline influenced failure to locate and mortality, but not refusal to participate. This finding provided some indication of what the effect on attrition might have been for mental disorders that developed during the follow-up.

Armed with such information about the potential for differential attrition, one can conduct a sensitivity analysis to gauge its effect (Greenland 1996). The risk ratios in various simulated scenarios are compared with the risk ratio in the actual study. This comparison indicates how much bias might have been introduced.

Consider a cohort study of the consequences of childhood exposure to head irradiation (table 13.1; Ron, Modan, Boice, Alfandany et al. 1988). The exposed group was Israeli children irradiated as a treatment for tinea capitis. The study found that these children had a higher risk of developing neural tumors than both their unexposed siblings and an unexposed comparison group of same-age children drawn from the national population registry. Some of the exposed children died from radiation-induced leukemias. The children who developed leukemia might also have been at most risk for neural tumors, if they had survived, because these children might have been susceptible to developing various kinds of cancer as a result of radiation exposure. We cannot adjust for this possibly differential attrition. Yet we may be interested in estimating what the effect of head irradiation on neural tumors might have been, in the absence of the competing risk of leukemia. To do so, we can compute a hypothetical result for the worst-case scenario. Suppose all the 14 radiation-exposed children who died of leukemia had instead lived on and developed neural tumors. Based on mortality data for the cohort (Ron, Modan, and Boice 1988), we estimate the risk ratio under this scenario to be 8.6, slightly higher than the reported risk ratio of 6.9.

Although we have introduced sensitivity analysis in the context of differential attrition, its use is by no means limited to this context. It is a widely applicable and useful tool in epidemiologic analysis (see Greenland 1996).

Potential Outcomes Approaches

We have limited our discussion to study outcomes that are missing because of cohort attrition, either loss to follow-up or competing risks. Outcome data may be missing for other reasons: for example, coding errors or incomplete data. For the purposes described here, study outcomes that are missing for other reasons can be handled in the same way.

It should also be noted, however, that in an emergent approach to statistical analysis and study design, attrition is subsumed within a much more general framework that has a different conceptual foundation than conventional methods. This schema is centered around a deeper concept of "missingness" or "potential outcomes." Though beyond the scope of this book, potential-outcomes approaches may lead to exciting developments in coming years; interested readers may refer to Gelman and Meng (2004) and Greenland (2004).

Conclusion

This chapter has provided a framework for the prevention and control of bias due to unequal attrition in cohort studies. Like the effects of third-variable confounding, the effects of unequal attrition can be limited by the design, as well as the analysis, of a cohort study. The most problematic kind of attrition is differential. This kind of attrition causes a bias that may not be remediable. We then resort to a sensitivity analysis to gauge the potential bias. In the next chapter, we proceed to differential misclassification, which, like differential attrition, may cause an intractable bias.

References

Badawi MA, Eaton WW, Myllyluoma J, Weimer LG, and Gallo J (1999). Psychopathology and Attrition in the Baltimore ECA 15-Year Follow-Up 1981–1996. *Soc. Psychiatry Psychiatr. Epidemiol* 34:91–98.

Bower C, Leonard H, and Petterson B (2000). Intellectual Disability in Western Australia. *J. Paediatr. Child Health* 36:213–215.

Boys A, Marsden J, Stillwell G, Hatchings K, Griffiths P, and Farrell M (2003). Minimizing Respondent Attrition in Longitudinal Research: Practical Implications from a Cohort Study of Adolescent Drinking. *J. Adolesc.* 26:363–373.

Clayton D and Hills M (1995). *Statistical Models in Epidemiology.* Oxford: Oxford University Press.

Conover S, Berkman A, Gheith A, Jahiel R, Stanley D, Geller PA, Valencia E, and Susser E (1997). Methods for Successful Follow-Up of Elusive Urban Populations: An Ethnographic Approach with Homeless Men. *Bull. N.Y. Acad. Med.* 74:90–108.

Cotter RB, Burke JD, Loeber R, and Navratil JL (2002). Innovative Retention Methods in Longitudinal Research: A Case Study of the Developmental Trends Study. *J. Child Fam. Stud.* 11:485–498.

Cottler LB, Compton WM, Ben Abdallah A, Horne M, and Claverie D (1996). Achieving a 96.6 Percent Follow-Up Rate in a Longitudinal Study of Drug Abusers. *Drug Alcohol Depend.* 41:209–217.

Coughlin SS and Beauchamp TL, eds. (1996). *Ethics and Epidemiology.* New York: Oxford University Press.

de Graaf R, Bijl RV, Smit F, Ravelli A, and Vollebergh WA (2000). Psychiatric and Sociodemographic Predictors of Attrition in a Longitudinal Study: The Netherlands Mental Health Survey and Incidence Study (NEMESIS). *Am. J. Epidemiol.* 152:1039–1047.

Eaton WW, Thara R, Federman B, Melton B, and Liang KY (1995). Structure and Course of Positive and Negative Symptoms in Schizophrenia. *Arch. Gen. Psychiatry* 52:127–134.

Esbensen FA, Miller MH, Taylor TJ, He N, and Freng A (1999). Differential Attrition Rates and Active Parental Consent. *Eval. Rev.* 23:316–335.

Essen-Möller E, Larsson H, Uddenberg CE, and White G (1956). Individual Traits and Morbidity in a Swedish Rural Population. *Acta Psychiatr. Neurolog. Scand. Suppl.* 100:1–160.

Fisher CB (2004). Informed Consent and Clinical Research Involving Children and Adolescents: Implications of the Revised APA Ethics Code and HIPAA. *J. Clin. Child Adolesc. Psychol.* 33:832–839.

Geerlings MI, Schmand B, Jonker C, Lindeboom J, and Bouter LM (1999). Education and Incident Alzheimer's Disease: A Biased Association Due to Selective Attrition and Use of a Two-Step Diagnostic Procedure? *Int. J. Epidemiol.* 28:492–497.

Gelman A and Meng X, eds. (2004). *Applied Bayesian Modeling and Causal Inference from Incomplete-Data Perspectives: An Essential Journey with Donald Rubin's Statistical Family.* Hoboken, N.J.: Wiley.

Greenland S (1996). Basic Methods for Sensitivity Analysis of Biases. *Int. J. Epidemiol.* 25:1107–1116.

Greenland S (2004). An Overview of Methods for Causal Inference from Observational Studies. In Gelman A and Meng X, eds., *Applied Bayesian Modeling and Causal Inference from Incomplete-Data Perspectives: An Essential Journey with Donald Rubin's Statistical Family, pp. 3–14.* Hoboken, N.J.: Wiley.

Hagnell O (1989). Repeated Incidence and Prevalence Studies of Mental Disorders in a Total Population Followed During 25 Years: The Lundby Study, Sweden. *Acta Psychiatr. Scand. Suppl.* 348:61–77.

Hagnell O, Lanke J, Rorsman B, and Ohman R (1986a). Predictors of Alcoholism in the Lundby Study. I. Material and Methods. *Eur. Arch. Psychiatry Neurol. Sci.* 235:187–191.

Hagnell O, Lanke J, Rorsman B, and Ohman R (1986b). Predictors of Alcoholism in the Lundby Study. II. Personality Traits as Risk Factors for Alcoholism. *Eur. Arch. Psychiatry Neurol. Sci.* 235:192–196.

Hagnell O, Ojesjo L, Otterbeck L, and Rorsman B (1994). *Prevalence of Mental Disorders, Personality Traits and Mental Complaints in the Lundby Study.* Stockholm: Scandinavian University Press.

Helgason T (1964). Epidemiology of Mental Disorders in Iceland. *Acta Psychiatr. Scand.* 40 (Suppl 173): 1–258.

Herman DB, Susser ES, Jandorf L, Lavelle J, and Bromet EJ (1998). Homelessness among Individuals with Psychotic Disorders Hospitalized for the First Time: Findings from the Suffolk County Mental Health Project. *Am. J. Psychiatry* 155:109–113.

Janssen I, Hanssen M, Bak M, Bijl RV, de Graaf R, Vollebergh W, McKenzie K, and van Os J (2003). Discrimination and Delusional Ideation. *Br. J. Psychiatry* 182:71–76.

Launer LJ, Dinkgreve MA, Jonker C, Hooijer C, and Lindeboom J (1993). Are Age and Education Independent Correlates of the Mini–Mental State Exam Performance of Community-Dwelling Elderly? *J. Gerontol.* 48:271–277.

Modan B (1987). Cancer and Leukemia Risks after Low Level Radiation—Controversy, Facts and Future. *Med. Oncol. Tumor Pharmacother.* 4:151–161.

National Institutes of Health (1979). *The Belmont Report: Ethical Principles and Guidelines for the Protection of Human Subjects of Research.* Bethesda, Md.: U.S. Department of Health, Education and Welfare.

National Institutes of Health, Director's Council of Public Representatives (2001). *Human Research Protections in Clinical Trials: A Public Perspective.* www.copr.nih.gov/reports/hrpct.asp.

Ribisl KM, Walton MA, Mowbray CT, Luke DA, Davidson WS, and Bootsmiller BJ (1996). Minimizing Participant Attrition in Panel Studies through the Use of Effective Retention and Tracking Strategies: Review and Recommendations. *Eval. Program Plann.* 19:1–25.

Roberts LW and Roberts B (1999). Psychiatric Research Ethics: An Overview of Evolving Guidelines and Current Ethical Dilemmas in the Study of Mental Illness. *Biol. Psychiatry* 46:1025–1038.

Ron E, Modan B, and Boice JD, Jr (1988). Mortality after Radiotherapy for Ringworm of the Scalp. *Am. J. Epidemiol.* 127:713–725.

Ron E, Modan B, Boice JD, Jr., Alfandary E, Stovall M, Chetrit A, and Katz L (1988). Tumors of the Brain and Nervous System after Radiotherapy in Childhood. *N. Engl. J. Med.* 319:1033–1039.

Schoevers RA, Beekman AT, Deeg DJ, Hooijer C, Jonker C, and van Tilburg W (2003). The Natural History of Late-Life Depression: Results from the Amsterdam Study of the Elderly (AMSTEL). *J. Affect. Disord.* 76:5–14.

Schulte PA, Hunter D, and Rothman N (1997). Ethical and Social Issues in the Use of Biomarkers in Epidemiological Research. *IARC Sci. Publ.* 313–318.

Steinberg KK (2001). Ethical Challenges at the Beginning of the Millennium. *Stat. Med.* 20:1415–1419.

Susser E, Moore R, and Link B (1993). Risk Factors for Homelessness. *Epidemiol. Rev.* 15:546–556.

Teplin LA, Abram KM, and McClelland GM (1996). Prevalence of Psychiatric Disorders among Incarcerated Women. I. Pretrial Jail Detainees. *Arch. Gen. Psychiatry* 53:505–512.

Torrey EF (1995). Jails and Prisons—America's New Mental Hospitals. *Am. J. Public Health* 85:1611–1613.

Vlahov, D (1994). The ALIVE Study. In Nicolosi A., ed., *HIV Epidemiology: Models and Methods*, 31–45. New York: Raven Press.

Wadsworth MEJ (1991). *The Imprint of Time: Childhood, History and Adult Life.* Oxford: Clarendon Press.

14 Differential Misclassification

Ezra Susser and Sharon Schwartz

The previous chapters dealt with characteristics of the people we recruited into the cohort and what we observed of their subsequent experience. We turn now to the way in which we label our observations. It is through our labeling of the experiences of the cohort members that they are classified in the cells of the fourfold table—exposed-diseased, exposed-nondiseased, unexposed-diseased, or unexposed-nondiseased. When we misclassify people, it is akin to shuffling them between these categories of the fourfold table.

This chapter addresses misclassification of the disease that is linked to the exposure, that is, misclassification of disease that is unequal for the exposed and the unexposed groups. This is the type of misclassification most relevant to cohort studies. In chapter 16, we discuss misclassification of the exposure that is linked to the disease, which is more relevant to case-control studies.[1]

We begin by describing common scenarios of differential misclassification in psychiatric research. Then, we consider the resulting bias and how we can limit it. We also discuss two special cases: third-variable effects and dependent nondifferential misclassification. Finally, we conclude this section on cohort studies and offer a segue to part IV, which addresses case-control studies.

Scenarios of Differential Misclassification

Some degree of disease misclassification occurs in virtually all cohort studies of mental disorders. Underascertainment is common. With end-of-study or periodic case ascertainment, individuals may fail to report disorders that occurred during the risk period. With ongoing case ascertainment by a registry, untreated cases are not ascertained.

---

[1] In some contexts, it is useful to describe the same problem in terms of *sensitivity* and *specificity* (defined in chapter 8). The sensitivity or specificity of the disease measure may be different for the exposed and unexposed. Conversely, the sensitivity or specificity of the exposure measure may be different for the diseased and nondiseased. In either case, the result will be differential misclassification.

Overascertainment occurs, as well. Symptoms can be misinterpreted; diagnostic thresholds, misapplied. In the United States, if (as has been alleged) clinicians prefer to assign diagnoses that are covered by their patients' insurance plans, studies relying on clinical records will overascertain these diagnoses.

We are concerned here, however, with circumstances in which the disease misclassification differs for the exposed and unexposed groups. We present four common scenarios of differential misclassification. These are not meant to cover all eventualities. Rather, they exemplify the situations that investigators need to consider in order to anticipate this kind of bias.

In the first scenario, the case finding is influenced by belief in the risk factor. A strong suspicion that the exposure is a cause of the disease is often the motivation for conducting a cohort study. A research team that believes in the risk factor may look harder for the disease among the exposed than among the unexposed. Such a belief may also be held by clinicians in the health system, as well as by the study participants, again resulting in more attention being paid to signs of disease in the exposed than in the unexposed. In this scenario, underascertainment is greater for the unexposed, and, perhaps, overascertainment is greater for the exposed. The observed effect of the exposure will be exaggerated.

This possibility is illustrated by successive cohort studies of Israeli children exposed and unexposed to head irradiation treatments for tinea capitis. As described in the previous chapter, an initial study showed that the exposed children had an increased risk of neural tumors (table 13.1; Ron et al. 1988). In response, the Israeli government passed legislation to compensate victims for any health effects. A later study examined whether the exposed children had an increased risk of schizophrenia (Gross et al. 2005), relying on the Israeli psychiatric registry for case detection. During the risk period for the schizophrenia study, however, Israeli clinicians and the study participants had been alerted to look for neuropsychiatric signs and symptoms in the exposed (but not the unexposed) cohort, creating the potential for higher case ascertainment in the exposed than in the unexposed. To check for bias, the authors examined secular trends, comparing results for periods before and after the legislation.

In the second scenario, the assessment instrument is more (or less) valid in the exposed than in the unexposed group. This scenario is particularly germane to research comparing mental disorders across cultural groups. The point is illustrated by an Australian study that compared Aboriginal and Caucasian children with respect to the prevalence of intellectual disability (table 14.1; Leonard et al. 2003). The study was based in the innovative registry system of western Australia described in the previous chapter. Although the authors found a higher prevalence of intellectual disability among Aboriginal children, they suggested that their result could partly reflect cross-cultural variation in case ascertainment. The assessment instruments were designed for use in the dominant Caucasian culture and were more likely to misclassify Aboriginal than to misclassify Caucasian children.

Cultural groups may differ appreciably in their interpretation of questions and in their tolerance for signs and symptoms. Writing about child mental

Table 14.1 Examples of Potential for Differential Misclassification in Cohort Studies

Sources	Study Description, Case Finding, and Misclassification Issue
Bromet et al. (2000)	*Study*: Kyiv Chornobyl Project
See also: Adams et al. (2002)	*Cohort (N = 600)*: Children exposed to the 1986 Chornobyl nuclear accident (in utero to age 15 months), living in Kyiv in 1997 (N = 300); unexposed were gender-matched classmates from the same school homeroom (N = 300). Psychological outcomes in exposed and unexposed compared.
	Case finding: Follow-up assessments (1997) included parent and child interviews, physical exams, teacher interviews; the second follow up study began in 2005.
	Misclassification issue: It proved infeasible to blind informants and interviewers to child's exposure status.
Leonard et al. (2003)	*Study*: Epidemiology of Intellectual Disability in western Australia.
See also: Bower et al. (2000)	*Cohort (N = 240,358)*: Live births in western Australia 1983–1992 surviving to Dec. 31, 1999; demographic characteristics obtained from Maternal and Child Health Research Database, and survivorship based on linked death registrations.
	Case finding: Outcome data obtained mainly from Disability Services Commission and Department of Education.
	Misclassification issue: Children from minority cultures, such as Aboriginal children, may be more likely to be misclassified as intellectually disabled, because of cultural differences in behavior and inappropriate tests.
Shaffer et al. (1985)	*Study*: National Collaborative Perinatal Project (NCPP)—New York-Columbia Site.
See also: Pine et al. (1997)	*Cohort (N = 180)*: Pregnancies enrolled at 12 sites in the NCPP 1959–1966; offspring followed in childhood ages 4 and 8 months; 1, 3, 5, and 7 years. The 180 subjects were selected from the 1962–1963 New York Columbia site birth cohort for follow-up at age 17. The exposed were 90 members with soft-signs on neurological exams at age 7; the unexposed were 90 age- and gender-matched members without soft-signs at age 7. Examined the relation of neurological soft-signs in childhood to psychiatric conditions in adolescence.
	Case finding: Neuropsychiatric assessments at age 17.
	Misclassification issue: Assessors were blinded to neurological soft-sign status at age 7. This was done to prevent them from paying greater attention to signs and symptoms in the exposed than in the unexposed.

health in India, for example, Savita Malhotra proposed that measurements of psychopathology in children might be influenced by cross-cultural differences in concepts and language, attitudes about what behaviors are normative, and the settings in which measures are taken (Malhotra et al. 1992). Since the reliability and validity of our outcome measurements will vary across cultural groups (Van Ommeren 2003) we should expect our case ascertainment to also vary.

This scenario also pertains more generally, however, to cohort studies. There are many other reasons for the validity of assessments to vary across exposure groups. It may even occur when the investigators and participants are blinded to the exposure status. The phenomenon was neatly demonstrated in the Amsterdam Study of the Elderly (Geerlings et al. 1999) described in the previous chapter (see table 13.1). This study examined whether low educational attainment was related to Alzheimer's disease. The authors used the Mini–Mental State Exam as one of two screening instruments to detect potential cases. The authors suspected that the Mini–Mental State Exam, which is used alone in some studies, would be less sensitive among people with high, as opposed to low, educational levels. For this reason, they had also included a second screening measure thought to be less influenced by educational level. Reporting their results, they showed that, using the Mini–Mental State Exam (MMSE) alone, they would in fact have obtained a stronger association between low education and Alzheimer's disease than they did by using both screening scales together.

In the third scenario, a perceived connection between the exposure and the outcome influences the propensity of the exposed group to reveal their disorder. This scenario is most likely to arise in cohort studies in which the exposure and the outcome have a strong emotional valence. This scenario is not uncommon in psychiatric epidemiology, where both exposure and outcome may carry a stigma.

The potential for this bias can be seen in cohort studies of prenatal maternal exposures as risk factors for neuropsychiatric disorders in children. On the one hand, an exposed mother may feel extremely anxious about whether her prenatal exposure harmed her child. This anxiety may lead her to observe and report her child's problems more than an unexposed mother. On the other hand, an exposed mother may fear that if her prenatal exposure appears to have damaged her child she may be stigmatized. For some highly stigmatized exposures such as cocaine use, she may even fear that the child could be taken away from her (Paltrow et al. 2000; Annas 2001). This fear may lead her to report her child's problems less than an unexposed mother.

In the fourth and final scenario, the study is actually designed so that the exposed and the unexposed are evaluated at a different time and in a different way. This design is common in studies built around unanticipated disasters. Often these studies have to be launched in a very short time frame that does not allow for construction of comparable exposed and unexposed cohorts.

With these constraints, a study of a disaster may resort to a rather crude comparison. For instance, the outcomes of people exposed to the disaster may be compared to the results of a previous study of another population. An additional problem in these studies is that there may be no data collected on the exposed group before the event, as is required to ensure that none of them has the study outcome at the start.

Studies with these limitations cannot be designated cohort studies. But studies of disasters generally include some of the elements of a cohort study, and they are of such vital importance in the search for causes of mental disorders that the designs they use merit careful consideration. They can usefully be considered alongside natural experiments. The investigators often attempt to approximate the features of a natural experiment, with varying degrees of success, depending upon the circumstances in which the study must be conducted.

An example is a study of the effects of 9/11—the September 11, 2001, terrorist attacks on the World Trade Center—on mental disorders among New York City public school children (Hoven et al. 2005). There were no data available on mental disorders among the schoolchildren before 9/11. The study was conducted 6 months afterward. The authors compared schoolchildren who had severe, moderate, and mild exposure to the event, but none of the schoolchildren in New York City was entirely unexposed to 9/11. For an unexposed group, the authors turned to a previous, cross-sectional study of child mental disorders in Stamford, Connecticut. This design presented two key difficulties. First, the comparison of the children who had different levels of exposure to 9/11 relied entirely on prevalence data collected 6 months after the event. Second, the comparison of the exposed groups with the unexposed Stamford children was fraught with uncertainty: the assessment procedures were not entirely identical, the cities were of a different scale, and the studies were done at different times.

Despite these difficulties, the study produced a coherent pattern of results. Among the New York City schoolchildren, the level of exposure to the event was strongly associated with anxiety or depressive symptoms (notably, agoraphobia and posttraumatic stress symptoms). The prevalence of mental disorders in the unexposed Stamford children was similar to that of the New York City schoolchildren who were mildly exposed. A parsimonious interpretation is that 9/11 had a substantial impact on psychiatric symptoms among New York City schoolchildren who had more than a mild exposure to the terrorist attacks.

Limiting the Bias

Cohort studies are exquisitely sensitive to differences in case ascertainment procedures for the two exposure groups. A twofold better case ascertainment in the exposed than in the unexposed group could produce a spurious risk ratio of 2. A mere 10 percent difference in case ascertainment across exposure groups could produce a spurious risk ratio of 1.1.

When the observed risk ratio is small (e.g., less than 1.3), it could be explained by some small difference in disease misclassification across the exposure groups. Small risk ratios are also more likely to reflect confounding, or unequal attrition. In fact, it has been suggested that small effects may lie beyond the resolving power of observational studies; one influential commentary argued that for very small magnitude associations "it is simply not possible to distinguish between bias and causation as explanations" (Shapiro 2000). A small-magnitude finding can be statistically significant and replicated in several large studies, yet be explained by a bias that is common to these studies.

Nonetheless, we can do much to limit the bias from differential misclassification. We depend mainly on anticipating and preventing it. We try to safeguard our study against any difference in case ascertainment between the exposed and unexposed groups.

A standard procedure for guarding against differential ascertainment is to ensure that the assessment of the outcome is done "blind" to the exposure status. This procedure prevents the assessors from looking harder for the disease in the exposed than in the unexposed (or vice-versa). Ideally, all those reporting or collecting diagnostically relevant information should be blind to exposure status. Thus, the influence of a belief in the hypothesized risk factor is minimized.

Carefully blinded assessments were used in a study of childhood neurological soft signs as a risk factor for young adult psychiatric outcomes (table 14.1; Shaffer et al. 1985). The study was based in a birth cohort. The exposed and unexposed groups were defined by the presence or absence of neurological soft signs at the age 7 follow-up. The psychiatric outcomes were ascertained by an in-depth assessment at age 17. Separate examiners were assigned to conduct adolescent, parent, and teacher interviews; all were blind to the presence or absence of neurologic soft signs in childhood. A committee of two psychiatrists and one psychologist, also blind to the exposure status, formulated the final diagnoses by consensus.

It is not always feasible, however, for the data collectors to be blinded. This pertains especially to special exposure cohort studies (described in chapter 10). Since these studies are built around a single exposure, the assessors are likely to be aware of the study hypothesis. In addition, the exposed and unexposed are often drawn from different populations. Sometimes exposure status is readily observable at interview or inadvertently revealed by the subject. Compounding the problem, the subjects themselves are not blinded; they are likely to be aware of their exposure and the purpose of the study, and their reporting may be influenced by it.

This can be illustrated in a study of the effects of the 1986 Chernobyl nuclear disaster on the mental health of children (table 14.1; Bromet et al. 2000). The exposed children were compared to a gender-matched unexposed group from the same schools in Kyiv, the city to which they had been evacuated. Although interviewers were rigorously trained to maintain the blind and systematically asked the children's mothers not to reveal their exposure status, they could not prevent the mothers of exposed children from revealing their experience of the nuclear disaster at the start of the interview.

It may still be possible to incorporate a check on the potential bias into the design. In a previous chapter (see table 10.3), we described a special exposure study that compared the parenting skills of "ex-care" women (reared in children's homes) and family-reared women. The study interviewers were not blinded. But the study also used blinded observers who made home visits to rate the interactions between the women and their children. The ex-care women showed poorer parenting on the blinded observational ratings, as well as on the interviewer ratings. The similarity of results from the two methods suggested that any bias in the interviewer ratings was small.

Difficult as it is to blind the assessors, it may be still harder, and sometimes impossible, to blind the study subjects. This problem arises in randomized trials of psychosocial interventions. Typically, these trials are single-blind, as opposed to double-blind. Thus, even in rigorous trials, the assessors are blinded to the subjects' exposure status (i.e., whether the subjects are in the experimental or control group), but the subjects are not. Generally, the subjects are also aware of the purpose of the intervention. Their reporting may be influenced by what they perceive to be the expectations of the researchers.

In any study, the precondition for devising effective safeguards is to identify the ways in which the exposed and unexposed cases might be ascertained differentially. We have described four common scenarios of differential ascertainment, but there are many others. Studies comparing the disease risk in men and women, for example, have to consider gender differences in the report of symptoms and use of treatments (Weissman and Klerman 1977). The pathways to case detection tend to be specific to the study at hand, reflecting the setting, as well as the exposure and disease, under investigation. Hence, it is essential to delineate at the design stage the factors likely to influence it. The exercise requires not only an appreciation of the study raters and the health system, but also an understanding of the subjective experience of the exposure and the illness among the study participants.

Ascertainment Effects of Third Variables

Sometimes a third variable influences case ascertainment within a cohort study. The third variable will then imitate a cause of the disease within the study. It helps determine whether an individual is labeled as a case or not. If the third variable is also associated with the exposure, it will imitate a confounder.

Suppose that in the study population the cases are more likely to be ascertained among women than among men, and that women are also more likely than men to have the exposure being investigated. Similar to confounding, these relationships will lead to bias in the observed association between the exposure and the study outcome.

In the United States, race is still associated with detection and treatment of a wide variety of diseases, reflecting a long history of racial discrimination (U.S. Office of the Surgeon General 2001; Smedley et al. 2003). This discrimination may pertain to a psychiatric disorder being investigated in a cohort study. It has been suggested, for example, that psychiatric diagnosticians may underascertain depression in black, as compared with white, patients (Strakowski et al. 2003). Accordingly, in a cohort study of depression, race may be associated with detection and diagnosis of the cases. If race is also associated with the exposure of interest, then race will be a third variable that mimics a confounder in the cohort study.

Unlike other forms of differential misclassification, this bias can be mitigated with use of the methods already described for confounders: once we have identified and measured such a third variable, we can use matching and adjustment to prevent and control the bias, just as we do for a confounder. It should be kept in mind, however, that adjustment will not remove the misclassification itself. It will only mitigate the effect of the difference in misclassification for the exposure groups. The remaining nondifferential misclassification can still bias the result, generally toward the null. In addition, if we do not have a reliable and valid measure of the third variable, there may be residual bias away from the null.

Unidentified or Unmeasured Variables

Although we can adjust for variables known to influence the ascertainment of the cases, the variables with the greatest impact on ascertainment may be largely unidentified or unmeasured. If the effect of these factors on ascertainment differs for the exposed and unexposed groups, they will mimic confounders and will be unadjusted. To the extent that this occurs, we in fact study the causes of developing the disorder *and* being ascertained as a case.

Several strategies are available for addressing this problem. One is to identify the factors influencing case ascertainment within the cohort, by executing a more intensive study of a subgroup of the cohort. Another is to match on some variable that represents many ascertainment factors taken together. In some instances, residency in the catchment area of a certain treatment facility may be such a variable. At present, however, most studies do not employ these strategies. We discuss this point further in chapter 18.

Dependent Nondifferential Misclassification

This type of misclassification occurs when the errors in the classification of disease status are linked to errors in the classification of exposure status. Epidemiologists do not usually consider dependant nondifferential misclassification along with differential misclassification. For epidemiologists, strictly speaking, the nondifferential misclassification of the exposure is correlated with the nondifferential misclassification of the disease (Kristensen 1992). Nonetheless, it leads to bias in much the same way as differential misclassification.

An example is social desirability. Persons who tend to offer socially desirable responses may have a higher threshold for revealing a stigmatized disease. This will create an apparent (artifactual) association between response style and disease. If the exposure is also a stigmatized, or undesirable behavior, these same people may have a higher threshold for revealing exposure status. This third variable, response style, will imitate a confounder. Although it may be associated with neither exposure nor disease, it is associated with exposure and disease reporting. Researchers sometimes try to adjust for response styles, using measures such as the Marlowe-Crowne Social Desirability Scale (Crowne and Marlowe 1964).

Social desirability can also lead respondents to provide positive responses they think the researcher desires. They may then overreport (rather than conceal) the exposure and the symptoms of the disease. This could again link exposure and disease errors. Therefore, like differential misclassification, dependent misclassification can bias the results either toward or away from the null value.

Conclusion

As we conclude the chapters on the cohort design, it may be helpful to draw attention to the main themes. First and foremost, the cohort study, by its design, helps to establish that the exposure is antecedent to the study outcome. Taking the approach of the cohort design to establish the temporal order means following the exposed and unexposed to determine the proportion who develop the study outcome in each group.

For the study to be valid, we want the exposed and unexposed to be fully comparable. However, we face sources of noncomparability at each turn. At the study outset, we immediately find ourselves confronted with differences between the exposed and unexposed on confounders that offer alternative explanations for an association between exposure and disease risk. As the study proceeds, we must contend with unequal attrition that further erodes the comparability of the exposed and unexposed. Although we try to limit these problems, we do not have the means to remove these effects; we can only collect the data required to adjust for them in our analyses. Moreover, we are beset by possible small differences in case ascertainment for the exposed and unexposed, which can cause appreciable artifacts. Faced with these realities, we may harbor some healthy doubt as to whether an association between the exposure and the disease in a cohort study truly reflects a causal connection between them.

Despite all these uncertainties, the cohort study has proved to be an ingenious device. While keeping to the same general theme, the design can take on many permutations, and has been used to investigate an extraordinarily wide range of exposures and diseases in all kinds of contexts. Cohort studies have produced numerous findings of great significance for the health of human societies. Furthermore, the longitudinal design carries the potential for extending epidemiology to examine over the life course the dynamic processes connecting the exposure to the outcome (see part VIII).

In fact, for most questions about the determinants of disease that vary within human populations, the cohort study is the most powerful device available. Although the randomized trial tends to produce more certain results, its application is necessarily restricted to a small fraction of the questions that can be addressed in the cohort design, and to a small fraction of the populations that can be enrolled in cohort studies (see part I). Like any powerful device, the cohort design has the potential for harm, as well as good, and we try to use it with care.

In the coming sections, we will see that all this uncertainty pertains not only to the cohort study; it is merely illuminated by the cohort design. A study comparing cases with controls is equally vulnerable, but in that design some of these problems are masked and thus harder to identify and remedy.

References

Adams RE, Bromet EJ, Panina N, Golovakha E, Goldgaber D, and Gluzman S (2002). Stress and Well-Being in Mothers of Young Children 11 Years after the Chornobyl Nuclear Power Plant Accident. *Psychol. Med.* 32:143–156.

Annas GJ (2001). Testing Poor Pregnant Patients for Cocaine—Physicians as Police Investigators. *N. Engl. J. Med.* 344:1729–1732.

Bower C, Leonard H, and Petterson B (2000). Intellectual Disability in Western Australia. *J. Paediatr. Child Health* 36:213–215.

Bromet EJ, Goldgaber D, Carlson G, et al. (2000). Children's Well-Being 11 Years after the Chornobyl Catastrophe. *Arch. Gen. Psychiatry* 57:563–571.

Crowne DP and Marlowe D (1964). *The Approval Motive.* New York: Wiley.

Geerlings MI, Schmand B, Jonker C, Lindeboom J, and Bouter LM (1999). Education and Incident Alzheimer's Disease: A Biased Association Due to Selective Attrition and Use of a Two-Step Diagnostic Procedure? *Int. J. Epidemiol.* 28:492–497.

Gross R, Sadetzki S, Modan B, Chetrit A, and Susser E (2005). Head Irradiation in Early Childhood and the Risk of Schizophrenia. New York: *Amer. Psychopathol. Assoc.* Poster presentation.

Hoven CW, Duarte CS, Lucas CP, et al. (2005). Psychopathology among New York City Public School Children Six Months after September 11th. *Arch. Gen. Psychiatry.* 62:545–552.

Kristensen P (1992). Bias from Nondifferential but Dependent Misclassification of Exposure and Outcome. *Epidemiology* 3:210–215.

Leonard H, Petterson B, Bower C, and Sanders R (2003). Prevalence of Intellectual Disability in Western Australia. *Paediatr. Perinat. Epidemiol.* 17:58–67.

Malhotra S, Malhotra A, and Varma VK (1992). *Child Mental Health in India.* Delhi: Macmillan India.

Paltrow LM, Cohen DS, and Carey CA (2000). Year 2000 Overview: Governmental Responses to Pregnant Women Who Use Alcohol or Other Drugs. *Women's Law Project: National Advocates for Pregnant Women.*

Pine DS, Shaffer D, Schonfeld IS, and Davies M (1997). Minor Physical Anomalies: Modifiers of Environmental Risks for Psychiatric Impairment? *J. Am. Acad. Child Adolesc. Psychiatry* 36:395–403.

Ron E, Modan B, Boice JD, Jr., Alfandary E, Stovall M, Chetrit A, and Katz L (1988). Tumors of the Brain and Nervous System after Radiotherapy in Childhood. *N. Engl. J. Med.* 319:1033–1039.

Shaffer D, Schonfeld I, O'Connor PA, Stokman C, Trautman P, Shafer S, and Ng S (1985). Neurological Soft Signs. Their Relationship to Psychiatric Disorder and Intelligence in Childhood and Adolescence. *Arch. Gen. Psychiatry* 42:342–351.

Shapiro S (2000). Bias in the Evaluation of Low-Magnitude Associations: An Empirical Perspective. *Am. J. Epidemiol.* 151:939–945.

Smedley BD, Stith AY, and Nelson AR, eds. (2003). Unequal Treatment: Confronting Racial and Ethnic Disparities in Health Care. *Washington, D.C.: The National Academies Press.*

Strakowski SM, Keck PE, Jr., Arnold LM, Collins J, Wilson RM, Fleck DE, Corey KB, Amicone J, and Adebimpe VR (2003). Ethnicity and Diagnosis in Patients with Affective Disorders. *J. Clin. Psychiatry* 64:747–754.

U.S. Department of Health and Human Services (2001). *Mental Health: Culture, Race, and Ethnicity—A Supplement to Mental Health: A Report of the Surgeon General.* Rockville, Md.: U.S. Department of Health and Human Services.

Van Ommeren M (2003). Validity Issues in Transcultural Epidemiology. *Br. J. Psychiatry* 182:376–378.

Weissman MM and Klerman GL (1977). Sex Differences and the Epidemiology of Depression. *Arch. Gen. Psychiatry* 34:98–111.

CASE-CONTROL DESIGNS IN PSYCHIATRIC EPIDEMIOLOGY

Logic of the Case-Control Design 15

Alfredo Morabia, Sharon Schwartz, and Ezra Susser

Case-control studies are commonly used in epidemiology and have been pivotal in many important public health breakthroughs (Paneth et al. 2004). The design was used, for example, to discover preventable causes of lung cancer (cigarette smoking; Doll and Hill 1952), sudden infant death syndrome (babies lying on their stomachs; Beal and Finch 1991), and HIV infection (unprotected sex; Jaffe et al. 1983).

In psychiatric research, however, the case-control study has been under-utilized. This statement may seem surprising, because the psychiatric litera-ture is replete with studies that compare cases with controls. Although this is true, the investigators doing such studies usually do not see the equivalence between their studies and the case-control studies done in epidemiology. Therefore, they do not recognize that they could make use of a powerful strategy with a developed technique.

This chapter explains the logic of the case-control strategy. We show how to conceptualize a case-control study as a condensed version of a cohort study. This relationship between the two designs is well established in epidemiology. It is not familiar, however, to many researchers in other fields.

In the next chapter, building on this logic, we discuss the central challenges to implementing a case-control study: selecting cases and controls from the same source population, establishing the temporal order of exposure and disease, and preventing a kind of differential misclassification in which the measurement of the exposure is linked to disease status. In chapters 17 and 18, we return to considering the logic of the design in more depth, and draw from it some practical guidelines for conducting case-control studies of mental disorders. Part V takes up the use of these guidelines in the context of biologi-cal psychiatry, one important domain where investigators often compare cases and controls but do not often utilize the principles developed for these designs in epidemiology.

Kinship of Cohort and Case-Control Studies

The case-control study appears at first glance to be precisely the converse of the cohort study. In a cohort study, we start with a group of people who are free of the disease and classify them as exposed or unexposed. We then compare the occurrence of disease in each exposure group. By contrast, in a case-control study, we select people with (cases) and without the disease (controls) and then compare prior exposure status in each outcome group.

But this appearance of contrast is deceptive. As we explained in chapter 6, the case-control and cohort designs are logically connected. In fact, the case-control design can be thought of as an efficient way to sample an underlying cohort. A case-control study can recreate the result that would have been obtained in a counterpart cohort study. Thus, the case-control and cohort studies can be seen as alternative pathways to reach the same endpoint. The case-control pathway is the more efficient: we attain the result in less time, with fewer study subjects, and at lower cost than in the cohort study. The design is particularly well suited for studying the causes of rare disorders, which pose difficulties for cohort studies because a very large population has to be followed to obtain sufficient numbers of cases.

On the other hand, the case-control approach is beset by more potential pitfalls and answers a narrower range of questions. It will yield the same result as the cohort study, as in principle it should, only when certain conditions are met. In addition, it yields only relative measures of effect, such as the odds ratio (see chapter 8).

The kinship between the two designs is most readily appreciated from the standpoint of the **nested case-control study**. This is a case-control study developed within a defined cohort, from which both the cases and the controls are selected. Understanding the nested case-control study helps uncover the logic of all types of case-control studies. Although initially we present this design as an intermediate step from the cohort to the case-control study, later in the chapter we show that the nested case-control study is an important design in its own right.

Nested Case-Control Study

The nested case-control study proceeds in the order that its name implies— we first create the nest, then select the cases, and lastly select the controls. The nest we create is a cohort study. An exposed and an unexposed group are followed over a specified time period (or risk period) to determine who develops the disease (the cases) and who does not (the noncases). Then we select the cases for the case-control study from the cases in the underlying cohort, or nest. Typically, we want to use all of the cases because they are relatively rare. We monitor the cohort members, and when someone gets the disease we select him or her as a case for our study.

Next the controls are selected from the noncases in the nest. Although, generally, the cases are scarce, potential controls are available in excess. The efficiency of the nested case-control study resides in using only a limited number of the available noncases as our controls yet obtaining an equivalent result to that of the cohort study.

How is it possible to obtain an equivalent result? In a case-control study, we cannot estimate the risk of disease in the exposed and in the unexposed as is required for the risk ratio. Nor can we estimate the odds of disease in the exposed and in the unexposed as required for the disease odds ratio. We can, however, estimate the odds of exposure in the cases and in the noncases as is required for the **exposure odds ratio** (i.e., the odds of exposure in cases divided by odds of exposure in noncases). This is sufficient because the disease odds ratio and the exposure odds ratio in the cohort are alternative ways of denoting the same effect (see chapter 8; see also the examples below). If we can estimate the exposure odds ratio, we have also estimated the disease odds ratio. The identity of these two odds ratios provides the key to the use of the case-control design.

In a nested case-control study, the odds of exposure in the cases is obtained directly (if the nested case-control study uses all the cases in the cohort). The odds of exposure in the noncases is estimated by drawing a sample of the noncases and using this sample to estimate the odds of exposure for all non-cases. So long as this sample—which we call our *control group*—gives us an accurate estimate of the odds of exposure in all the noncases, the odds ratio will be the same in our nested-case control as would be obtained from a study of the entire cohort. Yet we will have arrived at this result in a far more economical way, using only a fraction of the noncases.

Study Example

We can illustrate the equivalence of the results of the cohort and the nested case-control design, and the relative economy of the latter, using the data of the Prenatal Determinants of Schizophrenia Example (PDSE) study. We adopted the PDSE as an ongoing example partly because the data collected from this study allow for analysis by both the cohort and the nested case-control approaches. Thus, we can demonstrate how the cohort and the nested case-control designs can give equivalent results.

Before proceeding to the example, we should note that there are actually several variants of the case-control study and the odds ratio. In our example we use a design in which cases are collected in an ongoing way over the follow-up period. We compute the traditional odds ratio as described in chapter 8, based only on the individuals whose outcomes are known by the end of the study. In the context of a cohort study, this means that we exclude individuals lost to follow-up and competing risks. In the context of a nested case-control study, this means that the cases are compared with controls who do not have the disease at the end of the risk period. In chapter 18, we will introduce the **concurrent** or **incidence density odds ratio**, which enables us to use the information from the individuals who do not complete the study.

Recall that in the PDSE we examined exposure to high maternal body mass index as a risk factor for schizophrenia spectrum disorder (SSD) in a birth cohort (for a summary of the PDSE, see tables 10.6 and 10.7). Since we are computing the traditional odds ratio, we exclude the individuals lost to observation. In the PDSE, this means that we use the 60 cases ascertained over the entire period of follow-up and the 3,375 noncases who remained under observation at the end of the risk period.

Table 15.1 PDSE Cohort Study: Traditional Odds Ratio

	Schizophrenia Spectrum Disorder +	Schizophrenia Spectrum Disorder −	Total
Body mass index ≥ 27	A 13	B 347	360
Body mass index < 27	C 47	D 3,028	3075
Total	60	3,375	

$$\text{Disease odds ratio} = \frac{\text{Odds of disease in exposed}}{\text{Odds of disease in unexposed}}$$

$$= \frac{A}{B} \div \frac{C}{D} = \frac{13}{347} \div \frac{47}{3028} = \frac{39{,}364}{16{,}309} = \frac{AD}{BC} = 2.41.$$

$$\text{Exposure odds ratio} = \frac{\text{Odds of exposure in cases}}{\text{Odds of exposure in controls}}$$

$$= \frac{A}{C} \div \frac{B}{D} = \frac{13}{47} \div \frac{347}{3028} = \frac{39{,}364}{16{,}309} = \frac{AD}{BC} = 2.41.$$

$$\text{Disease odds ratio} = \text{Exposure odds ratio} = \frac{AD}{BC} = \frac{AD}{CB} = 2.41.$$

Note: The Prenatal Determinants of Schizophrenia Example (PDSE) cohort members were born in Oakland, California, during 1959–1967. They were enrolled in a health plan at the time of their birth, and cohort members who developed SSD were ascertained with use of the health plan registries for 1981–1997. The traditional odds ratio is computed with the 60 cases ascertained over the follow-up period, and the 3,375 noncases who were followed to the end of the study.

The results for the PDSE cohort study are displayed in Table 15.1 in a fourfold table. As explained in chapter 8, the odds of disease in the exposed can be computed from the fourfold table as A/B (13/347 = 0.0374639). The odds of disease in the unexposed can be computed as C/D (47/3028 = 0.0155217). Thus, the disease odds ratio is 0.0374639/0.0155217 = 2.41.[1] Table 15.1 also shows the computation of the exposure odds ratio from the cohort data (A/C divided by B/D) that is also 2.41.

The results for the PDSE nested case-control study are shown in Table 15.2. We used all the 60 cases of SSD in the cohort: 13 were exposed and 47 were unexposed. Hence A/C, the odds of exposure among the cases, is 13/47 = 0.2766.

To estimate B/D, the odds of exposure among the noncases, we drew a random sample of 360 controls (6 controls for one case) from the 3,375 non-cases. By random sample, we mean our procedure ensured that each of the 3,375 noncases had the same probability (360/3375 = 0.11) of being selected as a control. Among the 360 controls, 36 were exposed and 324 were unex-

---

[1] In the numeric calculations, we include the number of decimal places necessary for readers to reproduce our results.

Table 15.2 PDSE Nested Case-Control Study: Traditional Odds Ratio Using All Cases, and a Random Sample or Noncases as Controls

	Schizophrenia Spectrum Disorder +	Schizophrenia Spectrum Disorder −	Total
Body mass index ≥ 27	A 13	B 36	49
Body mass index < 27	C 47	D 324	371
Total	60	360	

$$\text{Exposure odds in cases} = \frac{13}{47} = 0.2766.$$

$$\text{Exposure odds in controls} = \frac{36}{324} = 0.1111.$$

$$\text{Exposure odds ratio} = \frac{0.2766}{0.1111} = 2.49.$$

posed. The odds of exposure among controls was 36/324, or 0.1111. The exposure odds ratio was 0.2766/0.1111 = 2.49.

The odds ratio of 2.49 obtained from the nested case-control study is close to that of 2.41 obtained from the cohort design in the same PDSE cohort. These results underscore the economy of the nested case-control study: 360 of the 3,375 noncases produced a result very similar to that of the cohort study.

Note that the exposure odds among the controls (36/324 = 0.1111) was only slightly lower than that among all the noncases (347/3028 = 0.1146; see table 15.1). This result illustrates that the exposure odds estimated from controls selected as a random sample from all the noncases will usually be quite similar to the exposure odds for all noncases. They will not usually be identical, however, because a random sample does not eliminate chance variation (Stuart 1984). The larger the size of the random sample, the more limited the chance variation, and the more precisely the exposure odds among the controls will estimate the exposure odds among all the noncases.

Selection Bias

We proposed at the outset of the chapter that the case-control study can produce the same odds ratio as the cohort study, but with the qualification that this will happen only when certain conditions are met. The most important condition is the absence of selection bias.

In a nested case-control study that uses all the cases in the cohort, this condition will be met when the controls are a fully representative sample of all the noncases. The term *fully representative* signifies specifically that the odds of exposure among the selected controls is the same as the odds of exposure among all noncases. Then, the exposure odds ratio will be the same as the disease odds ratio obtained from the cohort study that is the nest.

One approach to obtain a fully representative sample is random sampling. The proportion of all noncases selected for the random sample does not matter, as long as the selected noncases provide an accurate estimate of the odds of exposure among all noncases. As noted previously, however, selecting a larger sample will reduce random error and yield a more precise estimate.

Nested case-control studies, however, face constraints on adopting this procedure in its entirety. The study may not be able to use all of the cases, or all of the (selected) noncases. In some studies, for example, biological samples are required to measure the exposure, but are not available for all cases and noncases. In fact, virtually every investigation entails some such restrictions.

Under these conditions, the odds of exposure in the available cases may not be the same as in all the cases. Likewise, the odds of exposure in the available noncases may not be the same as in all the noncases. In the face of this potential bias, what can we do?

In order for the nested case-control study to produce the same odds ratio as the cohort study, we attempt to balance the odds for controls relative to cases. **Balancing the odds** means that whatever constraints we are under with regard to case availability, we should impose the same constraints when we select our control group. By balancing the selection of cases and controls, we seek to neutralize the potential for selection bias.

Balanced Odds

An odds ratio is a relationship between two odds, one in the numerator and the other in the denominator. By convention, in case-control studies the exposure odds for cases is the numerator, and the exposure odds for controls is the denominator. If the odds in either the numerator or the denominator is changed, we can still obtain the original odds ratio by changing the other odds in an equivalent way.

To illustrate this, we will use a hypothetical example. Suppose that in an underlying cohort or nest, one-half of all the cases are exposed, and one-fifth of all the noncases are exposed. In the cases, the odds of exposure is $0.5/0.5 = 1.0$; and in the noncases, it is $0.2/0.8 = 0.25$. The exposure odds ratio is $1.0/0.25$, or 4.0.

We conduct a nested case-control study in this cohort. The exposure is measured by analyzing stored blood samples obtained from the members of the cohort at the start of the follow-up. Only those cohort members who gave a blood sample can be utilized in our study. To complicate matters, the exposed cases were about twice as likely to have given blood as the unexposed cases. The odds of exposure for cases giving blood is 2.0, double the true odds of exposure of 1.0 for all cases. Let us examine two possible scenarios for the controls.

Suppose first that all of the individuals who became noncases gave blood and that we select a fully representative sample to be our controls. The odds of exposure in controls will be the same as for all noncases, 0.25. The resulting exposure odds ratio is 2.0/0.25 = 8.0, a serious overestimate of the true odds ratio of 1.0/0.25 = 4.0.

Now suppose that the exposed noncases were about twice as likely to have given blood as the unexposed noncases. The odds of exposure is 0.5 for noncases giving blood, double the true odds of exposure of 0.25 for all noncases. If we select a fully representative sample of noncases giving blood to be our controls, the odds of exposure in our controls will be 0.5. We arrive at an odds ratio identical (2.0/0.5 = 4.0) to the original result. In this scenario, we subjected the controls to the same selection as the cases, thereby balancing the odds.

In real studies, we cannot know all the selection processes for cases and for noncases. Nonetheless, it is sometimes reasonable to assume that persons, some of whom later became cases and some noncases, would have experienced equivalent selection processes. In regard to the example of stored blood samples, it may be reasonable to assume that "cases to be" and "noncases to be" from the cohort were equally likely to give blood samples, provided the blood was drawn before anyone developed the disease.

It is particularly important for investigators to avoid introducing any selection process that applies unequally to cases and controls. The restrictions that are applied to cases must also be applied to controls and vice-versa. If, for example, we exclude persons with comorbid disorders from the cases, we must also exclude them from the controls, and vice-versa. Thus, procedures that are the same for cases and controls are most likely to balance the odds.

Applications of the Nested Case-Control Design

We have used the nested case-control design to explain the logic of all case-control studies because the underlying cohort from which cases and controls are selected is visible. Thus, the relationship between the cohort and case-control designs, usually hidden in ordinary case-control studies, is in evidence. The nested design has, however, a strength and elegance in its own right: it captures the efficiency of the case-control study, while avoiding many of the vulnerabilities of ordinary case-control studies to be described. It exploits the innovation of the case-control design to the fullest extent possible.

We did conduct nested case-control studies within the actual PDS cohort. For example, one such study examined prenatal exposure to influenza as a risk factor for SSD (Brown et al. 2004). We thawed the archived prenatal maternal sera from the original cohort for 64 SSD cases and 125 controls and analyzed the sera for influenza antibodies. Exposure to maternal influenza in the first half of gestation was associated with a threefold increased risk of SSD. The use of the nested case-control design preserved the unreplenishable serum samples of thousands of cohort members for future studies and greatly reduced the costs of the study.

Table 15.3 Case-Control Studies Nested in Population Cohorts

Sources	Study Description and Findings
Cannon et al. (1999)	*Study hypothesis*: School performance in childhood as a risk factor for adult schizophrenia.
	Cohort (N = 97,600): All births in Helsinki 1951–1960.
	Cases (N = 400): Ascertained through national treatment registers (1969–1991); limited to those with Helsinki school records.
	Controls (N = 408): The next or previous Helsinki-born children with Helsinki school records.
	Finding: Cases and controls differed on nonacademic (handicrafts and sports) but not academic performance (ages 7–11).
Done et al. (1994)	*Study hypothesis*: Social maladjustment in childhood as a risk factor for hospitalized psychiatric disorders.
	Cohort (N = 17,414): Births in England, Scotland, and Wales during March 3–9, 1958; follow-up in 1965, 1969, 1974 and 1981.
	Cases (N = 154): Psychiatric admissions identified in the Mental Health Enquiry national register (1974–1986); neurosis $N = 79$, schizophrenia $N = 40$, affective psychosis ($N = 35$).
	Controls (N = 1,914): 10% random sample of noncases.
	Finding: Cases of schizophrenia and neurosis, but not affective psychosis, showed greater childhood social maladjustment than controls.

The nested design requires the existence of a suitable cohort from which to draw the cases and controls. For this reason, it is feasible only in special circumstances. Yet during the past decade, the nested case-control study has found important applications in psychiatric research, and the use of this design is increasing rapidly.

Two nested case-control studies are exhibited in table 15.3. One examined social maladjustment in childhood as a risk factor for adult psychiatric disorders (Done et al. 1994). It was nested in a birth cohort established in the United Kingdom in 1958, the National Child Development Study. People hospitalized with neurosis, schizophrenia, or affective psychosis—the cases— were compared with a control group comprising 10 percent of the noncases in the cohort. The other examined elementary school performance as a risk factor for schizophrenia (Cannon et al. 1999). The cohort comprised all people born in Helsinki, Finland, between 1951 and 1960. To obtain and review elementary school records was highly labor-intensive. Limiting the control group to a small fraction of the noncases in the cohort provided a great advantage in economy.

Generalizing to Any Case-Control Study

The logic of the ordinary case-control study is the same as that of the nested case-control study, with one additional complexity: the underlying cohort in which the cases and controls are nested and from which they are sampled is not visible. This underlying cohort must be imagined.

Suppose a cohort study is beset by a sudden destruction of information. Only a list of the cases remains. The control sample must be selected, as best one can, to represent the noncases in the cohort. This scenario in fact simulates the process of selecting controls for an ordinary case-control study. We must imagine the characteristics of a hidden cohort from which the cases have been drawn and select controls to represent such a population.

Examine the scenario in table 15.4. We aim to investigate exposure to sexual abuse in childhood as a risk factor for the development of anorexia nervosa. We collect data on a cohort of 20,000 people. However, before we can analyze the data, all the information is destroyed in a fire, except for the list of cases. To recreate the unknown results, we conduct a case-control study.

Capital letters denote the cells of the fourfold table (A, B, C, and D) in the underlying cohort (table 15.4A). This is the information that has been destroyed and is not available to us. As noted earlier, the odds ratio can be

Table 15.4 Hypothetical Case-Control Study of Exposure to Sexual Abuse in Childhood and Development of Anorexia Nervosa

A. UNDERLYING COHORT

	Anorexia Nervosa +	Anorexia Nervosa −	Total
Abused	A 150	B 9,850	10,000
Nonabused	C 50	D 9,950	10,000
Total	200	19,800	

$$\text{Exposure odds ratio} = \frac{A}{C} \div \frac{B}{D} = \frac{150}{50} \div \frac{9850}{9950} = 3.0.$$

$$\text{Disease odds ratio} = \frac{A}{B} \div \frac{C}{D} = \frac{150}{9850} \div \frac{50}{9950} = 3.0.$$

B. CASE-CONTROL STUDY FROM UNDERLYING COHORT: 10% OF NONCASES SELECTED AS CONTROLS

	Anorexia Nervosa +	Anorexia Nervosa −	Total
Abused	a 150	b 985	1,135
Nonabused	c 50	d 995	1,045
Total	200	1,980	

$$\text{Odds ratio} = \frac{a}{c} \div \frac{b}{d} = \frac{150}{50} \div \frac{9850 \times 0.1}{9950 \times 0.1} = 3.0.$$

expressed in two equivalent ways: either as the odds of exposure in the diseased (A/C) divided by the odds of exposure in the nondiseased (B/D), or as the odds of disease in the exposed (A/B) divided by the odds of disease in the unexposed (C/D). Both expressions reduce to the cross product AD/BC. If we were to study the entire cohort, the computed odds ratio would be $AD/BC = 3$ (table 15.4A).

We use lowercase letters (a, b, c, and d) to denote the corresponding cells of the fourfold table in our case-control study. Since the list of cases is complete, the ratio of exposed to unexposed among our cases (a/c) will equal the ratio of exposed to unexposed among all cases in the cohort (A/C), since they are the same people.

The controls are still to be selected from noncases. However, we have lost the information about the cohort. We cannot simply select a sample from the noncases, because we do not know who they are. We are compelled to imagine a preexisting lost cohort and take a sample for our controls. If we are skilled enough to imagine the cohort correctly and take a representative sample of the noncases for controls, the ratio of exposed to unexposed controls (b/d) will recreate the ratio of exposed to unexposed noncases in the cohort (B/D). We will recreate the odds ratio that would have been obtained with the entire underlying cohort. Table 15.4B illustrates this result for a 10 percent sample of the noncases.

Source Population

In a nested case-control study, the concepts of source population and study population (as defined in chapter 9) are meaningful and help identify sources of bias. We can trace the entire process of selection up to the final sample of cases and controls. First, in some studies, especially in psychiatric epidemiology, the source population may be selected from a naturally occurring population; for instance, the source population may be a random sample of people living in a community. Second, the study population for the cohort is selected from the source population; it comprises only the individuals who actually participate in the cohort study. Third, a subset may be selected from the total cohort to serve as the underlying cohort for the nested case-control study–for instance, those who gave blood samples. Fourth, from the underlying cohort, we derive the cases and controls.

In an ordinary case-control study, however, these distinctions are less readily applicable. Generally we attempt to directly visualize a naturally occurring source population from which the cases originate. In the next chapter, therefore, we will overlook these distinctions and use the term *source population* to refer to the population that gave rise to the cases. Nonetheless, it is important to be aware of these distinctions, and we will return to consider their implications in chapter 18.

Conclusion

The relation of the case-control to the cohort study is transparent for nested case-control studies. It is less so for ordinary case-control studies. Nonetheless, the same principles introduced for the nested case-control design apply to the more complex ordinary case-control study. Understanding how, in a nested case-control design, sampling can distort the exposure odds ratio also makes explicit the main assumptions of any case-control study and shows how violating the assumptions can create bias. In fact, in any case-control study we should always be undertaking the intellectual exercise of visualizing cases and noncases as being sampled from a source population (or underlying cohort), even if the cohort is hypothetical.

Finally, it should be kept in mind that noncomparability between the exposed and unexposed already present in the source population will be reproduced in a case-control study. We have discussed only how to avoid introducing further bias in the process of selecting cases and controls. The procedures used in case-control studies for dealing with noncomparability in the source population are discussed in chapter 18.

References

Beal SM and Finch CF (1991). An Overview of Retrospective Case-Control Studies Investigating the Relationship between Prone Sleeping Position and SIDS. *J. Paediatr. Child Health* 27:334–339.

Brown AS, Begg MD, Gravenstein S, Schaefer CA, Wyatt RJ, Bresnahan M, Babulas VP, and Susser ES (2004). Serologic Evidence of Prenatal Influenza in the Etiology of Schizophrenia. *Arch. Gen. Psychiatry* 61:774–780.

Cannon M, Jones P, Huttunen MO, Tanskanen A, Huttunen T, Rabe-Hesketh S, and Murray RM (1999). School Performance in Finnish Children and Later Development of Schizophrenia: A Population-Based Longitudinal Study. *Arch. Gen. Psychiatry* 56:457–463.

Doll R and Hill AB (1950). Smoking and Carcinoma of the Lung. *BMJ* 2:739–748.

Done DJ, Crow TJ, Johnstone EC, and Sacker A (1994). Childhood Antecedents of Schizophrenia and Affective Illness: Social Adjustment at Ages 7 and 11. *BMJ* 309:699–703.

Jaffe HW, Choi K, Thomas PA, et al. (1983). National Case-Control Study of Kaposi's Sarcoma and Pneumocystis Carinii Pneumonia in Homosexual Men: Part 1. Epidemiologic Results. *Ann. Intern. Med.* 99:145–151.

Paneth N, Susser E, and Susser M (2004). Origins and Early Development of the Case-Control Study. In Morabia A, ed. *History of Epidemiologic Methods and Concepts*, 291–311. Boston: Birkhauser.

Stuart A (1984). *The Idea of Sampling.* New York: Oxford University Press.

16 Applications of the Case-Control Study

Evelyn J. Bromet, Alfredo Morabia, Nancy Sohler and Ezra Susser

We have proposed that the case-control study offers a more efficient but more hazardous path to the same result as a cohort study. To explain the efficiency, we focused on its logic. To describe the hazards, we need to consider the practical problems of execution.

Implementing a case-control study presents three central challenges. The first is to select cases and controls from the same source population. The investigator attempts to visualize the population that gave rise to the cases, and to select the controls appropriately from this population. The second is to establish the temporal order of exposure and disease. As opposed to the cohort study, in the case-control study the antecedence of the exposure to the disease is not established by design. The third is to obtain an unbiased measure of the exposure with information retrieved retrospectively, after the outcome is already known. The retrospective measurement presents the problem that misclassification of the exposure can be linked to the disease status.

In this chapter, we illustrate how case-control studies of psychiatric disorders have attempted to meet these challenges. Building on this foundation of illustrative material, chapters 17 and 18 revisit some of the thorniest problems. The following part of the book (chapters 19–21) considers the case-control design in the context of biological studies in psychiatry.

Selection of Cases and Controls

The starting point for a case-control study is the selection of the cases. The controls are then chosen to represent the source population from which the cases arose. The selection of a case group is guided by three basic objectives.

First, we aim for incident or new onset rather than prevalent cases. For some disorders, like first-episode mania, this aim is easier to achieve because the onset is acute rather than insidious. For other disorders, like schizophrenia, it is more difficult because the prodromal period can be very long and the onset difficult to date. We may resort to an approximate definition of incident cases, substituting the time of the first treatment contact for the time of onset. In this context, a standardized assessment of the time between the true onset and the recruitment into the study can be important for interpreting the results (Hafner et al. 1992).

Second, in studies of mental disorders we aim for longitudinal diagnoses. Although new-onset cases are essential for causal inference, the psychiatric diagnoses people receive at the time of onset are often inaccurate. Longitudinal observation tends to clarify the nature of the patient's illness (Schwartz et al. 2000). For example, patients who initially receive a diagnosis of unipolar depression may later develop a manic episode, making it clear that they actually have a bipolar disorder. This adds some complexity to the selection of cases, since the study protocol needs to specify the amount of follow-up time and the sources of information that will be considered in the final diagnosis of a case.

Third, we aim to select the cases in a way that facilitates visualization of the population from which the cases are derived, in order to guide the selection of controls. Each of three approaches to case selection—population-based (table 16.1), facility-based (table 16.2), and mixed-origin (table 16.3)—has implications for visualization of this source population and therefore for control selection.

Population-Based Selection

Ideally, in a population-based case-control study, the cases are representative of all people with new onset of the disorder (incident cases) in a defined population over a specified time period. Although this ideal is rarely attained, reasonable approximations can be found. Pioneering this approach, R. G. Record and Thomas McKeown (1949, 1950) examined the causes of central nervous system malformations (table 16.1). Using the birth registers of the city of Birmingham, United Kingdom, they obtained cases by identifying all stillborn and infant deaths between 1940 and 1947 that were certified as due to central nervous system malformations. A systematic (one in 200) sample of the entire unaffected live- and still-born source population from the same city registers in the same years served as controls. In these data, an increased risk of malformation was associated with first parity and with previous malformations in offspring, but not with social status or viral infection during pregnancy. The study was limited to malformations that were fatal and, strictly speaking, used prevalent not incident cases in that the condition was present during gestation (Kline et al. 1989). Nonetheless, this innovative work set the stage for decades of subsequent research on congenital malformations (Leck 1996), as well as for the development of population-based case-control studies (Paneth et al. 2004).

Studies of mental disorders that approximate population-based case selection are usually based in registries and therefore are limited to treated cases. They also include studies of suicide based in a mortality index, with the limitation that not all suicides are recognized and recorded as such. Still another alternative is to derive the cases from a survey of mental disorders in a defined community, which allows for inclusion of untreated cases but captures mainly prevalent rather than incident cases.

A case-control study of obstetric complications as a risk factor for mania drew cases from the Dublin Psychiatric Case Register (table 16.1; Browne et al. 2000). This registry includes all contacts with psychiatric services in a well-defined area. Cases were all patients in the registry who were born in Dublin and were newly diagnosed with mania between 1972 and 1986. Controls were chosen from births in the same hospitals and years, matched on gender, maternal age, maternal parity, and paternal occupation. Similar proportions of obstetric complications were found in cases and controls.

Although population-based case selection means that the cases are ascertained in a well-defined population, this need not be a natural community such as a city or neighborhood. The population may also be defined as people sharing the same health services. In a precedent setting study, Shepherd et al. (1966) drew both the psychiatric cases and the comparison group from the service lists of general practitioners in the London area during the years 1961 and 1962 (table 16.1). They showed that treatment proportions for physical illness were higher in cases than in controls. Following and refining this precedent, many European studies of psychiatric disorders have been based in service lists of general practitioners.

Table 16.1 Case-Control Studies Using Population-Based Cases

Study	Study Description and Findings
Browne et al. (2000)	*Study question*: Obstetric complications as a risk factor for later mania.
	Cases (N = 76): Patients with mania diagnosed 1972–1986 identified in the Dublin Psychiatric Case Register and born in Dublin.
	Controls (N = 76): From persons born in same hospitals in Dublin in same years matched to cases on gender and other factors.
	Finding: Obstetric complications were not risk factors for later mania.
Record and McKeown (1949)	*Study question*: Risk factors for fatal congenital central nervous system (CNS) malformations.
	Cases (N = 755): All stillbirths and infant deaths due to CNS malformations recorded in municipal health department records, 1940–1947, Birmingham, United Kingdom
	Controls (N = 742): Every 200th live birth and stillbirth without CNS malformations registered during the same years.
	Finding: Parity and previous malformations in offspring were risk factors for CNS malformations.
Shepherd et al. (1966); Shepherd (1973)	*Study question*: Whether physical illness is more common among people with mental disorder.
	Cases (N = 2,049): Individuals with mental disorders were selected from a large representative group from a general practice.
	Controls (N = 6,894): Individuals without mental disorders were selected from the same general practice group.
	Finding: Treatment for some kinds of physical illness was more common in cases than in controls.

In the United States, an increasingly common approach is to identify cases from the registries maintained by a health insurance plan or health maintenance organization. An example is the Prenatal Determinants of Schizophrenia Example study described in the previous chapter. Under this design, cases may be identified either when they use one of the health plan's own services, or when they request reimbursement for use of another service.

Studies based in health services span a wide range. The cases may be workers referred to employee assistance programs in large corporations, children referred to school-based counseling programs, or college students treated at a student health center. These studies vary in the degree to which they conform to population-based case selection. The designation is most apt when virtually all the treated cases in the population covered by the health service can be identified.

In some contexts, this condition may be approximately met. General practitioners in a national health service, or certain kinds of prepaid health plans, might identify the vast majority of the treated cases among the enrolled population. In other contexts, however, it is not approximately met. People who could use psychiatric services based in workplaces or schools may instead go elsewhere to avoid being identified as having a mental disorder. In the United States, war veterans are entitled to health care programs offered by the Veterans Administration, but often choose to enroll in private health plans instead. When a study selects cases from a health service that identifies only some of the treated cases in the population covered, it conforms better to facility-based case selection.

Facility-Based Selection

Many investigators identify cases in clinics or hospitals without any well-defined catchment population. In these circumstances, visualizing the appropriate source population is much more difficult. We cannot enumerate the source population that controls should represent, and their selection accordingly becomes more complex.

Most often, the controls are patients admitted to the same clinic or hospital within the same period as the cases, but for a different disease. This approach assumes that patients admitted with the disease of the cases originate in the same source population as patients admitted with the disease of the controls. This assumption is not always realistic. The populations making use of the facility for different diseases may well be different. Consider U.S. teaching hospitals that treat both common and rare disorders. The catchment area for a common disorder is likely to be local. Renowned specialists in rare disorders, on the other hand, are likely to draw patients from across the United States, as well as other countries. Thus, the source populations for patients with a rare disorder and patients with a common disorder may be far from comparable even when both groups are treated in the same teaching hospital.

A multicenter case-control study of risk factors for injury from domestic violence exemplifies the challenges that researchers face (table 16.2; Kyriacou

Table 16.2 Case-Control Studies Using Facility-Based Cases

Study	Study Description and Findings
Graves et al. (1990)	*Study question*: Risk factors for Alzheimer's disease.
	Cases (N = 130): Patients diagnosed with Alzheimer's disease between 1980 and 1985 at two clinics.
	Controls (N = 130): Friends or nonbiological relatives of the cases.
	Finding: Head trauma was a risk factor for Alzheimer's disease (also family history; see chapter 30).
Kyriacou et al. (1999)	*Study question*: Risk factors for domestic violence.
	Cases (N = 282): Women who had been physically assaulted or injured by their male partners, recruited between 1997 and 1998 from eight university-affiliated emergency departments throughout the United States.
	Controls (N = 749): Consecutive female patients seen in the same emergency departments for other conditions (and with current or recent male partners, but no history of assault by these partners).
	Finding: Partner substance abuse and unemployment were risk factors for domestic violence.

et al. 1999). Cases were battered women intentionally injured by their male partners and treated in one of eight emergency departments across the United States. Controls were women seen for other reasons in the same emergency departments. The study found that the cases were more likely to be with partners who were substance abusers and unemployed than were the controls.

The study was well designed but still not immune to bias. Its validity rested on the assumption that women treated for these different conditions at the same emergency departments arose from the same populations. This assumption would be violated if the battered women (cases), desiring anonymity, avoided nearby emergency departments, whereas the women seen for other reasons (controls) did not.

Studies that use facility-based case groups sometimes use other kinds of control groups. In a study showing that head trauma was a significant risk factor for Alzheimer's disease, cases were identified at two clinics in Washington State (table 16.2; Graves et al. 1990). Controls were chiefly friends of the cases. Here the assumption is that the friends represent people who would use the same clinic if they developed Alzheimer's disease. (This design also matches controls to the social milieu of cases; see chapter 18.)

Such assumptions are difficult to verify. Nonetheless, an approach using explicit, if uncertain, assumptions about selection bias is much more likely to protect against it than an approach that altogether neglects the issue.

Mixed-Origin Selection

Some important psychiatric research questions require studies with case groups of mixed-origin for which it is virtually impossible to define any single, discrete source population. Such a case group might be clustered within a single locale but originate in diverse communities. We have described the potential diversity of a rare disease case group from a teaching hospital that might include cases from far-flung places. Similarly, a case group of runaway youth in an urban shelter for homeless children is likely to include children who migrated from many different communities. When one uses such case groups, the population that should be represented by the controls is far from evident.

A study of people with untreated drug abuse disorders in Rio de Janeiro, Brazil, exemplifies a mixed-origin case group (table 16.3; Lopes et al. 1996). Cases were recruited with the "snowball" method. Each case was asked to identify a friend case, that is, a friend who was a drug abuser not in treatment; the friend case was in turn asked to identify another friend case, and so forth. (Cases identified by this method are likely to be prevalent rather than incident cases.)

Given the heterogeneous population that gave rise to the cases in this study, the options for control groups were limited. The solution adopted was creative and as good as could be hoped for. The study used the same snowball method to identify friend-controls. Cases were also asked to identify noncase friends, and these noncase friends were in turn asked to identify other noncase friends. The findings suggested that prior alcoholism and early-onset psychiatric disorder were risk factors for later substance abuse.

Table 16.3 Case-Control Studies Using Mixed-Origin Cases

Study	Study Description and Findings
Lopes et al. (1996)	*Study question*: Psychiatric disorders and alcohol disorders as risk factors for drug abuse or dependence.
	Cases (N = 185): Persons abusing drugs and not in treatment, identified through a snowball approach, Jan.–July 1992 in Rio de Janeiro, Brazil.
	Controls (N = 185): Friends of drug abusers, who did not meet current or lifetime diagnostic criteria for drug abuse or dependence, also identified through a snowball approach.
	Finding: Prior alcohol dependence and early onset psychiatric disorder were risk factors for later substance abuse.
Susser et al. (1991)	*Study question*: Examined childhood experiences as risk factors for adult homelessness in psychiatric patients.
	Cases (N = 512): Three samples of homeless patients: (1) admitted to state hospital; (2) under psychiatric care in a shelter; (3) brought by outreach teams to a city hospital for involuntary admission.
	Controls (N = 271): Patients admitted to a state hospital who had never been homeless.
	Finding: Childhood experiences with foster care, group home placement, and running away, were risk factors for adult homelessness in psychiatric patients.

A study of adverse childhood experience as a risk factor for adult homelessness among psychiatric patients in New York provides another example (table 16.3; Susser et al. 1991). Although homelessness is not a disorder, the study can be framed as a comparison of cases (people with the outcome under study) with controls. To encompass various kinds of homelessness, the study included three case groups: patients brought to a city psychiatric hospital involuntarily after being assessed in the streets by special outreach teams, patients receiving psychiatric care in a municipal shelter, and patients reporting a history of homelessness on routine admission to a state psychiatric hospital. Only the latter case group yielded a corresponding control group: patients admitted to the state hospital without a history of homelessness. The other case groups were drawn from such diverse origins that there was no ready answer to control selection. A further constraint in this study was that the homeless patients were prevalent rather than incident cases of homelessness.

Establishing Temporal Order

The centrality of temporal order to causal inference can hardly be exaggerated. Unless the time sequence of associated variables can be established, which variable is the cause and which the effect remains open to question. We illustrated this point in part II, with the example of social class and schizophrenia.

In a cohort study, the temporal order of exposure and disease is inherent in the longitudinal construction of the design. The exposure will be on record before the advent (or at least the ascertainment) of the disease. In contrast, in a case-control study, the exposure is measured after the presence of disease is known. The exposure may plausibly be a consequence rather than a cause of the disease. Any case-control study sound enough to permit a causal inference must establish that the assumed cause preceded the assumed outcome.

Studies sometimes tailor the assessment of the exposure to reduce the potential for mistaking consequences for causes. This strategy was used in a study of stressful life events as a risk factor for depression (Brown and Harris 1978). Cases were women being treated for depression in hospitals and general practices in the neighborhood of Camberwell, London. (This otherwise well-conceived study used prevalent, as well as incident, cases.) Controls were selected from two random samples of women living in the Camberwell neighborhood. The investigators, well aware that adverse life events might be a consequence, as well as a cause, of depression, developed an interview protocol that restricted reports of life events to a defined interval: for cases, the year before the onset of depression; and for controls, the year prior to the interview. To assist recall, the interviewer established a timeline over the weeks of the relevant year, and the elicited events were anchored to the timeline. The interviews were tape recorded, and the actual coding of the nature and timing of events was done by raters who were blind to case-control status.

The findings pointed to the important role of threatening life events in the onset of depression in women who had three or more children under age 6 in the home, who lost a parent early in life, who had no male confidant, or who were not employed outside the home.

While temporal ordering is difficult in all case-control studies, diseases without clear onset, like many psychiatric disorders, exacerbate the problem. Many psychiatric disorders have an insidious onset, so the early manifestations may be present and precede the time of secure diagnosis by months or years. Before the disorder is diagnosable, premorbid signs and symptoms might in fact generate the exposure being investigated. Once the disorder is diagnosable, an interval may yet precede actual diagnosis. When, as is common, diagnosis depends upon treatment, such an interval might stretch into months or years. And when a study enlists prevalent cases, a further interval will separate the time of diagnosis from recruitment. Because the time frame over which the disease progresses from its first manifestation until disease detection is long, so too is the period of recall for the exposure and the disease onset. The potential for recalling incorrectly the timing of the exposure and disease onset further clouds the temporal order. These complexities are illustrated in figure 16.1.

The case-control study in Rio de Janeiro illustrates the difficulties of establishing the time order (table 16.3; Lopes et al. 1996). The researchers, interested in determining the relation of alcohol abuse or dependence to drug abuse or dependence, were aware that either disorder could be cause or consequence. If recall of the times of onset of the two conditions were hazy or faulty, the true time order could well be reversed. To determine the times of onset, the researchers relied on the Composite International Diagnostic Interview. Like most diagnostic interviews, this instrument has well-established reliability for diagnosis but not for time of onset. The necessary use of prevalent cases, as already noted, made the task still more difficult.

In the extreme, when a condition unfolds over the life course, without any clear transition between health and disease, the case-control study may be inapplicable. The time order of causes and manifestations cannot be mean-

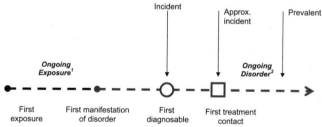

Figure 16.1 Interval from exposure to case ascertainment in a case-control study. Exposure is not assessed until the time of case ascertainment in a case-control study. The interval creates the potential for mistaking the temporal order of exposure and disease as explained in the text. (1) Exposure may be at one point in time, or it may be ongoing, possibly with cumulative effects. (2) Recovery from disorder may occur at any point after it is first diagnosable. Recovery may also be followed by relapse.

ingfully established. An example would be a study of a temperament characteristic that begins in early childhood but has different presentations over the life course.

Differential Misclassification

The exposure information in a case-control study can be collected by a variety of means, including interviews, reviews of existing records, analysis of biological samples, clinical examination, an array of focused special tests, or all of these combined. Whatever means are employed, the exposure information is retrieved after the disease outcome is known. Thus, the measurement of the exposure could be influenced by the presence or absence of the disease or its premorbid manifestations. This is the kind of potential differential misclassification most germane to case-control studies.

Differential misclassification represents an alternative explanation for an observed association between exposure and disease. It is analogous to the exposure's influencing the measurement of the outcome in a cohort study (see chapter 14). Indeed, it is simply the reverse; instead of the outcome measurement's being biased by knowledge of the exposure, the exposure measurement is biased by knowledge of the outcome.

Misclassification can be subtly intrusive in a case-control study. Disease status might lead to bias in measurement of the exposure in several ways. First, the investigator, believing that the exposure causes the disease, may look harder for the exposure in cases than in controls. To alleviate this problem, some studies devise a measurement protocol in which the exposure information is collected "blind" to the research hypothesis. To the extent possible, the exposure information should be collected blind to the presence or absence of disease in the study subject, as well.

Second, when exposure information is collected by interviews, **recall bias** may intrude: cases may be influenced by their disease experience to recall the nature or the timing of exposures differently from controls.[1] Diseased subjects tend to be eager to find a cause for their illness and may scrutinize memory for past exposure more intensively than controls. Their doctors, too, are likely to have prompted them to search their memory for exposure to known or suspected causes.

One way to limit recall bias is to choose controls from persons being treated for a disease other than the one being studied. Treated cases and treated controls are more likely to have undergone the same memory search process. For example, both cases and controls with (different) psychiatric disorders might scan their memories for adverse childhood experiences they suspect to be causes of psychological problems.

Third, the context or locale in which an interview takes place can affect the answers given to the interviewer. The context may well be determined by

---

[1] Recent findings in neuroscience suggest that some types of recall bias may have a neurobiological basis in the recreation and recategorization of groups of neurons following new experiences (Schacter 1996; Loftus 1997; Schacter 2001).

the presence of disease. For example, cases but not controls may have to be interviewed in the hospital rather than at home. Thus, conditions for interviewing should be as similar as possible for cases and controls. From this standpoint, patients under treatment are best compared with controls under treatment. Hospitalized controls can be interviewed like hospitalized cases; outpatient clinic controls, like outpatient clinic cases.

Fourth, the disorder being studied may itself impair the amount and accuracy of information provided about exposures. Many psychiatric disorders are associated with cognitive impairments or distortions. The study of head trauma as a risk factor for Alzheimer's disease provides an example (table 16.2; Graves et al. 1990). Since people with Alzheimer's disease were bound to have poor recollection of the exposure to head trauma, the authors turned to surrogate informants (usually spouses) to obtain the exposure history on cases and therefore used surrogate informants for the controls, as well.

In the extreme, in studies of completed suicide, no case is living to provide information. The investigator's only resort is to obtain the exposure information from records and from surrogate informants such as friends, relatives, or neighbors. In general, the same procedures should be used for the control group to ensure equivalence of the information for cases and controls. Thus, in a study of completed versus attempted adolescent suicide (Brent et al. 1988), the cases were compared with control youths hospitalized for suicide attempts. Exposure histories of both the cases and controls were obtained by means of so-called psychological autopsies, based on interviewing people who knew the (deceased) case or (living) control, in this study mainly parents. Compared to hospital controls, more of the suicide victims had a family history of bipolar disorder, no previous mental health treatment, and access to firearms in the home.

Differential misclassification of exposure can also work in the opposite direction. It can be responsible for masking or attenuating an association. This could happen, for example, if the cases, but not controls, are loath to report past exposures that could have been avoided. This type of misclassification would decrease the relationship between the exposure and disease.

Finally, it should always be kept in mind that if both cases and controls have inaccurate, but equal, recall of exposure, the resulting nondifferential misclassification can still bias measures of association toward the null value (see chapter 8). Indeed, equalizing the exposure measures for cases and controls by downgrading the quality of the measure in one group can increase nondifferential misclassification.

Conclusion

The case-control study is a powerful and effective design that can circumvent the inefficiencies of a cohort study. However, the efficiency comes at a cost. Difficulties in imagining and therefore sampling from the source population, establishing temporal order, and avoiding contamination of the exposure measure by the disease status pose challenges for the case-control design. In addition, because the study design begins with the selection of cases, unanticipated outcomes of the exposures cannot be examined. The exposure and disease under investigation, the specific causal ideas being tested, and the population under investigation can make these problems potent or benign. Each situation needs to be considered on its own merits. When the efficiency of the case-control study is unalloyed by additional biases it may be a virtually ideal design choice.

References

Brent DA, Perper JA, Goldstein CE, Kolko DJ, Allan MJ, Allman CJ, and Zelenak JP (1988). Risk Factors for Adolescent Suicide. A Comparison of Adolescent Suicide Victims with Suicidal Inpatients. *Arch. Gen. Psychiatry* 45:581–588.

Brown GW and Harris T (1978). *Social Origins of Depression: A Study of Psychiatric Disorder in Women.* New York: Free Press.

Browne R, Byrne M, Mulryan N, Scully A, Morris M, Kinsella A, McNeil TF, Walsh D, and O'Callaghan E (2000). Labour and Delivery Complications at Birth and Later Mania. An Irish Case Register Study. *Br. J. Psychiatry* 176:369–372.

Graves AB, White E, Koepsell TD, Reifler BV, van Belle G, Larson EB, and Raskind M (1990). The Association Between Head Trauma and Alzheimer's Disease. *Am. J. Epidemiol.* 131:491–501.

Hafner H, Riecher-Rossler A, Hambrecht M, Maurer K, Meissner S, Schmidtke A, Fatkenheuer B, Loffler W, and van der HW (1992). IRAOS: an Instrument for the Assessment of Onset and Early Course of Schizophrenia. *Schizophr. Res.* 6:209–223.

Kline J, Stein ZA, and Susser MW (1989). *Conception to Birth: Epidemiology of Prenatal Development.* New York: Oxford University Press.

Kyriacou DN, Anglin D, Taliaferro E, Stone S, Tubb T, Linden JA, Muelleman R, Barton E, and Kraus JF (1999). Risk Factors for Injury to Women from Domestic Violence against Women. *N. Engl. J. Med.* 341:1892–1898.

Leck I (1996). McKeown, Record, and the Epidemiology of Malformations. *Paediatr. Perinat. Epidemiol.* 10:2–16.

Loftus EF (1997). Creating False Memories. *Sci. Am.* 277:70–75.

Lopes CS, Lewis G, and Mann A (1996). Psychiatric and Alcohol Disorders as Risk Factors for Drug Abuse. A Case-Control Study among Adults in Rio De Janeiro, Brazil. *Soc. Psychiatry Psychiatr. Epidemiol.* 31:355–363.

Paneth N, Susser E, and Susser M (2004). Origins and Early Development of the Case-Control Study. In Morabia A, ed. *History of Epidemiologic Methods and Concepts.* Boston: Birkhauser, pp 291–312.

Record RG and McKeown T (1949). Congenital Malformations of the Central Nervous System: I. A Survey of 930 Cases. *Br. J. Soc. Med.* 3:183–219.

Record RG and McKeown T (1950). Congenital Malformations of the Central Nervous System: II. Maternal Reproductive History and Familial Incidence. *Br. J. Soc. Med.* 4:26–40.

Schacter DL (1996). *Searching for Memory.* New York: Basic Books.

Schacter DL (2001). *The Seven Sins of Memory: How the Mind Forgets and Remembers.* Boston: Houghton Mifflin.

Schwartz JE, Fennig S, Tanenberg-Karant M, Carlson G, Craig T, Galambos N, Lavelle J, and Bromet EJ (2000). Congruence of Diagnoses 2 Years after a First-Admission Diagnosis of Psychosis. *Arch. Gen. Psychiatry* 57:593–600.

Shepherd M (1973). The Prevalence and Distribution of Psychiatric Illness in General Practice. *J. R. Coll. Gen. Pract.* 23 (Suppl 2):16–22.

Shepherd M, Cooper B, Brown AC, and Kalton G (1966). *Psychiatric Illness in General Practice.* New York: Oxford University Press.

Susser ES, Lin SP, Conover SA, Struening EL (1991). Childhood Antecedents of Homelessness in Psychiatric Patients. *Am. J. Psychiatry* 148:1026–1030.

Choosing Controls

17

Sharon Schwartz, Alfredo Morabia, and Ezra Susser

This chapter sharpens the focus to a central pitfall of case-control studies in psychiatric research: selecting valid controls. We revisit the logic of control selection and the guideline of balancing the odds. We propose that this guideline can be used to operationalize the selection of controls in almost any context. We show a practical application by taking up the problem of control selection in the context of comorbid disorders, a central dilemma for psychiatric case-control studies.

Balancing the Odds

The odds ratio from a case-control study is the ratio of the exposure odds in cases (the numerator) to the exposure odds in controls (the denominator). Balancing the odds means that if we change the numerator we also change the denominator in an equivalent way. This will restore the odds ratio to its original value (see chapter 15).

The practical guideline for balancing the odds can be stated concisely as follows: impose the same restrictions on controls as were imposed on cases. We will develop more fully the rationale for this guideline to prepare the ground for practical application. To do so, we must revisit the issue of case ascertainment. This issue is salient in psychiatric research because for some mental disorders the ascertained cases may represent only a minority of the people who develop the disease.

Consider the study of obstetric complications as a risk factor for mania, described in the previous chapter (table 16.1; Browne et al. 2000). This was a population-based case-control study that drew cases from the Dublin Psychiatric Case Register and controls from individuals born in the same hospitals during the same years as the cases. Thus, the researchers attempted to draw the controls from the source population of the cases. The ascertained cases, however, were not all the individuals in Dublin who developed mania. They were restricted to those treated for mania. No equivalent restriction was placed on the controls to balance the odds. This would result in a bias if the exposure (obstetric complications) were associated with receiving treatment for the disorder (mania).

As explained in chapter 14, the same bias can affect cohort studies. In cohort studies with ongoing case ascertainment by a registry, the cases are ascertained as a result of their receiving treatment for their disorder. We usually cannot identify and measure the factors that determine whether an individual is treated for a disorder. Therefore, the outcome actually studied in such cohorts is developing the disease and being treated for it.

In a population-based case-control study, restriction to treated cases has similar implications. Typically, in this kind of case-control design we are actually studying risk factors for onset and treatment of the disorder. However, the source population is readily visualized, and the **ascertainment bias** is evident.

Now consider the facility-based case-control study of victims of domestic violence in the United States, which was also described in the previous chapter (table 16.2; Kyriacou et al. 1999). The study cases were battered women seen at eight emergency departments, and the controls were women treated for other conditions at the same emergency departments. Because cases and controls were being treated at the same emergency departments, this design potentially equated cases and controls on factors leading to treatment.

Under the facility-based design, however, it is difficult to visualize the source population for the cases, and one cannot be certain that cases and controls were selected into treatment in the same way. In this study of battered women, the investigators could not know all the factors determining which populations of women would be treated for which conditions at the specific emergency department where a case was ascertained. As explained in the previous chapter, it is possible that the cases and controls in this study were drawn from different populations even though they were treated at the same emergency departments. This possibility illustrates that, even though the facility-based design has the potential to equate cases and controls on selection into treatment, it is difficult to do so in practice, because different factors may select cases and controls into the same facility.

In such complex scenarios, the guidelines of balancing the odds help us to develop operational criteria for the selection of valid controls. By systematically considering the ways in which the cases were selected into treatment, we can derive criteria for controls that reproduce this selection process insofar as possible. We may even stipulate a selection for cases in order to reproduce the same selection for controls.

Suppose that in a study of battered women treated in an emergency department, we stipulated that all the cases must come from the local county. Since the cases would be restricted to one county, the controls would be selected with the same restriction. This procedure of balancing the odds would improve the chances of choosing controls that represent the source population of cases.

Controls as Potential Cases

In the process of applying this guideline, a subtle change in the meaning of a control group is introduced. Under this guideline, being a control represents the potential to be a case in the study, rather than simply the potential to develop the disease. Since the ascertained cases are restricted to persons with certain characteristics, the controls must be restricted in the same way to balance the odds.

Furthermore, by imposing this restriction we may accomplish something that a cohort study (and a population-based case-control study) limited to treated cases cannot achieve. Once the cases and controls are restricted on the factors influencing case ascertainment, these factors no longer influence the result for the odds ratio. By successfully balancing the odds in a case-control study, we can investigate the risk factors for developing the disease *per se*. We in effect remove the contribution of treatment and other ascertainment factors from the observed association between exposure and disease.[1]

At this point, we must caution that we do not recommend the use of the more complex case-control designs over the cohort and population-based case-control study. Although in principle balancing the odds will achieve this goal, the uncertainties are abundant and easily obscured. In general, it is preferable to use a more transparent design. It should also be kept in mind that many cohort studies are not limited to treated cases. Nonetheless, it is important to be aware of the potential advantages, as well as disadvantages, of case-control studies and to fully understand the implications of balancing the odds.

We are now ready to show how to apply the guideline to resolve a complex problem in control selection. To demonstrate its practical utility, we use it to answer a question that has perplexed investigators in psychiatric research: what is the appropriate strategy for control selection in a context of comorbidity?

Example of Comorbid Disorders

One of the prominent and problematic features of psychiatric disorders is that they are frequently comorbid (Boyd et al. 1984; Kessler 1997; Nemeroff 2002). For our purposes here, **comorbidity** means that in a population two disorders occur together in the same individual more often than expected by chance. Comorbidity has generated dilemmas not only for nosology and diagnostic assessment, but also for causal research. Psychiatric researchers have tried to adjust their selection of control groups to take account of comorbidity.

We will describe some current approaches to selection of controls in the context of comorbidity. Then we will apply the guideline of balancing the odds as an alternative approach. We will follow this with a hypothetical

---

[1] We note three caveats: (1) when simple restriction is extended to matching on selection factors, this has implications for the appropriate data analysis (see chapter 18); (2) we successfully distinguish the causes of the disease from the causes of ascertainment only to the extent that we successfully balance the odds (in practice, we never know if this was fully accomplished); and (3) if ascertainment is associated with disease subtype (e.g., a more serious form of the disease), the study results might apply only to the ascertained subtype.

numeric example that demonstrates the bias that can arise from current approaches. The example also shows that this bias can be avoided by the alternative approach of balancing the odds. We consider only comorbidity due to sharing a risk factor and defer to chapter 21 the discussion of control selection when there are other causes of comorbidity. For clarity, we use the term *case disorder* for the disorder being studied, and *comorbid disorder* for the disorder comorbid with the case disorder.

Current Approaches

A common strategy to handle comorbidity in psychiatric case-control studies is to exclude individuals with any psychiatric disorder from the control group. This ensures that the controls are free not only of the case disorder but also of any comorbid psychiatric disorder. We will refer to this kind of control group as a **well control** group.

The foremost rationale for using a well control group is that the inclusion of individuals with a comorbid disorder among the controls will make it more difficult to detect any difference in the frequency of the exposure between the cases and the controls. Indeed, excluding individuals with a comorbid disorder from the controls can accentuate differences between cases and controls. For example, the exposure may be a risk factor for a comorbid disorder, as well as for the case disorder. If so, the exposure frequency among people with this comorbid disorder will be greater than among the other noncases in the source population. Excluding individuals with the comorbid disorder from the controls will decrease the frequency of exposure among the controls and accentuate the difference in the frequency of exposure between cases and controls.

Does this argument warrant the use of well controls? Under the guideline of balancing the odds, the relevant question is, were individuals with comorbid disorders excluded from the cases? If the answer is no, then their exclusion from the control group is inappropriate. By reducing the exposure frequency in controls, the exclusion will create an artifactual difference in exposure frequency between cases and controls. In general, if the comorbid disorder is related to the exposure under investigation, this approach will lead to an overestimate of the odds ratio.

Another strategy employed in psychiatric research is to use a control group comprising only individuals being treated for a comorbid disorder. Sometimes this design is motivated by the belief that equating the cases and controls on as many factors as possible will enhance validity. This is the opposite strategy from well controls in that it excludes anyone without a specified comorbid disorder from the control group. We refer to this kind of control group as **unwell controls**.

The unwell control group also violates the guideline of balancing the odds. The relevant question is, did we exclude individuals without the comorbid disorder from the cases? If the answer is no, their exclusion from the controls is inappropriate. In general, if the comorbid disorder is related to the exposure under investigation, this type of control group will lead to an underestimation of the odds ratio.

To avoid misunderstanding, note that using individuals with another disorder for a control group can be an effective design, provided that the control disorder is unrelated to the exposure. This design can reduce ascertainment bias, because it is often reasonable to assume that the factors influencing the ascertainment of the case disorder also influence the ascertainment of the control disorder. In addition, using controls with another disorder may reduce differential misclassification of the exposure (see chapter 16).

Balancing the Odds

What is the appropriate strategy for control selection in a context of comorbidity? Under the guideline of balancing the odds, the answer to this question is as follows: impose the same restrictions as were imposed on the cases, no more and no less.

Generally, investigators disregard comorbid disorders in the selection of the cases. In these circumstances, we should also disregard them in the selection of the controls. On the other hand, in a study in which the cases are restricted to individuals without comorbid disorders, the same restriction should be imposed on the controls. This conclusion has important practical implications. It calls into question the use of well controls (also called supernormal controls), which is common in case-control studies of psychiatric disorders (Schwartz and Link 1989; Kendler 1990; see also Klein 1993). In biological studies, the use of well controls is widely purported to be a requirement for a valid study, and investigators who do not use well controls may be criticized for not doing so. Adding insult to injury, well controls require that a great deal of time and expense be devoted to screening potential controls to produce this bias. Similarly, it calls into question another practice, the use of unwell controls whose disorder may be associated with the exposure.

Numeric Example

We present a numeric example involving a comorbid disorder to demonstrate how well and unwell control groups lead to bias. The scenario builds upon the hypothetical example of a case-control study that was used in chapter 15 (see table 15.4).

The hypothetical study investigates whether exposure to sexual abuse in childhood is a risk factor for anorexia nervosa. The cases derive from an underlying cohort of 20,000, in which the probability of anorexia is .015 and .005 among those exposed and unexposed to childhood sexual abuse, respectively, and the traditional odds ratio is 3.0 (table 17.1A). We explicitly show the underlying cohort here because the bias is most easily seen in a scenario analogous to a nested case-control study.

We now complicate matters by introducing a comorbid disorder, depression, into the underlying cohort as shown in table 17.1B. In the new scenario, the risk of depression is 50 percent among the abused and 10 percent among the nonabused. In this scenario, anorexia is comorbid with depression because of the common shared risk factor of childhood sexual abuse.

Table 17.1 Effect of Using a Well Control Group: Hypothetical Example

A. RELATIONSHIP BETWEEN CHILD ABUSE AND ANOREXIA IN AN UNDERLYING COHORT

	Anorexia Nervosa +	Anorexia Nervosa −	Total
Abused	A	B	
	150	9,850	10,000
Nonabused	C	D	
	50	9,950	10,000

Probability of anorexia in the abused = .015 (150/10,000).
Probability of anorexia in the nonabused = .005 (50/10,000).

$$\text{Odds ratio} = \frac{A}{C} \div \frac{B}{D} = \frac{150}{50} \div \frac{9850}{9950} = 3.0.$$

B. HYPOTHETICAL UNDERLYING COHORT WITH COMORBID DISORDERS DISPLAYED

		Anorexia Nervosa +		Anorexia Nervosa −		Total
Abused		A	150	B	9,850	10,000
	Depressed +	75		Depressed +	4,925	5,000
	Depressed −	75		Depressed −	4,925	5,000
Nonabused		C	50	D	9,950	10,000
	Depressed +	5		Depressed +	995	1,000
	Depressed −	45		Depressed −	8,955	9,000

Depression among abused = 50% (5,000/10,000).
Depression among nonabused = 10% (1,000/10,000).

We will conduct three case-control studies that correspond to the three different strategies we have discussed for the selection of the controls. All three studies begin with the 200 cases of anorexia in the underlying cohort and sample the controls from the underlying cohort. We sample controls using a well control strategy in the first example, an unwell control strategy in the second, and a balanced odds approach in the third. We will compare the results from these three studies to see which is most successful in recreating the valid odds ratio. In portraying the results, we will use capital letters A, B, C, and D to denote the cells of the fourfold table in the underlying cohort, and lower case letters a, b, c, and d to denote the cells of the fourfold table in our case-control study.

Scenario Using Well Controls

We screen all the noncases in the cohort to identify individuals with the comorbid disorder (depression) and exclude these individuals from the control group. We take 20 percent of those who screened negative for controls. As shown in table 17.2, this control group comprises 985 abused and 1,791 nonabused individuals. It yields an odds ratio of 5.4.

Table 17.2 Case-Control Study Using Well Controls (Controls without Depression)

	Anorexia Nervosa +		Anorexia Nervosa −	
Abused	a	*150*	c	*985*
	Depressed +	75	Depressed +	0[a]
	Depressed −	75	Depressed −	985
Nonabused	b	*50*	d	*1,791*
	Depressed +	5	Depressed +	0[a]
	Depressed −	45	Depressed −	1,791

Nondepressed noncases: 4925 abused, 8955 nonabused (see table 17.1B).
Twenty percent selected as controls: 985 abused, 1791 nonabused.

$$\text{Case-control odds ratio} = \frac{a}{c} \div \frac{b}{d} = \frac{150}{50} \div \frac{4925 \times .2}{8955 \times .2} = \frac{150}{50} \div \frac{985}{1791} = 5.4.$$

$$\text{Cohort odds ratio (from table 17.1B)} = \frac{A}{C} \div \frac{B}{D} = \frac{150}{50} \div \frac{9850}{9950} = 3.0.$$

[a] Depressed noncases excluded from controls.

We would erroneously conclude that individuals exposed to sexual abuse in childhood are 5.4 times more likely to develop anorexia than the unexposed, when in fact the true odds ratio is only 3.0.

What went wrong? As can be seen by looking back at table 17.1B, by sampling as controls only those people without depression, we sampled 10 percent of the B cell (985 of 9,850) and 18 percent of the D cell (1,791 of 9,950). Thus, the ratio of exposed to unexposed controls (b/d = 985/1791) in the case-control study was less than the ratio of exposed to unexposed noncases (B/D = 9850/9950) in the underlying cohort. Indeed, the ratio of these sampling fractions (i.e., 10 percent/18 percent) indicates the amount of bias in the case-control odds ratio: 3.0, the true odds ratio, divided by 0.10/0.18 = 5.4. In other words, by including individuals with depression among the cases, while excluding them from the controls, we created an imbalance in the odds.

Scenario Using Unwell Controls

We compare those who developed anorexia (cases) with those who developed depression alone (controls). We use 10 percent of the noncase individuals with depression for controls. As shown in table 17.3, this control group comprises 492 abused and 99 nonabused individuals. It yields an odds ratio of 0.60.

From these data we would conclude that exposure to sexual abuse in childhood protects against anorexia. In this instance, by sampling as controls only those people with depression, we sampled 5 percent of the B cell (492 of 9,850) and one percent of the D cell (99 of 9,950). Thus, the ratio of exposed to unexposed controls (b/d = 492/99) in the case-control study was more than the ratio of exposed to unexposed noncases (B/D = 9850/9950) in the underlying cohort. As above, this sampling fraction (.05/.01) indicates the amount of bias in the odds ratio: 3.0, the true odds ratio, divided by .05/.01 = 0.60.

Table 17.3 Case-Control Study Using Unwell Controls (Controls with Depression Only)

	Anorexia Nervosa +		**Anorexia Nervosa −**	
Abused	a	150	b	492
	Depressed +	75	Depressed +	492
	Depressed −	75	Depressed −	0[a]
Nonabused	c	50	d	99
	Depressed +	5	Depressed +	99
	Depressed −	45	Depressed −	0[a]

$$\text{Case-control odds ratio} = \frac{a}{c} \div \frac{b}{d} = \frac{150}{50} \div \frac{492}{99} = 0.6.$$

$$\text{Cohort odds ratio (from table 17.1B)} = \frac{A}{C} \div \frac{B}{D} = \frac{150}{50} \div \frac{9850}{9950} = 3.0.$$

[a] Non-depressed noncases excluded from controls.

Table 17.4 Case-Control Study Using Cases and Controls Screened for Depression

	Anorexia Nervosa +		**Anorexia Nervosa −**	
Abused	a		c	
	Depressed +	0	Depressed +	0
	Depressed −	75	Depressed −	985
Nonabused	b		d	
	Depressed +	0	Depressed +	0
	Depressed −	45	Depressed −	1,791

Nondepressed cases: 75 abused, 45 nonabused (see table 17.1B).
Nondepressed noncases: 4,925 abused; 8,955 nonabused.
Twenty percent selected as controls: 985 abused; 1,791 non-abused.

$$\text{Case-Control odds ratio} = \frac{a}{c} \div \frac{b}{d} = \frac{75}{45} \div \frac{985}{1791} = 3.0.$$

Scenario Balancing the Odds

Since we included individuals with comorbid disorders in the case group, we also include them in the control group. As can be seen by referring back to table 15.4, using this approach, we will re-create the traditional odds ratio of 3.0, the same odds ratio as in the underlying cohort. An alternative way to balance the odds would be to exclude individuals with depression from both the case and control groups. As depicted in table 17.4, by imposing the restriction on cases and then applying it also to controls, we again re-create the traditional odds ratio of 3.0.

Conclusion

This chapter completes our discussion of the selection of controls for case-control studies under three simplifying conditions. The first is that there is no confounding in the underlying cohort that serves as the source population for the cases. The second is that there is no attrition in the underlying cohort. The third is that there is no differential misclassification. Under these conditions, the general principle for selection of controls is that they should be chosen to represent the exposure odds of the noncases in a real or imagined underlying cohort from which the cases are derived. If we achieve this, we obtain the true odds ratio of the underlying cohort.

In complex scenarios, we can operationalize this principle by following the guideline of balancing the odds. Thus, we impose on the controls the same restrictions that were imposed on the cases, no more and no less. The guideline facilitates resolving complicated questions about the selection of controls. It can also change the meaning of the study results in a subtle and potentially advantageous way by taking into account the factors that influence case ascertainment.

In real studies, these conditions rarely apply. We encounter confounding and unequal attrition in the underlying cohort. We may also encounter differential misclassification, which appears in reverse form in the case-control study. These have to be taken into account in the selection of controls, as well as in the analysis of the data. We will discuss how to do this in the next chapter, where we further refine our understanding of the case-control study.

References

Boyd JH, Burke JD, Jr., Gruenberg E, et al. (1984). Exclusion Criteria of *DSM-III*. A Study of Co-Occurrence of Hierarchy-Free Syndromes. *Arch. Gen. Psychiatry* 41: 983–989.

Browne R, Byrne M, Mulryan N, Scully A, Morris M, Kinsella A, McNeil TF, Walsh D, and O'Callaghan E (2000). Labour and Delivery Complications at Birth and Later Mania. An Irish Case Register Study. *Br. J. Psychiatry* 176:369–372.

Kendler KS (1990). The Super-Normal Control Group in Psychiatric Genetics: Possible Artifactual Evidence for Coaggregation. *Psychiatr. Genet.* 1:45–53.

Kessler RC (1997). The Prevalence of Psychiatric Comorbidity. In Weszler S and Sanderson WC, eds., *Treatment Strategies for Patients with Psychiatric Comorbidity*, 23–48. New York: Wiley.

Klein DF (1993). The Utility of the Super-Normal Control Group in Psychiatric Genetics. *Psychiatr. Genet.* 3:17–19.

Kyriacou DN, Anglin D, Taliaferro E, Stone S, Tubb T, Linden JA, Muelleman R, Barton E, and Kraus JF (1999). Risk Factors for Injury to Women from Domestic Violence against Women. *N. Engl. J. Med.* 341:1892–1898.

Nemeroff CB (2002). Comorbidity of Mood and Anxiety Disorders: The Rule, Not the Exception? *Am. J. Psychiatry* 159:3–4.

Schwartz S and Link BG (1989). The "Well Control" Artefact in Case/Control Studies of Specific Psychiatric Disorders. *Psychol. Med.* 19:737–742.

18 Comparability and the Case-Control Study

Alfredo Morabia, Sharon Schwartz, and Ezra Susser

The validity of a case-control study depends upon sampling controls from the noncases in an unbiased way, that is, independent of exposure status. Although this safeguard will prevent introducing bias when we select the controls, any bias already present in the underlying cohort will still be reflected in the case-control study. When the exposed and unexposed groups in the underlying cohort are not fully comparable as defined in part II, the resulting odds ratio will not reflect the causal effect of the exposure. It will be biased. In general, we handle the bias in parallel fashion for cohort and case-control studies. But the logical connections between the problem and its resolution are more difficult to see in the context of the case-control design.

This chapter will explain these connections and their practical implications for the selection of controls. We discuss in turn the main sources of noncomparability: confounding, unequal attrition, and differential misclassification. We will again use the nested case-control study to portray a logic that in large part also applies to the ordinary case-control study.

Confounding

In a case-control as in a cohort study, we use matching and statistical adjustment to minimize the effects of potential confounders. In both types of study, the purpose of matching is to safeguard the comparability of the exposed and unexposed. We next discuss the logic and practice of matching. We also more briefly discuss the logic of statistical adjustment (statistical methods are deferred to part VI).

Logic of Matching

In a cohort study, the purpose of matching is transparent: to make the exposure groups more comparable. Any difference in their disease risk is then more likely to reflect the exposure being investigated. In a case-control study, by contrast, the purpose is not at all transparent. The problem and the solution appear incongruous. The problem is the noncomparability of the exposed and unexposed, but the solution is to match the cases and controls.

To draw the missing logical connection, we can visualize the process as conducting multiple nested case-control substudies. Each substudy consists of cases and controls nested in a restricted portion of the underlying cohort in which there is no confounding. We do this by comparing the cases to controls within each stratum of the confounding variable. Then we average the results across the strata.

For example, suppose we conduct a nested case-control study within an underlying cohort in which gender is a confounding variable. That is, gender is a risk factor for the disease and the exposed and unexposed differ on gender (table 18.1A).

We therefore decide to match on gender. We can think of this as if we had two underlying cohorts, one male and one female. As illustrated in table 18.1B, within the male cohort, we conduct a substudy, in which we compare the exposure odds in the male cases to the exposure odds in the male controls (who represent the male noncases) to derive an odds ratio. In this instance, for each of the 114 male cases we randomly selected one male without the disease for a control. We did this by randomly selecting 114 men from the 886 nondiseased men depicted in table 18.1A. Note that when we select these men independent of their exposure status, we re-create the ratio of exposed to unexposed among the total group of nondiseased men. The odds ratio in males is 2.

Similarly, within the female cohort, we conduct a substudy. For each of the 22 female cases, we randomly selected one female for a control from among the 978 nondiseased females in the underlying cohort. We derive an exposure odds ratio for these women. Again, the odds ratio is 2. Then we take a weighted average of the two odds ratios. In this instance, since the odds ratio is 2 in men and 2 in women, the average is also 2. This ratio differs markedly, however, from the unadjusted odds ratio of 5.

We have just described a nested case-control study in which the investigators match on gender and compute an adjusted odds ratio. There are different methods for averaging across strata. A common approach, the Mantel-Haenszel summary odds ratio, is described in part VI.

Although the procedure removes the effect of the confounder, it simultaneously introduces new confounding. Since confounders are, by definition, associated with the exposure, when we select our controls according to confounder status we also, indirectly, select our controls according to exposure status. Thus, we violate our principle that controls should be selected independent of exposure status. This violation causes bias because when we make the controls more like the cases on the confounder we also make the controls somewhat more like the cases on our exposure. This effect is illustrated in column 1 of table 18.1C. After matching, the unadjusted odds ratio in the full sample of cases and controls is shifted toward the null.

The bias introduced by matching does not pertain within each substudy or stratum. Within a substudy where the cases and controls are all male (or female), the exposure of interest could not be related to being male (or female; see columns 2 and 3 of table 18.1C). The bias pertains only when the cases and controls from different strata are pooled together and the stratification is ignored (as in column 1).

Table 18.1 Matching in a Case-Control Study

A. GENDER DISTRIBUTION IN AN UNDERLYING COHORT

| | Total Underlying Cohort | | | | | |
| | Crude | | Male | | Female | |
	D+	D−	D+	D−	D+	D−
Exposed	112	888	108	792	4	96
Unexposed	24	976	6	94	18	882
Total	**136**	**1,864**	**114**	**886**	**22**	**978**
Odds ratio	5		2		2	

% Disease among males = 11.4.
% Disease among females = 2.2.

Ratio M/F among exposed = 9/1.
Ratio M/F among unexposed = 1/9.

B. MATCHING CASES ON GENDER

| | Total Underlying Cohort | | Male Cases with Male Controls | | Female Cases with Female Controls | |
	D+	D−	D+	D−	D+	D−
Exposed	112	888	108	103	4	2
Unexposed	24	976	6	11	18	20
Total	**136**	**1,864**	**114**	**114**	**22**	**22**
Odds ratio	5		2		2	

Average odds ratio = 2

C. ALL CASES AND ONE CONTROL PER CASE MATCHED BY GENDER

| | (1) Male Cases + Male Controls + Female Cases + Female Controls | | (2) Male Cases + Male Controls | | (3) Female Cases + Female Controls | |
	D+	D−	D+	D−	D+	D−
Exposed	112	105	108	103	4	2
Unexposed	24	31	6	11	18	20
Total	**136**	**136**	**114**	**114**	**22**	**22**
Odds ratio	1.4		2		2	

Thus, we can easily avoid the bias introduced through matching by conducting a stratified analysis to combine the unbiased results from the different substudies or strata. Alternatively, we could use a statistical modeling procedure. Because the purpose of matching in a case-control study is not easily understood, however, investigators sometimes make the mistake of ignoring the stratification and computing a crude odds ratio. It is important to use analytic techniques that adjust for the matched factor to neutralize the new confounding introduced by the matching process.[1]

Practice of Matching

In a case-control study, as in a cohort study, we can use either individual or frequency matching. In individual matching, controls are matched to each of the cases. For example, when one is matching on age and gender, if a case is a 35-year-old man, the control (or controls) chosen for that case will also be a 35-year-old man. Depending on how strictly the confounder needs to be controlled, we might allow matching within a range of values; in this instance, we might accept men ages 33 to 37. The case and the corresponding control (or controls) are considered as a set, which may be a pair (a case and one control), a triplet (a case and two controls), and so forth.

Frequency (or group) matching, on the other hand, consists of making the controls similar on average to the cases. Suppose we want to match on age and gender, and among our cases 25 percent are men ages 20–29, 25 percent are men ages 30–39, 25 percent are women ages 20–29, and 25 percent are women ages 30–39. Controls will be selected in such a way that 25 percent of them are also in each of these age-gender categories.

Costs and Benefits of Matching

The decision to match or not to match is made by weighing the benefits against the costs of the procedure in a particular study. The main benefit of matching is that it increases efficiency. By this the epidemiologist means that matching reduces the collection of unnecessary information. For the statistician, this means that, given the same sample size, the matched design yields an estimate with a smaller variance.

Table 18.2 shows a hypothetical case-control study of 100 cases and 100 controls in which we assume age is a confounder that needs to be controlled. The first column shows the age distribution observed in the study cases. None of the cases is younger than age 20, and most are between age 30 and 44.

Let us say we select the 100 controls randomly from the population at risk. The ages of our controls turn out to be evenly distributed across the 5-year age categories, as shown in the second column. Within age groups, the number of cases and controls are unbalanced, reducing efficiency. In the age group

---

[1] To avoid confusion, note that this is not necessary in a cohort study. Once the exposed and unexposed groups have been matched, we no longer need to adjust for the matched factor in the analysis to achieve the correct point estimate. Nonetheless, we need to consider matching to ascertain the correct standard error in a cohort study.

Table 18.2 Results from a Hypothetical Case-Control Study in which Controls Are Selected without Matching or Alternatively Are Matched to Cases on Age

Age	Unmatched Design		Matched Design	
	Cases	Controls	Cases	Controls
20 to 24	0	20[a]	0	0
25 to 29	1	20[b]	1	1
30 to 34	9	20	9	9
35 to 39	30	20	30	30
40 to 44	60	20	60	60
Total	100	100	100	100

[a] Controls that would be ignored in the stratified analysis.
[b] This analytic stratum would have a large variance because there is only one case.

20 to 24, where we have no cases, the 20 controls will not contribute to the analysis. In the age group 25 to 29, where we have only one case, the 20 controls will contribute very little to the analysis; with only a single case, the variance of the odds ratio in this age group will be large, no matter how many controls are used. In the age group 40 to 44, where we have 60 cases, the much smaller number of 20 controls is fewer than optimal for reducing variance.

Now let us match controls to cases on age, so that the 100 controls have the same distribution across age groups as the 100 cases, as shown in the third and fourth columns of table 18.2. We can now make more efficient use of the data collected. All of the controls contribute to the analysis, and in age groups where we have large numbers of cases we also have large numbers of controls. From an epidemiological perspective, all the data collected are useful. From a statistical point of view, given a sample size of 100 cases and 100 controls, this design gives us the most precise measure of effect.

Beyond its benefit for efficiency, matching is sometimes the only feasible way to remove confounding. This tends to pertain when the confounding variable has a very large number of categories. For example, when the confounder is the family of origin, the only feasible way to remove confounding may be to match cases to sibling controls. Similarly, when the confounder is a city block, it may be necessary to purposefully select controls who live on the same block as the cases.

On the other hand, matching may have substantial costs. Restricting eligibility means that many otherwise eligible subjects will be discarded. As a result, the study may take longer and the procedure of subject identification will be more cumbersome. In addition, because the cases and controls are made the same on the matching factor, such restriction prevents the investigator from examining whether the matching factor itself has any impact on the risk of disease.

Excess matching (or overmatching) can be deleterious and lead to loss of efficiency. Overmatching can occur when controls are matched to cases on a variable that is associated with the exposure but is not a confounder. The matching will therefore create a bias: an association between control selection and exposure, where beforehand there was no such association. The resulting bias requires an adjusted analysis for a variable that originally did not need to be controlled. In the end, there is a double loss of efficiency: time and energy have been wasted to proceed with a useless matching, and the adjusted analysis is statistically less efficient than the nonstratified one.

Overmatching is especially damaging when the matching factor mediates the effect of exposure on disease; that is, the causal pathway goes from exposure to matching factor to disease. Matching in this situation results in a clear loss of validity. Because controls were matched to cases on a variable that carries, totally or partially, the same information as exposure, the matched odds ratio will underestimate the true odds ratio, even if analytic techniques for matched designs are used.

Therefore, matching may make our study more efficient and is sometimes essential, but it can also prolong the study, increase its expense, constrain its scientific aims, and sometimes even undermine its validity. Matching should always be used with caution and with a well-considered rationale.

Logic of Statistical Adjustment

Statistical adjustment, either through stratification or statistical modeling, is another way to control for sources of noncomparability in a case-control study. As explained in chapter 13, statistical adjustment is logically equivalent to conducting substudies restricted to one value of the confounding variable and then averaging the results of the substudies. In this way, adjustment is quite similar to matching, except that the subjects are made comparable at the analytic rather than the selection stage of the study.

When a stratified analysis is used for adjustment, the substudy analogy is immediately apparent. The levels of the confounding variable or set of confounding variables define the strata. An odds ratio for the exposure-disease relationship is calculated within each stratum, and these stratum-specific odds ratios are combined with a Mantel-Haenzel or equivalent averaging procedure. This can be seen by reference to table 18.1A, where the odds ratio is correct within the stratum of males (odds ratio = 2) and within the stratum of females (odds ratio = 2), and a weighted average of these odds ratios would yield the correct odds ratio for the total cohort (odds ratio = 2).

In statistical modeling, the logic is essentially the same, although not as apparent. The methods used for adjustment are not unique to this design; they are similar to the methods used in cohort studies and are described in part VI.

Unequal Attrition

The traditional case-control study we have described so far is intrinsically unsuitable for taking account of unequal attrition in the exposed and unexposed groups in the underlying cohort. Preferably, one selects cases as they arise in the cohort, in order to obtain incident cases, among other reasons. The controls are selected, however, from the noncases still under observation at the end of the risk period. Thus, individuals lost to observation are excluded from the control group. They do not contribute to the result and may be considered as deleted from the study.

In part III we showed what happens in a cohort study with ongoing case ascertainment when the individuals lost to observation are deleted from the study, a procedure we termed restriction. This approach leads to a biased result (see chapter 13). The exact same reasoning pertains to the nested case-control (and to the ordinary case-control) study.

Concurrent Case-Control Study

The approach used to take account of unequal attrition in a case-control study is known as an **incidence density sampling** or **concurrent case-control study** (Morabia et al. 1995). It parallels the approach of survival analysis used in a cohort study, although, again, the connections are more difficult to see in the case-control design. The limitations of the approach also parallel the cohort study. We can remedy attrition that is merely unequal in the exposed and unexposed, but we cannot remedy attrition that is differential, as well as unequal, as defined in chapter 13.

In this approach, control selection occurs concurrently with case selection throughout the study. Every time a case is selected, one or more controls are selected from the population at risk at that moment in time, that is, from the population remaining disease-free and under observation. We will first show the procedure in an example and then explain how this procedure takes account of attrition in the underlying cohort.

We will compute an odds ratio based on concurrent sampling of controls, using the data of the Prenatal Determinants of Schizophrenia Example (PDSE) study. Recall that the PDSE examines whether high maternal body mass index is a risk factor for schizophrenia spectrum disorder in a birth cohort (see figure 10.1 and tables 10.6 and 10.7 for a summary of PDSE). All 60 cases in the PDSE cohort will be used. The exposure odds for the cases (i.e., exposed cases / unexposed cases) is $13/47 = 0.2766$.

We take a random sample of 6 individuals from the population at risk every time a case occurs. This yields a total of 360 concurrent controls for our 60 cases. The procedure is illustrated in table 18.3 for the first and the last of the 60 cases in the PDSE. For example, when a case occurred on May 18, 1981, there were 9,213 people still under observation who had not developed the disease. Six individuals were randomly selected from this group to serve as controls.

This procedure was repeated for every day on which a case arose. The resulting exposure odds for the controls (i.e., exposed controls / unexposed controls) was $= 38/322 = 0.1180$. The result for the concurrent odds ratio is exposure odds in cases (13/47) divided by exposure odds in controls (38/322) $= 0.2766/0.1180 = 2.34$.

A complete explanation of how concurrent sampling deals with attrition is beyond the scope of this book (see Rothman and Greenland 1998). To make the point accessible to readers, we will use the same device that was employed

Table 18.3 Concurrent Selection of Controls for First and Last Case in the PDSE Cohort

Date	N Cases with Onset on Date	Noncases under Observation on Date	Noncases Selected as Controls	Selection Probability for Controls
May 18, 1981	1	9,213	6	6/9,213 (0.65 per 1000)
Feb. 12, 1997	1	3,627	6	6/3,627 (1.65 per 1000)

to introduce survival analysis in a cohort study in chapter 13. We explained the logic of survival analysis in terms of three steps: (1) divide the risk period into many small time intervals, (2) compute a result for each interval (analogous to conducting a valid mini–cohort study for each time interval in which a case occurred), and (3) combine the results across the intervals.

The logic of concurrent sampling can be explained in a parallel fashion. We can think of the procedure in terms of the same three steps. First, we divide the risk period into very small time intervals. Second, we conduct a valid mini-case-control study for each time interval in which a case occurred. In a mini-case-control study using a single case, we select concurrent controls from among the remaining population at risk and compare the case with these controls. If the interval is very small, we can assume that there is no attrition in the underlying cohort within the interval. Therefore, the result for the mini-case-control study is valid in the sense that there is no bias due to unequal attrition. Third, we combine the valid results from these mini-case-control studies.

This logic also reveals that in concurrent sampling we are in essence matching controls to cases on follow-up time. Strictly speaking, therefore, each case with 6 controls comprises a matched set, since the cases and controls were matched on time. If the exposure is associated with observation time, the result should be computed with an analytic procedure that accounts for matching. Thus, we should employ an analytic procedure such as Mantel-Haenszel or statistical modeling to combine the results from the mini-case-control studies or case control sets.

Subtleties of Concurrent Sampling. In concurrent sampling, subjects can be selected as controls more than once. So long as they remain in the population at risk, they should remain in the pool of noncases from which the controls will be selected in the next informative time interval. In addition, and more surprising at first glance, individuals who are selected as controls can, at a later time, become cases in the same study. Just as in a cohort study each individual contributes person-time to the denominator until he or she becomes a case, so, too, in a case-control study individuals are eligible to be controls until they become cases. Analytic procedures should take such occurrences into account (Rothman and Greenland 1998).

Rate Ratio. There is also another way to see that the concurrent odds ratio takes account of attrition. The concurrent odds ratio ($OR_{concurrent}$) estimates the rate ratio in the underlying cohort (Miettinen 1976). As explained in chapter 13, the rate ratio takes account of attrition because it is based on person-time.

To simplify the explanation of this relationship between the $OR_{concurrent}$ and the rate ratio, we will use an argument that pertains to a special case: when the incidence rates in the exposed and the unexposed are constant over the risk period. It can be shown, however, that the relationship applies in general.

Let us first rewrite the equation for the rate ratio. As usually written, the numerator of the rate ratio is exposed cases / exposed person-time, and the denominator is unexposed cases / unexposed person-time. By simple algebra, the rate ratio can be rewritten with the numerator as exposed cases / unexposed cases, and the denominator as exposed person-time / unexposed person-time.

The equation for the $OR_{concurrent}$ is exposed cases / unexposed cases divided by exposed controls / unexposed controls. The numerator of the $OR_{concurrent}$ (exposed cases / unexposed cases) is identical to the numerator of the rewritten rate ratio.

What is less apparent but equally true, however, is that the $OR_{concurrent}$ denominator—the ratio of the exposed to the unexposed concurrent controls—is an estimate of the rate ratio denominator, the ratio of the exposed to the unexposed person-time. We can think of the concurrent controls as a sample of the person-time rather than the individual persons in the population at risk. The longer a person remains in the population at risk, the more person-time a subject contributes, and the greater the chance that he or she will be selected as a control in one or more of the intervals in which a case occurs (see table 18.3). Consequently, the ratio of exposed to unexposed concurrent controls will estimate the ratio of exposed to unexposed person-time in the cohort. Thus, the concurrent odds ratio will estimate the rate ratio.

Case-Base Design

In a traditional case-control study, we select the controls after all the cases arise, and in a concurrent case-control study we sample the controls when the cases arise. A third way to sample controls is before the cases arise.

In this **case-base** (or **case-cohort**) strategy, controls are sampled from the full underlying cohort defined at the beginning of the study. Thus, individuals lost to observation by the end of the study will have all been eligible to be selected as controls at the start of the study. This procedure provides a contrast with the traditional case-control study in which the individuals lost to observation are excluded from consideration.

The case-base design is not often utilized, because it presupposes that the underlying cohort is known and enumerated. It is very important in some contexts, however, such as in family-based genetic-association studies. Its use in genetic epidemiology will be explained in part VII.

Table 18.4 Numerator and Denominator of the Odds Ratio Computed in a Case-Control Study, According to the Sampling Scheme of Controls

Control Sample Scheme	Numerator	Denominator[a]	Estimated Effect
Traditional	Exposed cases/ unexposed cases	Exposed noncases[b]/ unexposed noncases	Traditional odds ratio
Concurrent	Exposed cases/ unexposed cases	Exposed person-time/ unexposed person-time	Concurrent odds ratio = rate ratio
Case-base	Exposed cases/ unexposed cases	Exposed cohort/ unexposed cohort	Case-base odds ratio = risk ratio

[a] In all 3 sampling schemes, validity of the observed odds ratio depends on random selection of controls from the denominator defined in the table. Under random selection of controls, the observed odds ratio may differ from the estimated effect, but only because of chance.

[b] As shown in chapter 15, noncases are individuals who remain disease-free after the cases have been selected, or, in other words, at the end of the risk period in the underlying cohort. Also shown in chapter 15, the traditional odds ratio in the case-control study estimates the traditional odds ratio in the underlying cohort.

The concurrent sampling of controls yields an odds ratio that estimates the rate ratio, whereas case-base sampling yields an odds ratio that estimates the risk ratio. This is because the ratio of exposed to unexposed controls will estimate the ratio of exposed to unexposed individuals in the baseline cohort, within the limits of sampling errors.

Thus, the $OR_{casebase}$ is as follows:

(exposed cases / unexposed cases) /
(exposed casebase controls / unexposed casebase controls).

This will estimate the quantity

(exposed cases / unexposed cases) / (exposed cohort / unexposed cohort).

This quantity can be rewritten as the risk ratio:

(exposed cases / exposed cohort) / (unexposed cases / unexposed cohort).

The components of the odds ratios for all three sampling schemes are summarized in table 18.4.

Comparison of Odds Ratios

We can compare the results from the traditional, concurrent, and case-base strategies by sampling controls in these three different ways in nested case-control studies in the PDSE cohort. To calculate each of the three odds ratios, all of the 60 cases were used, but different groups of controls were used. Consequently, the odds of exposure for the cases is constant (13/47), whereas the odds of exposure for controls is affected by the study design.[2]

---

[2] Again, for simplicity of exposition, we pool the controls in the concurrent case-control study, when, strictly speaking, these data should be analyzed as matched case-control sets.

Table 18.5 Number of Cases and Controls (by Exposure Status), and Odds Ratios Computed under Different Sampling Schemes in the PDSE Data

Sampling Scheme	Exposed Cases	Unexposed Cases	Exposed Controls	Unexposed Controls	Odds Ratio
Traditional	13	47	36	324	2.49
Concurrent	13	47	38	322	2.34
Case-base	13	47	39	321	2.28

The results are shown in table 18.5. In the PDSE data, where the disease was rare and overall attrition was high but unequal attrition was limited, the differences among these odds ratios are small.

Differential Misclassification

In a case-control study, there is a form of differential misclassification that does not emanate from noncomparability in the underlying cohort; disease status can influence the exposure measure. This type of differential misclassification is truly particular to the case-control design. In chapter 16 we discussed this kind of bias in some detail, including strategies to safeguard a study from it.

Here we turn to consider the implications for the case-control study of another kind of differential misclassification: differential misclassification in the underlying cohort. Misclassification of disease that is different for the exposed and unexposed (or ascertainment bias) will bias the risk ratio in the underlying cohort. Similarly, it can bias the odds ratio of a case-control study nested in the cohort. In part III, we described numerous scenarios in which ascertainment bias can arise in a cohort study. Some of these scenarios will generate an equivalent bias in the nested case-control study.

Consider a scenario of belief in the risk factor. The study subjects and their doctors suspect the exposure to be a cause of the disease and look harder for the disease in the exposed than in the unexposed. If this scenario pertained to the underlying cohort, it would also be reflected in the ascertainment of cases in the nested case-control study.

Matching on factors related to ascertainment can sometimes limit the bias. In fact, in a nested case-control study, matching on ascertainment factors is equivalent to balancing the odds to limit bias. As described in previous chapters, balancing the odds means that any factor that restricted the selection of the cases should also restrict the selection of the controls. Matching extends this notion to allow for multiple strata rather than simply restriction. For instance, cases and controls could be matched on a comorbid disorder, rather than excluding (or including) all cases and controls with a comorbid disorder. As explained, when we use matching, the data analysis should take the matching into account.

Extension to Ordinary Case-Control Study

We used the nested case-control study as a device to show that bias in the population that gave rise to the cases will be reflected in the result of the case-control study. The connections are easier to see in the nested design because the cases are derived from a fully enumerated underlying cohort. Nonetheless, the same connections pertain to ordinary case-control studies.

In regard to confounding and unequal attrition, the ordinary case-control study can be considered in the same way as the nested case-control study. All confounding and unequal attrition in the underlying cohort (of a nested case control) or the source population (of an ordinary case control) will produce bias in the odds ratio.

The bias of differential misclassification cannot be thought of in exactly the same way for the two designs. In the nested case-control study, the exposure is often measured with data or specimens collected before the onset of the disease. This practice makes it possible to prevent the classification of the exposure from being influenced by the disease status. For example, we can ensure that biological specimens are collected and analyzed "blind" to disease status. In the ordinary case-control study, in contrast, the exposure is measured after the disease has occurred. This makes it more difficult to prevent differential misclassification of the exposure that depends on disease status, discussed in detail in chapter 16.

Although noncomparability is most obvious in a nested case-control study where the cohort is enumerated, it is most pernicious in an ordinary case-control study, where it can be hidden. Indeed, in many case-control studies, because it is difficult to visualize the source population, it is also difficult to discern the bias that emanates from the source population. The most common use of the design is to compare the patients observed in a clinical setting with some other group, in order to illuminate the causes of their disease. The clinical setting is often a tertiary care center with no defined catchment population. How then can we verify that the controls were selected from the same source population as the cases, that we balanced the odds of selection for cases and controls, and that confounding and attrition in the source population were adequately controlled? When considered in light of these questions, the case-control study in a clinical setting may be appreciated as one of the most difficult of all designs in psychiatric research.

Conclusion

We have reiterated throughout this part of the book that a case-control study is not the mere comparison of some diseased and nondiseased people. The design is an elaborate attempt to re-create the conditions of a cohort study with an economy of time, subjects, and resources. This endeavor is now supported by a well-developed theory that we have reviewed in the last four chapters.

On finishing this part, consider the following problem and ponder whether you feel more empowered than before to address it. Suppose you want to conduct a case-control study of a newly recognized and defined psychiatric disorder of unknown etiology. It is extremely rare, and patients with this diagnosis will often be immediately transferred to a tertiary care referral hospital, where you will be able to identify and recruit them. How will you choose the controls? Will you select them from patients referred to these tertiary hospitals for other rare conditions, from neighbors of the cases, from siblings of the cases, from friends of the cases, or from residents of the neighborhoods surrounding the referral hospitals? Will you screen the controls to exclude persons with neuropsychiatric disorders? When will you select the controls? How will you measure the exposures without being influenced by knowledge of disease status?

This chapter also closes our presentation of the basic study designs of epidemiology. Although these designs are widely applicable for studying the causes of mental disorders, so far they have been applied in only a narrow realm. One of the challenges we now face is to extend their use, especially in studies of causes that are led by researchers from other disciplines, who are, naturally, unfamiliar with the epidemiologic perspective. Part V of this volume takes a step in this direction, examining the implications of the case-control design for research in biological psychiatry. We hope that this example will stimulate readers to carry these designs into many other domains.

Part VI will introduce methods for analyzing the data from risk factor studies. These studies are designed to select and distill the data relevant to answering questions about disease causation. The analytic methods allow for a further distillation. Statistics provide a way of organizing the data to reveal patterns that we can compare with predictions from our theories. There are many different statistical tools to select from and many different perspectives on the utility of these tools. The approaches described in part VI are those endorsed by most psychiatric journals and their statistical reviewers. Therefore, it is essential for readers to understand them. Among epidemiologists and a growing number of statisticians, a somewhat different perspective prevails. For example, leading epidemiologists do not concur with the practice of using p-values as a criterion to accept or reject a null hypothesis. More emphasis is placed on confidence intervals. In order for readers to make a reasoned choice, once they have understood the approaches in part VI, we suggest the following further readings: Cohen (1994), Poole (2001), Sterne and Davey Smith (2001), Rothman (2002), and Berkson (2003).

References

Berkson J (2003). Tests of Significance Considered as Evidence. Journal of the American Statistical Association 1942; 37:325–335. *Int. J. Epidemiol.* 32:687–691.

Cohen J (1994). The Earth Is Round ($p < .05$). *Am. Psychol.* 49:997–1003.

Miettinen O (1976). Estimability and Estimation in Case-Referent Studies. *Am. J. Epidemiol.* 103:226–235.

Morabia A, Ten Have T, and Landis JR (1995). Empirical Evaluation of the Influence of Control Selection Schemes on Relative Risk Estimation: The Welsh Nickel Workers Study. *Occup. Environ. Med.* 52:489–493.

Poole C (2001). Low *P*-Values or Narrow Confidence Intervals: Which Are More Durable? *Epidemiology* 12:291–294.

Rothman KJ (2002). *Epidemiology: An Introduction.* New York: Oxford University Press.

Rothman KJ and Greenland S (1998). *Modern Epidemiology,* 2nd ed. Philadelphia: Lippincott-Raven.

Sterne JA and Davey Smith G (2001). Sifting the Evidence—What's Wrong with Significance Tests? *BMJ* 322:226–231.

CASE-CONTROL DESIGNS IN BIOLOGIC PSYCHIATRY

Biologic Studies in Psychiatry

19

Jack M. Gorman and Ezra Susser

Although epidemiologic and biologic researchers share the common goal of finding causes of psychiatric disorders, they approach the task from different vantage points. As a result, they sometimes advocate conflicting approaches to the design of studies. Despite the rapid advances in both fields, dialogue between them remains limited. No doubt each of these fields still has much to learn from the other.

In this context, we examine how epidemiologists can contribute to the advance of biologic research. We focus on biologic studies in which cases are compared with controls, in part because one of the themes of this book is to facilitate the use of case-control designs in psychiatric research. We consider the process, as well as the content, of the exchange required. To be persuasive, epidemiologists will need not only to demonstrate the benefits of their approaches, but also to take into account the perspectives and research traditions of the listeners. Otherwise, suggestions may be inapplicable and will certainly be received without enthusiasm.

In this chapter, we first take the perspective of a biologic researcher. We point out the challenge of measuring the brain and how it sets the stage for research designs. Then we take the perspective of an epidemiologist. We suggest that biologic studies can be directly linked to epidemiology through consideration of the biologic factors being investigated within the same framework as other potential causes or risk factors for disease. We show how two classic biologic studies can be conceptualized as case-control studies.

Biologic Perspective

Biologic psychiatry is interested in defining the fundamental brain processes that subserve normal and abnormal human behavior and emotion. Thus, biologic assessments in neuropsychiatry are meant to open a window on the processes of the human mind. This is an extremely complex undertaking. We want to capture an ongoing brain process but have to rely on a snapshot at one moment in time. In addition, we measure only a surface manifestation of the underlying brain process. Notwithstanding the difficulties, these measurements are being continually refined, and biologic researchers have already begun to illuminate the pathophysiology of some psychiatric disorders.

Typically, researchers in biologic psychiatry are clinicians on a quest to understand the cause of a disorder they have encountered and treated. The investigator suspects that some aspect of brain function plays a role in causing the disorder. A study is typically designed to ask the following question: do the patients who have this disorder differ from a control group on a measure that reflects the suspected aspect of brain function?

Designing the study, the investigator confronts the central dilemma of this context: the conflicting imperatives of validity of measurement on the one hand, and sample size and selection on the other. This dilemma may be framed as "truth and consequences."

Truth and Consequences

Until recently, our ability to visualize brain processes was very limited. Most available measures in neuropsychiatry were indirect. Biologic researchers usually resorted to peripheral measures, such as assays of blood samples, that were believed to reflect brain activity but were not direct measures of the central nervous system. Peripheral biologic measures still play an important, if declining, role in biologic research.

We now have assessment procedures that directly visualize the brain and get us much closer to the processes of interest. These include, in addition to structural magnetic resonance imaging (MRI), the powerful new neuroimaging technologies like Positron Emission Tomography (PET), Single Photon Emission Computed Tomography (SPECT), and functional MRI and magnetic resonance spectroscopy (MRS). But these procedures are intensive, expensive to conduct, and sometimes invasive. The nature of the assessments limits the number and kind of individuals who are willing and able to undergo them, or who could ethically be asked to do so.

Studies may have to be conducted among patients in a specialty clinic or tertiary care hospital where the researchers and measurement technology are located. In this kind of setting, the patients may be derived from diverse populations and may have already had a variety of treatments in other settings. Typically, few are in their first episode of illness, and these few may be especially difficult to recruit, unable or unwilling to undergo intensive assessments.

Consequently, biologic researchers are "caught between a rock and a hard place." On the one hand, they may opt for indirect measures of uncertain validity, such as peripheral biologic measures of blood samples, or direct brain measures such as ordinary Computerized Tomography (CT) scans that have been routinized but are outmoded. On the other hand, they may choose to use more novel and intensive direct assessments that in practice constrain them to small numbers of cases who may be atypical. Novel assessments also impose constraints on the number and selection of the controls.

For most of us, the natural inclination is to try to get closer to the truth with more intensive measures. We accept what appears to be the inevitable consequence: a small study, atypical patients, and controls that do not provide an ideal basis for comparisons. We also accept that newly developed measures of the brain tend to be relatively untried and unstandardized. We expect that these measures will nonetheless yield new insights about biologic processes.

Epidemiologic Perspective

The epidemiologic perspective enables us to show that the general principles originally developed for risk factor investigations can be used to improve the design of biologic studies of causes. These principles are not rigid rules but can be used as a starting point for thinking about issues such as the selection of cases and controls in any given study. The more these principles are incorporated, the more rapidly biologic research will produce valid results.

By far the most common strategy for biologic research on causes is to compare a case group with a control group. We suggest that such studies can be considered as a special instance of the case-control design. The biologic measure is equivalent to the exposure measure in an ordinary epidemiologic case-control study. The biologic studies are usually led solely by biologic researchers and are not intended to be case-control studies. Yet the design is logically equivalent, and the appellation turns out to be strikingly apt.

As we will make clear, this is not merely a mental exercise. It has important practical implications. Accepting that these studies are actually case-control studies immediately suggests the issues that must be considered in study design and analysis.

Thus, in case-control studies, the method of selecting cases and controls is of paramount importance, providing the foundation for causal inference. In the selection of cases, biologic studies using prevalent instead of incident cases may find it difficult to determine whether the exposure predated the outcome. Almost all biologic researchers have faced the quandary of an association between a biologically measured factor and a disorder wherein it is unclear which one caused the other. In the selection of controls, biologic studies sometimes include decisions that appear to simplify the design but which actually introduce unnecessary complexity. An example is the exclusion of comorbid disorders from the control group (see chapter 21).

Sample size is also important because small-sample case-control studies tend to produce chance associations and fail to detect real ones (see part VI). The issues of sample selection and sample size are interrelated. In studies with small sample sizes and intensive measurements, the selection process becomes all the more important. Since each subject makes a substantial contribution to the result (as well as the cost) of the study, the subject must be selected so that the contribution is meaningful.

The use of measures that are reliable and comparable across studies is crucial to the interpretation of results from case-control studies. In biologic research on mental disorders, this criterion is difficult to meet and in fact is often not met. The problems are exacerbated by the complexity and novelty of the data. In the early applications of a procedure, we often have no standard precedent to follow, and the reliability of the measures is not established. The early MRI studies, for example, yielded thousands of data points that were summed and then used to measure the size of discrete brain structures. Cases and controls could be compared on many dimensions, using many procedures of analysis.

Although these principles are common to case-control studies in any domain, their application to this context is not easy and has to be weighed against other aspects of the study. Nowadays, biologic measures are routinely incorporated into epidemiologic research in other fields. But this experience is not directly applicable to biologic studies of mental disorders. A measure taken from a blood sample does not pose comparable difficulties to a measure of the brain.

Biologic Studies Reframed as Case-Control Designs

Two examples will be used to illustrate how biologic studies of mental disorders might be viewed as case-control designs. We will also use these examples to demonstrate the practical implications of doing so. We have chosen studies that have a well-deserved reputation as classics. Readers will then keep in mind that, though the methods of these (and any other) studies could be improved, they nonetheless produced durable and important results.

The first example is a study of abnormal smooth-pursuit eye movement and schizophrenia (table 19.1; Holzman et al. 1973). Under normal circumstances

Table 19.1 Classic Biological Studies Reframed as Case-Control Studies

Study	Study Description and Findings
Cleare et al. (1996)	*Study hypothesis*: Investigated role of serotonin dysfunction in the etiology of major depression.
	Cases (N = 19): Individuals with major depression, 12 female and 7 male.
	Controls (N = 19): Individuals without major depression matched for age, sex, and weight and (for women) menstrual status.
	Finding: Significantly lower prolactin and cortisol responses to d-fenfluramine in cases compared to controls.
Holzman et al. (1973)	*Study hypothesis*: Investigated whether individuals with schizophrenia exhibit alterations in smooth-pursuit eye-tracking patterns.
	Cases (N = 21): Patients with schizophrenia or schizoaffective disorder.
	Controls 1 (N = 33): Normal controls with no psychiatric disorder.
	Controls 2 (N = 12): Patients with another psychiatric disorder.
	Finding: More abnormal eye-tracking movement in cases than in controls.

(that is, in the absence of extreme fatigue, intoxicating substances, or certain medications), when an individual is asked to follow a target across a visual field the eyes move smoothly, tracing a sinusoidal curve. The investigators had reason to believe that such smooth-pursuit eye movement was selectively disrupted in a causal pathway leading to schizophrenia.

To examine this possibility, they chose a case group of 21 patients with schizophrenia or schizoaffective disorder and two control groups. One was a well control group of 33 individuals with no discernible psychiatric illness, and the other was an unwell control group of 12 patients being treated for a psychiatric disorder other than schizophrenia. Abnormal smooth-pursuit eye movement was more common in the cases than in either control group, suggesting that this brain function was indeed disrupted in schizophrenia.

The study question was whether an individual characteristic (smooth-pursuit eye movement) had a causal connection to a disorder (schizophrenia). To answer this question, the authors used a comparison of cases and controls. Thus, it is appropriate to view this study as a case-control design. This perspective is informative, because it enables us to evaluate the results and suggest further steps to clarify them. Consider, for example, the selection of the control groups. Based on the discussion introduced in chapter 17 and extended in chapter 21, it is likely that the comparison with the well control group overestimated the difference between cases and controls, whereas the comparison with the unwell control group underestimated it. The association was, in fact, stronger in the former than in the latter comparison. In this instance, the researchers were fortunate that the association proved robust. In other instances, however, the use of two control groups biased in opposite directions can be a recipe for an inconclusive result.

In the second example, the authors sought to determine whether an abnormality in central serotonergic neurotransmission was "the underlying biochemical deficit in depression" (table 19.1; Cleare et.al. 1996). This was a widely held hypothesis supported by evidence from a variety of sources. However, the results of previous clinical studies that attempted to directly test the hypothesis had been somewhat inconsistent.

The design the authors chose was to compare a case group with a control group. The 19 cases were patients who met criteria for a current diagnosis of major depression. The 19 matched controls were staff and student volunteers. The cases and controls were compared with respect to the responsiveness of the central serotonin neurotransmission system. This was measured by the change in serum levels of the hormones cortisol and prolactin in response to the serotonin stimulant d-fenfluramine. The results suggested a blunted response of cortisol and prolactin to d-fenfluramine in the cases compared with the controls. Thus, the study supported the hypothesis that reduced serotonergic activity in the brain is linked to depression.

In order to illustrate the ambiguities that are revealed in reframing biologic studies as case-control designs, we will consider this study from two different vantage points. From the first vantage point, the question being asked in this study corresponds to the motivating question of an ordinary case-control study. The investigators were looking for a causal connection between a characteristic of an individual (serotonergic abnormality) and the occurrence of a disorder (depression). Hence, the principles developed in the preceding sections are applicable to the evaluation of the study and to the interpretation of its results.

Drawing on these principles, the reader will note that the study was not limited to incident cases. This means that the serotonergic abnormality may have been a result rather than a cause of depression, or may have been related to the persistence or recurrence rather than the onset of depression. In addition, the data were not analyzed in the way that most directly addresses the causal question. To directly answer this question, we would compute an odds ratio to gauge the effect of the serotonergic abnormality on the disease risk. Instead, the study compared cases and controls with respect to the level of serotonergic activity, using an ANOVA analysis. Thus, by taking an epidemiologic perspective on this work, we can gain insight into the remaining questions and design more effective studies to answer them.

From the second vantage point, the question in this study was about the consequences of depression, or more precisely, the abnormal pathophysiology that characterizes depression after its onset. From this vantage point, it was not a study of causes. So it would not be appropriate to frame it as a case-control design.

Since the report was somewhat ambiguous about which of these two questions was being addressed, either vantage point could be legitimate. This same ambiguity is commonly found in biologic studies in psychiatry. It reflects our uncertainty about the pathophysiology, as well as the nosology, of mental disorders. The epidemiologic perspective compels us, however, to differentiate these questions and to spell out the implications for study design. Indeed, this would be a potentially important refinement in biologic studies in psychiatry, one that could be achieved only by epidemiologists and biologic researchers working together.

Integration

We have suggested that the case-control design is fundamentally the same, whether the study is designed by a biologic researcher, an epidemiologist, or anyone else. Though entirely logical, this integrative perspective has not been widely adopted in psychiatric research. Until recently, it faced social barriers to acceptance. Psychiatric researchers were emerging from a contentious era in which the relative importance of organic and nonorganic causes was hotly disputed. Epidemiologists were often identified with nonorganic sociologic or psychologic research. This debate has now been put to rest, with almost all parties accepting that the brain is the organ of the mind, and as such it is affected by the interplay of factors at many levels, including social experiences such as stigma and discrimination, psychologic states such as fear, biologic actions of neurotransmitters, and the regulation of genes. With these barriers behind us, the time is right for linking epidemiologic and biologic research. We should not think, however, that the process of integration will be simple. It will require both biologic and epidemiologic researchers to modify cherished concepts and methods.

It will also require some deep thinking about issues at the interface. One might ask, for example, whether biologic studies of pathophysiology are really seeking to establish causes in the sense that an epidemiologist perceives a cause. The abnormal function of a neurotransmitter might be considered as an integral part of the illness rather than either as a cause or a consequence of the illness. We suggest that in most instances the biologic factor is being considered as a cause, albeit one that is proximal to the illness. Nonetheless, there will be exceptions, and such issues cannot be glossed over. Confronting them directly and together represents the most effective if most challenging path to our common goal of discovering the causes of mental illnesses.

Conclusion

This chapter has argued that advantages can accrue from an interdisciplinary perspective. Although the purpose of this book is to demonstrate the uses of epidemiology, the benefits flow both ways. Epidemiologists have much to learn from biologic researchers. Studies jointly designed by biologic and epidemiologic researchers have the potential to propel us toward the discovery of causes.

By including acclaimed and groundbreaking biologic studies among our examples, we are attempting to show how epidemiologic principles can improve upon best practice in biologic psychiatry. We hope that this approach will make the potential benefits most compelling, especially for the upcoming generation of biologic researchers, whose studies will also benefit from our ever-improving understanding of the fundamentals of brain neurocircuitry and molecular function. In the next chapters, we suggest specific ways in which integrating epidemiologic methods into biologic studies could accelerate the discovery of causes.

References

Cleare AJ, Murray RM, and O'Keane V (1996). Reduced Prolactin and Cortisol Responses to d-Fenfluramine in Depressed Compared to Healthy Matched Control Subjects. *Neuropsychopharmacology* 14:349–354.

Holzman PS, Proctor LR, and Hughes DW (1973). Eye-Tracking Patterns in Schizophrenia. *Science* 181:179–181.

20 Choosing Cases in Biologic Psychiatry

Evelyn J. Bromet, Ezra Susser, Gary A. Heiman, and Jack M. Gorman

We have proposed that biologic studies comparing cases with controls often correspond well to the case-control design introduced in part IV. Now we show how this perspective can be useful for advancing biological psychiatry. To limit the scope, we focus this chapter on the selection and the definition of cases in biologic studies, and the next chapter on choosing controls.

Selection of Cases in Ordinary Case-Control Designs

As discussed in the previous chapter, biologic studies in psychiatry can often be viewed either as studies of the causes or as studies of the concomitant pathophysiology of a disorder. For now, we will view them as studies of causes, which means that they can be framed in the same terms as ordinary case-control studies. Later in the chapter, we will revisit this question and view them from the alternative perspective.

Epidemiologists attempt to meet three criteria when they are selecting cases for a case-control design (chapter 16): (1) ascertainment close to the time of onset, (i.e., incident cases), (2) diagnoses incorporating a longitudinal perspective, and (3) selection from a definable source population, such as a geographically defined community. Although a growing number of biologic studies attend to one or more of these guidelines, the nature and the pace of brain research have posed formidable barriers. The newest measurement procedures tend to be complex to administer and are often invasive, raising practical and ethical concerns in recruitment.

A report of an association of schizophrenia with hyperactive dopaminergic transmission at the D2 receptor illustrates both the promise and the dilemmas of using novel techniques in brain research to study causes (table 20.1; Abi-Dargham et al. 2000). The researchers devised a new strategy for using single photon emission tomography (SPECT) to gain insight into brain function. They first administered a dopamine-depleting agent, alpha methyl paratyrosine, to free the cellular receptor of dopamine. They then administered a highly selective radiotracer (IBZM) for the now unoccupied dopamine recep-

Table 20.1 Study Exemplifying Use of Novel Brain-Imaging Techniques

Study	Study Description and Findings
Abi-Dargham et al. (2000)	*Study question*: Investigated hyperactive dopaminergic transmission at the D_2 receptor in schizophrenia.
	Cases (N = 18): Untreated patents with schizophrenia ascertained from an inpatient psychiatric hospital.
	Controls (N = 18): Normal controls matched on age, gender, race, and parental socioeconomic level.
	Finding: IB2M SPECT results provide indirect evidence of hyperactive dopaminergic activity in cases in comparison to controls.

tor. The quantification of IBZM binding provided an indirect gauge of dopa-minergic activity before the depletion.

The assessments in this study were safe and well tolerated in the specialized setting in which they were administered. SPECT involves minimal radiation, the patients were all hospitalized, and alpha methyl paratyrosine administration tends to decrease psychotic symptoms because of its dopamine-depleting properties. Nonetheless, the assessments were time-consuming and intensive, and the safe use of these procedures depended on their administration by skilled investigators in a hospital ward with conditions designed specifically to facilitate biological research studies. Any patient recruited had to give informed consent to two brain imaging scans and two days of alpha methyl paratyrosine before treatment for his or her illness would be initiated. Combined with the complexity of the brain-imaging procedure, these requirements limited the study to 18 cases in a tertiary-care hospital. Although samples that are this small and highly selected are rarely seen in other contexts, they are not unusual in biologic psychiatry.

The accumulation of case-control studies of this type will naturally produce a mix of artifactual and true results. Patients recruited to specialized research units resemble a mixed-origin case group (chapter 16) in that they are drawn from multiple origins and arrive by multiple pathways. Therefore, it may be extremely difficult to visualize a source population and choose an appropriate control group. They are often prevalent cases, which makes it difficult to distinguish causes from effects of the disorder. The small sample sizes and the limited comparability of measures across studies add further uncertainty regarding the inferences and generalizability of the findings.

Thus, in the collective endeavor of searching for the causes of mental disorders, we need to balance two imperatives. On the one hand, it is essential to continually advance our understanding of the functioning of the brain. On the other hand, it is equally essential to select samples that allow for the drawing of sound conclusions. Biologic researchers tend to place the most value on obtaining more direct measurements of the brain and accept the consequence of small samples of the most accessible patients. Epidemiologists tend to argue that in studies with intensive and often novel assessments, the method of case selection and the sample size are all the more crucial for valid causal inference.

The better we balance these imperatives, the more rapid our progress will be. We suggest, therefore, that in planning any particular study we should evaluate the design from both perspectives. Depending upon the kind of conclusions we wish to draw, we may give more weight to one or the other perspective, but both are relevant to the design of almost any study.

In an early exploratory use of an entirely novel measure, a small sample of convenience may be quite appropriate, because of both practical and ethical considerations, and may yield useful preliminary results. Nonetheless, by considering the implications of the selection of cases (and of controls; see chapter 21) as discussed here, one may see ways to attain a better approximation to a well-selected sample, even under the practical constraints of the study. Once a measure becomes standardized and can be used safely in ordinary settings, larger studies using well-selected samples may be possible, or even mandatory, to test the preliminary findings and advance the field. To illustrate the possibilities, we describe some biological studies that have been innovative in attending to one or more of our three outlined criteria for case selection.

Biologic Studies Using Well-Selected Cases

The Markers and Predictors of Schizophrenia Project (Beiser et al. 1994) provides an example of a biologic study that applied these criteria. The cases were recruited at the time of their first psychotic episode. The initial assessment included both psychosocial and diagnostic information, as well as measures of smooth-pursuit eye movements, visibility of nail-fold plexus, and CT scans. Subsequent follow-up assessments were used to refine the diagnoses. People with psychosis were recruited from all sources of medical care—inpatient, outpatient, and general medical treatment providers—in Vancouver, British Columbia. Thus, the biologic data were obtained as close as possible to the onset of psychotic symptoms, longitudinal data could be incorporated into diagnoses, and the cases were drawn from a well-defined source population. A control group from the source population was also selected and assessed.

Another distinctive feature of this study is that it was designed to be suitable for both the investigation of causes (using a case-control design) and outcomes (using a clinical cohort design). The biologic and psychosocial measures taken at the initial assessment were analyzed in conjunction as predictors of outcome. For instance, an analysis of the predictors of 18-month occupational functioning included biologic variables such as smooth-pursuit eye movement, as well as psychosocial variables, such as premorbid social competence (table 20.2). However, the results afforded no simple interpretation, underscoring the complexity of the pathways and interactions among biologic and psychosocial predictors of outcome in schizophrenia.

An example of attention to mainly the first criterion, recent onset or incident cases, is a brain-imaging study of amygdala volume in depression (table 20.2; Frodl et al. 2002). Previous studies had been somewhat inconsistent and

Table 20.2 Studies Exemplifying Innovative Case Selection

Study	Study Description and Selected Findings
Beiser et al. (1994)	*Study question*: The study was suitable for investigating both causes and outcomes. The report cited here investigated both biologic and psychological predictors of occupational functioning at 18-month follow-up in individuals with a first-onset psychosis.
	Cases 1 (N = 33): Patients with first-onset schizophrenia drawn from a network of psychiatric and medical services in Vancouver.
	Cases 2 (N = 31): Patients with first-onset affective psychosis similarly obtained.
	Controls (N = 46): Age- and sex-matched normal controls drawn from family practices in low-income areas and unemployment centers.
	Finding: In schizophrenia, eye tracking, but not visibility of nail-fold plexus, was inversely related to occupational functioning at follow-up in the bivariate analysis, but the reverse was true in multivariate analyses that adjusted for initial occupational functioning. In affective psychosis, neither biological variable was significantly related to subsequent occupational functioning.
Frodl et al. (2002)	*Study question*: Investigated amygdala volume in individuals with a first episode major depression.
	Cases (N = 30): Inpatients with first episode major depression.
	Controls (N = 30): Healthy volunteers matched on age, gender, handedness and education and with no known neurologic or psychiatric disease in first degree relatives.
	Finding: Cases had increased amygdala volumes compared with controls.
Goetz et al. (2001)	*Study question*: 10–15 year follow-up of depressed adolescents and controls with baseline polysomnographic EEG recordings. Baseline study found no differences between cases and controls.
	Cases 1 (N = 28): Young adults who had major depression diagnosed in adolescence;
	Cases 2 (N = 25): Young adults who served as normal controls in the study in adolescence, but who had developed depression by the time of follow-up in young adulthood.
	Controls (N = 17): Depression-free normal controls.
	Finding: Baseline sleep patterns (sleep latency, sleep period time, REM latency, slow-wave sleep) were significantly more disturbed in the two depressed groups (combined) than in controls.

difficult to interpret, in part because they used prevalent cases. In contrast, the researchers in this study assembled a sample of patients hospitalized for their first episode of major depression. First admission is often used as a proxy for incident cases, although many first-admission cases may in fact have been ill for months and sometimes years. In this study, illness duration lasted from one month to 5 years (mean was about 6 months). Nevertheless, the procedure represented a substantial improvement on the common practice of using prevalent cases (e.g., consecutive admissions). This study found an increased amygdala volume in cases compared with controls.

An intriguing study of adolescent depression shows how the uses of longitudinal diagnosis can extend beyond the usual short-term follow-up assessment. Longitudinal information obtained at different stages of the life course proved crucial to defining case status. The study was built on the pioneering use of polysomnographic electroencephalogram (EEG) recordings in a study of childhood and adolescent depression (Puig-Antich et al. 1982). The initial study compared these cases with a control group but found no clear-cut differences. Later, another research group followed up the adolescents of the initial study, when they were young adults (table 20.2; Goetz et al. 2001). A number of control adolescents developed depression during the follow-up and were reclassified as latent depressive cases. A revised analysis compared both initial and latent depressed cases with the remaining controls on the original childhood EEG measure. The authors found several significant differences between the expanded case group and the control group, especially pertaining to sleep abnormalities during the first 100 minutes of the sleep period.

Definition of a Case in a Biologic Study

We have proposed that in epidemiologic studies of mental disorders it may be appropriate to tailor the definition of a case to the research question (chapter 9). For most mental disorders, diagnoses are based on thoughts, behaviors, and feelings, and we do not know how well these diagnoses correspond to an underlying pathophysiology. Although most studies adhere to the current nosology of the *DSM* or the *ICD* in defining the cases for a study, alternative approaches can be entirely legitimate.

In biologic studies, likewise, researchers have often taken the perspective that a diagnosis may not necessarily be the most useful definition of a case for the study. Next we discuss two consequences that follow from this perspective: the use of biologic markers, and the ambiguity about whether one is studying antecedents or consequences of a disorder.

Use of Biologic Markers

In order to attain a closer correspondence between an underlying pathophysiology and the cases being studied, biologic researchers increasingly turn to the use of biologic markers. In a given study, these physiological and molecular entities may serve as refinements, complements, or alternatives to conventional diagnostic criteria.

Biologic markers can be used in several different ways. One strategy is to apply a biologic marker to demarcate a subgroup of patients within a broad diagnostic category. The marker is used in combination with *DSM* or *ICD* diagnostic criteria to define the cases, in an attempt to select cases with a common pathophysiology. A notable early attempt to identify such a marker took the form of a study comparing cases with controls (table 20.3; Carroll et al. 1976). The authors assessed the cortisol response to dexamethasone as a biologic marker for endogenous depression, which was thought to be biologically distinct from other kinds of depression. They postulated that (1) abnormal hypothalamic pituitary axis (HPA) activity was a cause of endogenous depression, and (2) the dexamethasone test could be used as an indicator of the underlying abnormal HPA activity. They compared cases (endogenous depression) with controls (other psychiatric disorders including nonendogenous depression). Consistent with their hypothesis, an abnormal dexamethasone test result was associated specifically with endogenous depression. Subsequent research has failed to confirm the utility of the dexamethasone suppression test as a diagnostic tool because of a lack of specificity and sensitivity. Nevertheless, as a result of this work, a convincing body of evidence has been amassed showing that the neural systems that control the release of cortisol, beginning with corticotropin-releasing hormone, are abnormally regulated in patients with mood and anxiety disorders. This has led to attempts, still under investigation, to pharmacologically block the effects of a hyperactive HPA axis in patients suffering from depression.

Another strategy is to use a biologic marker to represent an intermediate step in one of the causal pathways to the disorder. Individuals with an intermediate outcome, though at high risk for the disorder, do not necessarily manifest the disorder per se. Nonetheless, this intermediate outcome may be used to define the cases in a study. Such an approach, in essence, attempts to reduce the complexity of psychiatric illness, by attending to one of the many biological processes that may be involved.

Perhaps the best-known kind of intermediate outcome in psychiatric research, selected so as to reflect genetic causes, is an endophenotype (see part VII; Gottesman and Shields 1982; Gottesman and Gould 2003). Event-related brain potentials illustrate a hypothesized endophenotype for alcoholism. Early on, studies related evoked brain potentials to alcoholism, and twin studies suggested that these evoked potentials were heritable traits (Begleiter et al. 1984; Rogers and Deary 1991). A subsequent study

Table 20.3 Study Exemplifying a Marker Differentiating Subgroups on a Biologic Process

Study	Study Description and Findings
Carroll et al. (1976)	*Study question*: Investigated whether the dexamethasone suppression test can discriminate endogenous depression from other disorders.
	Cases (N = 42): Individuals with "endogenomorphic" (unipolar and bipolar) depression.
	Controls (N = 42): Individuals with other psychiatric disorders, including schizophrenia, neurotic depression, anxiety disorder, personality disorder, and organic brain syndrome.
	Finding: Compared 24-hour plasma and urinary cortisol levels after a dose of dexamethasone. Found significantly higher 24-hour cortisol levels in the endogenous depression group.

specifically evaluated the P_{300} component of event-related brain potentials as a potential endophenotype. The authors concluded that the amplitude of the P_{300} waveform was lower in alcoholics than in nonalcoholics, lower in unaffected relatives of alcoholics than in relatives of controls, and lower in unaffected offspring of alcoholic fathers than offspring of controls (Hesselbrock et al. 2001). Basing their conclusions on these and past results, they suggested that this marker could indicate a genetically transmitted vulnerability to alcoholism. Some investigators are now using event-related potentials to define the outcomes in genetic linkage analyses (Almasy et al. 2001).

Intermediate outcomes are not used only in biological research and are not always necessarily represented by biological measurements. A neuropsychological battery to assess moderate cognitive decline, has been central to a method for obtaining an intermediate marker for Alzheimer's disease (Arnaiz and Almkvist 2003).

Interpretation of Results. When we suggested that diagnoses need not always be used to define a case, we also emphasized some important provisos (chapter 9). The "cases" in a study should be defined rigorously and explicitly and assessed with reliable instruments, and the results should be interpretable in relation to the diagnosable disorder. The interpretability is of particular import when a biologic marker is used to represent "cases" who have an intermediate outcome. By conventional criteria, individuals with the biologic marker may not have any diagnosable illness and may not even be symptomatic. How then do we interpret the result for the cases defined by the marker in terms of the disorder?

This is an area in which epidemiologic thinking can be useful to biologic researchers. Figure 20.1—adapted from an article on cancer epidemiology (Terry et al. 2000)—depicts the relationships expected among an exposure (cigarette smoking), an intermediate outcome (adenoma), and a disease (colorectal cancer). In this scenario, smoking causes a major increase in the risk of adenoma (risk ratio = 3.0), but only a minor increase in the risk of cancer (risk ratio = 1.3). It can be shown that, in general, as in this hypothetical example, the risk ratio for the intermediate outcome will be substantially larger than the risk ratio for the disease itself, provided two conditions are met. One is that the intermediate outcome is on the sole biologic pathway leading from the risk factor to the disease. The other is that this pathway accounts for only some of the cases of disease. Just such relationships have been postulated in psychiatric research. For example, where a prenatal insult is the exposure, ventricular enlargement represents an intermediate outcome, and schizophrenia is the disease.

We may draw three relevant conclusions from this work. First, examining the relation of an exposure to an intermediate outcome can be an effective strategy for the identification of causes. It may be much easier to detect the larger effect of the exposure on the intermediate outcome than the smaller effect of the exposure on the disease. This is because the power to detect an effect increases with the size of the effect as measured by the risk ratio (see part VI).

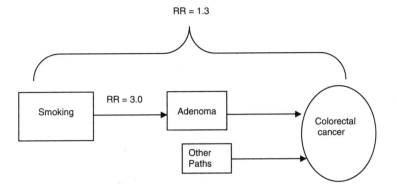

Smoking = exposure
Adenoma = intermediate outcome
Colorectal cancer = disease

Assumptions:
1) Risk of adenoma in unexposed = 15%
2) Overall risk of colorectal cancer = 3%
3) Prevalence of smoking = 50%
4) 50% of colorectal cancers arise from adenomas

Figure 20.1 A model illustrating that the risk ratio (RR) for the intermediate outcome can be much larger than the risk ratio for the disease.

Second, we should be careful not to misinterpret large risk ratios found for intermediate outcomes. In the scenario of figure 20.1, in accordance with the risk ratio of 3.0 between smoking and adenoma, we might legitimately infer that smoking is a cause of colorectal cancer. Its effect on the disease, however, would be a weak one; the risk ratio is a very modest 1.3. This is in part because in this scenario, the pathways via adenoma accounts for only about half the cases of colorectal cancer.

Third, the relationships depend in a systematic way on the assumptions made for the scenario. In figure 20.1, for example, the assumptions are that 50 percent of the disease occurs via the intermediate outcome and 50 percent via other pathways, and that 7 percent of those with the intermediate outcome progress to the disease. Attributing less than 50 percent of the disease to the intermediate outcome, or positing a weaker relationship of the intermediate outcome to the disease, would reduce the risk ratio to less than 1.3. Conversely, attributing more than 50 percent of the disease to the intermediate outcome, or positing a stronger relationship of the intermediate outcome to the disease, would increase the risk ratio to more than 1.3 (for further discussion, see Terry et al. 2000).

Thus, the correct interpretation of the results for an intermediate outcome in terms of the disease depends upon the causal process linking the intermediate outcome to the disease. This means that postulating causal pathways and examining the relationships among causes are essential parts of the study. Since the pathways are usually unknown, it may be wise to postulate several alternative scenarios and then examine how the different assumptions affect the interpretation, as in a sensitivity analysis (chapter 13).

Causes versus Concomitants

We proposed in the previous chapter that most biological studies compare cases and controls in order to elucidate causes and, therefore, can be conceptualized as case-control studies. Our discussion so far has been based on this premise. But many biological studies could also be characterized as investigations of the biological processes that are concomitant with or consequences of the disorder. In the previous chapter, we illustrated this with a study of serotonergic abnormality as the underlying biochemical deficit in depression, which could be seen as either a study of causes or a study of concomitants or consequences of depression. The IBZM study we have described (Table 20.1) provides an example of a study that might actually be closer to a study of concomitants or consequences than of causes.

The ambiguity arises in part because biological researchers tend to conceptualize the disorder in terms of pathophysiology, whereas current diagnostic criteria tend to be based on manifestations in thoughts, behaviors, and feelings. If one does not accept current diagnostic criteria and assessment methods as delineating the onset of the condition being investigated, it is difficult to make a distinction between proximal antecedents and early manifestations. In biological studies, therefore, it is not always clear whether the factor being investigated is best seen as an antecedent cause, as a concomitant pathophysiology, or as a consequence of a mental disorder.

The dilemma is well illustrated in a study of hippocampal volume in adolescent onset schizophrenia. The cases were 40 adolescent patients admitted with recent-onset schizophrenia, and the controls were recruited from the community via advertisement (Matsumoto et al. 2001). In contrast with previously reported findings on adults with first-admission schizophrenia, there were no significant differences in hippocampal volumes (after adjusting for whole brain volume) in these adolescent cases as compared with the controls. The authors suggested that the reduced hippocampal volume associated with schizophrenia in the previous studies of adults might not have preceded the illness, but rather might have been an early manifestation of the illness. That is, the hippocampal brain changes in schizophrenia may not be expressed until the brain developments that take place in late adolescence; therefore, they would be established by the time of a first-admission in adulthood but not by the time of a first-admission in adolescence. Implicit in this interpretation is the notion that schizophrenia is a neurodevelopmental disorder with varying manifestations over the life course. In other words, the condition may be present before the disorder can be diagnosed using current criteria, and before the brain changes that are often evident by the time of diagnosis in adulthood.

Nonetheless, the distinction cannot be entirely evaded, as it has implications for the design and interpretation of a study. Within the rubric of epidemiologic designs, studies of the causes of a disorder are case-control designs. Studies of the consequences of a disorder are clinical cohorts as defined in chapter 10.

Let us now take the view that biological studies are examining the concomitants or consequences of a disorder. What are the practical implications for the selection of cases? The biological processes associated with a disorder evolve over time. For long-term conditions, such as many psychiatric disorders, the changes may be substantial, even in the absence of treatment effects. Therefore, an overriding concern in the selection of cases for these studies is that the cases should be at a similar point in the course of illness. Incident cases are ideal, because they are close to onset and can be followed over time as a clinical cohort. But it is also appropriate, for this kind of study, to select cases at some other defined stage in the illness (e.g., 5–10 years or 25–30 years after onset). What one would want to avoid is selecting a case group that is heterogeneous in this respect.

As noted earlier, in many studies, the distinction is ambiguous. These studies might be thought of as hybrid designs that mix features of the case-control study and the clinical cohort study. The epidemiologic principles discussed here are, however, adaptable to this circumstance. The cases should ideally be incident cases under either perspective. The controls in such studies are used to determine whether the biological processes we observe are (or are not) related to the disorder, either as cause or consequence. In the main, the guidelines discussed in the next chapter are still applicable to selection of controls in the context of this ambiguity.

Conclusion

In biological studies comparing cases and controls, the principles developed by epidemiologists for the selection of cases in ordinary case-control studies can often be put in practice and substantially strengthen the design. However, these practices would impose unnecessary constraints on some biological studies in psychiatry, and their application must always be tailored to yield a net advantage. In regard to alternative approaches to defining cases, the interpretation of results from studies using biologic markers is an area in which epidemiologic concepts and methods can make a contribution to biological studies in psychiatry. Finally, although the epidemiologic perspective compels us to carefully consider the distinction between causes and consequences, sometimes in biological psychiatry the distinction between proximal antecedent and early manifestation has to be left ambiguous, and the principles of epidemiologic design can also be adapted to serve in this circumstance.

We have touched on but a few of the many issues involved in selecting and defining cases for biological studies of mental disorders. Our hope is that by opening this discussion, we will help to stimulate a wider dialogue between the disciplines. This would surely enrich both fields and hasten the discovery of causes of psychiatric disorders.

References

Abi-Dargham A, Rodenhiser J, Printz D, et al. (2000). Increased Baseline Occupancy of D_2 Receptors by Dopamine in Schizophrenia. *Proc. Nat.l Acad. Sci. USA* 97:8104–8109.

Almasy L, Porjesz B, Blangero J, et al. (2001). Genetics of Event-Related Brain Potentials in Response to a Semantic Priming Paradigm in Families with a History of Alcoholism. *Am. J. Hum. Genet.* 68:128–135.

Arnaiz E and Almkvist O (2003). Neuropsychological Features of Mild Cognitive Impairment and Preclinical Alzheimer's Disease. *Acta Neurol. Scand. Suppl.* 179:34–41.

Begleiter H, Porjesz B, Bihari B, and Kissin B (1984). Event-Related Brain Potentials in Boys at Risk for Alcoholism. *Science* 225:1493–1496.

Beiser M, Bean G, Erickson D, Zhang J, Iacono WG, and Rector NA (1994). Biological and Psychosocial Predictors of Job Performance Following a First Episode of Psychosis. *Am. J. Psychiatry* 151:857–863.

Carroll BJ, Curtis GC, and Mendels J (1976). Neuroendocrine Regulation in Depression. II. Discrimination of Depressed from Nondepressed Patients. *Arch. Gen. Psychiatry* 33:1051–1058.

Frodl T, Meisenzahl E, Zetzsche T, et al. (2002). Enlargement of the Amygdala in Patients with a First Episode of Major Depression. *Biol. Psychiatry* 51:708–714.

Goetz RR, Wolk SI, Coplan JD, Ryan ND, and Weissman MM (2001). Premorbid Polysomnographic Signs in Depressed Adolescents: A Reanalysis of EEG Sleep after Longitudinal Follow-Up in Adulthood. *Biol. Psychiatry* 49:930–942.

Gottesman II and Gould TD (2003). The Endophenotype Concept in Psychiatry: Etymology and Strategic Intentions. *Am. J. Psychiatry* 160:636–645.

Gottesman II and Shields J (1982). *Schizophrenia: The Epigenetic Puzzle*. Cambridge: Cambridge University Press.

Hesselbrock V, Begleiter H, Porjesz B, O'Connor S, and Bauer L (2001). P_{300} Event-Related Potential Amplitude as an Endophenotype of Alcoholism—Evidence from the Collaborative Study on the Genetics of Alcoholism. *J. Biomed. Sci.* 8:77–82.

Matsumoto H, Simmons A, Williams S, Pipe R, Murray R, and Frangou S (2001). Structural Magnetic Imaging of the Hippocampus in Early Onset Schizophrenia. *Biol. Psychiatry* 49:824–831.

Puig-Antich J, Goetz R, Hanlon C, Davies M, Thompson J, Chambers WJ, Tabrizi MA, and Weitzman ED (1982). Sleep Architecture and REM Sleep Measures in Prepubertal Children with Major Depression: A Controlled Study. *Arch. Gen. Psychiatry* 39:932–939.

Rogers TD and Deary I (1991). The P_{300} Component of the Auditory Event-Related Potential in Monozygotic and Dizygotic Twins. *Acta Psychiatr. Scand.* 83:412–416.

Terry MB, Neugut AI, Schwartz S, and Susser E (2000). Risk Factors for a Causal Intermediate and an Endpoint: Reconciling Differences. *Am. J. Epidemiol.* 151:339–345.

Choosing Controls in Biologic Psychiatry

21

Sharon Schwartz, Ezra Susser, and Jack M. Gorman

One of the most difficult—and intellectually intriguing—tasks of a biologic case-control study is the selection of the control group. The task is not only difficult but also quite hazardous. An inappropriate control group can mask the presence of a true association or create the illusion of an association when one does not exist.

The control group is always tailored to a particular study and therein lies the challenge. Choosing a control group depends on thinking through the implications of many other features of the study: the types of cases being selected, the biologic process being examined, and most critically, the specific hypothesis being tested. No criteria can be advanced to define the perfect control group, because there is no control group that is appropriate for all or even most case-control studies.

Nonetheless, it is possible to approach the task systematically. In previous chapters (part IV) we derived a practical guideline for making the best choice of a control group in an ordinary case-control study. In what follows, we demonstrate how it can be applied to biologic studies of causes.[1] We take up a central question, apply the guideline, and arrive at an answer that has important implications for biologic research. We hope to entice our readers to proceed similarly to address many other questions that arise about control groups in biologic studies.

The question we consider is whether or not the presence of a disorder other than the one being studied should influence the selection of an individual into the control group. We chose this question for several reasons. One is that this question is pervasive, as well as perplexing, in biologic psychiatry. Another is that current practices are prone to introduce artifact. Although we touched on this question in a previous chapter, the present discussion extends further, examining more varied and complex scenarios, and specifically focuses on biologic research.

---

[1] Although not discussed here, the guidelines are also useful for biologic studies in which the designation of the biologic factor as proximal antecedent or early manifestation is ambiguous.

We approach the question from the same two vantage points as previously. First, should we use a well control group, a control group that excludes people with other disorders? Second, should we use an unwell control group, a control group composed entirely of patients with other disorders? Answering these questions has implications for decisions about all other disorders in the control group, whether these disorders be comorbid with the study outcome or not. By *comorbidity* we mean a disorder that occurs together with the study outcome more often than would be expected based on chance alone (see chapter 17). Since comorbidity is a distinctive characteristic of psychiatric disorders, we pay special attention to it.

Practical Guideline

We begin by recapitulating the practical guideline for selection of controls which was derived in previous chapters. Here we present it concisely and overlook some nuances that are not required for the main argument.[2]

The selection of a control group in a case-control study depends on a thought experiment in which we conceptualize the case-control study as a condensed version of a cohort study. The cases and controls are thought of as deriving from a real or imagined underlying cohort. The cases are the people in the underlying cohort who develop the disease. The controls are a sample of the people in the underlying cohort who do not develop the disease. From this perspective, a control group should represent the exposure experience of the underlying cohort that gave rise to the cases. Note that the controls need not, and indeed should not, represent the general population, but rather the specific population that gave rise to the cases.

To choose a control group, the researcher needs to visualize this underlying cohort. Who are these people and where can they be located? Then the researcher needs to select controls from the underlying cohort such that the exposure odds in the controls will be the same as the exposure odds in the underlying cohort.

We derived a practical guideline for doing so: the same criteria should be applied to the selection of the controls as were applied to the selection of the cases. Our guideline suggests, for example, that the use of volunteer controls, common in biologic studies, can be problematic. Because biologic studies often require participants to undergo time-consuming, uncomfortable, or even invasive procedures, controls may be hard to find. Researchers often recruit controls through advertisements, sometimes from employees at the study institution. Although this procedure is reasonable from a practical and ethical standpoint, it implies different criteria for the entry of cases and controls into the study, which violates our guideline and can lead to biased results.

We now examine the implications of our guideline for the use of well controls and the use of unwell controls. For clarity of exposition, we rely on

---

[2] For example, we will assume here that the underlying cohort fully represents the source population.

hypothetical scenarios built to mimic the conditions of actual biologic studies.

Well Controls

The use of well controls means the researcher excludes from the control group individuals with disorders other than the one being investigated. This exclusion is frequently applied specifically to individuals with disorders the researcher suspects are comorbid with the study disorder. If we exclude people with other disorders from the control group, but not from the case group, however, we are applying different selection criteria to the case and the control groups. Thus, it is immediately apparent that this practice violates our practical guideline. Accordingly, we should expect it to introduce bias. In chapter 17, we showed that, in at least one scenario, it did.

Yet well controls are routinely used—and often recommended—for biologic case-control studies (Schwartz and Link 1989; Kendler 1990; Klein 1993). Generally, researchers screen potential controls for psychiatric disorders and sometimes even for elevated scores on symptoms scales, family history, and physical disorders. They include in the control group only well controls who have screened negative. They usually do not apply the same exclusions to the cases in the study.

The perception that well controls should be used has a powerful influence on the design of biologic research. Our ongoing Prenatal Determinants of Schizophrenia Example (PDSE; see tables 10.6 and 10.7) can be used to illustrate. A case-control neuroimaging study is nested within the actual PDS cohort (from which the PDSE is simplified to facilitate illustration). It was designed so that controls represent the individuals without schizophrenia spectrum disorders in the fully enumerated underlying PDSE cohort. Therefore, individuals with other psychiatric disorders were not excluded from the control group. In the initial review of the grant proposal, concerns were raised about this feature; not using well controls was considered a serious flaw in the design.

What would be the rationale for this view? The argument for well controls in biologic psychiatry is actually very reasonable. Researchers are cognizant of the potential overlap in the causes of diverse psychiatric disorders. It is often suspected that the biologic factor being investigated as a cause of the disorder under study may also play a role in other disorders. In this context, many biologic researchers argue much as follows: We should screen controls to exclude people with other psychiatric disorders. Otherwise, the presence of comorbid disorders in the control group would reduce the difference between cases and controls with respect to the biologic factor. This would make it more difficult to detect a true association between the biologic factor and the disorder under study.

Though apparently reasonable, the argument turns out to be mistaken. In order to demonstrate the mistake involved, we turn to a hypothetical example.

A Hypothetical Example

We have previously shown that the use of well controls introduces bias in one scenario (see chapter 17). But many scenarios have to be considered in the design of biologic studies. We describe a hypothetical example in which we can vary the features that may be particularly relevant to biologic studies. These features include the relationship between the exposure and the outcomes and other potential sources of comorbidity. For simplicity, we will assume that the exposure is never protective for the outcome under study.

The hypothetical example is shown in figure 21.1. It is fashioned after the neuroimaging case-control study in the PDS. Thus, we investigate the relation between ventricular enlargement and schizophrenia spectrum disorder, using a case-control study that is nested in a birth cohort. We will introduce a suspected comorbid disorder, substance use dependence, into this scenario. For brevity, we will often refer to ventricular enlargement as *exposure*, schizophrenia spectrum disorder as *study outcome*, and substance use dependence as *suspected comorbid disorder*. Whenever these terms are used for other purposes, it will be explicitly stated.

Figure 21.2 illustrates five possible effects of the exposure on the study outcome and suspected comorbid disorder. The exposure may be related to neither disorder, to both disorders in the same direction, to both disorders but in the opposite directions, to the suspected study outcome alone, or to the comorbid disorder alone. In the absence of other sources of comorbidity, we will observe comorbidity between study outcome and the suspected comorbid disorder only when the exposure is related to both in the same direction (scenario 2). When the exposure is related to the study outcome and the suspected comorbid disorder in opposite directions (scenario 3), the study outcome and the comorbid disorder will co-occur less often than would be expected based on their prevalences. In all other scenarios, the exposure does not cause comorbidity (scenarios 1, 4, and 5 in figure 21.2).

Figure 21.3 exhibits four other potential sources of comorbidity. Schizophrenia spectrum disorder and substance use dependence may also be

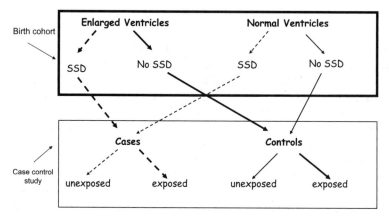

Figure 21.1 Underlying cohort for case-control study of ventricular enlargement and schizophrenia spectrum disorder. Adapted from Morabia (1997) with permission from Elsevier.

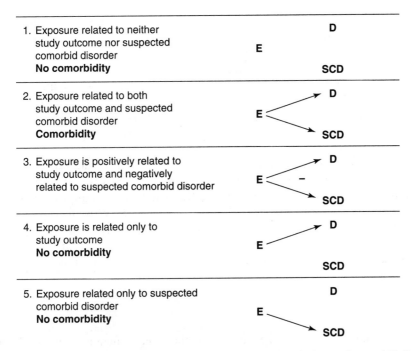

Figure 21.2 Relationship between exposure and study outcome and suspected comorbid disorder. E = exposure; D = study outcome; SCD = suspected comorbid disorder.

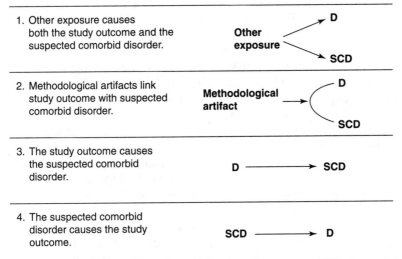

Figure 21.3 Other potential sources of comorbidity. D = study outcome; SCD = suspected comorbid disorder.

comorbid because in scenario 1 they share some other risk factor not reflected in ventricular enlargement—for example, some adverse childhood experience; because in scenario 2 a methodological artifact makes them appear to be comorbid (for example, having substance use dependence makes it more likely that an individual who does not have schizophrenia spectrum disorder will be misclassified as having it); because in scenario 3 schizophrenia spectrum disorder increases the risk of substance use dependence; or because in scenario 4 substance use dependence increases the risk of schizophrenia spectrum disorder.

Using a hypothetical example enables us to posit a true odds ratio, compute the odds ratios that would be obtained with well controls and without well controls, and compare these odds ratios with the true odds ratio. To illustrate how this is done, we consider in detail two scenarios. Since we have previously considered a scenario of true comorbidity (figure 21.2, scenario 2; see chapter 17), we consider here a scenario of no comorbidity and a scenario of artifactual comorbidity. Then we summarize the results that are obtained for all the scenarios.

Scenario of No Comorbidity

We consider the scenario in which ventricular enlargement is a true risk factor for substance use dependence, but not for schizophrenia spectrum disorder (see figure 21.2, scenario 5) and in which there is no other source of comorbidity between schizophrenia spectrum disorder and substance use dependence.

As depicted in figure 21.4, we have 100,000 exposed and 100,000 unexposed people with a disease risk of one percent in each group. The odds ratio between the exposure and the study outcome in the underlying cohort is 1.0, because the exposure is not a cause of the study outcome.

Since we are positing that the exposure is a cause of the suspected comorbid disorder, we assigned a risk of 50 percent for the suspected comorbid disorder in the exposed group and a risk of 10 percent for the suspected comorbid disorder in the unexposed group.

There is no association between the study outcome and the suspected comorbid disorder. Within the exposed group, the risk of the suspected comorbid disorder is 50 percent for people with and without the study outcome, and likewise, within the unexposed group the risk of the suspected comorbid disorder is 10 percent for people with and without the study outcome; hence, there is no actual comorbidity.

We first compute the odds ratio in a nested case-control study that follows our practical guideline for selection of the control group. The cases in our study are all of the individuals in the underlying cohort who develop the study outcome. The controls are a random sample of the noncases in the underlying cohort, say, 20 percent of those without the study outcome. By this procedure, we arrive at the true odds ratio of 1.0 (see odds ratio 2, figure 21.4).

We next compute the odds ratio in a nested case-control study that follows the well control approach (see odds ratio 3, figure 21.4). Again, the cases are

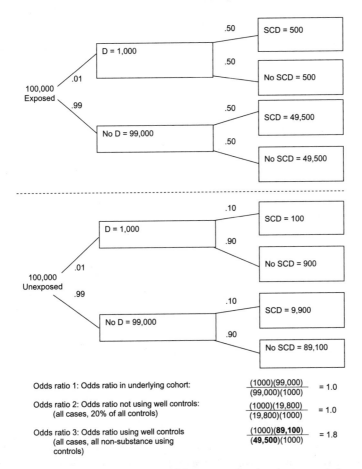

Odds ratio 1: Odds ratio in underlying cohort: $\dfrac{(1000)(99,000)}{(99,000)(1000)}$ = 1.0

Odds ratio 2: Odds ratio not using well controls: $\dfrac{(1000)(19,800)}{(19,800)(1000)}$ = 1.0
(all cases, 20% of all controls)

Odds ratio 3: Odds ratio using well controls $\dfrac{(1000)(\mathbf{89,100})}{(\mathbf{49,500})(1000)}$ = 1.8
(all cases, all non-substance using
controls)

Figure 21.4 Scenario of no comorbidity, in which exposure is related to suspected comorbid disorder (SCD) but not to study outcome (D). Well controls are indicated by boldface.

all those who develop the study outcome. But now we exclude individuals with the suspected comorbid disorder from the controls. We use as our controls all the noncases in the underlying cohort who do not have the suspected comorbid disorder. Thus we use 49,500 (99,000 – 49,500) exposed controls, and 89,100 (99,000 – 9,900) unexposed controls. We obtain an odds ratio of 1.8, much larger than the true odds ratio of 1.0.

In this scenario, using a well control group introduced bias. Not using a well control group led to the correct result. This exercise shows that well controls can cause bias even when the excluded disorder is not comorbid with the study outcome.

Scenario of Artifactual Comorbidity

We now consider a scenario that exactly parallels the first except for one feature: ascertainment bias. As depicted in table 21.1A, there is still no true comorbidity (the numbers in Table 21.1 derive from Figure 21.4). However,

Table 21.1 Scenario of Comorbidity in which the Ascertainment of the Study Outcome (D) Is Related to Suspected Comorbid Disorder (SCD)

A. Truth in the Underlying Cohort (100,000 Exposed and 100,000 Unexposed)

		D		No D
Exposed	SCD	500	SCD	49,500
	No SCD	500	No SCD	49,500
	Total	1,000	Total	99,000
Unexposed	SCD	100	SCD	9,900
	No SCD	900	No SCD	89,100
	Total	1,000	Total	99,000

$$\text{OR Exposed and D} = \frac{(1,000)(99,000)}{(99,000)(1,000)} = 1.0$$

B. Underlying Cohort with Ascertainment Bias

		D		No D
Exposed	SCD	1,000	SCD	49,000
	No SCD	500	No SCD	49,500
	Total	1,500	Total	98,500
Unexposed	SCD	200	SCD	9,800
	No SCD	900	No SCD	89,100
	Total	1,100	Total	98,900

$$\text{OR} = \frac{(1,500)(98,900)}{(98,500)(1,100)} = 1.4$$

C. Case-control Study with Well Controls from Underlying Cohort with Ascertainment Bias

		D		No D
Exposed	SCD	1,000	~~SCD~~	~~49,000~~
	No SCD	500	No SCD	49,500
	Total	1,500	Total	**49,500**
Unexposed	Substance use+	200	~~SCD~~	~~9,800~~
	No SCD	900	No SCD	89,100
	Total	1,100	Total	**89,100**

$$\text{OR} = \frac{(1,500)(\mathbf{89,100})}{(\mathbf{49,500})(1,100)} = 2.4$$

Note: Well controls in bold font. D = Study Outcome (Schizophrenia Spectrum Disorders); SCD = Suspected Comorbid Disorder (Substance Use).

because of ascertainment bias, there is now an apparent comorbidity between schizophrenia spectrum disorder and substance use dependence.

The apparent comorbidity emerges for the following reason. Among the 60,000 individuals with substance use dependence (50,000 and 10,000 unexposed in table 21.1A), one percent (600) are correctly diagnosed as having schizophrenia spectrum disorder; but an additional one percent, who do not have schizophrenia spectrum disorder, are also diagnosed as having it. Therefore, as shown in table 21.1B, we diagnose schizophrenia spectrum disorder in 1200 instead of 600 of the 60,000 individuals with substance use dependence. By contrast, among the 140,000 individuals without substance use dependence, only the one percent (1400) who are true cases are diagnosed. As a result of this bias, the risk of schizophrenia spectrum disorder appears to be twice as high among those with as among those without substance use dependence.

A study of the full underlying cohort would reflect this bias, yielding an odds ratio of 1.4, when the true odds ratio is 1.0 (figure 21.4). If we selected the controls in accordance with our guideline, taking a random 20 percent of the noncases, we would also obtain an odds ratio of 1.4. In other words, even following our guideline, and not using well controls, we would obtain a somewhat biased result. This bias would be due to differential misclassification that we cannot remove from the underlying cohort.

It is tempting to think that excluding individuals with substance use dependence from the control group would mitigate this bias. Nonetheless, our guideline argues against using well controls. Indeed, as can be seen in table 21.1C, using well controls exacerbates the problem, rather than solves it. Excluding individuals with substance use dependence from the control group, we obtain an odds ratio of 2.4, indicating a substantial bias above that caused by the initial misclassification. Thus, using well controls leads to more bias than not using well controls.

Other Scenarios

We have only approached two scenarios in detail here and one in a previous chapter. But the same approach can be taken to derive the results for all scenarios. These results are displayed in table 21.2.

The results show that, in virtually every scenario in which the exposure is related to the suspected comorbid disorder, the use of well controls will cause bias. These results pertain, in fact, to any disorder excluded from the well controls, whether or not its exclusion is motivated by suspected comorbidity. The one exception is that the use of well controls does not cause bias if the association between the exposure and the excluded disorder arises soley because the exposure causes the disorder of interest, which in turn causes the excluded disorder (the last column of row 4).

The use of well controls does not cause bias when the exposure under investigation is not associated with the excluded disorder. However, there is no situation in which well controls improve the validity of the results, and they almost always cause unnecessary expense and loss of power. This is true whether or not the excluded disorder is comorbid with the study outcome.

This result also pertains to other scenarios, not depicted here, in which well controls are used. For example, investigators sometimes exclude a disorder from the controls out of concern that the presence of the disorder in a control individual will bias the measurement of the exposure. Clearly, if this were true, the presence of the disorder in a case individual would also bias the measurement of the exposure. The result of excluding the disorder from

Table 21.2 Summary of Bias Caused by Using Well Controls in a Variety of Scenarios

Scenarios from figure 21.2	No Additional Sources of Comorbidity[a]	Comobidity Due to Other Risk Factor	Comorbidity SCD → D	Comorbidity D → SCD
Exposure related to neither D nor SCD	No bias	No bias	No bias	No bias
Exposure related to both D and SCD (same direction)	Bias	Bias	Bias	Bias
Exposure related to both D and SCD (negatively related to SCD)	Bias (negative direction)	Bias (negative direction)	Bias (negative direction)	Bias (negative direction)
Exposure related to D only	No bias	No bias	No bias	No bias
Exposure related to SCD only	Bias	Bias	Bias	Bias

Note: This summary assumes exposure is never protective for D (study outcome). SCD = suspected comorbid disorder.
[a] In this column there is no comorbidity unless the study outcome and the suspected comorbid disorder are both related to the exposure.

controls and not from cases would be differential misclassification of the exposure. On the other hand, excluding the disorder from both cases and controls would be perfectly legitimate and protect the study from such misclassification.

An irony in the use of well controls is that the situations in which this approach is most seductive are precisely the situations in which it causes bias. A well control group is most likely to be used when the investigator suspects a relationship between the exposure of interest and a comorbid disorder. This is the very situation in which the well control group will bias the results.

Our guideline also suggests, however, that if the cases are screened for the same (other) disorders as the controls, then the exclusion of these (other) disorders from both the case and control groups will not introduce bias. Such procedures are entirely legitimate. It should always be kept in mind, however, that because comorbidity is so common for psychiatric disorders, this approach can produce quite atypical case groups. The results from a study using such atypical cases and well controls may not generalize to more typical case groups and should be interpreted with caution.

Unwell Controls

We turn now to the use of a control group composed of patients with other disorders. For example, we may use patients with bipolar disorder as a control group in a study of schizophrenia spectrum disorder. As another example, we may use patients with depression as a control group in a study of anorexia nervosa. This is another common strategy in biologic studies. It is often but not always a reasonable one. We can use the epidemiologic vantage point to determine when this kind of control group will and will not lead to valid results. Once again, by thinking about sampling controls from an underlying cohort, we can see the implications of the choice.

Consider the same hypothetical example. We want to study the relation of ventricular enlargement to the risk of schizophrenia spectrum disorder in a scenario in which substance use dependence is comorbid with schizophrenia spectrum disorder. But this time we decide to use a sample of the cohort members treated for substance use dependence as our patient controls. This is equivalent to excluding from the control group all individuals who do not have substance use dependence or have not been treated for it. Since we are applying this exclusion to the control group but did not apply the same exclusion to the cases, we are once more violating our guideline.

What will this do to our results? If ventricular enlargement is associated with substance use dependence (or its treatment) in the underlying cohort, then this exclusion will inflate the proportion exposed in the control group. It will therefore artificially reduce the association between the exposure and schizophrenia spectrum disorder. On the other hand, if ventricular enlargement is unrelated to substance use dependence, then this exclusion has no impact on our result. It does not change the exposure odds in the control group, which we use to estimate the exposure odds among the noncases of the underlying cohort. Thus, within a nested case-control study, in some circumstances the use of patient controls carries potential for bias, and in other circumstances it does not cause bias but may confer no benefits.

In an ordinary case-control study, however, patient controls can confer benefits. Unlike a nested case-control study, for which cases are chosen from a delineated underlying cohort, an ordinary case-control study can mean difficulty in visualizing the underlying cohort. Most often in biologic studies, we recruit patients from a specialized treatment setting, and it may be virtually impossible to specify all the factors that selected the cases into this setting. A reasonable way to ensure that the selections imposed on the cases are also imposed on the controls is to use controls who were treated in the same location for a similar disorder. One assumes that the selection factors are approximately the same for two similar disorders. Therefore, by using patient controls, we may bring the selection of controls in closer approximation to our guideline.

To make a prudent decision, we need to weigh these points against each other. In particular, we need to make a judgment as to whether the exposures being investigated are likely to be associated with the disorder that defines the patient control group. If so, the potential for bias may be substantial.[3] Epidemiologists have devised strategies to shift the balance, so that the benefits of patient controls are more likely to outweigh the costs. One approach

---

[3] Nonetheless, this type of control can be effectively used as an adjunct to a valid control group to test for the specificity of effects.

is to have a control group consisting of people with a variety of different disorders. The mixture of disorders minimizes the likelihood that the selected disorders will be substantially related to the exposure under study.

This was the approach used in the study of endogenomorphic depression (table 20.3; Carroll et al. 1976) discussed in the previous chapter. The question posed in this study was whether abnormal hypothalamic pituitary adrenal (HPA) axis activity was related to endogenomorphic depression. To answer this question, the authors compared 42 individuals with endogenomorphic depression (cases) and 42 individuals ascertained from the same inpatient hospitals with other psychiatric disorders (controls).

The choice of cases and controls was actually quite complex. More specifically, the case group consisted of 34 patients with unipolar depression and 8 patients with bipolar disorder. Bipolar disorder was included because the authors considered endogenomorphic depression to be part of their condition. The control group consisted of 30 nondepressed patients (including 15 with schizophrenia, 2 with organic brain syndromes, 8 with anxiety neurosis, 3 with sociopathic personality disorder, and 2 with facial dyskinesias) and 12 patients with depressive neurosis. The researchers believed that depressive neurosis was fundamentally different from endogenomorphic depression and, in particular, not related to abnormal HPA activity. On this premise, it was reasonable to include patients with depressive neurosis in the control group.

The cortisol response to dexamethasone was used to indicate the presence or absence of abnormal HPA activity. The cases had significantly more abnormal responses to dexamethasone than the controls. In addition, none of the controls with depressive neurosis had an abnormal response.

The patient control group seems to many researchers to be the simplest possible control group. It turns out, however, to be one of the more complex, and its appropriate use requires a great deal of knowledge and discretion. Ideally, the patient controls should capture the effect of the treatment selection factors on the exposure-disease relationship, but should not have disorders that are associated with the biologic factor (exposure) being investigated. In practice, it is often a matter of degree; one aims for controls that have a large impact on reducing selection bias but introduce little other bias. The complexity of this decision well illustrates how epidemiologic thinking offers the biologic researcher a path through the maze of conflicting considerations in control selection.

Conclusion

Advances in biologic research are transforming our understanding of the pathophysiology of psychiatric disorders. Many of these contributions are being made with methods that are akin to those of risk factor epidemiology and, in particular, with comparisons of cases and controls that are equivalent to case-control studies. We have suggested in these chapters that epidemiologic and biologic researchers working together can sharpen the designs of these studies and further accelerate the pace of biologic research.

Thus, the development of the case-control study in epidemiology over the past 50 years has direct implications for biologic studies. We have demonstrated this point for the selection of cases and controls so as to produce a valid result, but it also pertains to other aspects of design. While epidemiology provides no rules that can be universally applied, it does provide guidelines to help us think through the problems in each specific study.

Biologic investigators will benefit directly and immediately. Better-designed case-control studies are better equipped to detect real effects and, at the same time, less likely to report artifactual findings. In the long term, however, the benefits will accrue equally to epidemiologists. As we have emphasized throughout this book, the more we understand the underlying biology of mental disorders, the more likely epidemiologists are to discover their causes and the means to prevent them.

References

Carroll BJ, Curtis GC, and Mendels J (1976). Neuroendocrine Regulation in Depression. II. Discrimination of Depressed from Nondepressed Patients. *Arch. Gen. Psychiatry* 33:1051–1058.

Kendler KS (1990). The Super-Normal Control Group in Psychiatric Genetics: Possible Artifactual Evidence for Coaggregation. *Psychiatr. Genet.* 1:45–53.

Klein DF (1993). The Utility of the Super-Normal Control Group in Psychiatric Genetics. *Psychiatr. Genet.* 3:17–19.

Morabia A (1997). Case-Control Studies in Clinical Research: Mechanism and Prevention of Selection Bias. *Prev. Med.* 26:674–677.

Schwartz S and Link BG (1989). The "Well Control" Artefact in Case/Control Studies of Specific Psychiatric Disorders. *Psychol. Med.* 19:737–742.

ANALYZING THE DATA

Gauging the Precision of Measures of Association

22

Melissa D. Begg and Michaeline Bresnahan

Epidemiologic study designs guide how we collect data to help us draw valid conclusions about underlying associations and causal relationships. The cohort study and the case control study, for example, are meant to evaluate the relationship between exposure and disease, to determine whether the exposure increases (or decreases) the risk of the disease. Statistics play a vital role in this process. Chapters 22–27 are intended to introduce a number of key statistical ideas and methods that will help you to better understand the literature in psychiatric epidemiology. The emphasis is, therefore, on conceptual understanding and interpretation, not on technical details, which are better covered in a textbook devoted entirely to statistics. At numerous points throughout these chapters, the interested reader is directed to alternative sources and texts for a more comprehensive treatment of the development and application of statistical methods.

The main goal in the statistical analysis of research data is to reduce a large number of data points to a small number of relevant, informative summary values. Chapter 8 addressed techniques for obtaining a simple measure to describe the association between exposure and disease. In this section, we make the transition from descriptive to inferential statistics. Inferential methods help us distinguish associations that are real from those that are due purely to chance. They also help us to distinguish causal associations from those due to confounding by other variables.

Chapter 8 described different techniques for gauging association between a binary outcome measure (say, disease presence or absence) and an exposure of interest. For each measure of association, or parameter, there is a theoretical quantity and corresponding sample value. The theoretical quantity reflects the true parameter value that exists in the target population. In contrast, the sample estimator is derived from a sample of subjects drawn from the target population. Our goal is to make inferences about the true parameter values by using our sample estimates of those values.

Consider, for example, the risk difference. If we were able to study the entire population of interest, we would be able to state definitively the true value of the risk difference, because we could calculate it directly with use of the observed values of the probability of disease given exposure status. In reality, it is not feasible to examine an entire population of subjects for any research question, unless that population is defined in such a limited way that the exercise becomes pointless. Even if we could examine, say, the entire population of pregnant mothers in the state of California during calendar year 2002, migration would occur in and out of state such that the true population itself would change; hence, our enumeration is unavoidably incomplete. Consequently, we work with estimators of population parameters that are derived from samples drawn from the population of interest.

Because they are based on data, sample estimators are random in nature. Multiple studies, even if conducted in identical fashion, will lead to multiple estimates of the parameter in question. To make judgments about the association, therefore, we have to take account of the contribution of chance, or sampling variability. This variation in sample estimators reflects the precision of an estimated association. The purpose of this chapter is to give guidance in how to quantify an estimator's precision.

One way to estimate the precision of a sample estimator would be to repeat the same study over and over again. This is, obviously, a clumsy way to approach the problem. Instead, we rely on known properties of the estimators (i.e., their sample distributions), established via statistical theory, in order to estimate variability from a single sample. This allows us to make statements about the precision of an estimator in a given study and, further, allows us to draw conclusions about the existence of an association between exposure and disease in the target population.

In this chapter we provide technical details for calculating the variability of the measures of association introduced earlier. Note that there is a distinction between variability of a measurement and variability of an estimator. If we have a set of observations on a particular variable, the **standard deviation** is the quantity that gauges the variability of that measurement from subject to subject in a population. Formulas for the standard deviation of an individual variable are available in introductory biostatistics textbooks (see, for example, Altman 1991). If, on the other hand, we use a set of observations to derive an estimate of an association parameter of interest (like the risk ratio or mean difference, for example), then the **standard error** is the quantity that gauges the variability of the estimator from sample to sample over repeated experiments of the same size. The formulas given below, therefore, are standard error formulas, since they describe the variability of sample estimators.

Variability of Measures of Association from a 2 × 2 Table

Consider again a cross-classification of a binary exposure by a binary disease outcome, as in table 22.1. The association between the exposure and disease can be described through one of the following measures of association: the risk difference (RD), the risk ratio (RR), and the odds ratio (OR). Methods for calculating estimates of these parameters were given in chapter 8. Statistical theory provides estimates of the variability of the sample estimators for each of these three parameters of interest. We summarize the relevant standard

Table 22.1 A Fourfold Table from a Cohort or Case–Control Study

	Diseased	**Non-diseased**	**Row Totals**
Exposed	a	b	m_1
Unexposed	c	d	m_2
Column totals	n_1	n_2	t

error formulas here; for a thorough discussion of their derivation and use, see Altman (1991), Agresti (1996), and Fleiss et al. (2003).

A scalar estimator for a parameter of interest is often referred to as a *point estimate*. Recall that the expression for the point estimate of the RD based on sample data is $[(a/m_1) - (c/m_2)]$. Principles from probability and statistical inference can be applied in order to derive an expression for the estimated variance of this statistic. The resulting standard error formula for the estimated RD is

$$\text{SE}\left(\hat{\text{RD}}\right) = \sqrt{\frac{ab}{m_1^3} + \frac{cd}{m_2^3}}.$$

We can use the point estimate of the RD, coupled with its standard error, to derive a range of plausible values, or **confidence interval**, for the true (population) RD. A confidence interval can be thought of as an enhancement of the point estimate. Rather than calculating a single estimate of the RD, we can calculate a range of values within which the population RD is likely to fall. The confidence interval, therefore, reflects not only our best guess as to the population RD (the point estimate), but it also points to the precision of our estimate. A confidence interval can be calculated at varying levels of surety; the most common choice is to report a 95 percent confidence interval. A 95 percent confidence interval can be interpreted to mean that, if we repeated our study many times, then 95 percent of the resulting confidence intervals for the RD (or any parameter of interest) would cover or include the true population RD. For an individual study, we say that we are "95 percent confident" that the population RD falls within the limits of our confidence interval. The precision or reliability of an individual estimator is clearly reflected by the confidence interval. A very wide confidence interval indicates that the effect estimate is imprecise, because the range of plausible values is large. A narrow confidence interval, on the other hand, indicates that we have a precise estimate, since the information points to a limited range of plausible values for the parameter of interest.

To calculate a confidence interval for the RD, we make use of the well-known fact that the RD estimator follows an approximate standard normal distribution in large samples. The normal (or Gaussian) distribution is the familiar bell curve described in many textbooks and research articles. This fact is enormously useful, because the properties of the standard normal distribution (i.e., a normal distribution with mean zero and variance one) are well established. For example, if a random variable follows a standard normal distribution, we know that approximately 95 percent of the observations from this distribution will fall within 1.96 standard deviations of its mean. This fact leads us to the following formula for a 95 percent confidence interval for the risk difference:

$$\hat{RD} \pm 1.96 \ SE(\hat{RD})$$

We should note that a confidence interval for a specific parameter of interest takes into account the random variability attributable to drawing a sample from a larger population. It is not, however, a measure of our confidence in the result in the most general sense. It cannot account, for example, for systematic errors due to biased sampling, poor research design, or confounding. A large sample may yield a very narrow yet inaccurate confidence interval for a measure of association, depending on the representativeness of the sample drawn.

Derivation of standard error formulas for the RR and OR is slightly more complicated, because the distributions of the ratio measures tend to be more skewed than the distribution of the RD. Recall that the possible range of values of the ratio measures runs from zero to positive infinity. Since this range has an unambiguous lower endpoint, but no upper endpoint, the distribution of either ratio measure (RR or OR) tends to be skewed to the right (i.e., the distribution has a long right tail, reflecting the possibility of very large values for the parameter). To make the problem of statistical inference for the RR and OR more tractable, we usually apply the logarithmic transform to these measures; that is, instead of working with these measures on their original scale, we take the natural log of each measure and work with that quantity. Omitting the details, we ask the reader to accept that the logarithmic transform of a ratio measure results in a statistic whose distribution better approximates the normal. Back-transformation via exponentiation allows us to express our results on the original scale for easier interpretation.

Remember the following formula for the estimator of the risk ratio: $\hat{RR} = (a/m_1)/(c/m_2)$. The standard error for the log of the risk ratio is given by

$$SE[\ln(\hat{RR})] = \sqrt{\frac{b}{am_1} + \frac{d}{cm_2}}.$$

A 95 percent confidence interval for the ln RR is then given by $\{\ln \hat{RR} \pm 1.96, SE[\ln(\hat{RR})]\}$. To obtain a 95 percent confidence interval for the RR, we exponentiate the endpoints of this interval, or apply the following formula directly:

$$\{\hat{RR} \exp(\pm 1.96 SE[\ln(\hat{RR})])\}.$$

The OR can be estimated by $\hat{OR} = ad/bc$. The standard error for the natural log of the OR, derived by Woolf (1955), is given by

$$SE[\ln(\hat{OR})] = \sqrt{\frac{1}{a} + \frac{1}{b} + \frac{1}{c} + \frac{1}{d}}.$$

A 95 percent confidence interval for the ln(OR) can be expressed as $\{\ln \hat{OR} \pm 1.96 SE[\ln(\hat{OR})]\}$, while the corresponding confidence interval for the OR can be computed as $\{\hat{OR} \exp(\pm 1.96 SE[\ln(\hat{OR})])\}$.

Sudden Infant Death and Maternal Schizophrenia: An Example

Consider the study reported by Bennedsen et al. (2001) examining the association between schizophrenia in mothers (the exposure) and reproductive outcomes in their offspring (congenital malformations, stillbirths, and infant deaths). In a cohort of 2230 singleton offspring of women diagnosed with schizophrenia, and a comparison group of 123,544 randomly selected singletons born during the same time period, 134 deaths from sudden infant death syndrome (SIDS) were identified. Are children of mothers with schizophrenia at higher risk of SIDS than children of mothers with no history of schizophrenia?

Bennedsen et al. reported the data in table 22.2 in the cohort for maternal schizophrenia and SIDS: since the study follows a cohort design, we can derive all three measures of association for binary data (RD, RR, and OR). We also calculate the corresponding confidence intervals for these parameters.

The estimated RD is 0.003481:

$$\hat{RD} = \frac{a}{m_1} - \frac{c}{m_2} = \frac{10}{2230} - \frac{124}{123,544} = 0.004484 - 0.001004 = 0.003481.$$

This estimate represents an absolute increase of 0.0035, or 0.35 percent, in the probability of SIDS associated with having a mother with schizophrenia. How precise is this estimate? Applying the formula for the standard error of the RD, we obtain

$$\mathrm{SE}\left(\hat{RD}\right) = \sqrt{\frac{ab}{m_1^3} + \frac{cd}{m_2^3}} = \sqrt{\frac{(10)(2220)}{(2230)^3} + \frac{(124)(123,420)}{(123,544)^3}} = 0.001418.$$

And so a 95 percent confidence interval for the population risk difference is given by

$$\hat{RD} \pm 1.96\,\mathrm{SE}(\hat{RD}) = 0.00348 \pm (1.96)(0.001418) = (0.000701, 0.006259).$$

We can, therefore, be 95 percent confident that the population RD falls within the limits of the confidence interval (0.0007 to 0.0063; or 0.07 to 0.63 percent), rounded to the fourth decimal place.

The estimated risk ratio is calculated to be 4.4678:

$$\hat{RR} = \frac{a/m_1}{c/m_2} = \frac{10/2230}{124/123,544} = 4.4678,$$

Table 22.2 SIDS Deaths among Offspring of Exposed and Unexposed Mothers from the Bennedsen Cohort (Bennedsen et al. 2001)

	Cases (SIDS)	Noncases	Total
Exposed (maternal schizophrenia)	10	2,220	2,230
Unexposed (no maternal schizophrenia)	124	123,420	123,544
Total	134	125,640	125,774

indicating a greater than fourfold increased risk of SIDS in exposed children as compared to unexposed children. Using the formulas provided for the standard error of the natural log of the estimated RR, we can construct a 95 percent confidence interval for the true RR:

$$SE\left[\ln\left(\hat{RR}\right)\right] = \sqrt{\frac{b}{am_1} + \frac{d}{cm_2}} = \sqrt{\frac{2220}{(10)(2230)} + \frac{123{,}420}{(124)(123{,}544)}} = 0.328037.$$

The natural log of the estimated RR is $\ln(4.4678) = 1.4969$. Therefore, a 95 percent confidence interval for the $\ln(RR)$ is given by:

$$\ln(\hat{RR}) \pm 1.96SE(\ln(\hat{RR})) = 1.4969 \pm 1.96(0.328037) = (0.8539, 2.1398).$$

Exponentiating the endpoints of this interval, we find that a 95 percent confidence interval for the RR spans from 2.35 to 8.50.

The estimated OR relating schizophrenia in the mother to SIDS in the offspring is

$$\hat{OR} = \frac{ad}{bc} = \frac{(10)(123{,}420)}{(2220)(124)} = 4.4834,$$

indicating the odds of SIDS, given a mother with schizophrenia, is greater than four times the odds of SIDS when a mother is without schizophrenia. The natural log of the OR is 1.5004. Using the formula provided for the standard error of the natural log of the OR, we find:

$$SE\left[\ln\left(\hat{OR}\right)\right] = \sqrt{\frac{1}{a} + \frac{1}{b} + \frac{1}{c} + \frac{1}{d}} = \sqrt{\frac{1}{10} + \frac{1}{2220} + \frac{1}{124} + \frac{1}{123{,}420}} = 0.329428.$$

A 95 percent confidence interval for the OR then follows as

$$\hat{OR}\exp[\pm 1.96SE(\ln(\hat{OR}))] = 4.4834\exp[\pm 1.96(0.329428)] = (2.3507, 8.5511),$$

so that a 95 percent confidence interval for the true OR ranges from 2.35 to 8.55, rounded to the second decimal place.

Interpretation of SIDS–Maternal Schizophrenia Example

All estimated measures of effect show significantly elevated risk of SIDS in children born to mothers with schizophrenia as compared to children born to mothers without schizophrenia. Interpretation of these findings, however, must be cautious. Important confounders of this association (e.g., smoking, prepregnancy maternal body mass index, and characteristics of delivery) were not controlled in the analysis presented here.

The methods introduced in this chapter assume independence among the observations, as one would obtain through simple random sampling. In the original study by Bennedsen et al. (2001), the study sample included data on multiple siblings within families. Because siblings cannot be considered independent, the authors relied upon specialized methods for nonindependent (clustered) data (Liang and Zeger 1986). Although for simplicity we did not employ these methods in our analysis, our findings are consistent with the (appropriately) adjusted findings reported by Bennedsen and colleagues.

Variability of Measures of Association for Continuous Exposures

In order to evaluate the association between a continuous exposure and the presence or absence of disease, suppose we calculate the difference in sample means between diseased and nondiseased groups. Just as there are standard error formulas that reflect the precision of measures of association for 2×2 tables, so, too, is there a standard error formula for the mean difference. This formula helps us to assess the precision of the mean difference estimator and allows us to calculate confidence intervals for the true difference in means between groups.

To begin, consider a set of values for a continuous exposure measure from one group of subjects. We can denote the individual observations as X_i, where i goes from one to N (the number of observations in the sample). Let μ represent the true population mean for the exposure variable of interest. The sample mean for the group is defined as

$$\hat{\mu} = \sum_{i=1}^{N} X_i/N = (X_1+X_2+X_3+ \cdots +X_N)/N$$

(where Σ indicates summation). The standard error formula for the sample mean from one group of observations ($\hat{\mu}$) is as follows:

$$SE(\hat{\mu}) = \sqrt{\frac{1}{N} \sum_{i=1}^{N} \frac{(X_i - \hat{\mu})^2}{(N-1)}}.$$

Now suppose we calculate the sample mean for diseased subjects ($\hat{\mu}_1$) and nondiseased subjects ($\hat{\mu}_2$). The following formula for the standard error for the difference in sample means, $\hat{\delta}$, assumes that the variability in measurements is unknown but equal across the two groups being compared:

$$SE(\hat{\delta}) = \sqrt{\left(\frac{1}{N_1} + \frac{1}{N_2}\right)} \sqrt{\frac{N_1(N_1-1)[SE(\hat{\mu}_1)]^2 + N_2(N_2-1)[SE(\hat{\mu}_2)]^2}{N_1+N_2-2}},$$

where subscripts 1 and 2 denote the diseased and nondiseased groups, respectively. The mean difference estimator follows a distribution known as Student's distribution with degrees of freedom equal to $(N_1 + N_2 - 2)$. Student's t distribution is symmetric like the normal, and it approaches the normal distribution as the sample size increases (see Rosner 1995 for further details). This allows us to compute a 95% confidence interval for the mean difference as: $\hat{\delta} \pm t_{df}SE(\hat{\delta})$, where t_{df} is the critical value from at t-distribution with degrees of freedom equal to df and upper (lower) tail area equal to 0.025 (for a total tail area of 0.05). Tables of critical values for the t-distribution can be found in most standard statistical textbooks (e.g., Altman 1991; Rosner 1994; Fleiss et al. 2003).

Perinatal Head Circumference and Violence in Schizophrenia: An Example

Consider Cannon et al.'s (2002) study examining perinatal and childhood risk factors for the outcome of violent and criminal behavior in schizophrenic subjects. In a population sample of 636 individuals with schizophrenia (born 1951–1960), the investigators identified 61 individuals with a criminal record.

Among the risk factors examined was head circumference at birth. Cannon et al. reported that the mean (and standard error) for head circumference among those with criminal records ($N_1 = 61$) was 35.3 cm (0.16 cm), whereas the corresponding figure for those without criminal record ($N_2 = 575$) was 34.9 cm (0.06 cm). The estimated difference in mean head circumference at birth, therefore, between the group with a history of criminal conviction and those without a history of criminal conviction can be computed as $\hat{\delta} = \mu_1 - \mu_2$ = 35.3 − 34.9 = 0.4 cm. How does this estimated mean difference relate to the mean difference in head circumference in the underlying population of individuals with schizophrenia? Applying our formula, we compute the standard error for $\hat{\delta}$ as

$$SE(\hat{\delta}) = \sqrt{\left(\frac{1}{N_1} + \frac{1}{N_2}\right)[N_1(N_1-1)SE(\hat{\mu}_1)]^2 + [N_2(N_2-1)SE(\hat{\mu}_2)]^2}$$
$$= 0.1916\,cm.$$

with $df = 61 + 575 - 2 = 634$, t_{df} can be approximated by the normal distribution critical value (1.96). The 95 percent confidence interval for the mean difference, then, is given by

$$\hat{\delta} \pm 1.96 SE(\hat{\delta}) = 0.4 \pm 1.96(0.1916) = (0.02, 0.78)\,cm.$$

Interpretation of Head Circumference–Violence Example

The data presented suggest that, among individuals with schizophrenia, head circumference at birth is, on average, 0.4 cm greater among those with criminal records than among those without criminal records. The 95 percent confidence interval for this difference suggests that the true increase in head circumference might lie in the range of 0.02 to 0.78 cm. A more detailed analysis, considering the impact of sex and other potential confounders of this association, is necessary to probe causal plausibility.

Conclusion

We use point estimates and confidence intervals to make judgments about the strength of an association between an outcome and an exposure of interest. To interpret our findings, we have to take account of the influence of chance (sampling variability) on the results we observe in our study sample. The methods presented in this chapter help us quantify the degree of uncertainty in our evaluation of a potential association.

The methods in the next chapter go beyond simple data description to help us determine whether an observed association is real (i.e., reflecting an association between exposure and outcome in the population at large), or not (perhaps the result of random fluctuation due to sampling variability). Statistical significance testing guides us in drawing conclusions about the associations that we observe. Like point estimates and confidence intervals, significance tests alone cannot tell us the "right" answer regarding distinction between causal and coincidental association. Rather, they tend, more often than not, to point us in the right direction.

References

Agresti A (1996). *An Introduction to Categorical Data Analysis.* New York: Wiley.

Altman DG (1991). *Practical Statistics for Medical Research.* London: Chapman & Hall.

Bennedsen BE, Mortensen PB, Olesen AV, and Henriksen TB (2001). Congenital Malformations, Stillbirths, and Infant Deaths among Children of Women with Schizophrenia. *Arch. Gen. Psychiatry* 58:674–679.

Cannon M, Huttunen MO, Tanskanen AJ, Arseneault L, Jones PB, and Murray RM (2002). Perinatal and Childhood Risk Factors for Later Criminality and Violence in Schizophrenia. *Br. J. Psychiatry* 180:496–501.

Fleiss JL, Levin B, and Paik MC (2003). *Statistical Methods for Rates and Proportions*, 3rd ed. New York: Wiley.

Liang KY and Zeger SL (1986). Longitudinal Data Analysis Using Generalized Linear Models. *Biometrika* 73:13–22.

Rosner B (1995). *Fundamentals of Biostatistics*, 4th ed. Belmont, Calif.: Duxbury Press.

Woolf B (1955). On Estimating the Relation between Blood Group and Disease. *Ann. Hum. Genet.* 19:251–225.

23 Using Significance Tests in Establishing Associations

Melissa D. Begg and Michaeline Bresnahan

Statistical significance testing can be viewed as a formal method for assessing the evidence with regard to a scientific conjecture. It reflects the degree to which we can be confident that an association observed in our study sample is also present in the target population.

Significance tests play a central role in psychiatric epidemiology—and, in fact, across the full gamut of human research. Given the omnipresence of statistical significance tests, it is essential for all investigators to understand the principles behind these tests and guidelines for their interpretation. The purpose of this chapter is to provide this background and to make recommendations for sensible evaluation of test results.

Throughout this chapter, keep in mind that tests of statistical significance comprise only one element in the evaluation of association between a chosen exposure and an outcome of interest. The result of a significance test must not be presented on its own; the estimated magnitude of association and corresponding confidence interval provide distinct, complementary information about the observed association and enable the reader to make sense of the reported test result. Furthermore, research norms in epidemiology place great emphasis on point estimates and confidence intervals. Proponents believe that increased emphasis on estimation promotes more thoughtful consideration of the magnitude and precision of the observed association, and helps researchers focus on the clinical and practical significance of a purported relationship. A thorough evaluation of any research finding must give due attention to both clinical import and statistical significance in order to draw the most accurate, defensible conclusions from a research study.

Remember that a statistical significance test does not necessarily give the right answer to a research question; rather it tends (more often than not) to steer researchers in the right direction. This is why in general no single research study can be used to establish causality. The results of any single study must be interpreted in the context of all other available research findings on the same topic. In this way, we further reduce the likelihood of incorrect inferences that might lead to inappropriate public health interventions.

Motivation

We begin with a hypothetical example to demonstrate the usefulness of statistical significance testing. Suppose that we have conducted a case-control study of maternal prepregnancy body mass index as a risk factor for diagnosis of a schizophrenia spectrum disorder (SSD) in the offspring. Further, suppose that the study design called for the recruitment of equal numbers of cases and controls, sampled independently, and that the observed proportions of subjects with high body mass index is 10 percent in the control group and 20 percent in the SSD case group. Note that these sample figures result in an estimated odds ratio of 2.25. What can we conclude from this study? Is there an association between body mass index and SSD risk?

When this question is posed in a classroom setting, most people ask to know the size of the case and control samples. When told that there are 10 cases and 10 controls, most are not convinced that a true association exists, given that the observed difference between the case and control groups amounts to only one more exposure among cases. When the hypothetical sample sizes are increased to 20 cases and 20 controls, the response is the same: they are unconvinced. Increasing the sample sizes to 50 and 50 changes the observed difference between the case and control groups to five more exposures among cases. At this point, the pendulum begins to swing toward concluding that the effect is real. By the time the sample size is increased to 100 cases and 100 controls, the majority of students are ready to claim that high body mass index is associated with higher risk of SSD. A few holdouts do not endorse the majority opinion until the sample size is increased to 200 cases and 200 controls.

This example demonstrates the need for statistical tools that move beyond measures of association. The demand to know the sample size before drawing a conclusion about the study's findings indicates a recognition that the weight of evidence depends on several factors, including the magnitude of the observed association, the size of the sample in which it is observed, and the precision of the estimate. Statistical significance testing provides a convenient way to formalize this process and to keep the process consistent from study to study and from researcher to researcher.

Construction of Statistical Significance Tests

Here we discuss how to use statistical significance testing to help us decide whether two or more groups are comparable with respect to a particular outcome (or exposure). A statistical significance test can be constructed in three steps. First, we must specify how the difference between groups will be measured. Second, we formulate the scientific conjecture in terms of a null hypothesis and an alternative hypothesis. Third, we need to construct a decision rule to allow us to say whether the data favor the null or alternative hypothesis.

Step 1. In order to discern whether an association is real, we must first determine how to operationalize it. For the moment, let us assume that we

Table 23.1 A Fourfold Table from a Cohort or Case-Control Study

	Diseased	Nondiseased	Row totals
Exposed	a	b	m_1
Unexposed	c	d	m_2
Column totals	n_1	n_2	t

are investigating a potential association between a binary outcome and a binary exposure measure, as in a case-control study (see table 23.1). Recall that the equivalence of the exposure odds ratio (OR) and the disease OR (see chapter 8) means that we can obtain valid estimates of the OR under either a cohort or a case-control design (for a full discussion of this issue, see chapter 8). Using the same notation for 2×2 tables introduced in chapters 8 and 22, we can estimate the OR relating exposure to disease status from the data as ad/bc. If there is no association between disease and exposure, the estimated OR should be approximately equal to one. If the OR is greater than one, it indicates a positive association between exposure and disease (i.e., the exposure is a risk factor for disease). If, on the other hand, the OR is less than one, it indicates a negative association (i.e., the exposure is protective against disease).

Step 2. The next step in constructing a statistical significance test is to specify null and alternative hypotheses. The null and alternative hypotheses are statements or assumptions about the true relationship between the exposure and outcome in the population at large. They are usually set so that they represent opposing conclusions—and the statistical significance test is the procedure by which we decide between them. The null hypothesis (denoted H_0) is so named because it typically expresses the status quo of no difference between the groups, or no association between disease and exposure. The alternative hypothesis (denoted H_A) usually states that the effect is not null; that, in fact, the groups differ and there exists an association between exposure and disease (without necessarily specifying whether this association is positive or negative). The null and alternative hypotheses are expressed in terms of the chosen measure of association. For our example, this is the OR:

$$H_0: \text{OR} = 1 \text{ (no association between exposure and outcome)}$$

versus

$$H_A: \text{OR} \neq 1 \text{ (exposure and outcome are related)}.$$

There can be a number of equivalent ways of expressing the null and alternative hypotheses for binary data. For example, we might replace the OR in these statements with the risk ratio (RR), if we have cohort data from which to estimate it. Similarly, we might reexpress the null hypothesis in terms of the risk difference (RD), again assuming that the study design permits estimation of the RD:

$$H_0: \text{RD} = 0 \text{ versus } H_A: \text{RD} \neq 0.$$

Any of the three choices for measuring association is appropriate, so long as the validity of the measure is supported by the design of the study (see chapter 8).

Step 3. Having formulated the question in terms of null and alternative hypotheses, we now face the problem of using the data to decide between the two. By calculating the selected measure of association, we can begin to explore whether the data are more consistent with the null hypothesis or with the alternative hypothesis. This evaluation, however, does not stop with the association measure. It is extremely rare to obtain an estimated OR of precisely 1.0, even if the true OR in the population is 1.0. Because of random variation, the sample estimate will differ somewhat from 1.0 even when the null hypothesis is true. Remembering that a sample estimate of the OR is a function of the data (and, therefore, a random quantity), we have to consider the precision of this estimate. A very small standard error for the OR estimator indicates that much information is available for estimating this effect. On the other hand, a relatively large standard error indicates that we lack information in our sample about the true OR in the population. As in the example of studying body mass index as it relates to SSD risk with 10 cases and 10 controls, our conclusions depend in part on the observed association but also must take account of the degree of precision of the estimate.

Therefore, as the third step in constructing a statistical significance test, in developing a rule for deciding whether the data favor H_0 or H_A, we make sure that it takes the level of precision into account. Let us define a test statistic T that is calculated from the data. T will be a function of the degree of association between exposure and outcome, as well as of the sample size and the prevalence of exposure and outcome. Generally speaking, test statistics are constructed such that large values of $|T|$ (where the vertical bars indicate absolute value) favor the alternative hypothesis, while small values of $|T|$ favor the null hypothesis. Although this information is helpful, it still does not constitute a decision rule. A decision rule is developed by our setting a value of $|T|$, called the critical value (c), above which we say that the data are more consistent with the alternative hypothesis. If, on the other hand, $|T|$ is less than the critical value, we say that the data are not sufficiently inconsistent with the null hypothesis for us to decide in favor of H_A. We can express this procedure in symbols as follows:

$$T \geq c \rightarrow \text{decide in favor of } H_A;$$

$$T < c \rightarrow \text{decide in favor of } H_0.$$

How do we choose c? Omitting the details, we use statistical theory to establish the properties of the test statistic under H_0; that is, statistical theory points to how the test statistic would behave (i.e., how large we might expect it to be) when the null hypothesis is true. Because the critical value is set according to expectations about the behavior of the test statistic on average, the results of the statistical significance test from a single sample may or may not be consistent with the truth in the population. In short, the statistical significance test might lead us to the wrong decision about whether of not chance accounts for the association between the exposure and disease in our data.

In order to describe the risks of an incorrect decision, it is necessary to introduce the concepts of type I and type II errors.

Errors in Tests of Statistical Significance

If we were to describe the behavior of a test statistic by cross-classifying the result of a test statistic based on a sample against the truth in the population at large, we would obtain table 23.2. The two cells on the main diagonal of the table display check marks, indicating that, in these instances, the sample-based test statistic leads us to the correct conclusion regarding the "truth" in the population. The off-diagonal cells, however, are those for which the test statistic leads us to the wrong conclusion. When the sample test statistic leads us to reject the null, when, in fact, the null hypothesis holds true in the population, we commit a type I error. In the language of diagnostic testing and misclassification that was introduced in chapter 8, a **type I error** is analogous to a false positive result, and the type I error rate is analogous to one minus the specificity. When the test fails to reject the null when the alternative is true, the result is a **type II error**. The type II error is analogous to a false negative result, so that the type II error rate is the analogue of one minus the sensitivity. The type I error rate is usually denoted by α, while the type II error rate is denoted by β. The quantity $1 - \beta$, or one minus the type II error rate, is known as the **power** of a test. It is more common to refer to a test's power than to its type II error rate.

Under ideal conditions, both the type I and type II errors would be minimized for a particular test procedure. This is, however, very difficult to achieve in practice. Typically, if we reduce the type I error by decreasing the likelihood of rejecting the null hypothesis, we encounter the additional effect of increasing the type II error. Conversely, if we seek to reduce the type II error by increasing the likelihood of rejecting the null, we simultaneously increase the type I error. Meeting both goals at once, therefore, seems impossible. It appears that, in order for us to proceed, one class of error must take precedence over the other.

The conventional strategy for statistical significance testing, as laid out by Neyman and Pearson (see Neyman and Pearson, 1967; Bickel and Doksum, 1977; Cox and Hinkley, 1974), is to set the type I error rate at an acceptable level and then choose a test procedure that maximizes power for a given α. This strategy is implemented by consideration of the distribution of test statistic T, assuming that the null hypothesis is true. The critical value is chosen

Table 23.2 Interpreting Findings from Tests of Significance

Test Result in the Sample	Truth in the Population	
	H_0 True	H_A Ture
$T < c$ (choose H_0)	√	Type II error
$T \geq c$ (choose H_A)	Type I error	√

such that the probability that T exceeds c is equal to α. The sample size is incorporated into this procedure in that the distribution of T under the null varies, depending upon the sample size (N).

The decision rule, then, amounts to gauging the size of the test statistic, T, against its expected size under the null hypothesis. For no good reason other than convention, the alpha level of a test (also known as its **significance level**) is typically set at 5 percent in the medical research literature. This means that if the null hypothesis is indeed true and there is no association between exposure and outcome in the population, then we must still expect to reject the null hypothesis in 5 percent of the research studies devoted to this question, simply by chance.

Definition and Role of the *p*-Value

As described so far, a statistical significance test compares the value of a test statistic to a critical value, yielding a dichotomous result. We either reject the null hypothesis at the 5 percent significance level or we do not. There remains a need to quantify the strength of a test result. That is, we want to be able to characterize the degree to which the data are (or are not) consistent with the null hypothesis. To fill this gap, investigators often report a *p*-value calculated from the test statistic. The **p-value** (short for probability value) is the probability of obtaining a test statistic $|T|$ as large or larger than that obtained from the sample data, assuming that the null hypothesis is true in the population. Whether the *p*-value is smaller or larger than the significance level (5 percent) is equivalent to whether the test statistic $|T|$ is larger or smaller than its corresponding 5 percent critical value, c.

Basing our decision rule on the *p*-value, therefore, is exactly the same as basing it on the size of $|T|$ in comparison with c. Unlike the comparison of $|T|$ to c, however, the *p*-value provides some measure of the strength of evidence from a study. The smaller the *p*-value is, the less likely it is that the results from the sample could have arisen from a population where the null hypothesis is true. For instance, a *p*-value of .01 indicates that we expect to obtain a test statistic as large (or larger) than that seen in our sample only one percent of the time when the null hypothesis is true. If the *p*-value is .003, then we expect to see results as or more extreme than those obtained from our sample in only 3 studies out of 1000 under the null hypothesis.

As stated, the procedure for conducting and interpreting a test of statistical significance is very clear. We reject the null hypothesis when the *p*-value is less than or equal to .05; we do not reject when p is greater than .05. There is a danger, however, in applying this rule too literally. While investigators may choose to use 5 percent as the significance level for a particular statistical test, we must acknowledge that there is very little difference between a *p*-value of .055 and one of .045. While the former clearly indicates that the value of the test statistic does not strictly exceed the critical value, the values of the two test statistics corresponding to these *p*-values are surely very, very similar. This kind of information should not be categorically dismissed as inconclusive. It is generally acceptable to describe test statistics with *p*-values very close to (but larger than) the nominal significance level as marginally significant. This avoids the problem of abandoning borderline research findings, which might cause subsequent researchers to neglect valuable information in the published literature.

Despite the valuable procedures and guidelines for testing as just described, we still have to acknowledge that in a given sample we cannot know whether or not the test statistic has led us to the correct conclusion (i.e., one that is consistent with the circumstances in the population). The most we can say is that the statistical properties of test statistics limit the likelihood of errors. A decision rule ensures that we will draw the correct conclusions most of the time throughout our careers, but does not ensure that we will be right in any particular instance. Above all, remember that the evaluation of an association involves a careful review of all the available data, including the test result, the estimated magnitude of effect, and its confidence interval.

Simple Test Procedures for Binary and Continuous Data

Now that the logic behind statistical significance testing and the computation of p-values is understood, let us consider some of the more commonly used procedures for comparing two groups. For a complete discussion of these procedures and their uses, please see a comprehensive, introductory textbook, such as Altman (1991).

Pearson's Chi-Squared Test for Comparing Proportions

Recall that several different study designs may yield results that can be summarized in a 2×2 table. For example, in a case-control study, we might cross-classify disease status (present/absent) and a binary exposure measure (exposed/unexposed). Alternatively, we might cross-classify a binary exposure and a binary outcome (affected/unaffected) in the context of a cohort study.

Although the design of the study governs which joint, conditional, and marginal probabilities are estimable, the study design does not impact the calculation of Pearson's chi-squared statistic for testing whether there is an association between exposure and outcome. Thus, the chi-squared test is valid under case-control, cohort, and cross-sectional study designs. It is also the appropriate statistic to apply without regard to the selected measure of association: risk difference (RD), risk ratio (RR), or odds ratio (OR). The null hypothesis for Pearson's chi-squared test is that there is no association between exposure and outcome. An equivalent expression for the null hypothesis is that the OR (or RR) is equal to one. This is also equivalent to stating that the risk difference is equal to zero. The alternative hypothesis states that the exposure and disease are associated, and that the OR (or RR) is not equal to one (or, equivalently, that the risk difference is not equal to zero).

The formula for the chi-squared statistic is as follows:

$$\chi^2 = \frac{t(ad - bc)^2}{m_1 m_2 n_1 n_2},$$

where quantities are defined as in table 23.1.

As with most test statistics, small values of χ^2 indicate that the data are consistent with the null hypothesis; large values reveal a lack of consistency with H_0. Under the null hypothesis (i.e., assuming OR = 1, RR = 1, or RD = 0), this statistic follows a chi-squared distribution with one degree of freedom. Critical values and *p*-values can, therefore, be computed by consulting a chi-squared table (available in most introductory statistics texts).

Example of Chi-Squared Test: Maternal Schizophrenia and Sudden Infant Death Syndrome (SIDS)

Recall the study by Bennedsen et al. (2001), introduced in chapter 22, which examines the association of maternal schizophrenia and risk of SIDS in the offspring (see table 23.3). To test this association, we can construct the following null and alternative hypotheses:

H_0: OR = 1 (no association between maternal schizophrenia and SIDS)

versus

H_A: OR ≠ 1 (maternal schizophrenia and SIDS are related).

Since both the exposure (schizophrenia in mother) and outcome (SIDS) are binary, we can use Pearson's chi-squared test to determine whether the data are consistent with the null hypothesis or the alternative. If the type I error is set at 5 percent, the critical value for the chi-squared distribution on one degree of freedom is 3.84. Pearson's chi-squared statistic can be computed as:

$$\chi^2 = \frac{t(ad - bc)^2}{m_1 m_2 n_1 n_2} = \frac{125774\big[(10)(123420) - (2220)(124)\big]^2}{(2230)(123544)(134)(125640)} = 24.93.$$

Compared to a chi-squared distribution with one degree of freedom, $p < .001$.

Interpretation of Chi-Squared Test Example

The large χ^2 value and corresponding *p*-value clearly indicate that observing a result as or more extreme than that observed in these data is highly unlikely (less than one in 1000) if there is truly no association between maternal schizophrenia and risk of death from SIDS in the target population. We reject the null hypothesis, therefore, and conclude that association exists between

Table 23.3 SIDS Deaths among Offspring of Exposed and Unexposed Mothers from the Bennedsen Cohort (Bennedsen et al. 2001)

	Cases (SIDS)	Noncases	Total
Exposed (maternal schizophrenia)	10	2,220	2,230
Unexposed (no maternal schizophrenia)	124	123,420	123,544
Total	134	125,640	125,774

maternal schizophrenia and SIDS. Note that the sign of the test statistic does not signify anything regarding the direction of the association between SIDS and schizophrenia; chi-squared statistics are always non-negative. To understand the nature of the relationship between SIDS and schizophrenia, we need to compute an estimate of the association between the two variables. From our earlier example in chapter 22, we know that the OR is estimated at approximately 4.5, indicating increased risk of SIDS among mothers with schizophrenia.

Student's t-Test for Comparing Means

Now suppose that the variable by which our two groups are to be compared is continuous. Student's t-test uses the fact that the sample mean is approximately normally distributed in large samples.

Before introducing the formula for the t-test, we must define some new notation. Suppose, for the sake of simplicity, that we are comparing mean exposure levels among diseased and nondiseased subjects in a case-control study. Let $\{X_{11}, X_{12}, X_{13}, \ldots, X_{1N_1}\}$ denote the observed exposure values in the case group, and let $\{X_{21}, X_{22}, X_{23}, \ldots, X_{2N_2}\}$ denote the exposures in the controls. The null hypothesis for Student's t-test is that the mean exposure level among cases (μ_1) is equal to the mean exposure level among controls (μ_2); or, equivalently, that the mean difference is zero. The alternative hypothesis states that the group means differ. In symbols, the null and alternative hypotheses can be expressed as:

$$H_0: \mu_1 = \mu_2 \text{ versus } H_A: \mu_1 \neq \mu_2.$$

The t-statistic is computed as

$$t = \frac{\hat{\mu}_1 - \hat{\mu}_2}{\sqrt{\left(\dfrac{1}{N_1} + \dfrac{1}{N_2}\right)}\sqrt{\dfrac{N_1(N_1-1)\left[SE(\hat{\mu}_1)\right]^2 + N_2(N_2-1)\left[SE(\hat{\mu}_2)\right]^2}{N_1 + N_2 - 2}}},$$

where $\hat{\mu}_j$, the group-specific estimate of the mean for cases ($j = 1$) or controls ($j = 2$), is computed as

$$\hat{\mu}_j = \sum_{i=1}^{N_j} X_{ji} / N_j,$$

and the group-specific standard error of the mean, $SE(\hat{\mu}_j)$, $j = 1, 2$, is given by

$$SE(\hat{\mu}_j) = \sqrt{\frac{1}{N_j} \sum_{i=1}^{N_j} \frac{(X_{ji} - \hat{\mu}_j)^2}{(N_j - 1)}}.$$

Student's t-statistic assumes that the variability in the exposure measurement is the same in cases and controls, but is unknown and must be estimated from the data.

As with most test statistics, large values of t indicate that the data are not consistent with the null hypothesis of equal means across disease groups.

Under the null hypothesis of equal means, Student's t-test follows a t-distribution with $(N_1 + N_2 - 2)$ degrees of freedom. A t-distribution is very similar to a standard normal distribution, except that it has fatter tails. As the sample size (and, therefore, the degrees of freedom) increases, the t-distribution gets closer and closer to a standard normal. Like the normal and chi-squared distributions, tables for the t-distribution are provided in most statistical texts. These tables can be used to determine critical values and p-values for a wide range of sample sizes.

Example of Student's t-Test: Head Circumference and Violence in Schizophrenia

Consider again the data reported by Cannon et al. (2002) and summarized in chapter 22. This study considered perinatal risk factors for criminal convictions among individuals with schizophrenia.

Using Student's t-test, we can formally evaluate the following hypotheses:

H_0: $\mu_1 = \mu_2$ (the mean birth head circumference is the same among cases and controls)

versus

H_A: $\mu_1 \neq \mu_2$ (the mean birth head circumference differs between cases and controls),

where cases are those with criminal records and controls are those without criminal records.

If we set alpha, the type I error rate, equal to 5 percent, then the critical value for the t-distribution with $N_1 + N_2 - 2 = 634$ degrees of freedom is 1.96. Substituting the sample values into the formula for the t-statistic, we find

$$t = \frac{35.3 - 34.9}{\sqrt{\left(\frac{1}{61} + \frac{1}{575}\right)}\sqrt{\frac{61(61-1)[0.16]^2 + 575(575-1)[0.06]^2}{61 + 575 - 2}}} = 2.0873.$$

According to the t-distribution on 634 degrees of freedom, we find that the p-value for this statistic is equal to .0373. Thus, if the null hypothesis is assumed to be true, we would obtain a result as or more extreme than that observed in the sample data fewer than 4 times out of 100. With this result, we would reject the null hypothesis and conclude that the data are more consistent with the alternative hypothesis. These data support the claim that mean head circumference at birth differs between schizophrenic subjects with and those without criminal records. Given that the mean difference is equal to 0.4 cm, we would further infer that head circumference is larger among those with criminal records than among those without records.

The formulas provided here assume that we are analyzing case-control data. If, in fact, we are analyzing mean measurements for a continuous outcome variable (e.g., severity of disease) among exposed (group 1) and unexposed (group 2) subjects in a cohort study, then we apply the same formulas, except that N_1 denotes the number of exposed subjects and N_2 denotes the number of unexposed subjects.

Conclusion

Tests of statistical significance help us to interpret the results of a research study. In combination with estimated measures of association (which point to strength of association), and confidence intervals (which point to the magnitude and precision of an estimated association), significance tests add to the weight of evidence on whether an observed relationship is more likely due to random fluctuation or to a true relationship between exposure and disease. Even if such a three-pronged analysis indicates that a finding is not due to chance, however, we still may not conclude that the association is causal in nature. For example, there may be a confounder that distorts the observed relationship between exposure and disease. The methods described in chapter 25 (stratification, statistical modeling, and matched analysis) can be used to examine the role of confounders in our effort to discern whether or not an observed association is causal. For more details, see the excellent texts by Altman (1991) and Fleiss et al. (2003).

We conclude with a caution. Note that the properties of the most commonly used statistical tests of association are based on large-sample approximations. This means that the distributions of these test statistics are derived as the sample size becomes infinitely large. In practice, therefore, the actual (finite) sample size must be large in order for the approximation to be accurate. Consequently, the performance of the test may be poor (e.g., the type I error rate may be higher than the specified level) when the sample size is small. Unfortunately, there is no simple, universal criterion for determining what makes a sample large enough, because the accuracy of the large sample approximation will also depend on the variability of the statistics and sample estimators in question, which vary from one instance to the next. To avoid incorrect inferences when faced with small samples, researchers often rely on exact nonparametric methods to evaluate statistical hypotheses. The enhanced availability of reliable, comprehensive exact statistical software packages, such as StatXact (2004), has enabled researchers to employ exact methods more regularly in their work. For a complete discussion of when and how to use exact statistical methods, see the texts by Edgington (1995), Manly (1997), Sprent and Smeeton (2000), Agresti (2002), and Good (2005).

Chapter 24 addresses the question of proper study planning to ensure adequate sample size, precision and power for statistical tests of association.

References

Agresti (2002). *Categorical Data Analysis*, 2nd ed. New York: John Wiley & Sons.
Altman DG (1991). *Practical Statistics for Medical Research*. London: Chapman & Hall.

Bennedsen BE, Mortensen PB, Olesen AV, and Henriksen TB (2001). Congenital Malformations, Stillbirths, and Infant deaths among Children of Women with Schizophrenia. *Arch. Gen. Psychiatry* 58:674–679.

Bickel PJ and Doksum KA (1977). *Mathematical Statistics: Basic Ideas and Selected Topics.* Oakland, Calif.: Holden-Day.

Cannon M, Huttunen MO, Tanskanen AJ, Arseneault L, Jones PB, and Murray RM (2002). Perinatal and Childhood Risk Factors for Later Criminality and Violence in Schizophrenia. *Br. J. Psychiatry* 180:496–501.

Cox DR and Hinkley DV (1974). *Theoretical Statistics.* London: Chapman & Hall.

Edgington ES (1995). *Randomization Tests*, 3rd ed. New York: Marcel Dekker.

Fleiss JL, Levin B, and Paik MC (2003). *Statistical Methods for Rates and Proportions*, 3rd ed. New York: John Wiley & Sons.

Good P (2005). *Permutation, Parametric and Bootstrap Tests of Hypotheses*, 3rd ed. New York: Springer-Verlag.

Manly BFJ (1997). *Randomization, Bootstrap and Monte Carlo Methods in Biology*, 2nd ed. London: Chapman & Hall.

Neyman J and Pearson ES (1967). *Joint Statistical Papers.* Cambridge: Cambridge University Press.

Sprent P and Smeeton NC (2000). *Applied Nonparametric Statistical Methods*, 3rd ed. London: Chapman & Hall.

StatXact: Statistical Software for Exact Nonparametric Inference, version 6 (2004). Cambridge, Mass.: Cytel Software.

24 Planning Studies: Estimating Power and Sample Size

Melissa D. Begg and Michaeline Bresnahan

Human research studies can be very difficult to conduct, very time-consuming to complete, and extremely costly. They require tremendous commitment from the investigators involved, as well as from all of the participants who contribute their time, their effort, and even their blood and other physical samples to further the cause of research. Given these considerations, investigators need to quantify, before embarking on a study, their ability to detect meaningful associations under the proposed study design. To this end, power and sample size calculations are essential to proper study planning.

Computing Power for a Given Sample Size

A power calculation consists of estimating, before conducting a research study, the probability of obtaining a significant test result from that study as it has been planned. In order to compute a power estimate, the investigator must specify the sample sizes of the two groups for comparison, the type I error rate (usually 5 percent), and the level of association that is expected if the alternative hypothesis is true (i.e., if the exposure and disease are associated). Naturally, it is difficult to specify the magnitude of the association between exposure and disease before the data have been collected. After all, if this were known at the start, there would be no need to conduct the study.

On the other hand, an investigator can make an educated guess as to the likely size of the association between exposure and outcome, a guess based on animal studies, prior research on the same question in humans, pilot data, or prior research on a similar question. Alternatively, researchers might posit the smallest level of association in the population that they would not want to miss in their sample. With regard to general trends, a larger sample size results in higher power, holding all else constant. A smaller (more restrictive) significance level means lower power when everything else is fixed. And the larger the magnitude of the hypothesized association, the higher the power for detecting a significant difference (i.e., for rejecting the null hypothesis) when all else is unchanged.

Recall that **power** is defined as the probability of rejecting the null hypothesis when the alternative hypothesis is true. In terms of the test statistic, power can be written (using notation from chapter 23) as

$$\text{Power} = \Pr(|T| \geq c \mid H_A \text{ is true}).$$

This expression for power points to the techniques used to compute it. Because power depends on the size of the test statistic in comparison to the critical value, we use the known distributional properties of the test under the alternative hypothesis to determine the likelihood that $|T|$ will exceed c.

Estimating Power for Binary-Response Data

Suppose that we are planning a study to investigate the association between a binary exposure and a binary outcome. The following formula gives the power for detecting a significant difference between two groups (either diseased and nondiseased subjects in a case-control study, or exposed and unexposed subjects in a cohort study), each of size n (for a total sample size of $2n$):

$$\text{Power} \cong \Pr\left(Z > \frac{z_{1-\alpha/2}\sqrt{\dfrac{2}{n}\bar{p}(1-\bar{p})} - (p_1 - p_0)}{\sqrt{\dfrac{1}{n}\left[p_1(1-p_1) + p_0(1-p_0)\right]}} \right).$$

In this formula, p_1 and p_0 represent the hypothesized probabilities of disease in the exposed group (subscripted 1) and unexposed group (subscripted 0), respectively, if this is a cohort study; and they denote the probabilities of exposure in the diseased and nondiseased groups if this is a case-control study. The term $\bar{p}$ represents the simple average of p_1 and p_0, $z_{1-\alpha/2}$ is the critical value for the test procedure of significance level α (e.g., $z_{1-\alpha/2} = 1.96$ when $\alpha = 0.05$), and Z is a standard normal deviate. Note that the formula assumes that p_1 is greater than p_0; if not, then we simply reverse the identities of the two comparison groups. The power of the test can be computed as the probability that a standard normal deviate is greater than the expression on the right side of the inequality in parentheses.

High Body Mass Index and Schizophrenic Spectrum Disorder (SSD): An Example

Consider a case-control study designed to evaluate the hypothesis that high prepregnancy maternal body mass index is associated with increased risk of SSD in the offspring. Suppose that we intend to recruit 100 cases and 100 controls, and we expect a high maternal body mass index prevalence of 10 percent among controls and 20 percent among cases. What is the power for testing for association between high maternal body mass index and offspring SSD risk under this study design?

Using our formula,

$$\text{Power} \cong \Pr\left(Z > \frac{1.96\sqrt{\frac{2}{100}(.15)(1-.15)} - (.20-.10)}{\sqrt{\frac{1}{100}[.20(1-.20)+.10(1-.10)]}} \right) = \Pr(Z > -.0205),$$

we find that the power of this test is equal to the probability that a standard normal random variable exceeds the value −0.0205. Comparing this value to published tables for the standard normal distribution, we find that the power is equal to about 51 percent. If we choose to go ahead with the study as currently planned, we have only about even odds of detecting the specified difference in exposure proportions. We may want to reconsider the study design, perhaps increasing the sample size to improve power. If we can recruit 200 cases and 200 controls, the power increases to 80 percent.

Estimating Power for Continuous-Response Data

As reviewed in the previous chapter, we may wish to compare two groups with respect to a continuous variable. In a case-control study, this amounts to comparing the mean exposure level in cases and controls. In a cohort study, we compare the mean response measurements in exposed and unexposed subjects. Under either design, the power calculation follows the same formula.

To simplify the presentation, let us assume that we are planning a case-control study. The formula requires four pieces of information to proceed: the significance level of the test statistic to be used (α), the sample size per comparison group (n), the difference in mean exposure levels of cases and controls that is anticipated under the alternative hypothesis ($\delta = \mu_1 - \mu_0$), and the standard deviation of the exposure measurement in a single sample (σ). Like the power formula for binary data, the formula for continuous data takes the form of a probability statement based on the distribution of a standard normal random variable:

$$\text{Power} = \Pr\left(Z \geq z_{1-\alpha/2} - \frac{\delta}{\sqrt{2\sigma^2/n}} \right).$$

Body Mass Index and Schizophrenia Spectrum Disorder (SSD): Another Example

Investigators plan a case-control study to evaluate a potential association between maternal body mass index, measured just before pregnancy, and the offspring's risk of SSD. Preliminary data indicate that the standard deviation of body mass index is approximately equal to $5\,\text{kg/m}^2$. The investigators speculate that the average body mass index among case women will be about $23\,\text{kg/m}^2$, while the average among controls will be about $21\,\text{kg/m}^2$. What is the power for detecting a difference of this size in a sample of 200 cases and 200 controls? Assume that the significance level of the test is 5 percent.

Substituting our hypothesized quantities into the expression already given,

$$\text{Power} = \Pr\left(Z \geq 1.96 - \frac{2}{\sqrt{2(5)^2/200}} \right) = \Pr(Z \geq -2.04)$$

we find that the power for this test is equal to the probability that a standard normal random variable exceeds -2.04. Using a normal table, this equates to a power of .9793, or almost 98 percent. This represents excellent power for detecting the anticipated difference in exposure levels between cases and controls.

Computing Sample Size for a Given Level of Power

Consider approaching the question of power from another direction. In ordinary circumstances, investigators are very unlikely to garner support for a study unless they can demonstrate that it is adequately powered. By convention, 80 percent power (or better) is deemed acceptable in most circumstances. If a study can be shown to have 90 percent power, it would be considered excellent. So, instead of computing power for a given sample size (which may or may not lead to a satisfactory result), investigators frequently compute the sample size required to achieve a prespecified level of power (say, 80 or 90 percent). For these calculations, the investigators must specify the type I error rate (usually 5 percent), the anticipated difference between the groups under the alternative hypothesis, and the desired power level. Given these three pieces of information, they can then apply standard formulas for computing n, the minimum sample size per group.

Estimating the Required Sample Size for Binary Data

Let us return to the previous example of planning a case-control study to evaluate the relationship between high maternal body mass index and offspring risk of SSD. Suppose that p_1 denotes the probability of exposure (high maternal body mass index) among cases, and p_0 denotes the probability of exposure among controls. If we want to conduct a significance test of the equality of these two proportions at significance level α and power $(1 - \beta)$, we should recruit n cases and n controls for study, where n per group is computed as

$$n = f(\alpha, \beta) \times [\{p_1(1 - p_1) + p_0(1 - p_0)\}/(p_1 - p_0)^2],$$

where $f(\alpha, \beta)$ is a known function of the type I error rate (α) and power $(1 - \beta)$. For a 5 percent–level test with 80 percent power, set $f(\alpha, \beta)$ equal to 7.9. For 90 percent power, set $f(\alpha, \beta)$ equal to 10.5. It is clear to see from the displayed equation that, as the difference between groups $(p_1 - p_0)$ increases, the required sample size decreases. Similarly, as desired power increases, the function $f(\alpha, \beta)$ increases, so the required n becomes larger.

Example

Suppose investigators plan a case-control study to evaluate a potential association between maternal body mass index (dichotomized as high or low) and the offspring's risk of SSD (present or absent). Summary data indicate that the prevalence of high maternal body mass index is 20 percent among cases, but only 10 percent among controls. What is the minimum sample size required in order to guarantee at least 90 percent power for detecting the specified association between maternal body mass index and SSD? Assume that the test will be conducted at the 5 percent significance level.

To compute the required sample size, we substitute the values $f(\alpha, \beta) = 10.5$, $p_1 = .20$, and $p_0 = .10$ into our equation:

$$n = 10.5 \times [\{.20(0.80) + .10(0.90)\}/(.20 - .10)^2] = 262.5$$

Thus, the investigators will need at least 263 subjects per group (263 cases and 263 controls) to achieve 90 percent power to detect a statistically significant difference between the two groups. Overall, the required sample size is 526.

Estimating the Required Sample Size for Continuous Data

We can also estimate a minimum sample size for detecting a statistically significant difference in mean levels of a continuous variable. In order to perform this calculation, we must specify significance level α, power $(1 - \beta)$, the size of the difference in means assuming that the alternative hypothesis is true, and the standard deviation (from a single sample) of the measure being evaluated. (We assume that the standard deviation of the measurement of interest is the same in the two groups being compared.) For example, imagine that we wish to compare SSD cases and controls with respect to average maternal prepregnancy body mass index, measured in kg/m^2. Suppose that μ_1 represents the mean exposure (maternal body mass index) among cases, and μ_0 represents the mean exposure among controls. Let δ represent the difference in means $(\delta = \mu_1 - \mu_0)$, while σ represents the standard deviation of body mass index measurements. Then the formula for the sample size per group is as follows:

$$n = f(\alpha, \beta) \times [2\sigma^2/\delta^2],$$

where $f(\alpha, \beta)$ is defined as before. Then we simply insert the f corresponding to the chosen α and β levels, as well as the hypothesized values for σ and δ (assuming H_A is true).

Suppose that the plan for the case-control study is modified so that cases and controls will be compared with respect to maternal body mass index on its original, continuous scale (kg/m^2). Preliminary data reveal that the standard deviation for body mass index is about $5\,kg/m^2$. Investigators speculate that the average maternal body mass index among cases is $23\,kg/m^2$, while the mean among controls is about $21\,kg/m^2$. Calculate the minimum sample size required to guarantee at least 90 percent power for detecting a statistically significant association between body mass index and SSD risk.

Set $f(\alpha, \beta) = 10.5$, $\delta = (23\,kg/m^2 - 21\,kg/m^2) = 2\,kg/m^2$, and $\sigma = 5\,kg/m^2$. Using our earlier expression for n,

$$n = 10.5 \times [2(5)^2/(2)^2] = 131.25.$$

Rounding up, we find that $n = 132$ is the smallest sample size per group (264 subjects overall) needed to assure us 90 percent power.

Issues in Power and Sample Size Calculations

It is important to remember that power and sample size calculations are no more than approximations. They give you a rough idea of whether your study design is reasonable, given expectations about the nature of the association between exposure and disease under the alternative hypothesis. Excessive attention to minute changes in the parameters to be specified is therefore unwarranted. Large changes to the parameters, however, can wield tremendous influence over the results, so it is essential that every assumption contributing to a power calculation be evaluated critically. In addition, there are occasions on which researchers may accept a lower-than-usual level of power for detecting differences. While 75–80 percent power is considered the bare minimum for most funded investigations, lower figures have been used in some studies, due to the urgency of the question and the window of opportunity for investigating it.

Please note that the formulas throughout this chapter assume equal numbers of subjects in the groups being compared (e.g., exposed and unexposed, case and control). In many instances, group sizes are unequal. For example, case-control studies often enroll more controls than cases because of financial or logistical considerations. In these instances, modified formulas for power and sample size calculations must be used. See other textbooks for more details (Breslow et al. 1980; Schlesselman 1982).

Investigators should expect reviews of any proposal to include a critical examination of the assumptions behind the power and sample size calculations. To prepare for this evaluation, the study's planners should be sure to consider four key power-related questions before submitting a proposal.

First, one has to assess whether the postulated magnitude of association is realistic. As can be seen from the many formulas given here, power looks better and the required sample size is smaller if we specify a very large difference between the two comparison groups. Although this option may appear attractive at first glance, remember that the reviewers may reject this assumption and conclude that the study investigators are ill informed, irrational, or (at worst) willfully deceptive. Specification of the size of the association between the exposure and outcome is typically the most difficult part of this process. The postulated effect often derives from smaller (and less reliable) studies, in a different patient population, perhaps looking at a different (but similar) exposure. The best strategy in presentation is to lay out the limitations of the power analysis in a straightforward fashion; it is also advisable to present power for a (limited) range of effect sizes under the alternative hypothesis. This effort indicates to a reviewer that the investigators are knowledgeable and realistic.

The second point to consider is the availability of resources. When calculating the required sample size, one has to ask whether the resources (in personnel, funding, and space) and the patient pool are large enough to support the recruitment and evaluation of $2n$ subjects. If all reasonable attempts at calculating power indicate that the minimum sample size exceeds the resources available for evaluation, the investigator is forced to reconsider the structure of the study. Corrective actions might include using less expensive measurement techniques, repeated testing to minimize the standard deviation of the measure of interest (if continuous), or even the adoption of a completely different study design (e.g., opting for a case-control design instead of a cohort design).

Third, the power calculations are done on the assumption that exposure and outcome are measured without error, but this is rarely the case. Random measurement error serves to decrease the precision of the measure of association, resulting in reduced power for detecting associations. Consequently, the statistical power of most studies is somewhat lower than expected. Although more accurate assessments may be more costly, and thereby constrain sample size, they may also enhance power by reducing error. Unfortunately, this point is often overlooked.

The final consideration is the availability of study participants. If the sample size is $2n$, investigators must provide a realistic estimate of the time required to recruit that number of participants to the study. This time requirement depends on the number of participants available, the proportion who are eligible for the study, and the expected likelihood of enrollment (i.e., the participation rate). Unless study planners can demonstrate the feasibility of the proposed study, reviewers are unlikely to support it. If the required number of participants cannot be achieved in a single institution, investigators may wish to consider a multi-institution effort.

Conclusion

This chapter has described some of the most basic and commonly used formulas for computing power and sample size. For additional reading on this subject, consult the following introductory, user-friendly discussions of the computation of power and sample size: Dupont and Plummer (1990), Fleiss, Levin, and Paik (2003), Pocock (1983), and Schlesselman (1982).

References

Breslow NE and Day NE (1980). *The Analysis of Case-Control Studies.* Lyon, France: International Agency for Research on Cancer.

Dupont WD and Plummer WD (1990). Power and Sample Size Calculations: A Review and Computer Program. *Controlled Clinical Trials* 11:116–128.

Fleiss JL, Levin B, and Paik MC (2003). *Statistical Methods for Rates and Proportions*. New York: Wiley.

Pocock SJ (1983). *Clinical Trials: A Practical Approach*. Chichester, England: Wiley.

Schlesselman JJ (1982). *Case-Control Studies: Design, Conduct, Analysis*. New York: Oxford University Press.

25 Adjustment for Covariates

Melissa D. Begg and Michaeline Bresnahan

Demonstrating an association between exposure and disease is only the first step towards causal identification. We must then attempt to rule out alternative explanations for observed associations. Although we would like to think that an observed association is due to our hypothesized exposure of interest, it is also possible that distortion caused by a confounding variable is responsible for all or part of this association. Furthermore, a confounder can conceal an association between an exposure and disease. Confounding, therefore, is a primary threat to establishing causation.

This chapter addresses the use of statistical analysis to rule out confounding as an alternative explanation. For example, consider our ongoing example of the association between maternal prepregnancy body mass index and risk of schizophrenia spectrum disorder (SSD) in offspring in the Prenatal Determinants of Schizophrenia Example (PDSE). It is possible that this relationship is distorted by a third factor (e.g., mother's age). Suppose, for the sake of argument, that advancing age in the mother is a true risk factor for SSD in her children, but body mass index is not. Also suppose that older mothers tend to have higher body mass index. If we examine the association between body mass index and SSD without consideration of mother's age, the resulting positive association we obtain would be the result of confounding. In this instance, we would want to account for the effect of maternal age before inferring that body mass index is a risk factor for SSD.

Because confounding can operate in any direction, it may lead us to exaggerate, understate, or even reverse the association of interest. The direction of the confounding effect can be difficult to predict, and the degree of distortion in the estimate can range from very modest to severe. Control for confounding can be attempted either during the design of a study (by pair-matching or frequency matching), or during the analysis by statistical adjustment.

The goal of statistical adjustment for confounders is to make the groups being compared as alike as possible with regard to everything except the factor of interest. For example, in a cohort study, we would want to make the exposed and unexposed subjects as alike as possible with respect to everything except the exposure of interest. As stated in earlier chapters, we use adjustment to help infer what would have been the difference in disease risk between the exposed and unexposed had there been no confounding. Then, if a difference between groups is observed, it is more likely due to the exposure of interest, not to other factors. This comparability of subjects across groups is the chief benefit of randomization in controlled trials, where participants are assigned at random to exposure groups so that there is more likely to be balance with regard to all risk factors, both known and unknown. Observational studies are more common in psychiatric epidemiology than are randomized trials, and are also more prone to confounding. It is therefore essential for proper inference in psychiatric epidemiology to apply methods to adjust for potential confounding in our pursuit of causal factors.

The purpose of this chapter is to introduce methods of statistical adjustment. Statistical adjustment is used to reduce the effects of confounders; or, more precisely, to infer what association would have been observed had there been no confounding. The main analytic methods for control of confounding include stratification, statistical modeling, and subgroup analysis. In this chapter, we first focus on stratification and regression analysis (a form of statistical modeling) as methods of analysis for unmatched samples. We then describe methods for analyzing matched data. Although matching to control for confounding is done before the data are collected, it is critically important that we apply statistical methods that account for the matching, because the analysis must correspond to the design to attain valid results. We consider subgroup analysis briefly at the end of the chapter.

An Adjusted Method for Gauging Association

Returning to the example of maternal body mass index and SSD risk, suppose that maternal body mass index is dichotomized as low versus high. The data might then be summarized in a 2×2 table cross-classifying body mass index by disease outcome (diagnosis of SSD versus not). In order to remove the potential effect of maternal age from this analysis, we might subdivide the participants under study into multiple strata defined by selected age ranges (say, maternal age 15–25, 26–35, 36–45, and 46+). We could then construct four separate 2×2 tables, cross-classifying body mass index status (low versus high) against SSD (present/absent) within each age stratum. The information contained in age stratum i (where $i = 1, 2, \ldots, k$) can be represented as in table 25.1.

Table 25.1 Cross-Classified Data from a Single Stratum (Stratum i) in a Cohort or Case-Control Study

	Diseased	**Nondiseased**	**Row Totals**
Exposed	a_i	b_i	m_{1i}
Unexposed	c_i	d_i	m_{2i}
Column totals	n_{1i}	n_{2i}	t_i

Let us suppose that we are interested only in the odds ratio, since this measure can be computed under either the cohort or case-control design. We could apply the methods for a single 2×2 table described in previous chapters to each stratum individually. This would yield an estimate and confidence interval for each stratum-specific odds ratio. Although this approach is useful to some degree, it does not address our need to summarize our findings on body mass index and schizophrenia risk across the age strata. It is desirable to somehow combine our stratum-specific findings to yield a unified result on the relationship between body mass index and schizophrenia, adjusted for the influence of mother's age. For this purpose, the methods proposed by Nathan Mantel and William Haenszel (1959) are perfectly suited.

The Mantel-Haenszel methods allow us to combine information across strata without pooling data across strata. This is a critical difference. Pooling the data (i.e., ignoring the strata) would yield an unadjusted assessment of association, potentially biased by the effect of mother's age. We would refer to the resulting effect estimate as *crude*, or *naïve*. The Mantel-Haenszel analysis combines information appropriately across strata, resulting in estimates that are adjusted for confounding by the stratum-defining variable. Note that Mantel-Haenszel methods that are based on the odds ratio are applicable to data from both case-control and cohort studies.

The Mantel-Haenszel summary odds ratio is calculated as a weighted average of the stratum-specific odds ratios, with weights that are calculated from the cell counts:

$$\hat{OR}_{MH} = \frac{\sum_{i=1}^{k} a_i d_i / t_i}{\sum_{i=1}^{k} b_i c_i / t_i}.$$

When there is a substantial difference between the unadjusted (pooled) odds ratio estimator and the adjusted (summary) odds ratio estimator, it is likely that the unadjusted estimator of the odds ratio has been distorted by confounding. In this case, we typically report that the adjusted estimate is a more valid reflection of the relationship between exposure and disease.

Approximate formulas for the standard error of log of the Mantel-Haenszel common odds ratio have been derived by Hauck (1979) and by Robins et al. (1986). These standard errors can be used to generate confidence intervals for the summary odds ratio (OR), and one or more versions of the standard error can be obtained in the commonly used statistical software packages. The specific formulas have been omitted here, but can be found in Fleiss et al. (2003), Schlesselman (1982), and Rothman and Greenland (1998).

Note that calculation of the Mantel-Haenszel summary OR may or may not be desirable when the stratum-specific ORs are very different from one another. We will see in chapter 27 that when the ORs vary greatly from stratum to stratum, the appropriate conclusion may be that there is effect modification or interaction; that is, the association between exposure and response varies by the level of the third factor. In these cases, calculation of a summary OR is not always desirable, since the effects being combined are not comparable. The formal assessment of interaction is introduced in chapter 27, and more complete discussions can be found in Jewell (2004), Fleiss et al. (2003), Schlesselman (1982), and Rothman and Greenland (1998).

An Adjusted Test of Significance

The simple chi-squared test procedure for binary data described in chapter 23 is sometimes characterized as crude, or unadjusted, because it makes no adjustment for the influence of potential confounders. Because of confounding, unadjusted tests of significance may result in misleading conclusions. Just as we used stratification to generate an adjusted measure of association, we can use stratification to conduct an adjusted test of significance. The Mantel-Haenszel test statistic summarizes the information across several 2×2 tables, yielding a single test statistic that assesses whether exposure and disease are associated after controlling (adjusting) for a third factor.

The null hypothesis for the Mantel-Haenszel statistic states that the common OR is equal to one (reflective of no association between exposure and response in any stratum). The alternative hypothesis, in contrast, states that the common OR differs from one. The formula for the Mantel-Haenszel statistic is

$$\chi^2_{\mathrm{MH}} = \frac{\left(\sum_{i=1}^{k} a_i - \sum_{i=1}^{k} m_{1i} n_{1i} / t_i \right)^2}{\sum_{i=1}^{k} \left(m_{1i} m_{2i} n_{1i} n_{2i} \right) / \left(t_i^2 \left(t_i - 1 \right) \right)}.$$

Under the null hypothesis, the distribution of χ^2_{MH} is chi-squared with one degree of freedom. This information allows us to calculate a p-value for the test.

Foreign Birth versus Nativity as Predictor of "Insanity": Mantel-Haenszel Example

Confounding effects are a central focus of an article reexamining the conclusions drawn by Edward Jarvis in *Insanity and Idiocy in Massachusetts 1855* (republished in 1971; Vander Stoep and Link 1998). In his landmark report, Jarvis identified all "insane" and "feeble-minded" persons living in Massachusetts. Note that the data reported are prevalence data.

In the recent article, the authors summarized the Jarvis data for "nativity" (i.e., place of birth) and insanity, as shown in table 25.2. The unadjusted OR estimated from these data is 1.2119, with 95 percent confidence interval extending from 1.1077 to 1.3259, suggesting an increased odds of insanity among foreign-born compared to native-born Massachusetts residents. It is important, however, to consider the potential influence of social class on these findings, since social class appears to be associated with both insanity and foreign birth in this population.

Table 25.2 Unstratified Data from the Jarvis Report

	Insane	Not Insane	Row Totals
Foreign born	625	229,375	230,000
Native born	2,007	892,669	894,676
Column totals	2,632	1,122,044	1,124,676

Table 25.3 Data from the Jarvis Report, Stratified on Social Class

	Stratum 1: Pauper Class		Stratum 2: Independent Class	
	Insane	Not Insane	Insane	Not Insane
Foreign born	581	9,090	44	220,285
Native born	941	12,513	1,066	880,156

To evaluate the influence of social class on the observed association between nativity and mental illness, we first stratify our sample according to a dichotomization of social class, following Jarvis: pauper class versus independent class. Nativity and insanity are cross-classified within each stratum of social class as appears in table 25.3. The analysis begins with computation of the stratum-specific ORs (and corresponding 95 percent confidence intervals). The estimated OR in the pauper class is 0.84993 (0.7638, 0.9458), and the estimated OR in the independent class is 0.1649 (0.1220, 0.2230). Although the crude analysis found an association between foreign birth and increased risk of insanity, the stratum-specific estimates suggest that the odds of insanity are lower among the foreign born compared with the native born. The difference between the crude analysis and the stratified analysis reflects confounding by social class of the relationship between insanity and nativity, since the crude OR indicates increased risk to foreign-born subjects compared to native-born subjects, whereas stratum-specific ORs reflect decreased risk.

To obtain a summary of the OR, combining evidence across social class strata, we compute the OR_{MH} estimator:

$$\hat{\text{OR}}_{\text{MH}} = \frac{\sum_{i=1}^{k} a_i d_i / t_i}{\sum_{i=1}^{k} b_i c_i / t_i} = \frac{\left[(581)(12,513)/23,125\right] + \left[(44)(880,156)/1,101,551\right]}{\left[(9090)(941)/23,125\right] + \left[(220,285)(1066)/1,101,551\right]}$$

$$= 0.5995,$$

with 95 percent confidence interval (0.5443, 0.6602), using the Robins-Breslow-Greenland standard error estimator.

We note that the estimated common OR, combining information across strata, shows foreign birth in comparison to native birth is protective against risk of severe mental illness, with odds of insanity reduced by almost half. A plausible range of values for the population OR spans from 0.54 to 0.66.

The next step in the analysis might be to formally test the association between nativity and insanity, adjusting for social class. To evaluate the null hypothesis of no association between nativity and insanity, assuming the same effect (i.e., a common OR) across strata (H_0: $OR_{common} = 1$) against the alternative hypothesis that there is an association between nativity and insanity in at least one stratum of social class (H_A: $OR_{common} \neq 1$), we compute the Mantel-Haenszel test statistic:

$$\chi^2_{MH} = \frac{\left(\sum_{i=1}^{k} a_i - \sum_{i=1}^{k} m_{1i} n_{1i}/t_i\right)^2}{\sum_{i=1}^{k} (m_{1i} m_{2i} n_{1i} n_{2i})/(t_i^2(t_i-1))}$$

$$= \frac{\{(581+44) - [(9671)(1522)/23{,}125 + ((220{,}329)(1110)/1{,}101{,}551)]\}^2}{\left[\dfrac{(9671)(13{,}454)(1522)(21{,}603)}{(23{,}125)^2(23{,}125-1)}\right] + \left[\dfrac{(220{,}329)(881{,}222)(1110)(1{,}100{,}441)}{(1{,}101{,}551)^2(1{,}101{,}551-1)}\right]}$$

$$= 104.1956.$$

Foreign Birth versus Nativity as Predictor of "Insanity": Interpretation of Mantel-Haenszel Test

Comparing this statistic $\chi_{MH} = 104.2$ to a chi-squared distribution with one degree of freedom, we find that the p-value is less than .001. Thus, we reject the null hypothesis in favor of the alternative; that is, there appears to be an association between nativity and insanity after adjusting for social class. Unlike the crude analysis, however, the direction of the association indicates a lower risk of insanity (summary $\hat{OR}_{MH} = 0.60$) among residents of Massachusetts who are foreign born as opposed to native born.

Note that the effect of social class in these data cannot be fully characterized as a simple case of confounding alone. Comparing the estimated OR for the pauper class to that for the independent class, we can see that the effect is much stronger in the independent class. In other words, the association between foreign birth and insanity is stronger in the independent class than in the pauper class. This might be construed as effect modification or interaction, as discussed in chapter 27.

Methods of Adjustment for Binary Data: Statistical Modeling

Mantel-Haenszel analysis is useful when one is evaluating a dichotomous (or dichotomized) exposure as a risk factor for a dichotomous outcome. It allows for adjustment for a multilevel categorical confounder. There may be times, however, when we need to adjust for a continuous confounder, or for several confounding variables simultaneously.

In these instances, a more flexible approach is required. Regression modeling is one such approach. In particular, logistic regression analysis is a technique that allows us to evaluate simultaneously the relationship of several exposure variables to a binary response. A further advantage of logistic regression is that it can accommodate continuous exposure variables. Finally, because of the equivalence of the disease OR and the exposure OR described previously, we can use logistic regression to model the odds of disease in cohort or case-control studies.

The Logistic Model Statement

A logistic model specifies that a function of the conditional probability of outcome (e.g., the probability of disease, given a set of exposure or predictor variables) is a linear function of the covariates (where the covariates might comprise the exposure of interest, as well as one or more confounding variables). Let p represent the conditional probability of disease, given a set of j exposure variables denoted by $X_1, X_2, \ldots, X_j$. The logistic model assumes that

$$\text{logit}(p) = \ln \frac{\Pr\left(\text{diseased} \middle| X_1 = x_1, X_2 = x_2, \ldots, X_j = x_j\right)}{\Pr\left(\text{nondiseased} \middle| X_1 = x_1, X_2 = x_2, \ldots, X_j = x_j\right)}$$

$$= \beta_0 + \beta_1 x_1 + \beta_2 x_2 + \ldots + \beta_j x_j.$$

As can be seen in the above equation, the *logit* of probability p is defined as the natural logarithm of the quantity p over one minus p (i.e., the *log odds*). The logit of p is assumed to vary linearly in the covariates X_1 to X_j, with the degree of variation governed by the beta terms (also known as *regression coefficients*).

The logistic model, then, is like the ordinary linear model for continuous data, except for the transformation of the response variable. One reason for the logit transform is to guarantee that the range of values yielded by the model is legitimate. For example, if we tried to model p as a linear function of the covariates,

$$p = \Pr(\text{diseased} \mid X_1 = x_1, X_2 = x_2, \ldots, X_j = x_j)$$
$$= \beta_0^* + \beta_1^* x_1 + \beta_2^* x_2 + \ldots + \beta_j^* x_j,$$

we might find that the model yields values for the estimated p^* that extend beyond the acceptable range; that is, we could estimate probabilities that are smaller than zero and greater than one. To avoid this problem, we transform p, using the logit function. Note that the range of the original probability is zero to one. The first step in the logit transform, taking $[p/(1 - p)]$, changes the range of the outcome variable to extend from zero to positive infinity. When we take the natural log of $[p/(1 - p)]$ in the second step of the transform, the resulting range of the outcome variable extends from negative infinity to positive infinity, eliminating the concern over the range of possible values for the linear predictor term. We can back-transform to obtain a model-based expression for p as follows:

$$p = \frac{\exp(\beta_0 + \beta_1 x_1 + \beta_2 x_2 + \ldots + \beta_j x_j)}{1 + \exp(\beta_0 + \beta_1 x_1 + \beta_2 x_2 + \ldots + \beta_j x_j)},$$

which always gives values for p that lie between zero and one.

Interpretation of the Regression Coefficients from a Logistic Model

Let us consider a logistic model with a single, binary predictor variable, X_1. Suppose that X_1 is coded as 1 for exposed, and 0 for unexposed. According to the model, the logit of the probability of disease for an exposed subject is equal to $\beta_0 + \beta_1$. For an unexposed subject, the logit is β_0. Taking the difference in these two expressions, we find that the logit of the probability of disease for an exposed subject minus that for an unexposed subject is equal to β_1. One of the properties of logarithms is that $\ln(a) - \ln(b) = \ln(a/b)$. Hence, β_1 is equal to the logarithm of the odds of disease for an exposed subject divided by the odds of disease for an unexposed subject. But this is exactly equal to the natural log of the OR, defined earlier. By this argument, then, each X-coefficient in a logistic regression model represents the log of an OR. The OR, then, can be obtained by exponentiating the appropriate regression coefficient (e^{β_j}) for covariate X_j.

For a binary exposure X_j, e^{β_j} represents the ratio of odds of disease for exposed subjects relative to unexposed subjects. For a continuous exposure variable, e^{β_j} represents the ratio of the odds of disease for a subject whose exposure level is one unit higher than another subject's. It follows from the model statement that the OR of disease for a k-unit difference in the continuous covariate is given by $e^{k\beta_j}$.

Note that if β_j, the coefficient for covariate X_j, is equal to zero, it translates to an OR of one, reflecting no association between the response variable and covariate X_j (regardless of whether X_j is categorical or continuous). When $\beta_j > 0$ (corresponding to an OR greater than one), higher levels of X_j are associated with increased risk of disease. When $\beta_j < 0$ (corresponding to an OR less than one), higher levels of X_j are associated with decreased risk of disease.

When we fit a logistic model with several covariates simultaneously, each regression coefficient can be considered "adjusted" for the effect of the other covariates (just as in a stratified analysis). So if we fit a logistic model for SSD as a function of dichotomized maternal body mass index and categorized maternal age, it would be appropriate to interpret the exponentiated regression coefficient for body mass index as the OR for high body mass index versus low body mass index in two women from the same age category.

Fitting Logistic Models

The logistic regression model just defined is a theoretical quantity. In practice, we do not know the true values of the beta terms (or regression coefficients). Instead, we use the data to derive estimates of the regression coefficients. The details behind the model-fitting procedure are beyond the scope of this discussion; we encourage interested readers to consult other sources for this information, including Schlesselman (1982), Fleiss et al. (2003) and Hosmer and Lemeshow (2000). It is sufficient for our purposes to say that we use the data to derive estimated regression coefficients, denoted as $\hat{\beta}_j$, for $j = 0, 1, 2, \ldots, k$ (where k is the number of x-variables in the model). These estimators, in turn, are used to derive estimates for the ORs.

Most computer software packages provide routines for fitting logistic regression models. Included in the typical output from a logistic model are the estimated regression coefficients (interpretable as log ORs), standard errors for the regression coefficients, and corresponding confidence intervals. Estimates and confidence intervals for the ORs can be readily obtained by exponentiating the regression coefficients and the endpoints of the reported confidence intervals. Some packages, including SAS, SPSS, and STATA, can perform the exponentiation and provide the OR estimates and confidence intervals directly. Tests of the statistical significance of each coefficient in the model are also included in the output. In order to assess whether the association between covariate X_j and response (disease) is statistically significant, we can compute the Wald test (or z-score) for that variable's regression coefficient. Remember that a regression coefficient of zero indicates that X_j and disease are independent. In order to formally assess the following hypothesis:

$$H_0: \beta_j = 0 \quad \text{versus} \quad H_A: \beta_j \neq 0,$$

we compute a z-score as $\hat{\beta}_j/\text{SE}(\hat{\beta}_j)$. Under H_0, this statistic follows a standard normal distribution, and we can use standard normal tables in order to generate a p-value. This test is considered crude, or unadjusted, if X_j is the sole predictor variable in the model; otherwise, we consider this test to be adjusted for the effects of the other covariates in the model.

Logistic regression modeling (and model fitting in general) is a complex topic and the appropriate use of these procedures requires far more background and detail than is furnished in this brief introduction. Our purpose has been to introduce readers to these approaches, and to connect them to the underlying logic of the study design. Hosmer and Lemeshow (2000) provide an excellent review of logistic regression modeling, including the theoretical basis for model fitting, techniques for model selection, goodness of fit of the model to the data, and the assessment of resulting effects.

Foreign Birth versus Nativity as Predictor of "Insanity":
Logistic Regression Example

Continuing with our previous example, a comparable assessment of the association between nativity and insanity, controlling for social class, can be achieved with logistic regression. In constructing a logistic model, one must consider three variables, each taking on two values: nativity (one if foreign born; zero if native born), social class (one if independent; zero if pauper), and outcome (one if insane; zero if not insane).

We fit two logistic models to these data: crude and adjusted. In the crude model (model 1), we regress the log odds of insanity on nativity only. In the adjusted model (model 2), we regress the log odds of insanity on nativity and social class.

Model 1 is as follows:

$$\text{logit}(p) = \ln \frac{\Pr\left(\text{insane}\middle| X_1 = \text{nativity}\right)}{\Pr\left(\text{not insane}\middle| X_1 = \text{nativity}\right)} = \beta_0 + \beta_1 X_1.$$

Table 25.4 Logistic Regression Analysis of the Jarvis Data

Model Covariates	Model 1		Model 2	
	Estimated Regression Coefficient (95% CI)	Estimated Odds Ratio (95% CI)	Estimated Regression Coefficient (95% CI)	Estimated Odds Ratio (95% CI)
Nativity	$\hat{\beta}_1 = 0.1922$ (0.1023, 0.2821)	$\exp(\hat{\beta}_1) = 1.2119$ (1.1077, 1.3259)	$\hat{\beta}_1 = -0.4849$ (−0.5787, −.3911)	$\exp(\hat{\beta}_1) = 0.6158$ (0.5606, 0.6763)
Social class			$\hat{\beta}_2 = 4.3449$ (4.2644, 4.4254)	$\exp(\hat{\beta}_2) = 77.082$ (71.120, 83.543)

Note: CI = confidence interval.

Model 2 is as follows:

$$\text{logit}(p) = \ln\frac{\Pr(\text{insane}\,|\,X_1 = \text{nativity}, X_2 = \text{social class})}{\Pr(\text{not insane}\,|\,X_1 = \text{nativity}, X_2 = \text{social class})} = \beta_0^* + \beta_1^* X_1 + \beta_2^* X_2.$$

The table 25.4 gives the estimated regression coefficients and ORs from two logistic models.

Foreign Birth versus Nativity as Predictor of "Insanity": Interpretation of Logistic Regression Models

In model 1, the logistic results are identical to those from the crude fourfold table analysis in our first example in this chapter. The unadjusted OR for nativity from both methods is approximately equal to 1.2, indicating an increase of 20 percent in the odds of insanity among foreign-born, as opposed to native, residents. The z-score for testing the statistical significance of the nativity effect is 4.19, with $p < .001$. The unadjusted model, therefore, indicates a statistically significant increase in the odds of insanity among foreign-born residents.

Model 2 adjusts for the effects of social class. The logistic results are closely comparable to those obtained from our Mantel-Haenszel analysis. The Mantel-Haenszel-adjusted estimate of the OR for nativity was 0.60, with 95 percent confidence limits of 0.54 to 0.66. The corresponding adjusted estimate from the logistic model is 0.62, with 95 percent confidence interval extending from 0.56 to 0.68. The z-score for nativity, controlling for social class, is −10.13, with $p < .001$. These analyses consistently demonstrate a reduction in risk of insanity among foreign-born residents of Massachusetts, after control for confounding by social class.

As noted earlier in our first example, we will see in chapter 27 that it may not be appropriate to characterize the effect of social class on the association between nativity and insanity as a simple case of confounding. Social class may in fact act as an effect modifier of the relationship between nativity and insanity.

Methods of Analysis for Matched Binary Data

Any statistical analysis plan must be appropriate to the design of the study. For instance, we have already discussed how study design governs which measures of association may be estimated under different sampling designs. This same principle applies when one is analyzing data from a matched study.

For simplicity, let us assume that we have collected data under a pair-matched design in which each case (or exposed) subject is matched on a number of potentially confounding factors with a corresponding control (or unexposed) subject. The similarity between matched subjects translates, typically, to positive correlation on the outcome measurement (say, exposure in a case-control study or disease in a cohort study). Simply put, two subjects from the same matched pair will tend to respond in a more similar way than two subjects from different matched pairs. This correlation influences the estimation of variability of the measure of association (e.g., the OR). If we fail to account for the correlation among matched subjects, our estimate of the standard error of the OR estimator will be incorrect. Biased standard errors result in invalid confidence intervals (i.e., confidence intervals will not have the specified coverage probability) and invalid test statistics (i.e., type I error rates will differ from the nominal level). On the other hand, if we employ analytic methods that respect the matched design, then we obtain valid inferences and avoid misleading results. Selected methods for analyzing matched data are described next.

McNemar's Methods for Pair-Matched Data

The best way to think about pair-matched data is to remember that different pairs are independent, while the individual members of a single pair are not. A valid way to analyze the data, then, is at the level of the pair. Suppose, using the example of the PDSE, that we have data from a matched case-control study of prenatal (first-trimester) exposure to influenza infection as a risk factor for SSD. Cases and controls are pair-matched on date of birth (+/− one month), gender, number of prenatal blood draws (an indicator of level of prenatal care), and duration of follow-up. We then record, for each individual, whether or not the mother experienced influenza infection during the first trimester of pregnancy. If we simply record the exposed proportions separately for cases and controls, then the matching is lost. We cannot reconnect the case and control members of each pair. Instead, we should record the outcome for each pair of individuals. We record the number of pairs for which both subjects were exposed (a), the number of pairs for which neither subject was exposed (d), the number of pairs for which the case was exposed but the control was not (b), and the number of pairs for which the control was exposed but the case was not (c), as in table 25.5.

Table 25.5 represents the typical presentation of pair-matched data with a binary response. In the table, t represents not the number of *individuals* under study, but the number of *pairs* under study. It follows that the number of individuals is $2t$. Because this format is so different from the typical format

Table 25.5 Conventional Display for Matched Case-Control Data

Case	Control		
	Exposed	**Unexposed**	
Exposed	a	b	
Unexposed	c	d	
			t

for a 2×2 table, we cannot apply the methods described earlier in this chapter for dichotomous data. Instead, we apply the methods proposed by Quinn McNemar (1947) for paired data.

The McNemar methods provide a way to estimate the OR relating exposure to outcome, using paired data. If the data are summarized in the matched-pair format just delineated, then the McNemar OR, $\hat{OR}_{Mc}$, is estimated as b/c. We can calculate a standard error for the log OR estimator as $\sqrt{(1/b)+(1/c)}$. Using the fact that the logarithm of the OR estimator is approximately normally distributed, we compute a 95 percent confidence interval for the OR by calculating a confidence interval for the log OR and exponentiating the endpoints, or by taking $\{\hat{OR}_{Mc} \exp(\pm 1.96 SE[\ln(\hat{OR}_{Mc})])\}$. Like any other OR, the McNemar OR can be interpreted as the odds of disease in the exposed divided by the odds of disease in the unexposed, regardless of study design, because of the equivalence of the disease OR and the exposure OR.

In addition to giving a method for estimating the OR and corresponding 95 percent confidence interval, McNemar also provided a test of the statistical significance of the association. The null hypothesis for McNemar's test states that the OR relating exposure to disease is one; the alternative states that the OR differs from one. The test statistic takes the form

$$\chi^2_{MC} = \frac{(b-c)^2}{(b+c)}.$$

Under the null hypothesis of no association between exposure and disease, McNemar's statistic follows a chi-squared distribution on one degree of freedom. Critical values and p-values, then, can be obtained from published tables for the chi-squared distribution.

Head Trauma and Alzheimer's Disease: An Example of McNemar's Test

Consider a matched case-control study on the association between head trauma and Alzheimer's disease as described previously in chapter 16 (Graves et al. 1990). Cases with Alzheimer's disease were ascertained from a geriatric psychiatric clinic and a Veteran's Administration hospital. Because the case participants were cognitively impaired, surrogate informants were identified from whom information on history of head injuries was obtained. Pair-matched controls without evidence of memory loss, of the same sex and approximately the same age as each case, were ascertained from friends of

Table 25.6 Matched Case-Control Data from Graves

Case	Control		
	Exposed **(Head Trauma)**	**Unexposed** **(No Head Trauma)**	
Exposed (head trauma)	3	28	
Unexposed (no head trauma)	8	91	
			130

the case participant or case surrogate. To ensure comparability of information on cases and controls, exposure information on history of head trauma was obtained from surrogates for controls, as well. One hundred thirty pairs of cases and controls with appropriate surrogates were identified.

The raw data are shown in table 25.6.

Using the formula introduced, we estimate the OR relating head trauma to risk of Alzheimer's disease as $\hat{OR} = b/c = 28/8 = 3.5$. The standard error for the natural log of the OR estimator is equal to

$$\text{SE}\left(\ln\left(\hat{OR}\right)\right) = \sqrt{(1/b) + (1/c)} = \sqrt{(1/28) + (1/8)} = 0.4009.$$

Thus, a 95 percent confidence interval for the natural log of the OR can be computed as

$$\ln(\hat{OR}) \pm 1.96\text{SE}(\ln(\hat{OR})) = \ln(3.5) \pm 1.96(0.4009) = (0.4670, 2.0385).$$

It follows that a 95 percent confidence interval for the OR is calculated as $(\exp(0.4670), \exp(2.0385)) = (1.5952, 7.6792)$.

To test the statistical significance of this relationship, we can use the chi-squared procedure proposed by McNemar. The test statistic equals

$$\chi^2_{\text{MC}} = \frac{(b-c)^2}{(b+c)} = \frac{(28-8)^2}{(28+8)} = 11.1111,$$

with a corresponding p-value of .0009 (based on a chi-squared random variable with one degree of freedom).

The matched pairs analysis indicates that the odds of Alzheimer's among victims of head trauma is more than three times higher than the odds when there is no head trauma. From the test statistic, we know that this finding is statistically significant ($p < .001$).

Derivation of McNemar's Methods

There are several ways to derive McNemar's estimator for the OR and the test statistic. Perhaps the most instructive is by way of the Mantel-Haenszel procedures. If we were to allow each matched pair to comprise a single stratum in the Mantel-Haenszel framework, then the resulting Mantel-Haenszel OR and test statistic would be identical to the McNemar OR and test statistic. Both approaches lead to precisely the same formulas.

While this is an interesting observation, it is also a very useful one. Specifically, recognizing the equivalence between the McNemar and Mantel-Haenszel methods for one-to-one matching leads to methods that are appropriate for more general matching (i.e., matching of one case to several controls; or multiple cases to multiple controls, with varying numbers of members per matched set). If we define each stratum as the membership of a single matched set, then we can apply the Mantel-Haenszel formulas to derive estimates of the OR, confidence intervals, and test statistics that both account for the matching and are adjusted for the confounding effects of the matching variables.

More Advanced Methods for Analyzing Matched Binary Data

The simple McNemar methods suffice, in many instances, for the description of association estimated from pair-matched data. There will be times, however, when additional covariate adjustment is desired. For example, in the example of the matched case-control study of maternal influenza and offspring SSD risk, we may wish to control for mother's age, in addition to the matching factors. Although we did not match on maternal age in the design phase of the study, we might still want to adjust for it in the analysis stage. If the data were independent, we could fit a logistic regression model to make the adjustment. Because the data are pair-matched, this approach is inappropriate, because it ignores the correlation between the two members of each pair. One solution to this problem is to use a specialized logistic regression technique, known as *conditional logistic regression*, in order to conduct the adjusted analysis.

The conditional logistic regression model is identical in spirit to the ordinary logistic model, but the estimation routine acknowledges the membership of each matched pair so that the resulting standard errors are corrected for intrapair correlation. Like ordinary logistic regression, conditional logistic regression provides estimates of the relevant ORs, their standard errors, and confidence intervals. Interpretation of these parameters is precisely the same as for the ordinary logistic model. The regression coefficients from the conditional model (like those from the ordinary model) represent log ORs, so that OR estimators may be obtained by exponentiation. Because the regression coefficients are approximately normally distributed, we are able to use the standard approach (estimate plus or minus 1.96 times the standard error) to obtain 95 percent confidence limits. Again, exponentiation of the endpoints of a confidence interval for the log OR gives a valid confidence interval for the OR itself. Similarly, tests of H_0: $\beta_j = 0$ versus H_A: $\beta_j \neq 0$ can be computed as $\hat{\beta}_j / SE(\hat{\beta}_j)$, which follows a standard normal distribution under H_0.

Many statistical software packages can fit conditional logistic models. The only additional information that must be provided is a "set membership" variable that reveals which individuals belong to which matched sets. Hosmer and Lemeshow (2000) provide an excellent introduction to conditional logistic regression analysis.

Applications to More General Clustered Study Designs

In our discussion of analytic methods for matched data, we emphasized the importance of choosing a method of analysis that accounts for the intra-pair correlation induced by the matching process. This concept applies to any study design in which the observations cluster together (i.e., are not sampled independently). For example, we can view data on siblings from different families as a type of "matched" data. Even though we do not assign individuals to their matched sets (i.e., families) in family studies, the members of the set (siblings in the family) are certainly not independent, because they are closely "matched" on a host of measured and unmeasured factors. A valid analysis recognizes the dependence among siblings within a family, just as we must acknowledge the correlation between members in a matched pair. The methods described here (McNemar's approach, the Mantel-Haenszel methods, and conditional logistic regression) may be useful for analyzing other sets of correlated (or clustered) data. A detailed discussion of the topic of correlated data analysis is beyond the scope of this book. The text by Davis (2002) is an excellent source for further reading.

Methods of Adjustment for Binary Data, Based on Subgroup Analysis

If our aim is to evaluate the effect of one exposure on the outcome after removing the influence of another variable, then subgroup analysis seems a natural solution. By separating out different subgroups of subjects (as defined by level of the confounding variable or effect modifier), we can evaluate the effect of the primary exposure of interest on outcome without concern for the effect of the third variable.

There are two problems with this approach. First, in order to be able to subdivide the sample into subgroups and effectively evaluate associations within a subgroup, a very large sample is required. Otherwise, the subgroups are so small they prevent meaningful statistical analysis. Second, the primary benefit of subgroup analysis is its primary drawback: we obtain separate estimates of effect for a number of different subgroups. Although there are occasions on which this is desirable (e.g., when interaction exists; see chapter 27), it is typically undesirable to present a number of different effect estimates as a means of adjustment for confounding when one is summarizing a research study. The primary purpose of a statistical analysis is to take a large number of data points and reduce them to a small number of relevant, informative summary statistics. A multiplicity of reported effect estimates, then, can be a barrier to effective communication of results.

Conclusion

This chapter has introduced a number of approaches for statistical adjustment. When applied to observational psychiatric data, these methods can lead to a better understanding of the interrelationships between exposures of interest, disease outcomes, and the role of potential confounding variables.

In contrast with crude (unadjusted) analyses, adjusted analyses take account of the effects of other variables that may influence the observed association between the primary exposure and outcome of interest. Careful evaluation of confounders can result in more robust inferences, leading to enhanced understanding of disease mechanisms, better therapeutic interventions, and more effective public health prevention strategies.

Confounding is one type of bias that we encounter in analyzing epidemiologic data. The methods discussed in this chapter, such as logistic regression modeling, help us address this problem. Subgroup analysis is another such method of statistical adjustment that helps us understand the influence of other variables on the estimated association between exposure and disease. This approach not only reveals confounding, however, but also enables us to identify interaction among variables of interest. Another potential source of bias is that of unequal attrition over time in follow-up studies. Clearly, duration of follow-up will influence a subject's cumulative risk of developing disease while under observation, with longer follow-up translating to potentially greater risk. Thus, when individuals under study are being followed for differing lengths of time to ascertain disease status, we must take proper account of duration of follow-up in order to make valid inferences. We use survival analytic methods, as described in the next chapter, to evaluate associations using time-to-event data.

References

Agresti A (1996). *An Introduction to Categorical Data Analysis*. New York: Wiley.

Davis C (2002). *Statistical Methods for the Analysis of Repeated Measurements*. New York: Springer-Verlag.

Fleiss JL, Levin B, and Paik MC (2003). *Statistical Methods for Rates and Proportions*. New York: Wiley.

Graves AB, White E, Koepsell TD, Reifler BV, vanBelle G, Larson EB, and Raskind M (1990). The Association between Head Trauma and Alzheimer's Disease. *Am J Epidemiol* 131:491–501.

Hauck, WW (1979). The Large Sample Variance of the Mantel-Haenszel Estimator of a Common Odds Ratio. *Biometrics* 35:817–819.

Hosmer DW and Lemeshow S (2000). *Applied Logistic Regression*, 2nd ed. New York: Wiley.

Jarvis E (1971). *Insanity and Idiocy in Massachusetts: Report of the Commission on Lunacy, 1855*. Cambridge, Mass.: Harvard University Press.

Jewell N (2004). *Statistics for Epidemiology*. New York: Chapman & Hall/CRC.

Mantel N and Haenszel N (1959). Statistical Aspects of the Analysis of Data from Retrospective Studies of Disease. *J. Natl. Cancer Inst.* 22:719–748.

McNemar Q (1947). Note on the Sampling Error of the Difference between Correlated Proportions of Percentages. *Psychometrika* 12:153–157.

Robins J, Breslow N, and Greenland S (1986). Estimators of the Mantel-Haenszel Variance Consistent in Both Sparse Data and Large-Strata Limiting Models. *Biometrics* 42:311–323.

Rothman KJ and Greenland S (1998). *Modern Epidemiology*, 2nd ed. Philadelphia: Lippincott-Raven.

Schlesselman JJ (1982). *Case-Control Studies: Design, Conduct, Analysis*. New York: Oxford University Press.

Vander Stoep A and Link B (1998). Social Class, Ethnicity, and Mental Illness: The Importance of Being More Than Earnest. *Am. J. Public Health* 88:1396–1402.

26 Event Time Analysis

Melissa D. Begg and Michaeline Bresnahan

This chapter describes statistical methods for taking account of **unequal attrition**, that is, different follow-up times across exposed and unexposed groups in a cohort study. As discussed in previous chapters, differences between the exposure groups in the duration of follow-up time can introduce bias into measures of the association between exposure and disease.

For example, suppose we wish to compare disease risk among exposed and unexposed subjects. Suppose, further, that all the subjects in the exposed group are followed for 10 years, whereas the unexposed are followed for only 2 years. Clearly, subjects who are followed longer have a greater risk of developing disease while under observation, regardless of any effect of the exposure. In this way, unequal follow-up time can obscure the relationship between exposure and disease. When these conditions pertain, we can use statistical procedures to try to approximate what the result would have been if follow-up time had been the same across exposure groups. This chapter describes statistical methods for taking account of different follow-up times.

In this chapter we consider methods for analyzing time to an event as an outcome in its own right. Most of the methods of analysis presented up until this point have considered only binary outcomes (e.g., presence or absence of disease). In contrast, this chapter defines the outcome as the *time until disease onset*. From this perspective, a nondiseased subject in our study is not a control as in a case-control study, but someone who has not yet developed disease.

To analyze disease incidence data from this perspective, we rely on methods that come under the interchangeable headings of survival analysis, time-to-event analysis, or failure-time analysis. Although we chose the more common term, survival analysis, in Part III, here we will choose the label event time analysis to underscore the fact that the endpoint of interest is not necessarily death or failure of some kind. It can represent diagnosis of disease, recurrence of symptoms, response to treatment, full remission, or discontinuation of therapy.

Elements of an Event Time Analysis

To conduct an event time analysis, a researcher must specify the following three items:

1. A clearly defined starting point for commencement of follow-up (e.g., birth, first episode of illness, start of treatment, or time of randomization);
2. A clearly defined outcome event (e.g., death, disease onset, or remission of symptoms);
3. A consistent metric for calculating time elapsed from the starting point until the occurrence of the outcome event (e.g., days, weeks, years).

Suppose, for illustrative purposes, that the exposure of interest is binary in nature (say, exposed versus unexposed). Then we might want to compare the average event time in the exposed subjects to that of unexposed subjects. Under the simplest possible study design, we might set out to record event times on a randomly selected group of subjects from the exposed population and another group selected from the unexposed population. We would follow these groups until each and every subject experienced the event of interest. The mean (or median) event time in the exposed group could be compared to the mean (or median) event time in the unexposed group.

There is a serious problem, however, with this design. Often the distribution of event times is heavily skewed to the right, meaning that very large values for the event time can be observed. If our study design dictates that we must follow every last subject until he or she experiences the event, the study may have to continue for an unmanageably long period of time. Compounding this problem is the fact that participants can withdraw or be lost to follow-up before the study's formal conclusion. There may also be losses due to competing risks (e.g., when a participant dies from a disease other than the one being investigated) before the end of the study (see part III).

For these reasons, event time data are rarely fully observed. Rather, we have complete follow-up at the time of analysis on only a proportion of participants (for whom we can record event time explicitly), and partial follow-up for the remainder (for whom we can specify only a lower limit for the true, but unobserved, event time). This partial follow-up is referred to as **censoring** in the statistical literature. The key to successful analysis of event time data is to properly account for both types of information (event times and censoring times).

Note that methods for analyzing event times and censoring times presume that censoring is noninformative, or independent of event occurrence; that is, for an event time analysis to yield a valid result, we must be willing to assume that participant withdrawals and losses to follow-up are unrelated to the risk of the event. If this assumption is wrong, then our estimates will be biased. Because censoring prevents our seeing the actual event times for a proportion of individuals, there is no way to verify this assumption in practice. Critical evaluation of the assumption, therefore, must be based on conjecture and a frank assessment of the potential for informative censoring (i.e., when the risk of censoring is related to the risk of event occurrence).

Appropriate methods for event time data recognize the importance of accommodating differing durations of follow-up. We introduce several such methods.

Basic Features of Event Time Data

A typical time-to-event data set includes a mix of observed event times and censoring times for the subjects under study. We use these data in order to (1) describe the disease incidence or cumulative incidence for a particular group of subjects or cohort; (2) assess whether an exposure can prolong or curtail time until disease onset; and (3) relate a set of subject characteristics to time until disease onset, with a view to obtaining better estimates of prognosis or a better understanding of disease etiology. The standard analysis is framed around the survival distribution, defined as the probability that a subject's event time (T) exceeds some specified value (t), and is denoted by

$$S(t) = \Pr(T > t).$$

Clearly, the survival distribution function is defined only for nonnegative values of t (i.e., there can be no negative survival times). At $t = 0$, the survival probability equals 100 percent, because all subjects begin the study without yet having experienced the event of interest (e.g., they are disease-free at baseline). $S(t)$ decreases over time, with zero being its lowest possible value. Estimation of the **survival curve**, $\hat{S}(t)$, is usually the first step in analyzing event times. The survival curve estimate gives the proportion of subjects who remain event-free at any point in time. Its complement, $1 - \hat{S}(t)$, therefore, is an estimate of the cumulative incidence or risk of the event up to time t.

Describing Disease Onset: Estimating the Survival Curve

A comparison of event incidence (and cumulative incidence) across groups begins by generating an estimate of the survival curve for each group. The most commonly used method for estimating survival curves was proposed by Edward L. Kaplan and Paul Meier (1958). The Kaplan-Meier method dictates dividing follow-up time into a series of contiguous, nonoverlapping intervals, I_j. For each interval, we calculate the number of subjects *at risk* (i.e., still being followed and still event-free) just before the start of the interval (n_j), and the number who fail (or have an event) in the interval (d_j). The probability of surviving beyond the start of the interval conditional on surviving to the start of the interval is then given by

$$\frac{n_j - d_j}{n_j}.$$

The probability of surviving a series of consecutive intervals can then be obtained by simply multiplying the interval-specific conditional survival probabilities. Therefore, the cumulative incidence over a series of consecutive intervals is computed as ($1 -$ cumulative survival probability).

Before the introduction of the Kaplan-Meier estimator, data analysts grappled with the problem of interval selection. Kaplan-Meier provided an innovative solution, defining the intervals in accordance with the observed event times in the sample. Kaplan and Meier were able to show that this approach leads to the maximum likelihood estimator for $S(t)$, which has many desirable statistical properties.

To compute the intervals, one ranks the observed distinct event times from smallest to largest. The intervals are then defined as extending from the jth smallest event time to the $(j+1)$th smallest event time. The estimated survival probability is held fixed from the start of one interval until the start of the next; hence, the Kaplan-Meier survival curve is a step function, with steps extending from one observed event time until the next larger observed event time. Although the value of $\hat{S}(t)$ does not change when a censoring occurs, censored values are not ignored in this calculation. Rather, notice that n_j, the number at risk just before interval j, counts those subjects who have not yet failed and who are not yet censored just before the start of the interval. Since n_j appears in the numerator and denominator of the calculation of the interval-specific survival probability, withdrawals and losses to follow-up impact all subsequent interval-specific survival probabilities. Of course, continuous follow-up of all subjects still at risk in the study is required to implement this analysis.

Most biomedical software programs can produce the Kaplan-Meier estimator. To generate a single Kaplan-Meier curve, the user must provide two pieces of information: a variable with the follow-up times, and an indicator variable that reveals whether the subject was censored (usually coded as zero) or observed to have the event (usually coded as one). These two variables are sufficient for the computer to generate a single curve. Once obtained, the output can be used to estimate survival probabilities at specific follow-up times (e.g., 3 months, one year, or 5 years), as well as the median survival time (time t_{50} such that half the subjects will have experienced the event before t_{50}; half, afterward) or any other survival percentile. If the user wishes to generate separate curves according to the value of another variable (say, exposed versus unexposed), then that other categorical variable must also be included in the data set so that the computer can determine group membership and generate the group-specific Kaplan-Meier estimators.

Psychosocial Intervention and Cancer Recurrence: An Example of the Kaplan-Meier Method

Consider a study examining the influence on cancer recurrence and survival of a 6-week psychosocial intervention (structured group meetings focused on health education, stress management, coping skills enhancement, and psychological support) among melanoma patients (Fawzy et al. 2003). The investigators followed patients with stage I malignant melanoma from time of surgery until recurrence, death, or study drop out, up to a maximum of 10 years. Thirty-four participants were randomized to the psychosocial intervention (exposed), and 34 participants were randomized to control or no intervention (unexposed). For the purposes of this example, we focus only on time from surgery until death, recorded in months.

The investigators report that 11 of the 34 exposed patients (32 percent) and 9 of the 34 exposed patients (26 percent) died over the 10-year follow-up

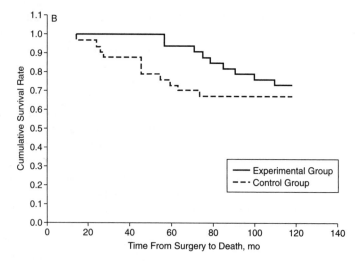

Figure 26.1 Survival probability for patients with malignant melanoma after psychosocial intervention versus control. Copyright © 2003, American Medical Association. All rights reserved.

period. From this information alone, it does not appear that the intervention had a substantial effect on survival. This analysis, however, fails to account for duration of follow-up, which can have a substantial impact on the findings.

The event-time analysis begins by estimating survival (or one minus the cumulative incidence) probabilities over the course of follow-up (i.e., from zero to 120 months), using the Kaplan-Meier method. For comparison of survival across the two exposure groups, two separate survival curves can be produced, and corresponding parameters (e.g., median survival or one-year survival) can be contrasted (see figure 26.1). We see that the estimated survival probability in the experimental group consistently exceeds that in the control group throughout the 10-year follow-up period.

Comparing Survival by Exposure Status: The Logrank Statistic

Chapter 23 described several significance tests for assessing whether an observed difference between exposure groups is likely due to chance, or due to another explanation (e.g., a true causal relationship). While the chi-squared test can be used to assess the equivalence of two proportions, the logrank test can be used to assess the equivalence of two survival curves. The logrank test moves beyond comparing simple proportions in order to account for differing follow-up times among exposed and unexposed study participants.

The logrank statistic achieves this goal by making comparisons only among subjects who have been followed for equal periods of time. To see this, suppose that we want to compare two groups: exposed and unexposed. Like the Kaplan-Meier estimator, the logrank procedure takes advantage of the

Table 26.1 Table Format for Interval i, Used in Calculating the Logrank Statistic

Interval i	Developed Disease	Did Not Develop Disease	Row Totals
Exposed	a_i	b_i	m_{1i}
Unexposed	c_i	d_i	m_{2i}
Column totals	n_{1i}	n_{2i}	t_i

observed event times in both groups in order to define a series of contiguous, nonoverlapping follow-up intervals for analysis. Just before the start of each interval, we enumerate the individuals still under study and at risk of disease. We create a 2×2 table for each interval, cross-classifying exposure status by disease onset, as indicated in table 26.1.

Within each table, we can then compare the exposure status for the (one or more) individuals who develop disease at the start of the interval to those individuals who are still under observation and disease-free throughout that interval. In order to combine information across all the observed event times (i.e., across all the tables), we can use the formulas for the Mantel-Haenszel test (see chapter 25). The formula for the logrank statistic is as follows:

$$\chi^2_{LR} = \frac{\sum_{i=1}^{k}(a_i - (m_{1i}n_{1i}/t_i))^2}{\sum_{i=1}^{k}(m_{1i}m_{2i}n_{1i}n_{2i})/(t_i^2(t_i - 1))}.$$

The null hypothesis for the logrank statistic asserts that the survival distribution in the exposed group is equal to the survival distribution in the unexposed group. Under the alternative hypothesis, the survival distributions differ. When the null hypothesis is true, the distribution of χ^2_{LR} is chi-squared with one degree of freedom. This information allows us to calculate a p-value for the test.

Psychosocial Intervention and Cancer Recurrence: An Example of the Logrank Statistic

Again consider the study of a psychosocial intervention among melanoma patients (Fawzy et al. 2003). From the curves in figure 26.1, we see that the survival probability in the experimental group consistently exceeds survival in the control group throughout the whole follow-up period. To assess whether this difference is statistically significant, the authors computed the logrank statistic. This statistic evaluates the null hypothesis that survival in the intervention and control groups are equal throughout the entire follow-up period against the alternative that survival in the intervention and control groups differ. For these data, the investigators found that the difference was not statistically significant ($p = .39$ by the logrank test).

Note that the general form of the logrank procedure allows for comparison of more than two exposure groups. In this case, the degrees of freedom for the test statistic are equal to the number of exposure levels minus one. Formulas for the more general case are omitted here, but an excellent review of this procedure can be found in Collett (1994).

The Kaplan-Meier estimator and the logrank test allow us to compare the time to disease onset across two or more groups of subjects. More complex methods are required if we wish to evaluate the influence of several variables at once on the distribution of event times; these methods are described next.

Adjusting for Multiple Covariates: The Proportional Hazards Model

Proportional hazards regression is a technique for assessing the impact of a number of categorical and continuous predictor variables on event times. Like the Kaplan-Meier and logrank methods, proportional hazards regression analysis defines the follow-up intervals according to the observed event times in the sample. Just before the start of each interval, we enumerate the individuals who are still under study and disease-free. The constellation of exposure variables for the individuals experiencing the event is compared to the average exposure variables for all individuals still event-free and at risk just before the event occurs. In this way, we compare only those individuals who have survived for equal periods of time, thus removing any bias introduced by unequal durations of follow-up.

The proportional hazards model is built around the hazard rate or incidence rate, denoted by $h(t)$, which represents each individual's instantaneous risk of event onset at any time t over the course of follow-up. Note that the hazard rate can be derived from the survival function, $S(t)$, and vice-versa. The parameters from a proportional hazards model can be evaluated as comparisons of hazard rates from different exposure groups.

Under the proportional hazards model, the hazard rate for a subject with a specific set of covariate values is expressed as

$$h(t \mid X_{1i} = x_{1i}, X_{2i} = x_{2i}, \ldots, X_{pi} = x_{pi}) = h_0(t)\exp(\beta_1 x_{1i} + \beta_2 x_{2i} + \ldots + \beta_p x_{pi}),$$

where $h_0(t)$ represents the (perhaps hypothetical) event hazard rate for a subject whose covariate values are all equal to zero. A parametric-style analysis would specify a particular distribution for the event time distribution and would fill in its formula for $h(t)$ in the expression. However, there are many plausible choices for event time distribution functions, and it is often difficult to ascertain which distribution is most appropriate for the data in hand. The preferred route is to conduct a semiparametric analysis, in which we leave the hazard function unspecified, and focus exclusively on the estimation of the beta parameters (regression coefficients). Cox (1972, 1975) gives the rationale and procedure for doing so, establishing the enormously useful and popular proportional hazards regression methods used in epidemiology, medicine, and other disciplines.

In order to compare event rates in individuals with different covariate values, we take the ratio of two hazard rates as specified in the model. For example, suppose there is only one predictor, exposure, defined as one if the subject is exposed and zero otherwise. Then the hazard rate for an exposed subject takes the form

$$h(t \mid X_{1i} = 1) = h_0(t)\exp[\beta_1 \times 1] = h_0(t)\exp(\beta_1),$$

while the hazard rate for an unexposed subject is equal to

$$h(t \mid X_{1i} = 0) = h_0(t)\exp[\beta_1 \times 0] = h_0(t).$$

The ratio of these two hazards, then, reduces to $\exp(\beta_1)$. The form of the model guarantees the cancellation of the $h_0(t)$ term, thereby allowing us the flexibility to avoid a fully parametric analysis. The hazard ratio, or incidence rate ratio, compares the event rate among exposed subjects to that among unexposed subjects. Its range is from zero to positive infinity. If $\exp(\beta_1)$ is greater than one, then the rate of, say, disease onset is greater among exposed subjects. If $\exp(\beta_1)$ is less than one, then exposure reduces the rate of disease onset. The ratio is precisely equal to one when the event rates in the exposed and unexposed groups are identical.

Note that the formulation of the model demands that the ratio of hazard functions for, say, exposed and unexposed subjects is the same over the entire follow-up period. This is not equivalent to saying that the hazard (or incidence) rates are constant over time; rather, the model assumes that the ratio of incidence rates is constant over time. This assumption, naturally, may not be met in a given data set. If the true incidence rate ratio varies over time, the summary hazard ratio from a proportional hazards model may or may not represent a reasonable approximation to the degree of association between exposure and event onset (much as the Mantel-Haenszel summary odds ratio may not adequately describe the relationship between a binary exposure and disease when interaction is present, as discussed in chapters 25 and 27). For a thorough discussion of the implications of the failure of the proportional hazards assumption, and a review of methods for evaluating it, see Kalbfleisch and Prentice (1980), Hosmer and Lemeshow (1999), and Collett (1994).

The proportional hazards model can also be used to evaluate the influence of a continuous predictor variable on event time. Suppose that X_{1i} represents age in years at the start of follow-up. Then $\exp(\beta_1)$ can be interpreted as the hazard ratio comparing the event rate in a subject who is $(s + 1)$ years old to that in a subject whose age is s at baseline. As for binary exposure variables, this incidence rate ratio is assumed to remain constant throughout the entire period of follow-up. Depending on the scale of the continuous measurement, we may wish to estimate the hazard ratio for a larger (or smaller) difference in the covariate value. For example, the hazard ratio corresponding to a 10-year age difference would be represented by $\exp(10\beta_1)$.

When the proportional hazards model includes more than one predictor variable, then each regression coefficient may be interpreted as adjusted for the levels of the other covariates. For example, suppose we wish to evaluate the effect of maternal prepregnancy body mass index on the rate of development of schizophrenia spectrum disorders (SSD), using data from the Prenatal Determinants of Schizophrenia Example. Body mass index is coded as *low*, *normal*, *high*, or *very high*. We want to control for mother's age (in years) at the time of the birth, because it may confound the relationship between maternal body mass index and offspring SSD risk. If we fit a model with both predictor variables, then the estimated hazard ratio for each body mass index category (relative to the referent group) can be interpreted as the estimated effect of body mass index for two children whose mothers were of the same age (but different body mass index categories), thus reducing potential confounding due to maternal age. At the same time, of course, by using an event time analysis we have also removed potential bias due to differences in duration of follow-up.

Most statistical software programs provide routines for fitting a proportional hazards model. The user must provide a variable containing the follow-up times, an indicator variable for event/censored, and the variable, or variables, containing the predictor information. The output from a proportional hazards model provides the estimated regression coefficients ($\hat{\beta}_1, \hat{\beta}_2, \ldots,$ $\hat{\beta}_p$), their corresponding standard errors, and 95 percent confidence intervals. Note that the regression coefficients are interpretable as log hazard ratios. The point estimates (and corresponding confidence interval limits) must be exponentiated to obtain estimates of the hazard ratios. Some packages perform the exponentiation automatically or offer it as an option in the model statement.

Finally, observe that a hypothesized coefficient value of zero indicates no association between the corresponding predictor variable and time to disease. Consequently, the effect of an individual predictor variable can be tested by our computing the ratio of its estimated regression coefficient to its standard error. Using results from the theory of statistical inference, we can then generate a p-value by comparing the value of this statistic to tables for the standard normal distribution.

Psychosocial Intervention and Cancer Recurrence: An Example of Proportional Hazards Regression

Proportional hazards regression analysis was used to compare the exposed and unexposed groups in the already described study of melanoma recurrence and psychosocial intervention (Fawzy et al. 2003). Because prognosis of melanoma is known to vary with certain patient and disease characteristics, the investigators chose to conduct an adjusted analysis using proportional hazards regression. Although randomization helps protect against covariate imbalance, it does not guarantee that the intervention and control groups will be comparable on all other factors, especially in a relatively small sample. To control for potential confounding of the association between intervention and survival, the investigators fit a model for time until death as a function of treatment assignment, sex of the patient, and Breslow depth (a characteristic of the tumor).

Table 26.2 shows selected output from the proportional hazards model. The point estimate for the hazards ratio for treatment is approximately 0.35 with 95 percent confidence interval (0.12, 0.99). We interpret this result to mean that the rate of death from melanoma is only 35 percent as great among intervention patients as among control patients, adjusted for sex and Breslow

Table 26.2 Output from a Proportional Hazards Regression Model for Time until Death as a Function of Intervention Group, Sex, and Breslow Depth

Covariate	Estimated Regression Coefficient (95% CI)	Estimated Hazard Ratio (95% CI)	z-Score	p-Value
Intervention (1 if treated; 0 if control)	−1.055 (−2.102, −0.008)	0.348 (0.122, 0.992)	−1.976	.048
Breslow depth (1 if >1.5 mm; 0 otherwise)	0.852 (0.458, 1.246)	2.344 (1.581, 3.476)	4.239	<.001
Sex (1 if male; 0 if female)	1.955 (0.703, 3.207)	7.064 (2.019, 24.72)	3.059	.002

depth. This reduction in the death rate associated with treatment is statistically significant ($p = .048$) when we control for Breslow depth and sex. Recall that the difference in death rates was not significant in the unadjusted analysis. In this instance, it would probably be prudent to do some further analysis (perhaps separately in men and women, or separately by Breslow depth) to further understand the confounding influences of these other characteristics on the relationship between treatment and death.

Conclusion

A complete event time analysis will comprise multiple components, including Kaplan-Meier curves, logrank statistics, adjusted and unadjusted estimates of rate ratios and their confidence intervals, and adjusted tests of statistical significance from proportional hazards regression models. Each component delivers valuable and complementary information to allow the researcher to make the best use of the available data. The Kaplan-Meier estimator describes the distribution of survival times across exposure groups. The logrank statistic provides a way to assess statistical significance of a difference in survival curves. Estimated rate ratios and confidence intervals from the proportional hazards model describe the magnitude of association between exposure and disease incidence, before and after adjustment for potential confounders. And the results of the regression model test procedures reveal the statistical significance for the observed associations when controlled for one or more confounding variables. These methods can prove most useful when one is trying to identify risk factors for the onset of mental illness.

This chapter has provided a brief introduction to the concepts and methods for event time analysis. For further reading, there are many good sources. Altman (1991) gives a simple, one-chapter introduction to survival analysis that is more complete than that offered here. The textbooks by Collett (1994) and Hosmer and Lemeshow (1999) give a much more complete introduction with an emphasis on applications. Cox and Oakes (1984) and Kalbfleisch and Prentice (1980) give detailed, theoretical discussions of statistical techniques for event time analysis.

References

Altman DG (1991). *Practical Statistics for Medical Research*. London: Chapman & Hall.

Collett D (1994). *Modelling Survival Data in Medical Research*. London: Chapman & Hall.

Cox DR (1972). Regression Models and Life Tables (with Discussion). *J. R. Stat. Soc. Ser. B* 74:187–220.

Cox DR (1975). Partial Likelihood. *Biometrika* 62:269–276.

Cox DR and Oakes D (1984). *Analysis of Survival Data*. London: Chapman & Hall.

Fawzy FI, Canada AL, and Fawzy NW (2003). Malignant Melanoma: Effects of a Brief, Structured Psychiatric Intervention on Survival and Recurrence at 10-year Follow-Up. *Arch. Gen. Psychiatry* 60:100–103.

Hosmer DW and Lemeshow S (1999). *Applied Survival Analysis: Regression Modeling of Time to Event Data*. New York: Wiley.

Kalbfleisch JD and Prentice RL (1980). *The Statistical Analysis of Failure Time Data*. New York: Wiley.

Kaplan EL and Meier P (1958). Nonparametric Estimation from Incomplete Observations. *J. Am. Stat. Assoc.* 53:457–481.

Assessing Heterogeneity of Effects

27

Alfredo Morabia and Michaeline Bresnahan

In chapter 23, we explored one way of isolating the effect of a variable from other exposures associated with the same outcome. We saw how to measure an average effect across strata of one or several confounders. But sometimes an average effect can mask the fact that the effect of the studied variable differs across subgroups of the population. Consider the extreme but plausible situation in which the average effect of a psychotropic medication is null because it mixes a protective effect in half of the population (e.g., men) and a deleterious in the other half (e.g., women). Thus, theoretical considerations or discoveries in the data analysis can lead us to go beyond average effects and investigate whether the association of an exposure with the studied outcome varies according to the level of another variable, that is, whether there is heterogeneity of effect.

Take our ongoing example of the association between maternal prepregnancy body mass index and risk of schizophrenia spectrum disorder (SSD) in the Prenatal Determinants of Schizophrenia Example. In chapter 22, we showed that we could separate the effect of body mass index from that of mother's age by subdividing the subjects under study into multiple strata defined by selected maternal age categories (i.e., 15–25, 26–35, 36–45, and 46+) and then combining the information across strata, using the Mantel-Haenszel procedure. We obtained a single summary estimate of the odds ratio of body mass index and SSD adjusted for mother's age, which estimated the average effect of body mass index on SSD across mother age groups.

Now we can ask a more refined question: does the effect of body mass index vary depending on age? Suppose that the stratum-specific odds ratios (ORs) relating body mass index to schizophrenia risk were computed as OR = 4.5 for mothers aged 15–25, OR = 2.7 for mothers aged 26–35, OR = 1.6 for mothers aged 36–45, and OR = 1.0 for mothers over 45. These results would indicate that the strength of the association between body mass index and schizophrenia changes with mothers's ages. The effect of body mass index would be heterogeneous across mothers' age groups.

The heterogeneity of effect is usually referred to in epidemiology as an **interaction** or **effect modification** between two factors. Factor A is said to interact with factor B in its association with disease D. Alternatively, we can

319

say that factor B *modifies* the effect of factor A on disease D (or A modifies the effect of factor B). Since there are several different measures of effect (e.g., risk differences, risk ratios, and odds ratios), the heterogeneity will always refer to a specific type of effect: heterogeneity of risk differences, heterogeneity of risk ratios, or heterogeneity of odds ratios. We cannot assume that the absence of interaction for one measure of association implies the absence of interaction for the other measures of association. In fact, the reverse is typically closer to the truth. Homogeneity of risk differences almost invariably implies heterogeneity of risk ratios, and, vice-versa, homogeneity of risk ratios almost always implies heterogeneity of risk differences.

The purpose of this chapter is to introduce methods frequently used in epidemiology to assess statistical heterogeneity of effect in the studied sample. As in the case of confounding, the main analytic methods include stratification and statistical modeling. We first define additive and multiplicative interaction. Then we describe methods based on stratification: comparing homogeneity across strata of the effect modifier, comparing the expected and observed joint effect of two factors, or using graphical representation of interaction. We also briefly indicate methods that allow us to test the statistical significance of apparently heterogeneous effects. Finally, we introduce statistical modeling of interaction by logistic regression. We defer the discussion of interaction from a conceptual standpoint to part VIII of this book.

Additive versus Multiplicative Interaction

As noted, there are two types of statistical interaction, depending on the effect that is estimated. Effect modification of the risk difference (absolute effect) corresponds with additive interaction. Effect modification of the risk ratio or odds ratio (relative effect) corresponds with multiplicative interaction.

Additive Interaction

The risk difference (RD) is the excess of risk in those exposed to the cause under study, compared to the risk in the unexposed: $RD = Risk_{exposed} - Risk_{unexposed}$. Suppose that we conducted a cohort study and used the RD to measure the association of two factors, A and B, with the outcome of interest. A and B are noninteracting if the risk difference for those exposed to both A and B ($RD_{a,b}$, using as reference the risk in those exposed to neither A nor B, $R_{-,-}$) is the sum of the risk difference for those exposed to A in the absence of B ($RD_{a,-} = R_{a,-} - R_{-,-}$), and the risk difference for those exposed to B in the absence of A ($RD_{-,b} = R_{-,b} - R_{-,-}$). In this instance, $RD_{a,b} = RD_{a,-} + RD_{-,b}$.

In contrast, there is additive interaction between A and B when the observed risk difference for those exposed to both A and B, the joint risk difference, does not equal the sum of the individual risk differences for A and B: $RD_{a,b} \neq RD_{a,-} + RD_{-,b}$. The joint risk difference can be greater than the sum of the individual risk differences ($RD_{a,b} > RD_{a,-} + RD_{-,b}$). This situation is commonly referred to in the epidemiologic literature as additive synergy (and sometimes as positive additive interaction). The joint risk difference can also be smaller than the sum of the individual risk differences ($RD_{a,b} < RD_{a,-} + RD_{-,b}$), which is referred to as additive antagonism (or negative additive interaction).

Multiplicative Interaction

Using the risk ratio (RR) as our measure of association implies that the risk in the exposed is a multiple of that in the unexposed: $Risk_{exposed} = Risk_{unexposed} \times RR$. The same multiplicative relation applies to the joint effect of two factors. If A and B are noninteracting, their joint effect should be the simple product of their individual effects. The RR for A and B ($RR_{a,b}$; relative to the risk in those exposed to neither A nor B, $R_{-,-}$) will be the product of the individual RR of A in the absence of B ($RR_{a,-} = R_{a,-} \div R_{-,-}$) and the individual RR of B in the absence of A ($RR_{-,b} = R_{-,b} \div R_{-,-}$). In this instance, $RR_{a,b} = RR_{a,-} \times RR_{-,b}$.

There is multiplicative interaction between A and B when the RR for those exposed to both A and B, the joint RR, differs from the product of the individual RR for A and B: $RR_{a,b} \neq RR_{a,-} \times RR_{-,b}$. The joint RR can be greater than the product of the individual risk ratios ($RR_{a,b} > RR_{a,-} \times RR_{-,b}$). This situation is commonly referred to in the epidemiologic literature as **multiplicative synergy** (and sometimes as positive multiplicative interaction). The joint RR can also be smaller than the product of the individual RRs ($RR_{a,b} < RR_{a,-} \times RR_{-,b}$), which is referred to as **multiplicative antagonism** (or negative multiplicative interaction). For simplicity, in this chapter we adhere to this common terminology and defer to part VIII a discussion of what terminology might be most meaningful and appropriate.

Assessment of Interaction for Binary Data

We will now describe several techniques to assess interaction between two factors and an outcome. They are all equivalent and simply different approaches to assessing heterogeneity of the risk differences and risk ratios just described.

To illustrate these techniques, we will use an example adapted from a report based on the Dunedin study, a birth cohort described in chapter 9. This report investigated the interaction between a functional polymorphism in the promoter region of the serotonin transporter (5-HTT) gene and the number of stressful life events (occurring after the 21st birthday and before the 26th birthday) on the occurrence of past-year depression at age 26 (Caspi et al. 2003). Table 27.1 presents the data, using a typical $2 \times 2 \times 2$ tabulation allowing for the assessment of interaction.[1]

---

[1] Note that for ease of discussion we limit the comparison to four or more stressful life events versus no stressful life events. The original article includes comparisons to one, two, and three stressful life events, as well.

Table 27.1 Risk of Past-Year Depression at Age 26 According to Genotype and Stressful Life Events

Short Allele[a] (*G*)	Life Events[b] (*E*)	Risk[c] (*R*) Stratum	Risk (%)
No (−)	No (−)	$R_{-,-}$	10
No (−)	Yes (*E*)	$R_{-,E}$	17
Yes (*G*)	No (−)	$R_{G,-}$	10
Yes (*G*)	Yes (*E*)	$R_{G,E}$	33

[a] Short allele of the *5-HTT* promoter polymorphism.
[b] Four or more stressful life events between the ages of 21 and 26 versus no stressful life events.
[c] Risk of past-year depression at age 26.
Source: Adapted from Caspi et al. (2003).

Table 27.2 Information Needed to Assess Interaction by Comparing the Effect of One Factor across Strata of the Other Factor

Factor A	Factor B	Risk	Risk Difference (RD)	Risk Ratio (RR)
No (−)	No (−)	$R_{-,-}$	0 Referent for A absent stratum	1
No (−)	Yes (+)	$R_{-,b}$	$RD_{B[A\ is\ absent]} = R_{-,b} - R_{-,-}$	$RR_{[A\ is\ absent]} = R_{-,b} \div R_{-,-}$
Yes (+)	No (−)	$R_{a,-}$	0 Referent for A present stratum	1
Yes (+)	Yes (+)	$R_{a,b}$	$RD_{B[A\ is\ present]} = R_{a,b} - R_{a,-}$	$RR_{[A\ is\ present]} = R_{a,b} \div R_{a,-}$

Assessing Interaction by Stratification

Stratification is a very intuitive way of assessing interaction, because it directly indicates whether the effect of factor A across strata or levels of factor B is homogeneous or not. In the presence of interaction, the effect of A will differ across strata of B.

Let us apply this form of analysis to our working example. Table 27.2 shows the results of a stratification of effects (RD and RR for factor B).

Let us look for effect modification by presence of the short allele (G) on the association between stressful life events (E) and risk of depression. In our working example, we have heterogeneous RDs for life events: $RD_{G\ is\ absent} = 0.17 - 0.10 = 0.07$, and $RD_{G\ is\ present} = 0.33 - 0.10 = 0.23$; and heterogeneous RRs: $RR_{G\ is\ absent} = 0.17 \div 0.10 = 1.7$, and $RR_{G\ is\ present} = 0.33 \div 0.10 = 3.3$. Both the RD and the RR are heterogeneous: for both measures of association, the effect of E when G is present is larger than the effect of E when G is absent.

The interaction is said to be **quantitative (or ordinal)** when the stratum-specific effect differs by magnitude but not by direction, as in our example, in which stressful events increase the risk of major depression in both genotypic groups, but to a greater degree among the short-allele carriers. There are situations, however, in which the heterogeneity is **qualitative (or disordinal)**; that is, the same exposure can be protective in one stratum of the other factor but deleterious in the other.

Table 27.3 Steps to Assess Interaction by Comparing the Observed with the Expected Joint Effect of Two Factors on a Given Outcome

Step Number	Correction
1	What is the individual effect of cause A in the absence of exposure to cause B?
2	What is the individual effect of cause B in the absence of exposure to cause A?
3	What is the observed joint effect of A and B?
4	What is the expected joint effect of A and B in the absence of interaction?
5	Is the observed joint effect similar to the expected joint effect in the absence of interaction?

Comparing Expected and Observed Joint Effects

Another way of assessing the heterogeneity of effect is to compare the joint effects of the two factors observed in the data to the joint effect that would be expected if their two effects were noninteracting. Table 27.3 summarizes the five steps comprising this approach.

As stressed already, a key issue in assessing interaction is the selection of the measure of association. If we follow these five steps to analyze the data in table 27.1 to evaluate whether the effects of E and G are simply additive, the appropriate measure of effect is the RD, and we get the following answers: first, $RD_{E,-} = 0.07$; second, $RD_{-,G} = 0$; third, observed $RD_{E,G} = 0.23$; fourth, expected $RD_{E,G} = 0.07 + 0 = 0.07$; and fifth, the observed $RD_{E,G}$ is larger than the expected, suggesting that there is additive interaction.

Now, let us reanalyze the same data to evaluate whether the effects of E and G are multiplicative. Here, we compute the RRs and get the following answers: first, $RR_{E,-} = 1.7$; second, $RR_{-,G} = 1.0$; third, observed $RR_{E,G} = 3.3$; fourth, expected $RR_{E,G} = 1.7 \times 1.0 = 1.7$; and fifth, the observed $RR_{E,G}$ is larger than the expected, indicating multiplicative interaction.

Note that the assessment of interaction with this approach can also be applied to case-control study data. For additive interaction, we substitute the excess OR: OR -1.0, for the RD.[2] For multiplicative interaction we simply substitute OR for the RR. It should be noted that these substitutions are reasonable only when the OR is a close approximation of the RR. This will occur if the outcome is rare; if the controls have been sampled from the base, as in a case-base case-control study; or if the controls have been sampled concurrently to case occurrence (see chapter 18). When the OR is not a close approximation of the RR, the overestimation of the RR will differ across strata of the effect modifier. The biased, heterogeneous ORs may give the impression that there is multiplicative interaction when in reality there is none. This circumstance in which ORs are heterogeneous but

[2] This can be seen by simply dividing each component of the risk difference by the risk in the referent group. For example, the risk difference for the G group is $R_{G,-} - R_{-,-}$. Dividing each component by $R_{-,-}$ we get $R_{G,-}/R_{-,-} - R_{-,-}/R_{-,-} = RR_{G,-} - 1$.

underlying RRs are not has been referred to as the *interaction fallacy* (Morabia et al. 1997).

Graphical Assessment of Interaction

The heterogeneity of effect can also be depicted graphically, as in figure 27.1. Values of factor A are on the *x*-axis; risk is on the *y*-axis. Two lines are drawn on the graph. The first depicts the relation of the first exposure (here, number of stressful life events) and the outcome (risk of depression) in the absence of the second exposure (the short allele of the *5-HTT* gene). The second line depicts the relation of the first exposure (here, number of stressful life events) and the outcome (risk of depression) in the *presence* of the second exposure (here, the short allele of the *5-HTT* gene).

There is interaction whenever the two lines are not parallel on the chosen outcome scale, that is, the arithmetic scale for RD and logarithmic scale for RR. Figure 27.1 shows that the two lines are divergent both on the arithmetic and on the logarithmic scale, indicating both additive and multiplicative interactions.

Interaction Magnitude

The magnitude of the interaction can be expressed as the difference of absolute effects or the ratio of relative effects of one factor across strata of a second factor. For example, if the second factor is B, the magnitude of interaction can be expressed as $RD_{B\ present} - RD_{B\ is\ absent}$, or $RR_{B\ is\ present} \div RR_{B\ is\ absent}$, or $OR_{B\ is\ present} \div OR_{B\ is\ absent}$. In our working example, the magnitude of the interaction can be expressed as the extent to which the genotype modifies the effects of stressful life events: $RD_{G\ is\ present} - RD_{G\ is\ absent} = 0.23 - 0.07 = 0.16$,

Arithmetic Scale for Risk Differences

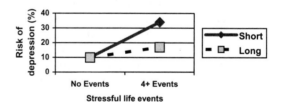

Logarithmic Scale for Relative Risks

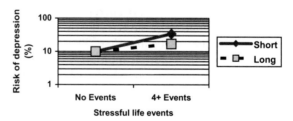

Figure 27.1 Risks associated with no or 4+ stressful events, by short or long allele genotype of the *5-HTT* gene.

or $RR_{G \text{ is present}} \div RR_{G \text{ is absent}} = 3.3 \div 1.7 = 1.9$. As we will see, the magnitude of the interaction can also be quantified by the beta coefficient for the interaction term in a regression model.

The interaction magnitude is a unique expression of the relationship among the three studied factors (e.g., A, B, and Y = outcome). In other words, A modifies the effect of factor B just as much as B modifies the effect of factor A. We have the following equalities:

$$(RD_{B \text{ when A is present}} - RD_{B \text{ when A is absent}}) = (RD_{A \text{ when B is present}} - RD_{A \text{ when B is absent}})$$

and

$$(RR_{B \text{ when A is present}} \div RR_{B \text{ when A is absent}}) = (RR_{A \text{ when B is present}} \div RR_{A \text{ when B is absent}}).$$

In our example, we have

$$(RD_{G \text{ when E is present}} - RD_{G \text{ when E is absent}}) = (RD_{E \text{ when G is present}} - RD_{E \text{ when G is absent}})$$
$$= 0.16$$

and

$$(RR_{G \text{ when E is present}} \div RR_{G \text{ When E is absent}}) = (RR_{E \text{ when G is present}} \div RR_{E \text{ when G is absent}})$$
$$= 1.9.$$

Statistical Tests for Interaction

A thorough review of statistical methods for evaluating interaction is beyond the scope of this brief introduction. See Fleiss et al. (2003), Agresti (1996), Schlesselman (1982), Hosmer and Lemeshow (2000), Rothman and Greenland (1998) and Jewell (2004) for further details.

We will, however, illustrate here some of these techniques. For this purpose, we revisit an example used in chapter 25. This example was based on a report reexamining the conclusions drawn by Edward Jarvis in *Insanity and Idiocy in Massachusetts 1855* (republished in 1971; Vander Stoep and Link 1998). We used Jarvis's data for "nativity" (i.e., place of birth) and "insanity" stratified by social class to estimate ORs, as shown in table 25.3. We saw that the estimated ORs were 0.85 and 0.16, respectively, in the pauper and independent classes. We concluded from our previous analyses that the relationship among social class, nativity, and insanity could not be fully characterized as an instance of confounding, because the estimated ORs were not homogeneous for the pauper and the independent classes. The protective effect of foreign birth against insanity is much stronger in the independent class (0.16) than in the pauper class (0.85).

Test of Homogeneity

Even though the effect of nativity looks stronger in the independent class than in the pauper class, it is useful to formally test whether the two stratum-specific ORs are homogeneous. To evaluate the null hypothesis of homogeneity of the ORs in the two strata of social class (H_0: $O\hat{R}_1 = O\hat{R}_2$) against the alternative hypothesis that the ORs are different (H_A: $O\hat{R}_1 \neq O\hat{R}_2$), we may compute the

Woolf test of homogeneity, using the Mantel-Haenszel summary OR estimator:

$$\chi^2_{\text{woolf}} = \Sigma\, v_i^{-1}\, (\ln \hat{OR}_i - \ln \hat{OR}_{MH})^2 = 111.35,$$

where $\hat{OR}_i$ is the estimated odds ratio in the ith stratum; $\hat{OR}_{MH}$ is the Mantel-Haenszel estimate of the common OR, and v_i is the estimated variance of the natural logarithm of $\hat{OR}_i$ (given by the sum of the reciprocals of the 4 cell-counts in the ith stratum).

Comparing this statistic ($\chi^2_{\text{woolf}} = 111.35$) to a chi-squared distribution with one degree of freedom, we find that the p-value is less than .001. Thus, we reject the null hypothesis in favor of the alternative; that is, there appears to be heterogeneity of the ORs.

In this example, we had sufficient statistical power to reject the null hypothesis of OR homogeneity because the sample size and the interaction magnitude were large. Often we lack statistical power to assess interaction. Note also that the interaction was assessed on a multiplicative scale. However, since the relationship was greater than multiplicative it is also greater than additive (see Part VIII).

Logistic Regression

A comparable assessment of the interaction between nativity and social class can be achieved with the use of logistic regression. In chapter 25 we saw that in the construction of a logistic model there are three variables to consider, each taking on two values: nativity (one if foreign born; zero if native born); social class (one if independent; zero if pauper), and outcome (one if insane; zero if not insane). To test for interaction, we need to add a fourth variable, which is the product of nativity and social class:

$$\text{logit}(p) = \beta_0 + \beta_1 A + \beta_2 B + \gamma AB$$

Table 27.4 explains why the addition of the product of the two variables allows us to test for interaction. Let us reexpress table 27.2, but using the coefficients of the logistic regression model. Remember that the βs represent log odds of the outcome Y.

Table 27.5 gives the estimated regression coefficients and ORs for this logistic model. We will now use the coefficients given in table 27.5 to compute the ORs as in table 27.4. In the model with interaction, the logistic ORs for nativity are $\exp(-0.1625) = 0.85$ and $\exp(-0.1625 + -1.639) = 0.16$ respectively for the pauper and the independent classes. Recall that in the crude $2 \times 2 \times 2$ stratified analysis (table 25.3) the estimated ORs were the same, that is, 0.85 and 0.16 for the pauper and independent classes. Based on the stratified analysis, the estimated magnitude of the interaction is $0.16 \div 0.85 = 0.19$. This is the same as the logistic OR associated with the interaction term $\gamma = 0.1940$. Indeed, a χ^2 test on the coefficient of the interaction term is a formal test of the statistical significance of the multiplicative interaction. In this example it yields a $p < .0001$ (computation not shown). The confidence interval also tells us that the plausible values of the interaction magnitude range between 0.14 and 0.27.

Table 27.4 Information Needed to Compute the Stratum-Specific Odds Ratios on the Basis of the Coefficients of the Logistic Regression Model Involving a Product Term between A and B

Factor A	Factor B	Risk	Terms of the Model that Are not Null	Log Odds Ratio[a]	Odds Ratio[a]
No (−)	No (−)	$R_{-,-}$	β_0	Reference	Reference
No (−)	Yes (+)	$R_{-,b}$	$\beta_0 + \beta_2$	$\log OR_{A \text{ is absent}}$ $= (\beta_0 + \beta_2) - \beta_0$ $= \beta_2$	$\exp(\beta_2)$
Yes (+)	No (−)	$R_{a,-}$	$\beta_0 + \beta_1$	1	Reference
Yes (+)	Yes (+)	$R_{a,b}$	$\beta_0 + \beta_1 + \beta_2 + \gamma$	$\log OR_{A \text{ is present}}$ $= (\beta_0 + \beta_1 + \beta_2$ $+ \gamma) - (\beta_0 + \beta_1)$ $= \beta_2 + \gamma$	$\exp(\beta_2 + \gamma)$

−, means not exposed.
[a] The OR can be obtained by exponentiation of the log OR.

Table 27.5 Logistic Regression Analysis of the Jarvis Data, with Interaction

Model Covariates	Estimated Regression Coefficient (95% CI)	Estimated Odds Ratio (95% CI)
Nativity	$\hat{\beta}_1 = -0.1625$ (−0.2694, −0.05571)	$\exp(\hat{\beta}_1) = 0.8499$ (0.7637, 0.9458)
Social class	$\hat{\beta}_2 = -4.128$ (−4.218, −4.039)	$\exp(\hat{\beta}_2) = 0.0161$ (0.0147, 0.0176)
Interaction	$\hat{\gamma} = -1.639$ (−1.959, −1.319)	$\exp(\hat{\gamma}) = 0.1940$ (0.1409, 0.2671)

Note: CI = confidence interval.

Conclusion

This chapter has introduced common terminology for additive and multiplicative interaction and has described approaches to assessing them. It also briefly has introduced ways of testing the statistical significance of multiplicative interaction. We will revisit the assessment of interaction from a more conceptual perspective in the last part of the book (chapter 33).

It is very tempting to search for heterogeneous effects in a sample, be it on the basis of genetic or social differences, but we caution that it is not a straightforward endeavor. First, in order to achieve adequate statistical power, the sample size for detecting interaction effects usually has to be very large (see Smith and Day 1984). Second, interaction or effect modification observed in the data do not necessarily correspond to some underlying, true *causal* interactions. Spurious heterogeneity of effects may result from errors in the study design or variable measurement.

Nonetheless, the presence of statistical interactions should be interpreted as a warning that a summary effect across all population subgroups may not be sufficiently specific to describe the association under study: the summary or average effect combines subgroup-specific effects across strata of the effect modifier that can be substantially heterogeneous. In these situations, it may be most informative to report results separately for each subgroup. We must remember, however, that what we consider heterogeneity is effect-measure-specific. In chapter 33, we will discuss ways to reconcile our conceptual and statistical ideas about interaction.

References

Agresti A (1996). *An Introduction to Categorical Data Analysis.* New York: Wiley.

Caspi A, Sugden K, Moffitt TE, Taylor A, Craig IW, Harrington H, McClay J, Mill J, Martin J, Braithwaite A, and Poulton R (2003). Influence of Life Stress on Depression: Moderation by a Polymorphism in the *5-HTT* Gene. *Science* 301:386–389.

Fleiss JL, Levin B, and Paik MC (2003). *Statistical Methods for Rates and Proportions.* New York: Wiley.

Hosmer DW and Lemeshow S (2000). *Applied Logistic Regression,* 2nd ed. New York: Wiley.

Jewell N (2004). *Statistics for Epidemiology.* New York: Chapman & Hall/CRC.

Morabia A, Ten Have T, and Landis JR (1997). Interaction Fallacy. *J. Clin. Epidemiol.* 50:809–812

Rothman KJ and Greeland S (1998). *Modern Epidemiology.* Philadelphia: Lippincott-Raven.

Schlesselman JJ (1982). *Case-Control Studies: Design, Conduct, Analysis.* New York: Oxford University Press.

Smith PG and Day NE (1984). The Design of Case-Control Studies: The Influence of Confounding and Interaction Effects. *Int. J. Epidemiol.* 13:356–365.

Vander Stoep A and Link B (1998). Social Class, Ethnicity and Mental Illness: The Importance of Being More Than Earnest. *Am. J. Public Health* 88:1396–1402.

THE SEARCH FOR GENETIC CAUSES OF MENTAL DISORDERS

Integrating Epidemiology with Genetics

28

Mary-Claire King, Habibul Ahsan, and Ezra Susser

At this point in the book, we begin to move beyond the conventional domain of risk factor epidemiology. The study of genetic causes has been given short shrift or entirely omitted from most epidemiology textbooks. As a basic science of public health, however, epidemiology needs to incorporate the full range of determinants of human health. It is increasingly clear that understanding genetic, as well as nongenetic, causes of disease is vitally important to public health research and practice (Merikangas and Risch 2003a). Thus, epidemiologists require a unified logical framework for studying causes, be they environmental or genetic, or some combination of the two.

The search for genetic causes is especially compelling for psychiatric disorders (Plomin et al. 2000; Tsuang and Tohen 2002). Evidence accumulated over the past 50 years demonstrates that genetic causes play a role in many mental disorders. Applying modern tools to identify these genetic causes holds promise for major discoveries (Insel and Collins 2003).

We propose that finding genetic causes of mental disorders will also provide a key to finding nongenetic causes. We would be more likely to detect an environmental cause if we could study the individuals whose genetic makeup renders them vulnerable to its effects. The converse is also true. We would be more likely to find a genetic cause if we could study the individuals who have the environmental exposure required for this genetic vulnerability to lead to a disease. Thus, integrating research on genetic and environmental causes would be mutually beneficial.

The Breakthrough of Genomics

Genetic epidemiology has been defined as "the study of the role of genetic factors and their interaction with environmental factors in the occurrence of disease in human populations" (Khoury et al. 1993, p. 3–4). Although genetic epidemiology is still relatively young (Morton and Chung 1978; King et al. 1984; Beaty and Khoury 2000; Khoury and Little 2000), its growth has been very rapid, and it has already undergone a series of transitions. In this chapter, we provide an overview of these transitions, bearing in mind that the field is still evolving. Readers unfamiliar with the specific designs mentioned here will find them described in the following chapters.

By the time genetic epidemiology emerged, a sophisticated concept of genetic causation had already been developed. Toward the end of the 19th century, Sir Francis Galton, a cousin of Charles Darwin and progenitor of statistical genetics (as well as of eugenics), proposed that hereditary transmission was reflected in quantitative (continuous) traits such as height (Galton 1894; Gillham 2001). Only 30 years before, Gregor Mendel had discovered that in peas hereditary transmission was reflected in qualitative (discontinuous) characteristics such as alternative colors, but his work was unknown to Galton. Upon the rediscovery of Mendel's work in the early 1900s, a debate raged between biometricians such as Karl Pearson, who found evidence for quantitative (continuous) inheritance (Pearson and Lee 1903), and Mendelian geneticists such as William Bateson, who found evidence for qualitative (discontinuous) inheritance (Bateson 1909). Both groups claimed the mantle of Galton. Sir Ronald Fisher resolved the debate by demonstrating that the Mendelian mode of inheritance was compatible with both quantitative and qualitative variation (Fisher 1918; Fisher 1930; Box 1978). Many small, particulate effects could appear in sum as a hereditary quantitative trait such as height. At the same time, a single inherited particulate effect could also appear as a hereditary qualitative trait such as eye color.

By analogy, it was logical that a specific genetic factor could influence the risk of disease in a variety of ways. It could have a small effect on the risk of a disease, as one of many factors that determined a quantifiable liability to disease. Alternatively, it could have a powerful, virtually determinate effect, as a mutation that nearly always produced the disease. Or the influence could be something in between.

Genetic epidemiologists were equipped from the start with these sophisticated concepts of causation. By the 1960s, while it was evident that some diseases were largely attributable to single-gene effects, models for polygenic diseases had also been developed (Falconer 1965; Gottesman and Shields 1967). These multifactorial models generally posited that an individual's liability to disease reflected the contribution of many genetic and nongenetic factors, and that disease occurred when the liability exceeded a threshold.

Still, the inadequacy of tools available for genetic analysis constrained the applications of these models. Investigators collected data on disease in families to study familial aggregation (see chapter 30); studied twins to estimate the genetic contribution to disease (see chapter 31); studied adopted children to separate the contributions of genes and environment (Rosenthal and Kety 1968; Fieve et al. 1975; see also chapter 10); evaluated patterns of genetic transmission in families, using **segregation analysis** (Morton and Chung 1978; Beaty and Khoury 2000; Khoury and Little 2000); and conducted early genetic linkage and association studies on extended kindreds (e.g., Baron et al. 1987). Much was achieved. But until the development of new technology, the identification of disease genes was limited.

The development of increasingly powerful tools for collecting and analyzing genetic data drove the evolution of these research designs. In the 1980s and early 1990s, **genetic linkage studies** became more and more successful. Linkage studies seek to identify genetic markers on chromosomes that cosegregate with a disease within pedigrees in which the disease is transmitted in a Mendelian pattern (see chapter 32). A genetic marker cosegregating with disease provides a clue to the chromosomal location of a causal gene. The power of this approach was vastly increased by new methods for identifying variable DNA sequences that could serve as genetic markers. An early success with Huntington's disease demonstrated the power of the approach (Gusella et al. 1983). Within a short time, genetic linkage was used to map and eventually identify specific genes for hundreds of diseases. These genes were generally "major genes," which are virtually necessary and sufficient for disease. Such genes are amenable to mapping by linkage studies because they fully explain coinheritance of markers with the disease within pedigrees (see chapter 32).

By contrast, with a few notable exceptions (Hall et al. 1990), linkage studies were singularly unsuccessful in finding the genetic causes of common multifactorial diseases. Thus, the historic division between the Mendelian and the biometric perspective resurfaced in somewhat different form in the practice of genetic research (Risch 2000). Scientists rapidly discovered the genetic causes of diseases that are transmitted on a single gene (like the color of Mendel's peas) and therefore segregate in Mendelian fashion within pedigrees (Online Mendelian Inheritance in Man [OMIM]). But they were stymied in the search for genetic causes of **complex diseases** influenced by many small contributions from multiple genetic (and environmental) factors.

Before the turn of the century, however, progress of the human genome project and emerging technology created new possibilities for research on complex diseases. As the sequencing of the human genome progressed, scientists were equipped to rapidly sequence individual genes and their millions of allelic variations. This led to a renaissance of association studies. In **genetic association studies**, cases and controls are compared with respect to the presence or absence of a genetic factor (cohort designs are now also used; see chapter 29). Association studies could be used to examine whether specific genetic alleles—including those with functional consequences that are considered normal—were associated with risk of disease (Risch and Merikangas 1996). This kind of genetic cause can be considered as a genetic risk factor, and questions about the relation of a genetic allele to disease risk can be posed, and answered, within the framework of risk factor epidemiology.

In fact, genomics has opened up a new frontier for the application of risk factor designs. With the completion of the human genome project (International Human Genome Sequencing Consortium 2001), the next challenge is to understand how the now fully sequenced genes, their variations, and the proteins they encode affect disease risk in human populations. In this endeavor, the methods developed by risk factor epidemiology are increasingly useful, even essential.

Identification of a Genetic Risk Factor

Studies today of genetic risk factors are usually directed toward finding genetic causes of complex disorders believed to have multiple genetic, as well as environmental, causes. This places much of current human genetic research squarely within the realm of the risk factor concepts and methods we have described in the earlier parts of the book. Nonetheless, studies of genetic risk factors cannot simply be slotted into the designs developed to investigate environmental risk factors. Unlike environmental risk factors, genes are transmitted from parents to offspring in identifiable and determined patterns. Of course, culture and other environmental factors are also transmitted in families (Feldman and Cavalli-Sforza 1984); the difference is that patterns of cultural transmission are not determined. Epidemiologic risk factor designs require some modification for application to genetic studies. Furthermore, strategies for investigating genetic alleles that originated in human genetics had to be reconceptualized later through the lens of epidemiology (King et al. 1984; Weissman et al. 1986; Susser and Susser 1988).

A distinctive feature of genetic studies is that the identification of a genetic risk factor may logically begin with a family, the genetic equivalent of an epidemiological cluster. A family can be thought of as a kind of natural experiment, illuminating a genetic cause that is otherwise hard to detect (see chapter 10). Although a disease may be complex and heterogeneous in the population as a whole, in some unusual pedigrees a specific genetic cause may be responsible. This may provide a clue to guide subsequent studies in detecting a genetic risk factor of general importance. Presently, the trend is to use linkage, association, and other strategies in conjunction to map and identify causative genes that may have either modest or large effects (see chapter 33).

The discovery of the *APOE4* allele as a risk factor for Alzheimer's disease exemplifies how cases clustered in pedigrees can lead the way to a genetic risk factor. Initially, the researchers sought to find a gene with a very major influence, rather than a modest influence, on Alzheimer's disease. Accordingly, they carried out genetic linkage analysis in a series of pedigrees with familial Alzheimer's disease (Pericak-Vance et al. 1991). Their findings were at first inconclusive and puzzling. They did not find strong evidence for linkage anywhere in the genome, but they did find weak evidence for linkage on chromosome 19. Previous linkage findings had been reported only for early-onset familial Alzheimer's disease, whereas this signal seemed to derive only from the pedigrees with the more common late-onset Alzheimer's disease. Because Alzheimer's disease did not seem to be inherited in a strictly Mendelian fashion in these pedigrees, the investigators had evaluated linkage with use of the **affected pedigree member** (APM) method. This approach is appropriate for complex traits; it includes everyone's genotypes but phenotypes only of the affected relatives (i.e., those with Alzheimer's disease).

These initial findings generated broad interest when, shortly thereafter, the gene coding for apolipoprotein E was located within this region of chromosome 19 (the gene is denoted *APOE*; the encoded protein, ApoE). There was independent evidence that the ApoE protein was associated with senile plaques, a neuropathologic hallmark of Alzheimer's disease (Katzman 1986). These findings stimulated the researchers to examine the association between genetic alleles of *APOE* and Alzheimer's disease (Strittmatter et al. 1993). They found that the allele *APOE4* was more than three times as common among Alzheimer's cases in the pedigrees than in an unrelated control group.

We will return to this example in more detail in the next chapter. For now, we note that the process began with a search for linkage in a family study. Then an initial association study was conducted with cases from the pedigrees. It was motivated by an a priori hypothesis about a genetic allele known to correspond to a functional difference in a protein with a potential role in the disease. Only after this study did researchers turn to prototypical case-control genetic association studies to confirm and extend the evidence for the risk factor (Poirier et al. 1993). It is now widely accepted that individuals with the *APOE4* allele of the *APOE* gene have a substantially increased risk of Alzheimer's disease (Pastor and Goate 2004). However, many cases of the disease occur without the allele (it is not necessary), and many individuals with the allele do not get the disease (it is not sufficient). In a subset of the Framingham Study cohort followed for dementia up to 1992, carrying an *APOE4* allele was a strong risk factor for Alzheimer's disease (e.g. RR = 3.7 for *APOE3/APOE4* heterozygotes as opposed to those with no *APOE4* allele). Nonetheless, one-half of the individuals who developed Alzheimer's disease did not carry an *APOE4* allele, and 90 percent of those who did carry an *APOE4* allele had not developed Alzheimer's disease by age 80 (Myers et al. 1996). The allele represents one of the first and best-established genetic risk factors for a common complex disease.

Because most people with a single copy of the *APOE4* allele do not develop Alzheimer's disease, *APOE4* is not a highly penetrant allele for the disease. Penetrance refers to the age-specific risk of developing disease, given the presence of the associated allele. *APOE4* is, however, quite a strong risk factor for Alzheimer's disease. In principle, a similar process could lead to discovery of other alleles with less severe effects.

Genetic Research on Mental Disorders

As we have emphasized in earlier chapters, it is difficult to demarcate valid diagnostic categories for mental disorders. They are expressed in thoughts, behaviors, and feelings; are often comorbid with one another; and may change their manifestations over the life course. With notable exceptions, such as Alzheimer's disease, our present-day diagnoses do not correspond to a well-defined pathophysiology.

The conundrums of psychiatric diagnosis are not insuperable. With the rapid progress of neuroscience and biological psychiatry, we are gaining insights into the pathophysiology of mental disorders, facilitating the discovery of causes. For most disorders, however, we are unlikely to achieve more than a partial understanding in the near future. The brain is the most complex and highly differentiated organ. The relationships between pathophysiology and our thoughts, behaviors, and feelings are bound to be extremely complex.

This complexity of diagnosis poses a formidable challenge to genetic research on mental disorders. In genetic parlance, the problem resides in the definition of the phenotype. The term **phenotype** refers to the observable trait or disease for which one seeks a genetic cause.

The results of genetic studies, especially genetic linkage studies, can be exquisitely sensitive to classification of the phenotype (Hodge and Greenberg 1992). A famous example is a genetic linkage study of bipolar disorder conducted among the Old Order Amish, a genetically isolated religious sect in Pennsylvania, descended from 30 progenitors who emigrated from Europe in the 18th century. Genetic linkage analysis of a large Amish pedigree yielded evidence that a gene for bipolar disorder was linked to markers on chromosome 11 (Egeland et al. 1987). As the first study to report linkage for a mental illness using variable DNA sequences as genetic markers, it generated much excitement. But later the linkage result proved false when one of the unaffected persons in the pedigree developed bipolar disorder and another was diagnosed with depression (Kelsoe et al. 1989). Thus, changes in the disease classification of even a few individuals in key pedigrees may have profound effects on linkage results.

Of necessity, then, psychiatric geneticists have paid very careful attention to the measurement and classification of phenotypes. The chances of finding genetic effects depend on choosing phenotypes that reflect underlying genotypes. In part for this reason, genetic research on mental disorders has developed three distinctive features.

First, **family history (or familial aggregation) studies** remain important to genetic research (Gottesman 1991; Kendler 2005).[1] Today these studies are rarely required for their original purpose, which was to establish the possibility of genetic causation of a disorder. However, they are needed for other purposes, one of which is to guide the definition of traits or disorders as phenotypes in genetic research (see chapter 30). Often, traits exhibiting strong familial aggregation are more closely related to genotype.

Second, **twin studies of heritability** remain useful. Rather than examining the relation of a specific gene to a specific disorder, heritability studies examine the relation of genotypic variation to phenotypic variation. Classical heritability methods enable one to infer how much of the observed variation in the phenotype (e.g., IQ) is explained by variation in the entire (unobserved) genome. Current methods of heritability analysis can incorporate specific observed genes into the analysis. In general, highly heritable traits are more closely tied to an underlying genotype (see chapter 31). Recent developments of heritability methods have been derived mainly from studies of complex behavioral and cognitive traits associated with mental disorders (Plomin et al. 2000). The methods have also been applied to mental disorders themselves (Kendler 1997). Although heritability estimates are by no means confined to studies of mental traits and disorders, there may be no other field in which they have such an influential role. It is likely that they will continue to be important in genetic research on psychiatric disorders, even if it were for no other purpose than to refine the outcomes used.

---

[1] We use the term *family history study* throughout this volume as synonymous with *familial aggregation study*. It does not imply any particular method of collecting data, such as the *indirect family history method*.

Third, genetic studies of psychiatric traits increasingly focus on endophenotypes, that is, possible intermediate, disease-associated phenotypes that can be studied in place of the psychiatric disorders themselves (Gottesman and Gould 2003). It has been suggested that the use of endophenotypes may be a central feature of genetic research on mental disorders in the coming decade (Insel and Collins 2003). Endophenotypes for psychiatric disorders are usually based on physiologic or neuropsychologic assessments. These measures are thought to be more closely tied to pathophysiology than are the more readily observable thoughts, behaviors, and feelings used for psychiatric diagnosis. In addition, it is usually assumed—though rarely demonstrated—that the genetic causes of the endophenotype are simpler and less heterogeneous, and therefore easier to detect, than the genetic causes of the disease. A principal advantage of an endophenotype is that, unlike clinical diagnoses, it may be quantifiable on all or most individuals, thereby in principle increasing the statistical power of genetic studies. The most useful endophenotypes are those that can be reliably measured, are strongly associated with the disease, and cosegregate with the disease within families.

The rationale for using an endophenotype was well articulated by a research team that used working memory deficit as an endophenotoype for schizophrenia (Weinberger et al. 2001). The authors posited that schizophrenia represents the confluence of several syndromes, each with its own genetic determinants. The authors also posited that it would be unlikely that a single genetic determinant would have a very large effect on the risk of the disorder. It might be possible, however, to detect a gene that influenced the risk of one of the component syndromes. Converging lines of evidence suggested that abnormal information processing in the prefrontal cortex, a core biological feature of schizophrenia, may be one such syndrome. The abnormality is reflected in deficits in working memory, which can be measured on neuropsychological tests such as the Wisconsin Card Sort. This reasoning led the authors to investigate the genetic basis of working memory deficits as an endophenotype. Their results suggested that a common genetic polymorphism—the *Val* allele of the Val158Met polymorphism in the catechol-o-methyl-transferase (*COMT*) gene—may be strongly associated with working memory deficits yet weakly associated with schizophrenia. Illustrating the difficulties of using endophenotypes, subsequent studies confirmed the association at this allele with working memory deficits, but not with schizophrenia (Williams et al. 2005).

These distinctive features are reflected in the choice of topics and examples in the chapters that follow. We devote considerable attention to defining the appropriate phenotypes for genetic research. In addition, we devote full chapters to heritability and family history studies.

In accord with the book as a whole, our emphasis rests heavily on exposing the logic of the designs. We do not discuss statistical modeling. We also do not review the present state of knowledge. For reviews of genetic findings on psychiatric disorders, see McGuffin et al. (2002), O'Donovan et al. (2003), Merikangas and Risch (2003b), and Owen et al. (2004). We use examples of gene-environment interactions in some of the chapters, but defer full discussion of this topic to part VIII.

To limit the scope, we are selective rather than inclusive, covering only the topics we deem most essential to the development of a common framework for genetic and epidemiologic research. Some important designs fall beyond this scope, such as adoption studies and studies of discordant monozygotic twins (for an excellent discussion of these approaches, see Rutter et al. 2001). We note some of the uses of studies of functional genomic and epigenetic studies in chapter 33.

Finally, in order to focus on developing a unified framework for studies of environmental and genetic factors, we do not address the many issues that arise in the collection of data needed to arrive at a valid result. Good research in this field requires thorough consideration of potential sources of bias in the ascertainment of cases, the selection of controls, the diagnostic assessments, and other areas. Our extensive review of these issues for cohort and case-control studies in previous chapters is largely applicable to genetic epidemiology studies, but it is also important to consider these issues in the specific context of genetic research. For a discussion of these issues in genetic epidemiology studies, we refer readers to Khoury et al. (1993) and Haines et al. (1998). For brief overviews, see Ottman and Susser (1992), and Fyer and Weissman (1999).

Conclusion

We believe that research on genetic causes depends on understanding both the biology of genes and the strategies for detecting causes in human populations. Ideally, studies will be conducted by teams that combine genetic and epidemiologic expertise. The chapters that follow offer readers a platform from which they can approach these studies as epidemiologists. We hope that this vantage point will enable readers to develop in a variety of directions, forming productive partnerships with geneticists, learning how to conduct genetic epidemiology studies and contributing to the further development of this rapidly evolving field.

References

Baron M, Risch N, Hamburger R, Mandel B, Kushner S, Newman M, Drumer D, and Belmaker RH (1987). Genetic Linkage Between X-Chromosome Markers and Bipolar Affective Illness. *Nature* 326:289–292.

Bateson W (1909). *Mendel's Principles of Heredity.* Cambridge: Cambridge University Press.

Beaty TH and Khoury MJ (2000). Interface of Genetics and Epidemiology. *Epidemiol. Rev.* 22:120–125.

Box JF (1978). *R. A. Fisher: The Life of a Scientist.* New York: Wiley.

Egeland JA, Gerhard DS, Pauls DL, Sussex JN, Kidd KK, Allen CR, Hostetter AM, and Housman DE (1987). Bipolar Affective Disorders Linked to DNA Markers on Chromosome 11. *Nature* 325:783–787.

Falconer DS (1965). The Inheritance of Liability to Certain Diseases, Estimated from the Incidence among Relatives. *Ann. Hum. Genet.* 29:51–76.

Feldman MW and Cavalli-Sforza LL (1984). Cultural and Biological Evolutionary Processes: Gene-Culture Disequilibrium. *Proc. Natl. Acad. Sci. USA* 81:1604–1607.

Fieve RR, Rosenthal D, and Brill H, eds. (1975). *Genetic Research in Psychiatry.* Baltimore: Johns Hopkins University Press.

Fisher RA (1918). The Correlation Between Relatives on the Supposition of Mendelian Inheritance. *Trans. Roy. Soc. Edinb.* 52:399–433.

Fisher RA (1930). *Genetic Theory of Natural Selection.* Oxford: Oxford University Press.

Fyer AJ and Weissman MM (1999). Genetic Linkage Study of Panic: Clinical Methodology and Description of Pedigrees. *Am. J. Med. Genet.* 88:173–181.

Galton F (1894). *Natural Inheritance.* New York: Macmillan.

Gillham NW (2001). *A Life of Sir Francis Galton: From African Exploration to the Birth of Eugenics.* New York: Oxford University Press.

Gottesman I (1991). *Schizophrenia Genesis: The Origins of Madness.* New York: Freeman.

Gottesman II and Gould TD (2003). The Endophenotype Concept in Psychiatry: Etymology and Strategic Intentions. *Am. J. Psychiatry* 160:636–645.

Gottesman II and Shields J (1967). A Polygenic Theory of Schizophrenia. *Proc. Natl. Acad. Sci. USA* 58:199–205.

Gusella JF, Wexler NS, Conneally PM, et al. (1983). A Polymorphic DNA Marker Genetically Linked to Huntington's Disease. *Nature* 306:234–238.

Haines JL and Pericak-Vance M, eds. (1998). *Approaches to Gene Mapping in Complex Human Diseases.* New York: Wiley-Liss Publishing.

Hall JM, Lee MK, Newman B, Morrow JE, Anderson LA, Huey B, and King MC (1990). Linkage of Early-Onset Familial Breast Cancer to Chromosome 17q21. *Science* 250:1684–1689.

Hodge SE and Greenberg DA (1992). Sensitivity of Lod Scores to Changes in Diagnostic Status. *Am. J. Hum. Genet.* 50:1053–1066.

Insel TR and Collins FS (2003). Psychiatry in the Genomics Era. *Am. J. Psychiatry* 160:616–620.

Katzman R (1986). Alzheimer's Disease. *N. Engl. J. Med.* 314:964–973.

Kelsoe JR, Ginns EI, Egeland JA, et al. (1989). Re-evaluation of the Linkage Relationship between Chromosome *11p* Loci and the Gene for Bipolar Affective Disorder in the Old Order Amish. *Nature* 342:238–243.

Kendler KS (1997). The Genetic Epidemiology of Psychiatric Disorders: A Current Perspective. *Soc. Psychiatry Psychiatr. Epidemiol.* 32:5–11.

Kendler KS (2005). Psychiatric Genetics: A Methodologic Critique. *Am. J. Psychiatry* 162:3–11.

Khoury MJ, Cohen BH, and Beaty TH (1993). *Fundamentals of Genetic Epidemiology.* Oxford: Oxford University Press.

Khoury MJ and Little J (2000). Human Genome Epidemiologic Reviews: The Beginning of Something HuGE. *Am. J. Epidemiol.* 151:2–3.

King MC, Lee GM, Spinner NB, Thomson G, and Wrensch MR (1984). Genetic Epidemiology. *Annu. Rev. Public Health* 5:1–52.

International Human Genome Sequencing Consortium. (2001). Initial Sequencing and Analysis of the Human Genome. *Nature* 409:860–921.

McGuffin P, Owen MJ, and Gottesman I (2002). *Psychiatric Genetics and Genomics.* Oxford: Oxford University Press.

Merikangas KR and Risch N (2003a). Genomic Priorities and Public Health. *Science* 302:599–601.

Merikangas KR and Risch N (2003b). Will the Genomics Revolution Revolutionize Psychiatry? *Am. J. Psychiatry* 160:625–635.

Morton NE and Chung CS (1978). *Genetic Epidemiology.* New York: Academic Press.

Myers RH, Schaefer EJ, Wilson PW, et al. (1996). Apolipoprotein E Epsilon4 Association with Dementia in a Population-Based Study: The Framingham Study. *Neurology* 46:673–677.

O'Donovan MC, Williams NM, and Owen MJ (2003). Recent Advances in the Genetics of Schizophrenia. *Hum. Mol. Genet.* 12(Spec. 2):R125–R133.

Online Mendelian Inheritance in Man (OMIM), http://www.ncbi.nlm.nih.gov/omim.

Ottman R and Susser M (1992). Data Collection Strategies in Genetic Epidemiology: The Epilepsy Family Study of Columbia University. *J. Clin. Epidemiol.* 45:721–727.

Owen MJ, Williams NM, and O'Donovan MC (2004). The Molecular Genetics of Schizophrenia: New Findings Promise New Insights. *Mol. Psychiatry* 9:14–27.

Pastor P and Goate AM (2004). Molecular Genetics of Alzheimer's Disease. *Curr. Psychiatry Rep.* 6:125–133.

Pearson K and Lee A (1903). On the Laws of Inheritance in Man. *Biometrika* 2:357–462.

Pericak-Vance MA, Bebout JL, and Gaskell PC, Jr., et al. (1991). Linkage Studies in Familial Alzheimer Disease: Evidence for Chromosome 19 Linkage. *Am. J. Hum. Genet.* 48:1034–1050.

Plomin R, DeFries J, McClearn GE, and McGuffin P (2000). *Behavioral Genetics,* 4th ed. New York: Freeman.

Poirier J, Davignon J, Bouthillier D, Kogan S, Bertrand P, and Gauthier S (1993). Apolipoprotein E Polymorphism and Alzheimer's Disease. *Lancet* 342:697–699.

Risch N and Merikangas K (1996). The Future of Genetic Studies of Complex Human Diseases. *Science* 273:1516–1517.

Risch NJ (2000). Searching for Genetic Determinants in the New Millennium. *Nature* 405:847–856.

Rosenthal D and Kety SS (1968). *The Transmission of Schizophrenia.* Oxford: Pergamon Press.

Rutter M, Pickles A, Murray R, and Eaves L (2001). Testing Hypotheses on Specific Environmental Causal Effects on Behavior. *Psychol. Bull.* 127:291–324.

Strittmatter WJ, Saunders AM, Schmechel D, Pericak-Vance M, Enghild J, Salvesen GS, and Roses AD (1993). Apolipoprotein E: High-Avidity Binding to Beta-Amyloid and Increased Frequency of Type 4 Allele in Late-Onset Familial Alzheimer Disease. *Proc. Natl. Acad. Sci. USA* 90:1977–1981.

Susser M and Susser E (1988). Separating Heredity and Environment: Research Designs and Strategies. In Henderson and Burrows, eds. *Handbook of Social Psychiatry,* 117–134. New York: Elsevier.

Torrey EF, Bowler AE, Taylor EH, and Gottesman II (1994). *Schizophrenia and Manic-Depressive Disorder.* New York: Basic Books.

Tsuang M and Tohen M (2002). *Textbook In Psychiatric Epidemiology,* 2nd ed. New York: Wiley.

Weinberger DR, Egan MF, Bertolino A, Callicott JH, Mattay VS, Lipska BK, Berman KF, and Goldberg TE (2001). Prefrontal Neurons and the Genetics of Schizophrenia. *Biol. Psychiatry* 50:825–844.

Weissman MM, Merikangas KR, John K, Wickramaratne P, Prusoff BA, and Kidd KK (1986). Family-Genetic Studies of Psychiatric Disorders. Developing Technologies. *Arch. Gen. Psychiatry* 43:1104–1116.

Williams HJ, Glaser B, Williams NM, Norton N, Zammit S, MacGregor S, Kirov GK, Owen MJ, and O'Donovan MC (2005). No Association Between Schizophrenia and Polymorphisms in COMT in Two Large Samples. *Am. J. Psychiatry* 162:1736–1738.

Genetic Association Studies

29

Habibul Ahsan, Gary A. Heiman, and Ezra Susser

The goal of genetic association studies is to investigate the effects of genotypic variation on disease risk. These designs are built on a concept of a genetic cause that closely resembles the concept of a risk factor in epidemiology. Moreover, they correspond well to designs previously articulated by risk factor epidemiologists. Thus, the concepts and methods of risk factor epidemiology are particularly useful in this context.

Genetic association studies allow one to test whether individuals with a specific genetic allele (exposed) have a higher disease risk than those without the allele (unexposed; Risch and Merikangas 1996; Cardon and Bell 2001). The presence or absence of an allele is defined by the DNA sequence of a candidate gene or marker. If a disease is caused by the interplay of multiple genetic and nongenetic factors, then the genetic allele being investigated may be one of many factors that increase the disease risk. This is essentially the same as the concept of a risk factor in epidemiology. We have merely restated it to explicitly encompass genetic, as well as nongenetic, risk factors.

Like other risk factors, a genetic risk factor can be examined by either cohort or case-control designs, and also by their variants known as family-based designs. We will describe each of these approaches below, drawing attention to similarities and differences from studies of nongenetic risk factors. At the outset, we note three important differences.

First, in almost all circumstances, genotype (allelic status) is determined biologically before birth and is permanent (except for somatic mutations in individual cells). It is reasonable to assume that the allele (exposure) was antecedent to the disease, regardless of the time at which the allele was measured. Therefore, a pivotal feature of cohort studies—that the exposure is known to be antecedent to the disease—generally pertains to both cohort and case-control studies of genetic association.

Second, confounding in genetic association studies takes a distinctive form, based on differences in individuals' ancestry. This form of confounding is referred to as **population stratification**. It occurs because frequencies of most alleles vary across populations. Allele frequency differences across populations are virtually nonexistent at some genes and genetic markers and very large at others. Any social grouping—for example, ethnicity, neighborhood of residence, occupation, religion, or caste—that is associated with both genetic ancestry (allele frequency) and disease risk represents a potential confounder of associations between an allele and a disease. In a particular study, the potential for bias will reflect the historical demography of the population used in the study.

As an example of population stratification, consider the possibility of confounding by ethnicity. Ethnicity is most often defined as the cultural subgroup with which one identifies (e.g., "native Dutch" in Holland, or "Chinese-American" in the United States). Because ethnicity is often associated with genetic ancestry, it may also be associated with allele frequencies. Ethnicity may also be associated with the disease being studied, because ethnic groups may differ on multiple environmental risk factors, as well as on multiple (other) disease-causing alleles. Thus confounding by ethnicity could produce an apparent association between the allele and the disease. Note that "ethnicity" in this context may be a proxy for multiple specific environmental and genetic confounders, so that a crude matching on ethnicity may not entirely remove the confounding.

Third, an association between an allele and a disease may reflect either the causal effect of the specific allele being examined or of another allele in the same chromosomal region. The latter possibility arises because of a phenomenon called **linkage disequilibrium** (described in chapter 32). Many genetic association studies are actually designed to examine associations between numerous presumably noncausal alleles from many different chromosomal regions and disease. An association of disease with one of these noncausal alleles may indicate the chromosomal region in which the causal allele is located and thereby aid in its identification. We discuss this strategy in chapter 33. The present chapter focuses on studies that examine genetic alleles for which the investigator hypothesizes a causal effect.

Cohort Design

A cohort study can be used to examine the effect of a genetic allele on disease risk in much the same way it is used to examine the effect of a nongenetic exposure. One compares the disease risk for exposed individuals (those who carry the specified allele) and unexposed individuals (those who do not carry the specified allele). In evaluating the results, as in any cohort study, we consider differences between the exposed and unexposed that may produce spurious associations and, in particular, confounding (see chapter 12), unequal attrition (see chapter 13), and differential misclassification (see chapter 14).

The use of a cohort to study a genetic association is illustrated by a report on genetic susceptibility to depression that was based on the follow-up of the Dunedin birth cohort at age 26 (table 29.1; Caspi et al. 2003). As described in chapter 10, the Dunedin birth cohort has been assessed at multiple time points during childhood and young adulthood. In this report, the genetic exposure was defined as the genotype of the serotonin transporter gene (*5-HTT* or *SLC6A4*). The serotonin transporter is involved in the reuptake of serotonin at brain synapses and therefore may play an important role in mood

Table 29.1 Example of a Study of Genetic Association within a Cohort

Source	Study Description and Selected Findings
Caspi et al. (2003)	*Study*: Investigated the relation between the short and long alleles of the serotonin transporter gene and depression at age 26 years.
	Hypothesized a gene-environment interaction. After exposure to stressful life events, susceptibility to depression would vary by allelic status.
	Cohort (N = 1,037): Used a birth cohort in Dunedin, New Zealand (described in chapter 9; see table 9.1). This analysis was restricted to 847 non-Maori cohort members with complete follow-up data at age 26.
	Finding: Individuals with a short allele were more susceptible to depression after exposure to life events. Homozygotes for the short allele appeared more susceptible than heterozygotes.

Note: The data were derived from a cohort, but the study had features of a case-control, as well as a cohort, design.

regulation. Genotype was defined at a **functional polymorphism** in the promoter region of the gene, assessed as the short (s) and long (1) allelic variants. The *s* allele is associated with lower transcriptional efficiency.[1] Among the 847 cohort members used in the analysis, 17 percent were s/s, 51 percent were s/1, and 31 percent were 1/1.

The authors hypothesized a gene environment interaction; after one's exposure to stressful life events, his or her susceptibility to depression would vary according to allelic status. (We used this same example to illustrate the analysis of interaction in chapter 27.) The results were consistent with this hypothesis. Among individuals who reported no stressful life events, individuals with an s allele (s/s or s/1) were not more likely than 1/1 individuals to develop depression. In the subgroup of individuals who reported four or more stressful life events, however, individuals with an s allele were about twice as likely as 1/1 individuals to develop depression (33 percent compared with 17 percent).

In addition, there appeared to be some gradation of effect among those with an s allele. The s/s individuals were more susceptible than the s/1 individuals to develop depression after stressful life events. This gradation argues against a dominant mode of transmission of disease susceptibility, under which heterozygotes (s/1) and homozygotes (s/s) should have similar disease risk.

The association between allelic status and risk of depression was weak and nonsignificant in the cohort as a whole. Detection of the allelic effect depended upon identifying the subgroup with an environmental exposure that served

---

[1] The polymorphism in the promoter region of the *5-HTT* gene is located approximately 1000 DNA base pairs upstream of the transcription initiation site and is composed of 16-base-pair repeated elements. The polymorphism consists of an insertion or deletion of 44 base pairs (three copies of the repeat element). The short allele is associated with lower transcriptional efficiency of the promoter compared to the long allele.

as a causal partner to the genetic allele. Associations found only among sub-groups are notoriously inconsistent across studies, and often turn out to be artifactual (Cardon and Bell 2001). However, it is also true that this pattern of results should be expected for common alleles. They will often have weak effects, which may be detectable only after their causal partners are identified (Risch 2000; Terwilliger and Weiss 2003). Although the Dunedin result must be considered preliminary, pending testing in other studies, it is consistent with the study hypothesis.

The Dunedin investigators reduced the potential for confounding by strati-fication in their New Zealand population by excluding individuals reporting Maori ethnicity (7 percent) from the analysis. The potential for unequal attri-tion was limited by the virtually complete follow-up at age 26 (96 percent). The potential for differential misclassification was not as well addressed, and the authors did not fully utilize the cohort design in this report; the exposure to life events (from age 21 to age 26) and the outcome of depression (in the past year) were both obtained in the age 26 assessment, as would be done in a case-control study.[2] Notwithstanding these limitations, the study was one of the first to use data on both environmental and genetic exposures in a well-characterized cohort to analyze a common genetic allele as a risk factor for a mental disorder.

Although as yet there are few examples of full-fledged cohort studies of genetic association in psychiatric research, the design will surely be widely used in coming years. Even now, investigators are genotyping large popula-tions, establishing procedures to ascertain diseases in these populations, and linking the genomic data with the disease outcomes. An example is the European Prospective Investigation into Cancer and Nutrition (EPIC study, one of the largest cohort studies ever conducted. Started in the early 1990s, EPIC has recruited 400,000 individuals through 22 collaborating centers in nine European countries. The data being collected include exten-sive questionnaires on environmental risk factors, banked DNA samples, and disease onset information (Riboli 1992; Margetts et al. 1997). Although the primary focus is cancer, an extension to psychiatric disorders has begun (Surtees et al. 2006).

The cohort strategy is certainly alluring, especially for mental disorders, where the design may allow for better characterization of the phenotype. Longitudinal data can be used to obtain more valid diagnoses and to charac-terize diagnostic subtypes that may be genetically distinct. Cohort studies are also valuable for establishing the temporal order between environmental exposure and disease when nongenetic risk factors must also be related to the disease, as in studies of gene-environment interactions.

---

[2] As a result of this procedure, the temporal order was determined by subjects' recall of the timing of life events and depression, as would be done in a case-control study. This recall also created the potential for the kind of differential misclassification that is germane to case-control studies. The presence of depression could have affected the reporting of either the timing or the occurrence of life events, so the misclassification of the exposure could have differed for cases and noncases. But unless related to allelic status, the potential differential misclassifica-tion would be unlikely to explain the finding of gene-environment interaction.

However, the cohort strategy can be very expensive. It is too early to judge whether cohort studies will lead to major genetic discoveries that would not have been found with case-control designs. This is of particular concern because most difficulties of case-control genetic association studies, discussed next, also pertain to cohort studies.

Case-Control Design

Unlike cohort studies, case-control studies of genetic alleles and psychiatric illnesses are already numerous. In a case-control study, the investigator compares the proportion of cases with a specified allele (exposed) to the proportion of controls with the same allele.[3] As described for the Dunedin study, researchers may also differentiate individuals who are homozygous and heterozygous for the specified allele as highly and moderately exposed, respectively.

The case-control approach was used to establish the association between Alzheimer's disease and the *APOE4* allele. As described in the previous chapter, the link between APOE locus and Alzheimer's disease was initially found in a genetic linkage study (Pericak-Vance et al. 1991). The authors then compared 83 cases from their American families with 91 controls from a different genetic study in France (Strittmatter et al. 1993). The frequency of the *APOE4* allele was 0.52 among cases (based on 83 cases) and 0.16 among controls (based on 91 controls), a significant difference.[4]

Within a very short time, a Canadian research group documented the same association in a case-control study with less potential for confounding (table 29.2; Poirier et al. 1993). The 91 cases were patients referred to a Montreal cognitive disorders clinic and diagnosed with Alzheimer's disease. The 74 controls were spouses of Alzheimer's patients and elderly volunteers. The *APOE4* allele frequency was 0.38 among the cases, compared with 0.12 among controls. The authors noted that in the previous study from the United States the pedigrees were of several ancestries and the control group was French, creating potential for confounding by population stratification. Nonetheless, the results of the two studies were similar, suggesting that *APOE4* was a risk factor in the populations studied. After a decade of further work, *APOE4* is firmly established as a risk factor for Alzheimer's disease (Pastor and Goate 2004).

Few other genetic risk factors for psychiatric disorders have been firmly established by case-control studies. Overall, the results of such studies have been inconsistent (Hirschhorn et al. 2002; Ioannidis et al. 2003). For example, a series of studies examined the relationship between alcoholism and the *A1* allele of the gene encoding the dopamine D2 receptor. The initial study was

---

[3] To differentiate this strategy from the family-based study, the case-control study in this context is sometimes referred to as a *population-based genetic association study*. We avoid this term, because genetic association studies of psychiatric disorders are rarely population-based in the sense of drawing a representative sample from a well-defined population (see part IV).

[4] They reported allele frequencies, rather than genotypes, since there were no *APOE4* homozygotes.

Table 29.2 Examples of Case-Control Studies of Genetic Association

Sources	Study Description and Selected Findings
Blum et al. (1990)	*Study*: Compared alcoholic and nonalcoholic individuals for the presence of the *A1* allele of the dopamine D2 receptor gene. For this purpose, obtained postmortem brain tissues from the National Neurological Research Bank.
	Cases (N = 35): Postmortem diagnoses of alcohol abuse or dependence by two psychiatrists, based on review of all available data.
	Controls (N = 35): Postmortem nonalcoholic diagnoses by two psychiatrists, based on review of all available data. Similar to cases on age, sex, and race.
	Finding: 69% of cases versus 20% of controls had the *A1* allele.
Poirier et al. (1993)	*Study*: Compared individuals diagnosed with probable Alzheimer disease and normal controls for the presence of *APOE4* allele.
	Cases (N = 91): Patients referred to a Montreal cognitive disorders clinic and diagnosed with Alzheimer's disease.
	Controls (N = 74): Healthy spouses of Alzheimer's patients and elderly volunteers, matched for age of cases.
	Finding: The frequency of *APOE4* allele was 3.11 times higher in cases than in controls (0.38 versus 0.122).

motivated by evidence that the dopamine D2 receptor plays a role in the reward system that maintains addictive behaviors. The researchers compared DNA samples from postmortem brain tissue of 35 individuals with alcoholism (cases) and 35 nonalcoholics (controls) for the presence of the *A1* allele (table 29.2; Blum et al. 1990.)[5] They found that 24 (69 percent) of the alcoholics but only 7 (20 percent) of the controls carried the *A1* allele. Numerous studies attempted to replicate this finding, with mixed results. Some interpreted the evidence as strongly supporting association (Cloninger 1991; Noble 2000), whereas others suggested that the associations were probably artifactual (Gelernter et al. 1993; Ioannidis et al. 2003).

To reduce potential confounding in genetic association studies by population stratification, more rigorous studies match cases and controls at least on ethnic group. But same ethnicity does not ensure same ancestry. The potential for residual bias after matching on ethnicity was illustrated by a study of diabetes among Native American (Pima and Papago) populations (Knowler et al. 1988). The authors described an apparently strong association between immunoglobulin *Gm* alleles and diabetes mellitus (prevalence ratio 0.27; 95 percent confidence interval 0.18–0.40). They then showed that the association was entirely due to population stratification. Although the study participants all identified themselves as Native American, participants varied in numbers

---

[5] Although brain tissue of deceased subjects was used in this study, blood samples are generally used for genotyping in association studies, because DNA is the same in all tissues.

of white versus Native American ancestors. After the researchers stratified for the number of Native American versus white ancestors, the genetic association vanished. The confounding had arisen because the number of Native American ancestors was related to both frequency of the *Gm* genotype and to prevalence of diabetes mellitus.

A second reason for inconsistency is the low prior probability that any given genetic allele will be a cause of the disorder. Once investigators depart from a limited number of well-founded a priori hypotheses and begin testing very large numbers of alleles for potentially causal associations, it is inevitable that many of the initial reports of positive results will turn out to be false positives.

A third reason for inconsistency may be an overreliance on significance tests to distinguish true from false results. In large studies, very small associations that are statistically significant may be due to bias, including population stratification bias (Heiman et al. 2004). Emerging analytic methods for detecting population stratification bias appear to be less dependable in studies of small effects (Cardon and Bell 2001). Conversely, in small studies, true associations between allele and disease may not be statistically significant. A nonsignificant association is often interpreted as absence of association, but this interpretation is not correct (Gigerenzer et al. 1989; Cohen 1994). Confidence intervals for effect size often overlap for significant and nonsignificant studies of the same association (for elaboration of this point, see Rosenthal et al. 2000.)

A fourth reason for inconsistency is not related to artifact but to true heterogeneity of genetic causes. For some diseases, many different alleles can produce similar phenotypes, either by disrupting the same gene at different points, or by disrupting different genes in the same biological pathway. In different populations, different alleles leading to the same phenotype may appear. It is, then, unlikely that studies done in different populations will consistently detect an effect of any one such allele, even with large sample sizes. When the effect of the allele also depends on the presence of an environmental exposure, it is even more unlikely.

All these sources of inconsistency may also affect cohort studies of genetic risk factors. In fact, the example of residual confounding was from a longitudinal study of diabetes in Native Americans. One approach to minimize the effect of population stratification bias is the use of family-based designs, many of which are variants of the case-control study.

Family-Based Designs

Family-based genetic association studies are a collection of strategies for matching cases and controls on family of origin (Khoury and Flanders 1995; Gauderman et al. 1999). Family-based approaches may select siblings, cousins, or other family members as controls. By matching on family of origin, these designs effectively control population stratification bias.

An example is the case–unaffected sibling control design. We begin by selecting cases, and choose their unaffected siblings as controls (Gauderman et al. 1999; Siegmund et al. 1999; Thomas 2004). A case with a Puerto Rican father and a Norwegian-American mother would be matched to unaffected siblings. Case and controls thus share the same ancestry. We then compare allelic distributions between cases and their sibling controls.

A study of associations between variants in monoamine oxidase (*MAO*) genes and bipolar disorder illustrates how a family-based approach may correct for unforeseen biases in an ordinary case-control association study (Parsian and Todd 1997). MAO, a key enzyme for the metabolism of monoamines, has two subunits, A and B, encoded by two different (but adjacent) genes on the X chromosome. Previous case-control association studies had reported that certain alleles of *MAOA* and *MAOB* were associated with affective disorders (Lim et al. 1994; Kawada et al. 1995). Following this lead, researchers examined the association between *MAOA* and *MAOB* genetic alleles and bipolar disorder, genotyping 83 people with bipolar disorder (cases) and 84 unrelated controls. As in previous studies, the cases differed significantly from the controls with respect to the frequency of certain *MAOB* (though not *MAOA*) alleles.

In addition, however, these researchers conducted a complementary family-based study, using the **case-parent triad** design (described in the next section). In this family-based study, the authors found no evidence for associations between either *MAOA* or *MAOB* alleles and bipolar disorder. Their interpretation was that the case-control study using unrelated controls had produced an artifactual result for *MAOB* alleles, because of population stratification bias.

A family-based design does not necessarily require any departure from the ordinary logic of a case-control study. Controls are often selected to match cases on social, ethnic, or geographic background, among other factors. They can also be selected to match cases on family of origin.

But some family-based designs extend beyond simple matching. Innovative approaches include the case-parent triad (see Ahsan et al. 2002) and the kin-cohort design (Gail et al. 1999). Nonetheless, all of these approaches can be usefully conceptualized in terms of risk factor designs, while taking into account the genetics that underlie them. This conceptualization enables us to distill a bewildering variety of emerging strategies into a few essential core designs whose principles are understood. To demonstrate this point, we focus on the case-parent triad design.

Case-Parent Triad Design

The case-parent triad design can be conceptualized as a case-base (or case-cohort) study. As described in chapter 18, in a case-base study the controls are selected as a random sample of the total cohort at the start of the follow-up. The odds ratio is, as always, computed as the exposure odds in cases divided by the exposure odds in controls. Under this procedure for control selection, the odds ratio will equal the risk ratio (except for random error). This equality of odds ratio and risk ratio marks the case-base study as a hybrid. It does not pertain to ordinary case-control studies, in which the odds ratio is not identical to the risk ratio and generally overestimates it.

It is not immediately apparent that the case-parent triad design is equivalent to the case-base design. In a case-parent triad study, the genotypes of the parents of the cases are used to derive the genotypes of the source population of the cases. Thus, the control group is generated from the parents, rather than being sampled from the cohort at the start of follow-up. The case-parent triad originated from human genetics. When incorporated into genetic epidemiology, it was initially considered an ordinary case-control study and only recently explicitly considered as a case-base design (Ahsan et al. 2002). We will first use a hypothetical example to introduce the case-parent triad and to demonstrate its equivalence to the case-base design, and then discuss an application.

Case-Parent Triad as Case-Base Design

Like any risk factor study, the case-parent triad investigates the relation of an exposure (presence of an allele) to a disease. We will designate the hypothesized disease susceptibility allele as A and the normal (or wild-type) allele as B. There may be many normal alleles, but we will call them all B for simplicity. The goal is to estimate the risk ratio for the disease in relation to allele A.

In the case-parent triad design, we begin by selecting individuals with the disease who will be the cases. Then each case is matched with his or her mother and father. The mother and father could each have one of three genotypes: AA, AB, or BB. In its simplest form, the case-parent triad study includes only the cases with AB × BB parents. This parental genotype is said to be fully informative because we know which parent can contribute an A allele to the child and that the prior probability of transmission is 50 percent.

Figure 29.1 depicts a hypothetical birth cohort of 100,000 children with AB × BB parents. Fifty percent (50,000) of children inherit allele A, and 50

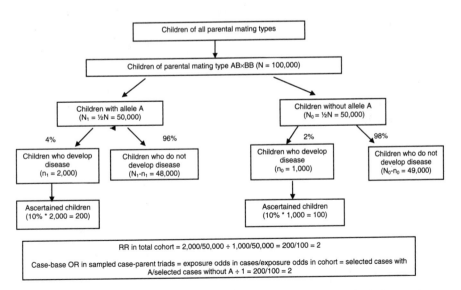

Figure 29.1 Estimating risk ratio from the case-parent triad design: hypothetical example.

percent do not, as expected from the laws of Mendelian transmission. The total number of children who develop the disease is 3,000; among those with allele A, 2,000 (4 percent) develop the disease, whereas among those without allele A, 1,000 (2 percent) develop the disease. The risk ratio is 4 percent/2 percent = 2.

We will now obtain the risk ratio in this cohort by using a case-parent triad design. If the case-parent triad design is a case-base study, then the odds ratio can be computed as the exposure odds in a random sample of cases divided by the exposure odds in a random sample of the total cohort, and this odds ratio will equal the risk ratio (except for random error). We will adopt this approach to compute the odds ratio in our example and see whether it yields a risk ratio of 2, which we know to be the true risk ratio.

As shown in figure 29.1, for our case-parent triad study, we begin as always by selecting the cases. We draw a 10 percent random sample of 300 from the 3,000 cases in the cohort. Since 2,000 of all the 3,000 cases in the cohort carry the A allele, we expect that 200 of our 300 cases will carry the A allele. Using our 300 selected cases, we estimate the exposure odds in the cases. The odds is the number of cases with the A allele divided by the number without the A allele, i.e., 200/100 = 2.

But we do not draw a random sample of the total cohort. We do not assess any of the remaining 2,700 cases or the 97,000 noncases in the cohort. How, then, can we compute the exposure odds in a random sample of the total cohort as required to compute an odds ratio?

Using the basic laws of Mendelian transmission, we estimate the odds of exposure in the total cohort in accordance with the parental genotypes. In the present scenario, where all of the birth cohort derive from AB × BB parents, under Mendelian transmission on average 50 percent of children carry the A allele and 50 percent do not.[6] Therefore, we expect the numbers of exposed and unexposed to be equal, and the exposure odds in the total cohort to be equal to one. Thus, we can estimate the exposure odds in the total cohort *without* selecting any sample for study.

We can now compute our estimate of the odds ratio and compare it with the true risk ratio. The exposure odds in our selected cases divided by the exposure odds in the total cohort is 2/1 = 2, which is equal to the true risk ratio.

This hypothetical example is built on the conditions that the selected cases are a random sample of all cases, with AB × BB parents. All parents need to be typed to identify the informative ones. Under these conditions, the exposure odds in our selected cases will estimate the exposure odds among all cases, and the exposure odds in the total cohort is expected to be equal to one. As a result, the exposure odds in our selected cases will estimate the case-base odds ratio, which is always equal to the risk ratio. Thus, we can correctly estimate the risk ratio simply by studying our selected cases.

---

[6] Although this is generally true, it is possible that some alleles may deviate from these transmission probabilities. These deviations have been referred to as *transmission distortions* (see Whittemore et al. 2004).

Other Mating Types

The simplifying condition of fully informative mating types is not required for the use of the case-parent triad design to estimate the risk ratio from the vantage point of a case-base design. Cases who are offspring of other mating types can also contribute to the result for the risk ratio as long as one parent is heterozygous (AB).

When we include cases who are offspring of other mating types, the exposure odds in the total cohort is not expected to be equal to one. For example, for cases with AB × AB parents, 75 percent of the offspring would receive an A allele, and 25 percent would not, so that the exposure odds derived from their parental genotypes would be 75 percent/25 percent = 3. Provided one knows the genotypes of the parents, however, the results from cases of different mating types can be combined to compute the risk ratio.

Although this approach to computing the risk ratio clarifies the nature of the design, case-parent triad studies do not often use it in practice. Investigators increasingly utilize statistical modeling to incorporate data from all mating types, include multiple affected siblings, distinguish heterozygote (AB) from homozygote cases (AA), and impute the allelic status of subjects for whom blood samples are missing (Thomas 2004). These methods bring many advantages and confer greater statistical power. However, they are less transparent.

Example of a Case-Parent Triad Study

To illustrate both the practical difficulties and the potential value of the case-parent triad method, we consider a study of the relationship of panic disorder to polymorphism in the gene *COMT*, which encodes catechol-O-methyltransferase (table 29.3; Hamilton et al. 2002). *COMT* has an important role in the metabolism of catecholamine neurotransmitters, which are

Table 29.3 Example of a Case-Parent Triad Study of Genetic Association

Source	Study Description and Selected Findings
Hamilton et al. (2002)	*Study*: Using a case-parent triad design, investigated the association between the transmission of the *COMT Val/Met* alleles and panic disorder.
	Subjects: 249 individuals from 83 triads consisting of panic disorder proband, mother and father. Probands diagnosed by experienced interviewers using semistructured interviews. The triads included two overlapping sets derived from two sources: (1) families used in a genetic linkage study where more than one case could be ascertained from a family and (2) same as above but only one case per family, and supplemented with cases from other sources.
	Finding: Association between the high-activity *COMT Val* allele and panic disorder in the first set of triads (only *p*-values were reported: $p = .03$) but not in the second set.

potentially important to several psychiatric disorders. The *COMT* protein sequence is polymorphic at amino acid residue 158 (i.e., *Val158Met*), yielding two proteins that differ in enzymatic activity. Enzymatic activity is highest among *Val/Val* homozygotes, intermediate for *Val/Met* heterozygotes, and lowest for *Met/Met* homozygotes. The *COMT Val158Met* polymorphism has been studied as a candidate for several mental disorders, including alcoholism (Wang et al. 2001) and schizophrenia (Egan et al. 2000), as well as panic disorder.

In this study, the investigators hypothesized a priori that one of the *COMT* alleles would be associated with panic disorder, although they felt there were not good grounds for specifying whether the *Val* or the *Met* carriers would be more likely affected. In their study population, the frequencies of the *Val* and *Met* alleles were similar to reports from European populations, each approximately 50 percent (Palmatier et al. 1999). As the authors noted, when both of the alleles at a biallelic site are common, an effect of one of the two alleles on an uncommon disorder could only be a modest one in the total population and might be difficult to detect.

Two different and overlapping sets of case-parent triads were used in this study. The first, larger set drew the cases from pedigrees used in these authors' linkage study of panic disorder, in which they had identified a linkage signal in the region on chromosome 22 harboring the *COMT* gene. In this first set of triads, a single pedigree could contribute more than one case, which were therefore not independent of one another. The second, smaller set of triads was limited to one case from each of the pedigrees used in the linkage study and supplemented by cases derived from other sources. Senior clinical investigators diagnosed all cases according to the *DSM III-R*.

The two sets of triads were analyzed separately with computer software available at the time. (With methods now available, the data could have been analyzed with use of all the triads in a single analysis.) In the analysis of the first set, the authors found a significant association between the transmission of the high-activity *Val* allele and panic disorder. Curiously, when male and female cases were examined separately, the association was evident only among female cases. In the analysis of the partly overlapping and somewhat smaller second set, however, there was no significant association between the *Val* allele and panic disorder.

The reason for the discrepant results between the two sets could not be determined. In light of our previous discussion of genetic heterogeneity, however, the discrepancy is perhaps not surprising. The first set of triads was not only larger, but also more homogeneous, including multiple cases from the pedigrees in which a linkage signal had been identified. One would be less likely to detect an association in the more heterogeneous second set of triads, which also included cases derived from other sources (personal communication, Hamilton SP 2004). Subsequently, another (case-control) study reported a significant association between the high-activity *Val* allele and panic disorder, only among women (Domschke et al. 2004). Although any causal inference is premature, this result lends some support to the result from the first set of triads.

Case-Control versus Case-Parent Triad

In recent years, the relative merits of the case-control and case-parent triad designs have been hotly disputed. The debate has focused on these two approaches because they are currently the most widely used. But the points raised are of much more general relevance and pertain to choosing among the wide variety of genetic association designs that are becoming available: cohort designs, case-control designs, case-parent triad designs, and other family-based designs.

On one hand, the case-parent triad design eliminates population stratification bias. It also can be extended to the examination of parent-of-origin effects, such as imprinting. On the other hand, the case-control study facilitates collecting large samples and examining genetic and nongenetic effects, and their interactions within the same study. There are also many practical differences to be weighed in any particular context; for example, the case-parent triad study requires genotyping of two parents for each case, whereas the case-control study requires recruitment and full assessment, including genotyping, of an appropriate control group.

The primary motivation for the case-parent triad design—to avoid population stratification bias—was recently called into question with the argument that distortion of the effect estimate because of a single population-stratification confounder will tend to be modest (Wacholder et al. 2000). Although this may sometimes be true for a single confounder, it is a hazardous premise, especially for studies of modest effects (see chapter 12). In epidemiologic studies, multiple confounders, or a poorly measured strong confounder, do sometimes lead to spurious results. With respect to population stratification, one cannot discern the strength or nature of the effects of ancestry. The study of diabetes and immunoglobulin genotype among Native Americans was an example of this problem.

Others have proposed that the magnitude of bias due to population stratification in a particular study can be estimated with "genomic controls" and structured analysis of association (Devlin and Roeder 1999; Pritchard and Donnelly 2001; Rosenberg et al. 2002; Gorroochurn P et al. 2006).[7] If these analytic methods were to suggest that population stratification bias was not a problem in a specific case-control study, it would also suggest that in this instance the case-parent triad design was not necessary. Of course, one would need to have the cases and controls available to carry out this analysis. As yet, these analytic methods have not been fully tested. In addition, they have been taken up mainly to guide the setting of the threshold or *p*-value for claiming a positive result in a case-control study, rather than for producing

---

[7] One use of genomic controls involves genotyping a panel of unlinked genetic markers scattered in different parts of the genome, in addition to the alleles of interest. Absent population stratification bias, these unlinked markers should not be associated with being a case or control. Therefore, they serve as a genomic control for gauging the potential bias and adjusting for it. Note that these markers are not *controls* in the sense we have used the term in this book, but rather a way to estimate the potential for stratification bias. See Thomas (2004) for a clear explanation of these and other approaches. Note also that these methods have not yet been fully tested, suggesting a need for caution in their use (Spence et al. 2003).

unconfounded effect estimates (Freedman et al. 2004; Marchini et al. 2004).

In our view, both designs can be appropriate for detection of allelic effects. When it is feasible to collect a large enough number of triads, the case-parent triad design is preferable. Genotyping large populations provides the basis to conduct studies of this kind for some disorders. An example pertaining specifically to psychiatric disorders is a new Norwegian birth cohort of 100,000 (Magnus 2003), in which blood samples from mother, father, and child are being archived. This birth cohort is designed to investigate genetic and non-genetic risk factors for psychiatric (as well as other) disorders. The ongoing collection of longitudinal data should add to the power of the study by more precisely defining the phenotypes.

Ordinary case-control studies may be more appropriate if the sample size required is very large, or if the number of triads is constrained. Very large sample sizes are needed if the anticipated effect is small or the frequency of the allele is low (see Risch 2000). The number of triads is limited if parents are unavailable and parental DNA samples were not archived, as often happens in studies of late-life disorders. Careful collection of data on factors that may be related to ancestry will help safeguard against population stratification bias. Cases and controls may then be matched insofar as possible on ancestry, and the effect estimated may be adjusted for potential confounding. Methods such as genomic controls may usefully supplement but not supplant these safeguards.

We believe that any one of the designs described here—cohort, case-control, and family-based—may be the right choice in a particular context. There are also other variants that exploit our knowledge of genetic transmission to increase statistical power, such as studies that include cases from multigenerational pedigrees or multiple affected siblings in the same family.

Selection Bias

Although the current debate on case-control and case-parent triad designs draws attention to their differences, some of their similarities are equally important. In both designs, we still have to address other sources of bias, particularly selection bias. It is possible that an allele could reduce survival before the onset of the disease. Then the ascertained cases may underrepresent the frequency of the allele among cases. Conversely, an allele might increase the duration of the disease and, thereby, its ascertainment. Then the ascertained cases may overrepresent the frequency of the allele among cases.

Another possibility is that various alleles may be related to mild or severe forms of a disease. For example, Gaucher disease is a lysosomal storage disorder caused by numerous genetic mutations in the *GBA* gene. Depending upon the mutation, or mutations, involved, it may range from a mild nonneuronopathic disorder to severe disease with progressive neurologic symptoms (Montfort et al. 2004). In such instances, the mild cases may sometimes be undetected, and a study based on hospital or clinic cases may fail to detect any role for the mutations that cause the mild cases.

The validity of results will rest on the validity of the assumption that exposed and unexposed cases have the same probability of being selected for the study. As always, appropriate design and interpretation of the study depend on appreciating the possibilities for selection bias from the source population, as described in part IV. When it is feasible, restriction to incident cases selected with consistent and complete diagnostic protocols may constrain the potential for selection bias.

The Case-Only Design for Interaction

The **case-only design** is a strategy often employed to screen for gene-environment interactions in genetic association studies. As its name implies, the case-only design includes only individuals who have the phenotype under study (cases). Each individual is categorized in terms of both genetic exposure (present versus absent) and environmental exposure (present versus absent). Nowadays, the genetic ex-posure is usually measured by the presence versus absence of a specific disease-related genetic allele. (When disease-related alleles have not yet been identified, the genetic exposure may be measured by a proxy, such as the presence versus absence of a family history of disease.)

To screen for interaction, an odds ratio is computed as follows: the numerator is the odds of having the environmental exposure, given the presence of the genetic exposure, and the denominator is the odds of having the environmental exposure, given the absence of the genetic exposure. This odds ratio can be interpreted as an estimate of the interaction effect under a multiplicative model as described in chapter 27. An odds ratio that is appreciably greater than one indicates that the environmental factor modifies the risk ratio for the genetic effect, and, equivalently, the genetic factor modifies the risk ratio for the environmental factor (Khoury and Flanders 1996; Schmidt and Schaid 1999; Gatto et al. 2004).

Certain assumptions are necessary for a case-only study to provide a valid estimate of multiplicative interaction. Most important, the genetic and environmental factors must be unassociated in the source population that gave rise to the cases in the study. When this assumption is reasonable, the method is suitable for detecting large interaction effects, though likely to miss modest ones (i.e., those that are evident under an additive but not a multiplicative model; see chapter 36).

This design is increasingly applied in lieu of the case-control design for evaluating gene-environment interaction. It can also be used to evaluate interactions between two genetic exposures and, in theory, between two environmental exposures. Recent work has clarified the nature of the design, the potential for bias, and the means of adjusting for bias (Gatto et al. 2004). Two key points emerge from this work. First, the association between the genetic and environmental exposure in the source population should not be gauged by measuring this association in a control group, an approach suggested in earlier literature. Second, if the variables that account for the association between the genetic and environmental exposure in the source population can be specified and measured, then adjusting for these variables in the analysis can remove the bias and yield a valid result. In any particular study, using sensitivity analyses, one can assess whether the case-only design will yield a valid result for interaction under various hypothetical scenarios.

Multiple Testing

Genomic technologies now permit an investigator to identify all the genetic variation in any gene of interest in any study subject. For both genetic and epidemiologic hypotheses, this wealth of information raises the question of which variation is likely to be meaningful for disease.

Statistical analysis alone does not offer an efficient way to answer this question, because the number of different alleles is vast, so the number of individual tests is far too large to extract meaningful results. Various approaches have been suggested to address this problem. Evaluating alleles of functional significance is certainly a wise first step (Tabor et al. 2002). Considering genes, rather than alleles, as the unit of evaluation has been proposed (Neale and Sham 2004). A further grouping of the genes known to be involved in a biologic process has also been suggested (Thomas 2004). Other possibilities include dividing a sample into a *discovery series,* in which all variation is determined and the most promising associations are identified, with or without depending on *p*-values, and a *validation series,* in which only the few most promising associations are tested. We will discuss the issue of multiple comparison more fully in chapter 33.

Concordance of Genetic and Nongenetic Causes

Genetic findings that complement nongenetic risk factors can strengthen causal inference (for a classic example, see Goldstein et al. 2001). Suppose that, in a series of epidemiologic studies, we consistently find that not taking a certain vitamin is associated with increased risk of a disease. However, we still suspect that these results could be due to intractable confounding, because taking a vitamin may be associated with so many other health-conscious behaviors. Now suppose that having a certain genetic allele results in lower enzymatic activity in a biological pathway which is impeded by lack of this vitamin. If having this genetic allele is also associated with increased risk of disease, it would support the previous hypothesized effect of low vitamin intake on disease risk.

In chapter 6, we described a series of cohort and case control studies that suggested that periconceptual folate supplements reduced the risk of neural tube defects. Due in part to the potential for confounding, these studies were inconclusive. We now know that being homozygous for a certain genetic polymorphism (*MTHFR 677 C* to *T*) can have biological effects similar to that of low folate intake, for example, elevated homocysteine levels. We also know that mothers with the *MTHFR TT* genotype have an increased risk of having a child with a neural tube defect. If these genetic findings had been available to complement the cohort and case control studies, they would have substantially strengthened the evidence for a causal link. (The causal link was ultimately established by randomized clinical trials of periconceptual folate supplementation; see chapter 6).

With the rapid advance of genomics, epidemiologists have begun to systematically search for genetic association results that may be informative for causal inference about hypothesized nongenetic risk factors (Davey Smith and Ebrahim 2003; Davey Smith and Ebrahim 2004).[8] The underlying premise is that genetic association studies have one of the essential elements of a natural experiment (chapter 10): individuals cannot choose their genetic alleles. In some contexts, this feature makes it possible to isolate the effects of (the genetic substitute for) the exposure of interest from the most important potential confounders.

Conclusion

The study designs for examining genetic associations can be understood with the concepts of risk factor epidemiology that enable us to distill the complex array of genetic and other designs into a relatively few fundamental approaches. A unified approach to the study of genetic and nongenetic causes confers an enormous advantage in scope and flexibility. Valuable epidemiologic tools for genetic studies include, but are not limited to, the understanding of confounding and effect estimates. At the same time, we emphasize that the designs require modification and adaptation for the context of genetic research.

To fully understand the causes of complex psychiatric disorders, we need to go beyond establishing genetic risk factors one at a time and elucidate the interplay among the various factors in a causal pathway (see part VIII). This is especially true for the interaction among combinations of genetic and environmental factors. Although it is a far more complex undertaking, developing a unified approach to the study of genetic and nongenetic risk factors represents a first and necessary step toward this goal.

Acknowledgments

We are grateful to Drs. Abby J. Fyer, Steven P. Hamilton, James A. Knowles, and Myrna M. Weissman, for providing us with the case-parent triad data from their study of panic disorder (grants MH 28274 and MH 37592). This work was supported in part by grants CA 69398 (HA), DAMD 170010213 (HA).

---

[8] This approach has been referred to as "Mendelian randomization" in recent literature. The term is used because according to Mendel's laws, the parental allele which is transmitted to an offspring is a stochastic or random event. To avoid misinterpretation, however, it should be noted that "randomization" only pertains to transmission of alleles within family based designs.

References

Ahsan H, Hodge SE, Heiman GA, Begg MD, and Susser ES (2002). Relative Risk for Genetic Associations: The Case-Parent Triad as a Variant of Case-Cohort Design. *Int. J. Epidemiol.* 31:669–678.

Blum K, Noble EP, Sheridan PJ, Montgomery A, Ritchie T, Jagadeeswaran P, Nogami H, Briggs AH, and Cohn JB (1990). Allelic Association of Human Dopamine D2 Receptor Gene in Alcoholism. *JAMA* 263:2055–2060.

Cardon LR and Bell JI (2001). Association Study Designs for Complex Diseases. *Nat. Rev. Genet.* 2:91–99.

Caspi A, Sugden K, Moffitt TE, et al. (2003). Influence of Life Stress on Depression: Moderation by a Polymorphism in the *5-HTT* Gene. *Science* 301:386–389.

Cloninger CR (1991). D2 Dopamine Receptor Gene Is Associated but Not Linked with Alcoholism. *JAMA* 266:1833–1834.

Cohen J (1994). The Earth Is Round (*p* < .05). *American Psychologist* 49:997–1003.

Davey Smith G and Ebrahim S (2003). "Mendelian Randomization": Can Genetic Epidemiology Contribute to Understanding Environmental Determinants of Disease? *Int. J. Epidemiol.* 32:1–22.

Davey Smith G and Ebrahim S (2004). Mendelian Randomization: Prospects, Potentials, and Limitations. *Int. J. Epidemiol.* 33:30–42.

Devlin B and Roeder K (1999). Genomic Control for Association Studies. *Biometrics* 55:997–1004.

Domschke K, Freitag CM, Kuhlenbumer G, et al. (2004). Association of the Functional *V158M* Catechol-O-Methyl-Transferase Polymorphism with Panic Disorder in Women. *Int. J. Neuropsychopharmacol.* 7:183–188.

Egan MF, Goldberg TE, Gscheidle T, Weirich M, Bigelow LB, and Weinberger DR (2000). Relative Risk of Attention Deficits in Siblings of Patients with Schizophrenia. *Am. J. Psychiatry* 157:1309–1316.

Freedman ML, Reich D, Penney KL, et al. (2004). Assessing the Impact of Population Stratification on Genetic Association Studies. *Nat. Genet.* 36:388–393.

Gail MH, Pee D, and Carroll R (1999). Kin-Cohort Designs for Gene Characterization. *J. Natl. Cancer Inst. Monogr.* 26:55–60.

Gatto NM, Campbell UB, Rundle AG, and Ahsan H (2004). Further Development of the Case-Only Design for Assessing Gene-Environment Interaction: Evaluation of and Adjustment for Bias. *Int. J. Epidemiol.* 33:1014–1024.

Gauderman WJ, Witte JS, and Thomas DC (1999). Family-Based Association Studies. *J. Natl. Cancer Inst. Monogr.* 26:31–37.

Gelernter J, Goldman D, and Risch N (1993). The *A1* Allele at the D2 Dopamine Receptor Gene and Alcoholism. A Reappraisal. *JAMA* 269:1673–1677.

Gigerenzer G, Swijtink Z, Porter T, Daston L, Beatty J, and Kruger L (1989). *The Empire of Chance: How Probability Changed Science and Everyday Life.* Cambridge: Cambridge University Press.

Goldstein J, Hobbs H, and Brown M (2001). Familial Hypercholesterolemia. In Scriver C, Beaudet A, Sly W, and Valle D, eds., *The Metabolic and Molecular Bases of Inherited Disease*, 8th ed., pp. 1981–2030. New York: McGraw-Hill.

Gorroochurn P, Heiman GA, Hodge SE, and Greenberg DA (in press). Centralizing the Non-central Chi-square: A New Method to Correct for Population Stratification in Genetic Case-Control Association Studies. *Genetic Epidemiology.*

Hamilton SP, Slager SL, Heiman GA, et al. (2002). Evidence for a Susceptibility Locus for Panic Disorder Near the Catechol-O-Methyltransferase Gene on Chromosome 22. *Biol. Psychiatry* 51:591–601.

Heiman G, Hodge S, Gorroochurn P, and Greenberg D (2004). Effect of Population Stratification on Case-Control Association Studies. I. Elevation in False Positive Rates and Comparison to Confounding Risk Ratios (a Simulation Study). *Hum. Hered.* 58:30–39.

Hirschhorn JN, Lohmueller K, Byrne E, and Hirschhorn K (2002). A Comprehensive Review of Genetic Association Studies. *Genet. Med.* 4:45–61.

Ioannidis JP, Trikalinos TA, Ntzani EE, and Contopoulos-Ioannidis DG (2003). Genetic Associations in Large versus Small Studies: An Empirical Assessment. *Lancet* 361:567–571.

Kawada Y, Hattori M, Dai XY, and Nanko S (1995). Possible Association between Monoamine Oxidase A Gene and Bipolar Affective Disorder. *Am. J. Hum. Genet.* 56:335–336.

Khoury MJ and Flanders WD (1995). Bias in Using Family History as a Risk Factor in Case-Control Studies of Disease. *Epidemiology* 6:511–519.

Khoury MJ and Flanders WD (1996). Nontraditional Epidemiologic Approaches in the Analysis of Gene-Environment Interaction: Case-Control Studies With No Controls! *Am. J. Epidemiol.* 144:207–213.

Knowler WC, Williams RC, Pettitt DJ, and Steinberg AG (1988). *Gm3;5,13,14* and Type 2 Diabetes Mellitus: An Association in American Indians with Genetic Admixture. *Am. J. Hum. Genet.* 43:520–526.

Lim LC, Powell JF, Murray R, and Gill M (1994). Monoamine Oxidase A Gene and Bipolar Affective Disorder. *Am. J. Hum. Genet.* 54:1122–1124.

Magnus, P. The Norwegian Mother and Child Cohort Study (Protocol) (2003). http://www.fhi.no/dav/D66DB9C31F.pdf.

Marchini J, Cardon LR, Phillips MS, and Donnelly P (2004). The Effects of Human Population Structure on Large Genetic Association Studies. *Nat. Genet.* 36(5):512–517.

Margetts BM and Pietinen P, eds. (1997). *Int. J. Epidemiol.* 26:S1–S189.

Montfort M, Chabas A, Vilageliu L, and Grinberg D (2004). Functional Analysis of 13 *GBA* Mutant Alleles Identified in Gaucher Disease Patients: Pathogenic Changes and "Modifier" Polymorphisms. *Hum. Mutat.* 23:567–575.

Neale BM and Sham PC (2004). The Future of Association Studies: Gene-Based Analysis and Replication. *Am. J. Hum. Genet.* 75:353–362.

Noble EP (2000). Addiction and Its Reward Process through Polymorphisms of the D2 Dopamine Receptor Gene: A Review. *Eur. Psychiatry* 15:79–89.

Palmatier MA, Kang AM, and Kidd KK (1999). Global Variation in the Frequencies of Functionally Different Catechol-O-Methyltransferase Alleles. *Biol. Psychiatry* 46:557–567.

Parsian A and Todd RD (1997). Genetic Association between Monoamine Oxidase and Manic-Depressive Illness: Comparison of Relative Risk and Haplotype Relative Risk Data. *Am. J. Med. Genet.* 74:475–479.

Pastor P and Goate AM (2004). Molecular Genetics of Alzheimer's Disease. *Curr. Psychiatry Rep.* 6:125–133.

Pericak-Vance MA, Bebout JL, Gaskellpe Jr et al. (1991). Linkage Studies in Familial Alzheimer Disease: Evidence for Chromosome 19 Linkage. *Am. J. Hum. Genet* 48:1034–1050.

Poirier J, Davignon J, Bouthillier D, Kogan S, Bertrand P, and Gauthier S (1993). Apolipoprotein E Polymorphism and Alzheimer's Disease. *Lancet* 342:697–699.

Pritchard JK and Donnelly P (2001). Case-Control Studies of Association in Structured or Admixed Populations. *Theor. Popul. Biol.* 60:227–237.

Riboli E (1992). Nutrition and Cancer: Background and Rationale of the European Prospective Investigation into Cancer and Nutrition (EPIC). *Ann. Oncol.* 3:783–791.

Risch N and Merikangas K (1996). The Future of Genetic Studies of Complex Human Diseases. *Science* 273:1516–1517.

Risch NJ (2000). Searching for Genetic Determinants in the New Millennium. *Nature* 405:847–856.

Rosenberg NA, Pritchard JK, Weber JL, Cann HM, Kidd KK, Zhivotovsky LA, and Feldman MW (2002). Genetic Structure of Human Populations. *Science* 298:2381–2385.

Rosenthal R, Rosnow RL, and Rubin DB (2000). *Contrasts and Effect Sizes in Behavioral Research: A Correlational Approach.* Cambridge: Cambridge University Press.

Schmidt S and Schaid DJ (1999). Potential Misinterpretation of the Case-Only Study to Assess Gene-Environment Interaction. *Am. J. Epidemiol.* 150:878–885.

Siegmund KD, Gauderman WJ, and Thomas DC (1999). Association Tests Using Unaffected-Sibling versus Pseudo-Sibling Controls. *Genet. Epidemiol.* 17(suppl 1): S731–S736.

Spence MA, Greenberg DA, Hodge SE, and Vieland VJ (2003). The Emperor's New Methods. *Am. J. Hum. Genet.* 72:1084–1087.

Strittmatter WJ, Saunders AM, Schmechel D, Pericak-Vance M, Enghild J, Salvesen GS, and Roses AD (1993). Apolipoprotein E: High-Avidity Binding to Beta-Amyloid and Increased Frequency of Type 4 Allele in Late-Onset Familial Alzheimer Disease. *Proc. Natl. Acad. Sci. USA* 90:1977–1981.

Surtees PG, Wainwright NW, Willis-Owen SA, Luben R, Day NE, and Flint J (2006). Social Adversity, the Serotonin Transporter (5-HTTLPR) Polymorphism and Major Depressive Disorder. *Biol. Psychiatry* 59:224–229.

Tabor HK, Risch NJ, and Myers RM (2002). Opinion: Candidate-Gene Approaches for Studying Complex Genetic Traits: Practical Considerations. *Nat. Rev. Genet.* 3:391–397.

Terwilliger JD and Weiss KM (2003). Confounding, Ascertainment Bias, and the Blind Quest for a Genetic "Fountain of Youth." *Ann. Med.* 35:532–544.

Thomas DC (2004). *Statistical Methods in Genetic Epidemiology.* New York: Oxford University Press.

Wacholder S, Rothman N, and Caporaso N (2000). Population Stratification in Epidemiologic Studies of Common Genetic Variants and Cancer: Quantification of Bias. *J. Natl. Cancer Inst.* 92:1151–1158.

Wang T, Franke P, Neidt H, Cichon S, Knapp M, Lichtermann D, Maier W, Propping P, and Nothen MM (2001). Association Study of the Low-Activity Allele of Catechol-O-Methyltransferase and Alcoholism Using a Family-Based Approach. *Mol. Psychiatry* 6:109–111.

Whittemore AS, Halpern J, and Ahsan H (2004). Covariate Adjustment in Family-Based Association Studies. *Genet. Epidemiol.* 28(3):244–255.

Modern Family History Studies

30

Regina Zimmerman, Habibul Ahsan, and Ezra Susser

For many decades, when little information was available on specific genes, examining whether a disease clustered or aggregated in families was a first step toward establishing a role for genetic causes (King et al. 1984). The approach was referred to as a familial aggregation study and was a staple of human genetic research. A finding of familial aggregation would be followed by studies designed to separate the contributions of heredity from those of environment, and to identify a pattern of genetic transmission (for a good account in the psychiatric literature, see Gottesman and Shields 1982).

In this chapter, we describe first the uses and then the designs of family history (or familial aggregation) studies in modern genetic research. Family history studies continue to play a central role (Merikangas 2005), but now they are undertaken to establish more than the familial aggregation of a disease. Current applications span a wide range, from refining phenotypes to targeting preventive interventions. Although the term familial aggregation is still commonly used to refer to these studies, we prefer the more generic term family history study, because it is more compatible with what is now understood to be the common logic underlying the designs, and because it helps to underscore that these studies are now being used for so many other purposes.

Current Uses of Family History Studies

Family history studies are guided by a very broad concept of genetic causation. All genetic causes are combined into a pooled genetic component. Although, or perhaps because, these studies rely upon such a broad concept of genetic effects, they retain an important role in genetic epidemiology.

Underlying their various uses is the idea that a family history of a phenotype—which may or may not be a disease—can be examined as a risk factor for that phenotype (Weissman et al. 1986; Susser and Susser 1987; Susser and Susser 1988; Khoury et al. 1993). If the phenotype is a disease, a cohort study defines each individual as exposed or unexposed, in accordance with the presence or absence of a family history of disease, and then compares the disease risk in the exposed and unexposed groups so defined. A case-control study compares cases and controls with respect to family history of disease (exposure).

Highly familial phenotypes usually have strong genetic causes, although many nongenetic risk factors also run in families. For example, dietary practices are highly familial, but usually for cultural, not genetic, reasons (McGuffin and Huckle 1990). Conversely, if a phenotype is not familial, it does not necessarily imply that there is no role for genes (Cui and Hopper 2000). For example, Down's syndrome is genetic, caused by triploidy of chromosome 21, that is usually *de novo* and maternal. Typically, the disease is not present in the ancestors of the cases and there are no offspring. Similarly, age-associated *de novo* point mutations in paternal germ lines have been shown to cause some neuropsychiatric disorders (Rousseau et al. 1994; Fletcher and Marsden 1996; Crow 1997) and are being investigated as causes of others (Malaspina et al. 2001); in such instances the disease will not be present in ancestors.

We describe here some of the contributions family history studies currently make to psychiatric research, including refining phenotypes used as outcomes in genetic studies, targeting preventive interventions, characterizing genetic effects, and exploring gene-environment interaction, as well as the original purpose of establishing familial aggregation of a disease. The procedures for implementing these family history studies in the field do not fall within our scope (defined in chapter 28). It should be noted, however, that certain features characterize the most robust studies. These features include an attempt to interview all available relatives, rather than relying upon one family member to provide information about other relatives; keeping interviewers blind to the exposure group when they are assessing the disease outcomes in a cohort study; keeping interviewers blind to the disease status of the cases and controls when these interviewers are assessing disease in case or control relatives (i.e., the exposure) in a case-control study; and avoiding selective ascertainment, such as overrepresentation of families with multiple affected members (for suggested reading, see chapter 28).

Refining Phenotypes

First, family history studies may suggest a phenotype that is genetically transmitted and is broader than the core diagnosable disorder. For example, family history and adoption studies established that a spectrum of conditions cluster in the families of individuals with schizophrenia (Kety et al. 1976). As a result, some pedigree linkage studies of schizophrenia assess a range of conditions defined as schizophrenia spectrum disorder (Kendler et al. 1995). Researchers thus avoid misclassifying individuals with schizophrenia spectrum disorders as entirely unaffected, which would undermine efforts to detect genetic linkage. Similarly, recent studies have suggested that a spectrum of conditions clusters in families of individuals with autism, including Aspergers syndrome (Bolton et al. 1994; Piven et al. 1997).

Second, family history studies permit one to identify a subgroup of cases in which genetic causes are powerful. These families will likely be the most informative in the discovery of the genes responsible for the disease. For example, familial aggregation studies of epilepsy showed that genetic effects were likely to be greatest for epilepsy with onset before age 35 and occurring in the absence of postnatally acquired brain insults (Ottman et al. 1996a; Ottman et al. 1996b; Ottman et al. 1998). These two criteria were used to identify families for subsequent genetic linkage studies, and a single family containing 11 individuals meeting the criteria was found. Analyses of epilepsy phenotypes in this family led to further refinement of the phenotype and definition of a new epilepsy syndrome characterized by temporal lobe seizures with auditory features (Winawer et al. 2000). Later, linkage analysis and mapping led to identification of the *LGI1* gene as a cause of this form of epilepsy (Kalachikov et al. 2002).

Third, family history studies can clarify whether or not comorbid disorders should be grouped together as a phenotype for genetic research. A familial aggregation study of panic disorder and depression defined three mutually exclusive groups of cases—panic only, depression only, and panic plus depression—as well as a fourth group of normal controls (Weissman et al. 1993). The prevalences of panic and depression among the relatives of the four groups suggested that, despite the frequent comorbidity, these disorders are genetically transmitted independently in families. Based on these results, panic and depression would not be grouped together in genetic research.

Fourth, family history studies can be employed to establish and refine endophenotypes. As described previously (chapter 28), endophenotypes are traits presumed to reflect genetic susceptibility to a diagnosable disorder. Studying the endophenotype rather than the disorder is intended to streamline the search for a specific genetic determinant. Highly familial traits tend to be the most useful endophenotypes, because such traits are most likely to have a strong genetic basis. A well-designed family history study offers a rigorous approach to examining the familial clustering of a potential endophenotype. Family history studies were used, for example, to establish that event-related brain potentials clustered in families and could serve as an endophenotype for alcoholism (see chapter 20). As yet, few endophenotypes in psychiatric research have been as carefully evaluated to gauge familial transmission.

Targeting Preventive Interventions

Family history is an "exposure" that synthesizes a great deal of information about many genetic and environmental familial causes of a mental disorder (Merikangas 2005). It can be extremely useful. For example, one application is to identify people at high risk for a psychiatric disorder. With appropriate cautions regarding privacy and other ethical concerns, some of these individuals may be targeted for preventive interventions.

In the field of drug addiction, it is feasible to develop psychosocial preventive interventions for high-risk individuals identified early in their life course, before developing drug problems (Ialongo et al. 1999). In this era of genomics and proteomics, it is not unrealistic to think that pharmacologic preventive interventions could also be developed for a subset of these individuals. Drug addiction is a heterogeneous disorder with many environmental causes and probably also many genetic causes. The nature of the causes varies across settings. It is therefore unlikely that any one susceptibility gene for drug addiction would efficiently identify large numbers of very high risk individuals as potential subjects for preventive intervention. The far more accessible measure of family history of drug addiction may better serve the purpose.

Likewise, a family history of depression may be useful for identifying high-risk children. Some studies suggest that being the child of a depressed parent and the grandchild of a depressed grandparent signifies a very high risk for developing psychopathology of various kinds (Weissman et al. 1997; Warner et al. 1999; Weissman et al. 2005). A family history of depression in parents and grandparents is an exposure that is often feasible to measure, and could be used to identify very high risk children potentially in need of monitoring and preventive interventions. Even after specific genes for psychiatric diseases are identified, family history studies will continue to be useful in guiding which family members should undergo and benefit from genetic testing.

Characterizing Effects of Disease Genes

After discovery of a disease-causing gene, investigators characterize its impact in order to draw implications for disease prevention. Initially, these studies may focus on understanding the variety and frequency of mutant alleles of the gene and the associated disease risks. Later, studies may attempt to identify nongenetic causes that could be modified to reduce disease risk among genetically susceptible individuals. As many more genetic effects are discovered, this domain of genetic epidemiology is likely to become increasingly important. Although gene characterization studies can directly examine the gene as a risk factor, the research tends to be multifaceted and interwoven with family history approaches.

To exemplify the advanced stages of gene characterization, we look outside of psychiatric research and turn to research on the *BRCA1* and *BRCA2* genes for breast cancer. A recent study identified 1,008 cases of incident breast cancer among Ashkenazi Jewish women in New York (King et al. 2003). Of these, 104 cases carried a high-risk *BRCA1* or *BRCA2* mutation.[1] The researchers studied the relatives of these 104 cases, collecting data on both genotype and disease history.

Of the 104 index cases with mutations, 52 had no history of breast (or ovarian) cancer in their mothers or sisters. The absence of a family history in these 52 cases might suggest that the effect of the mutation on breast cancer was somewhat lower within the families of these cases. Further detailed studies of these families did not, however, support this interpretation; absence of family history simply reflected paternal inheritance and/or small family size.

---

[1] Specifically, one of three ancient mutations that had been previously described in this population; two were in the *BRCA1* gene, and one was in the later identified *BRCA2* gene.

Next, the researchers explored whether or not the effect of these mutations had changed over time. The data revealed a clear historical trend. Mutation carriers born before 1940 had a lower risk of breast cancer at each age than those born after 1940: that is, they were less likely to have developed breast cancer by any given age. The data also suggested that physical activity in youth had a protective effect. It appeared that the historical trend could be explained in part by a decline in physical activity across the generations. Since physical activity among young women is modifiable, this may prove to be a useful clue to somewhat modifying disease risk among genetically susceptible women.

Exploring Gene-Environment Interactions

Finding environmental causes of mental disorders will depend in part on identifying individuals genetically vulnerable to environmental effects. This means examining whether or not the effects of an environmental exposure differ according to the presence or absence of genetic alleles. We described an example from the Dunedin study in the previous chapter (see table 29.1). When the subjects were divided according to the presence or absence of a specific genetic allele (the s allele), the effect of life events on depression was evident only among the individuals who carried this allele.

Although perhaps ideal, this direct approach is not often feasible, because most genes underlying vulnerability to environmental stimuli are not yet identified. We can, however, use family history data to provide some indication of the presence or absence (or the degree) of genetic influence on a trait.[2] The strategy allows for exploratory analyses that may provide important clues to gene-environment interactions.

Family history data were used for this purpose in a longitudinal study in Denmark of individuals who had two parents, one parent, or no parent with a schizophrenia spectrum disorder (Parnas et al. 1993). Obstetric data were obtained from midwifery records. The study assessed the effects of family history and of birth complications on the outcome of structural brain abnormalities (the sample was too small to examine the outcome of schizophrenia). The results suggested that there was a positive interaction between family history and birth complications on some brain abnormalities, notably ventricular enlargement, which are associated with schizophrenia.

Establishing Familial Aggregation

Today, complex traits are generally assumed to be influenced by genetic makeup, but the family history study is still useful for gauging the size of the family history effect. As we next describe the designs of family history studies, we give examples of studies used for this purpose.

---

[2] Especially with extension to second- and third-degree relatives, more than one relative may have the disorder. The family history exposure might then be considered as a continuous variable.

The Designs of Family History Studies

In a family history cohort study, as in any cohort study, one begins with disease-free individuals, defines each individual as exposed or unexposed (based on the presence or absence of a family history of disease, usually in first-degree relatives), and then compares the subsequent risk of the disease in the exposed and unexposed groups. When feasible, this design is well suited to most questions posed by family history studies. Nonetheless, the cohort design is not often used in family history studies. It tends to be difficult to implement and takes a long time to complete.[3]

Table 30.1 shows a cohort study that investigated the relation of parental to offspring alcohol use (Gleiberman et al. 1991). Three member sets of father, mother, and young adult son or daughter were assessed in 1960. The offspring were assessed again in 1977 when their age was similar to their parents' age in 1960. For illustration, we focus on exposure to high-volume drinking fathers.[4] (The number exposed to high-volume drinking mothers was very small.) The drinking patterns of offspring exposed and unexposed to high-volume drinking fathers were similar in 1960 (6% versus 5% became high-volume drinkers), but differed in 1977 (33% versus 18% became high-volume drinkers). The result is intriguing in that the effect of paternal family history increased over the adult life course of the offspring.

In a case-control family history study, one begins with cases and controls as the index subjects. As in any case-control study, these are thought of as

Table 30.1 Example of a Family History Study with a Cohort Design

Source	Study Description and Selected Findings
Gleiberman et al. (1991)	*Study*: Investigated the relation of parental to offspring drinking in a subsample of the Tecumseh, Michigan, longitudinal study. The sample comprised 190 three-member sets of father, mother, and adult son or daughter. All three members were interviewed about drinking patterns in 1960; the offspring were interviewed again about drinking patterns in 1977. Here we restrict attention to the outcome of high-volume drinking, defined in this study as more than two drinks daily for men and more than one drink daily for women. We compare high-volume drinking in offspring exposed and unexposed to high-volume drinking fathers.
	Exposed (N = 18): Father reported high-volume drinking in 1960.
	Unexposed (N = 172): Father did not report high-volume drinking in 1960.
	Finding: The exposed and unexposed offspring did not differ in high-volume drinking in 1960 (6% versus 5%), but did differ in 1977 (33% versus 18%).

[3] In theory, a family history cohort study could be designed as a historical cohort study (defined in chapter 10), which would greatly reduce the time required to complete it. In practice, this is rarely done, because investigators are reluctant to rely entirely on historical records of disease for ancestors to define the exposed and unexposed groups.

[4] To prevent misinterpretation, we note that while high-volume drinking is a health outcome of interest, it does not signify abuse or dependence.

being derived from a real or imagined underlying cohort (chapter 15).[5] Each case and control is defined as exposed or unexposed, according to the presence or absence of a family history of disease (usually in first-degree relatives). In a case-control study, one can answer this question: how much does having a family history of disease increase the odds of developing the disease? This is a key question for genetic counselors and clinicians, and for the design of preventive interventions.

A study that compared people with Alzheimer's disease with matched controls is shown in table 30.2 (Graves et al. 1990). We previously used this study to exemplify the case-control design (chapter 16) and the analysis of matched data (chapter 25), but focused on the finding that head trauma was a risk factor for Alzheimer's disease. The cases and controls were also assessed for the presence (or absence) of family history, defined as having (or not having) a first-degree biological relative with dementia. The odds ratio was 2.2, indicating that having a family history of dementia was also a risk factor for Alzheimer's disease.

A third design, which we term the **reconstructed cohort** (Susser and Susser 1989), is a hybrid. This design begins with cases and controls as the index subjects. The cases and controls are used, however, to define their relatives as exposed or unexposed, and the data are analyzed in the form of a cohort study. The cohort of relatives is reconstructed in the sense that these persons

Table 30.2 Example of a Family History Study with a Case-control Design

Source	Study Description and Selected Findings
Graves et al. (1990)	*Study*: Compared Alzheimer's disease cases and normal controls with respect to presence or absence of dementia in first-degree relatives.
	Cases (N = 130): Individuals diagnosed with Alzheimer's disease between 1980 and 1985 at two hospitals in Washington state. Information was obtained from surrogate respondents (i.e., spouses and children).
	Controls (N = 130): Friends or nonbiological relatives of cases matched on age and sex. Information was obtained from surrogate respondents; control surrogates were matched to case surrogates on relationship to study subject.
	Finding: Having a first-degree relative with dementia was a risk factor for Alzheimer's disease (OR = 2.21).

Note: OR = odds ratio.

[5] Note that for a family history case-control study to be nested in a family history cohort study it must use the same definition of family history as the cohort study. For example, if in the cohort study the family history exposure is defined as disease in one or both parents, then in the case-control study it must be defined likewise as disease in one or both parents. Similarly, if the family history is defined as disease in first-degree relatives in the cohort study, then it must be defined likewise as disease in first-degree relatives in the case-control study. When the same definition of exposure is used, the cohort and case-control studies are counterparts as in any other context and will produce the same result for the odds ratio (Zimmerman 2003).

are included in the study (that is, constructed as a cohort) because of their related index case or control. The disease status of the index study subject defines the exposure status (presence or absence of a family history) of each person in his or her family. In sum, researchers use the same people as in the case-control study, but the cases and controls define exposure and their relatives are the exposed and unexposed cohorts.

Two recent examples of reconstructed cohort studies are shown in table 30.3. One of these studies found a fourfold elevated risk of obsessive-compulsive disorder among case relatives, as compared to control relatives (Nestadt et al. 2000). The other found a threefold elevated risk of substance use disorders among case relatives, as compared to control relatives (Merikangas et al. 1998).

What is achieved by looking at case and control relatives as the exposed and unexposed groups of a reconstructed cohort study? One advantage over the case-control study is that we can answer a wider range of questions, obtaining risks, risk ratios, and odds ratios. It is possible to estimate the absolute risk of disease, given exposure (or lack of exposure), which can be very useful to medical follow-up and design of interventions. Another advantage is that the investigator can make use of survival analysis, which is not applicable in case-control studies. In the case-control approach, differences in age between case and control relatives can lead to differences in detection of the family history exposure for cases and controls, or differential misclassification (chapter 16). Similarly, absent adjustment, differences in family size

Table 30.3 Examples of Family History Studies with a Reconstructed Cohort Design

Sources	Study Description and Selected Findings
Nestadt et al. (2000)	*Study*: Compared first-degree relatives of OCD cases and normal controls with respect to risk for OCD.
	Exposed (N = 343): First-degree relatives of 80 cases with OCD. Cases were ascertained from five specialty OCD treatment clinics in the Baltimore, MD, and Washington, DC, area.
	Unexposed (N = 300): First-degree relatives of 73 controls. Controls selected via random-digit dialing from the same area and matched to cases on sex, race, and age and whether medical care had been received in the preceding year.
	Finding: the prevalence of OCD was higher in relatives of OCD cases than in the relatives of normal controls (11.7% vs. 2.7%).
Merikangas et al. (1998)	*Study*: Compared first-degree relatives of individuals with substance use disorder (i.e., drug and alcohol) and normal controls with respect to risk of substance use disorders.
	Exposed (N = 1,012): First-degree relatives of 238 cases with a substance use disorder recruited from outpatient substance disorders clinics in greater New Haven, CT, area.
	Unexposed (N = 255): First-degree relatives of 61 controls selected via random-digit dialing from same area as cases.
	Finding: The prevalence of substance use disorders was higher in the relatives of cases than in the relatives of controls (9.1% vs. 3.1%).

for cases and controls can lead to differential misclassification. On the other hand, the reconstructed cohort study uses a single individual (case or control) to measure the family history exposure, whereas the case-control study uses all first-degree relatives to measure the family history exposure; in this sense, the measure of exposure in the case-control study is more precise if family size and age structure are the same (Zimmerman 2003).

An advantage of the reconstructed cohort over the ordinary prospective cohort study is that the reconstructed cohort study is easier to implement and can be completed in a much shorter time. In addition, it is generally feasible to include several generations in the reconstructed cohort. Ancestors, siblings, and descendants of the cases and controls can all be included. On the other hand, the design is not as tight or transparent as an ordinary cohort study, in which one first defines the exposed and unexposed groups, and then follows them over a specified time period.

Relationships among the Designs

Despite its potential advantages, the use of the prospective cohort study is limited because of time, expense, and feasibility. Most often, the choice is between the reconstructed cohort study and the case-control study. We have noted that the same people are used in the reconstructed cohort and the case-control designs but that the analysis is different. The results are usually but not necessarily similar. Therefore, it is important to understand the relationship between these analytic approaches.

We posit a nested case-control design, in which we use all the cases from a longitudinal cohort study and select the controls as a random sample of the noncases in the cohort. Suppose we select from the underlying cohort the 10 female cases and 10 female controls exhibited in figure 30.1. We accurately determine the presence or absence of disease in their biological parents and siblings. Each case and control has one male and one female sibling.

Analyzing these simple data in the form of a case-control study, we would examine whether the odds of a positive family history (exposure) among index cases differs from the odds of a positive family history (exposure) among index controls. If we define a positive family history (i.e., being exposed) as having any parent or sibling affected, the traditional odds ratio is 6 (figure 30.1). As in any case-control study, we would expect this odds ratio to be the same, within sampling variation, as the odds ratio in the underlying cohort from which the cases and controls were derived.

Now suppose we analyze the same data in figure 30.1 as a reconstructed cohort study. Note that the cases and controls define both their parents and siblings to be exposed or unexposed. This may appear to violate the requirement that exposure antedate disease. However, it does not, as the disease status of the study subjects is being used as a proxy for the ongoing presence (or absence) of the genetic factor in the family (Susser and Susser 1989). The odds ratio for the reconstructed cohort is 5.6, and the risk ratio is 5 (figure 30.1).

The odds ratios for the case-control and reconstructed cohort study are different. Although we are analyzing the same people, they are in different

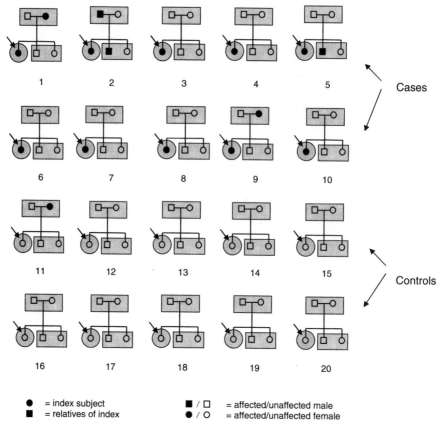

Analyzed as a case control study
- 10 cases: 4 "exposed" (i.e., have an affected relative) (#1, #2, #5 and #9)
- 10 controls: 1 is "exposed" (i.e., has an affected relative) (#11)

	Diseased	Non-diseased	Total		
Exposed	4	1	5	OR =	6.0
Unexposed	6	9	15		
	10	10	20		

Analyzed as a reconstructed cohort study
- 40 cohort members are "exposed" (i.e., relatives of index cases): 5 have disease
- 40 cohort members are "unexposed" (i.e., relatives of index controls): 1 has disease

	Diseased	Non-diseased	Total		
Exposed	5	35	40	OR =	5.6
Unexposed	1	39	40	RR =	5.0
	6	74	80		

Figure 30.1 Analysis of the same data as a case-control and a reconstructed cohort study. Hypothetical study with 20 female index subjects (10 cases, 10 controls). Both parents and two siblings of each index subject were assessed.

roles. Thus, the family members who define exposure and those who define disease outcome are reversed. The index cases and controls, who represent the outcome in the case-control study, represent the exposure in the reconstructed cohort. The relatives, who define the exposure in the case-control study, define the outcome in the reconstructed cohort.

The reconstructed cohort is a legitimate cohort, but it is *not* the underlying cohort in which the case-control study is nested (Zimmerman 2003). The expected odds ratio for the case-control study is the same as for its underlying cohort, but that underlying cohort is not the reconstructed cohort. Hence, the odds ratios from these two analytic approaches are not necessarily the same.

In choosing the most appropriate analysis, the investigator will need to weigh many factors. The reconstructed cohort study would be used to answer questions that require computation of risks, as well as risk ratios. When odds ratios are of interest, both approaches may be used and the two results may be compared. The reconstructed cohort odds ratio may be either smaller or greater than the case-control odds ratio, depending upon the degree of genetic heterogeneity, the magnitude of genetic versus environmental effects, other factors that influence the clustering of disease in the families of the index subjects, and the different precision with which the family history exposure is measured in the two designs, as has been explained (Zimmerman et al. 2003).

One also considers the many practical issues in implementing these studies that could lead to bias (Ottman and Susser 1992; Haines et al. 1998; Fyer and Weissman 1999), and the analysis of family history data, not discussed here, including computation of confidence intervals for measures of effect, accounting for correlated outcomes within a family (see chapter 25), and, when appropriate, statistical modeling, such as survival analysis (see chapter 27; for a good discussion of analytic methods, see Thomas 2004). The best choice may not be clear-cut. What is most important is that the investigator understand the relationship between the two designs, which makes it possible to weigh these various factors within a logical framework.

We have discussed these designs with the presumption that the same phenotype is used to define both the risk factor (family history) and the outcome. It is also possible, of course, to conduct family history studies in which the phenotype defining the risk factor is not the same as the phenotype defining the outcome. This has been done in some nonpsychiatric illnesses—for example, in examining the phenotype of colorectal polyp in relation to family history of colorectal cancer (Ahsan et al. 1998). This may also be done in a study of a spectrum of genetically related conditions, or in a study designed to clarify the relationship between a putative endophenotype and a disorder.

Conclusion

Family history studies are now used for a much wider range of purposes than in the past. In this chapter, we have discussed their usefulness for refining phenotype definitions, targeting preventive interventions, characterizing genetic effects, and exploring gene-environment interaction. These are in addition to their original role in genetic research, which was to examine whether diseases aggregate in families. We have also elaborated their relationship to the risk factor designs described in previous chapters.

Family studies rely on a broad concept of genetic effects. They do not differentiate genetic and nongenetic contributions to familial clustering. Despite or perhaps because of these features, they make a unique contribution to understanding the genetic causes and the prevention of complex psychiatric diseases.

References

Ahsan H, Neugut AI, Garbowski GC, Jacobson JS, Forde KA, Treat MR, and Waye JD (1998). Family History of Colorectal Adenomatous Polyps and Increased Risk for Colorectal Cancer. *Ann. Intern. Med.* 128:900–905.

Bolton P, Macdonald H, Pickles A, Rios P, Goode S, Crowson M, Bailey A, and Rutter M (1994). A Case-Control Family History Study of Autism. *J. Child Psychol. Psychiatry* 35:877–900.

Crow JF (1997). The High Spontaneous Mutation Rate: Is It a Health Risk? *Proc. Natl. Acad. Sci. USA* 94:8380–8386.

Cui J and Hopper JL (2000). Why Are the Majority of Hereditary Cases of Early-Onset Breast Cancer Sporadic? A Simulation Study. *Cancer Epidemiol. Biomarkers Prev.* 9:805–812.

Fletcher NA and Marsden CD (1996). Dyskinetic Cerebral Palsy: A Clinical and Genetic Study. *Dev. Med. Child Neurol.* 38:873–880.

Fyer AJ and Weissman MM (1999). Genetic Linkage Study of Panic: Clinical Methodology and Description of Pedigrees. *Am. J. Med. Genet.* 88:173–181.

Gleiberman L, Harburg E, Di Franceisco W, and Schork A (1991). Familial Transmission of Alcohol Use: IV. A Seventeen-Year Follow-Up on the Relationships between Parent and Adult Offspring Alcohol Use; Tecumseh, Michigan. *Int. J. Epidemiol.* 20:441–447.

Gottesman II and Shields J (1982). *Schizophrenia: The Epigenetic Puzzle*. Cambridge: Cambridge University Press.

Graves AB, White E, Koepsell TD, Reifler BV, van Belle G, Larson EB, and Raskind M (1990). A Case-Control Study of Alzheimer's Disease. *Ann. Neurol.* 28:766–774.

Haines JL and Pericak-Vance M, eds. (1998). *Approaches to Gene Mapping in Complex Human Diseases*. New York: Wiley-Liss Publishing.

Ialongo NS, Werthamer L, Kellam SG, Brown CH, Wang S, and Lin Y (1999). Proximal Impact of Two First-Grade Preventive Interventions on the Early Risk Behaviors for Later Substance Abuse, Depression, and Antisocial Behavior. *Am. J. Community Psychol.* 27:599–641.

Kalachikov S, Evgrafov O, Ross B, et al. (2002). Mutations in *LGI1* Cause Autosomal-Dominant Partial Epilepsy with Auditory Features. *Nat. Genet.* 3:335–341.

Kendler KS, Neale MC, and Walsh D (1995). Evaluating the Spectrum Concept of Schizophrenia in the Roscommon Family Study. *Am. J. Psychiatry* 152:749–754.

Kety SS, Rosenthal D, Wender PH, Schulsinger F, and Jacobsen B (1976). Mental Illness in the Biological and Adoptive Families of Adopted Individuals Who Have Become Schizophrenic. *Behav. Genet.* 6:219–225.

Khoury MJ, Cohen BH, and Beaty TH (1993). *Fundamentals of Genetic Epidemiology*. Oxford: Oxford University Press.

King MC, Lee GM, Spinner NB, Thomson G, and Wrensch MR (1984). Genetic Epidemiology. *Annu. Rev. Public Health* 5:1–52.

King MC, Marks JH, and Mandell JB (2003). Breast and Ovarian Cancer Risks Due to Inherited Mutations in *BRCA1* and *BRCA2*. *Science* 302:643–646.

Malaspina D, Harlap S, Fennig S, Heiman D, Nahon D, Feldman D, and Susser E (2001). Advancing Paternal Age and the Risk of Schizophrenia. *Arch. Gen. Psychiatry* 58:361–367.

McGuffin P and Huckle P (1990). Simulation of Mendelism Revisited: The Recessive Gene for Attending Medical School. *Am. J. Hum. Genet.* 46:994–999.

Merikangas K (2005). Bridging Genetics and Epidemiology of Mental Disorders. In Zorumski CF and Rubin EH, eds., *Psychopathology in the Genome and Neuroscience Era*. Arlington, VA: American Psychiatric Publishing.

Merikangas KR, Stolar M, Stevens DE, Goulet J, Preisig MA, Fenton B, Zhang H, O'Malley SS, and Rounsaville BJ (1998). Familial Transmission of Substance Use Disorders. *Arch. Gen. Psychiatry* 55:973–979.

Nestadt G, Samuels J, Riddle M, Bienvenu OJ, III, Liang KY, LaBuda M, Walkup J, Grados M, and Hoehn-Saric R (2000). A Family Study of Obsessive-Compulsive Disorder. *Arch. Gen. Psychiatry* 57:358–363.

Ottman R, Annegers JF, Risch N, Hauser WA, and Susser M (1996a). Relations of Genetic and Environmental Factors in the Etiology of Epilepsy. *Ann. Neurol.* 39:442–449.

Ottman R, Lee JH, Hauser WA, Risch N (1998). Are Generalized and Localization-Related Epilepsies Genetically Distinct? *Arch. Neurol.* 55:339–344.

Ottman R, Lee JH, Risch N, Hauser WA, and Susser M (1996b). Clinical Indicators of Genetic Susceptibility to Epilepsy. *Epilepsia* 37:353–361.

Ottman R and Susser M (1992). Data Collection Strategies in Genetic Epidemiology: The Epilepsy Family Study of Columbia University. *J. Clin. Epidemiol.* 45:721–727.

Parnas J, Cannon TD, Jacobsen B, Schulsinger H, Schulsinger F, and Mednick SA (1993). Lifetime *DSM-III-R* Diagnostic Outcomes in the Offspring of Schizophrenic Mothers. Results from the Copenhagen High-Risk Study. *Arch. Gen. Psychiatry* 50:707–714.

Piven J, Palmer P, Jacobi D, Childress D, and Arndt S (1997). Broader Autism Phenotype: Evidence from a Family History Study of Multiple-Incidence Autism Families. *Am. J. Psychiatry* 154:185–190.

Rousseau F, Bonaventure J, Legeai-Mallet L, Pelet A, Rozet JM, Maroteaux P, Le Merrer M, and Munnich A (1994). Mutations in the Gene Encoding Fibroblast Growth Factor Receptor-3 in Achondroplasia. *Nature* 371:252–254.

Susser E and Susser M (1989). *Familial Aggregation Studies. A Note on Their Epidemiologic Properties*. *Am. J. Epidemiol.* 129:23–30.

Susser M and Susser E (1987). Indicators and Designs in Genetic Epidemiology: Separating Heredity and Environment. *Rev. Epidemiol. Sante Publique* 35:54–77.

Susser M and Susser E (1988). Separating Heredity and Environment: Research Designs and Strategies. In Henderson AS and Burrows GD, eds., *Handbook of Social Psychiatry*, 117–134. New York: Elsevier.

Thomas DC (2004). *Statistical Methods in Genetic Epidemiology*. New York: Oxford University Press.

Warner V, Weissman MM, Mufson L, and Wickramaratne PJ (1999). Grandparents, Parents, and Grandchildren at High Risk for Depression: A Three-Generation Study. *J. Am. Acad. Child Adolesc. Psychiatry* 38:289–296.

Weissman MM, Merikangas KR, John K, Wickramaratne P, Prusoff BA, and Kidd KK (1986). Family-Genetic Studies of Psychiatric Disorders. Developing Technologies. *Arch. Gen. Psychiatry* 43:1104–1116.

Weissman MM, Warner V, Wickramaratne P, Moreau D, and Olfson M (1997). Offspring of Depressed Parents. 10 Years Later. *Arch. Gen. Psychiatry* 54:932–940.

Weissman MM, Wickramaratne P, Adams PB, Lish JD, Horwath E, Charney D, Woods SW, Leeman E, and Frosch E (1993). The Relationship between Panic Disorder and Major Depression. A New Family Study. *Arch. Gen. Psychiatry* 50:767–780.

Weissman MM, Wickramaratne P, Nomura Y, Warner V, Verdeli H, Pilowsky DJ, Grillon C, and Bruder G (2005). Families at High and Low Risk for Depression: A 3-Generation Study. *Arch. Gen. Psychiatry* 62:29–36.

Winawer MR, Ottman R, Hauser WA, and Pedley TA (2000). Autosomal Dominant Partial Epilepsy with Auditory Features: Defining the Phenotype. *Neurology* 54:2173–2176.

Zimmerman R (2003). Familial Aggregation Study Designs: Causes of Discrepancies in Case Control and Reconstructed Cohort Effect Estimates. Doctoral Dissertation, Columbia University, 126pp. UMI Microform 3071403.

Twin Studies of Heritability

31

Sharon Schwartz and Ezra Susser

Effective partnerships between epidemiologists and geneticists require careful consideration of heritability studies, a central tool for investigating the causes of disease in human populations. Although the heritability study has been applied in many health domains, the application to mental health has been the most far-reaching. Indeed, a discipline of **behavioral genetics** has emerged that specializes in applying these designs to study the causes of mental traits and disorders.

Although the concepts underlying heritability studies can be traced back over a century, study designs to assess heritability crystallized in parallel with population-based risk factor designs in the 1960s and thereafter. An early wave of studies using these designs provided compelling evidence for genetic effects on many diseases (e.g., on schizophrenia, as reviewed by Gottesman and Shields, 1982). Recently, another wave of findings has suggested that genetic influences are even more wide-ranging and powerful than was previously understood (Rutter 2004).

Behavioral geneticists have also generated significant, if controversial, findings on nongenetic causation. Findings from heritability studies of twins have been interpreted to mean that shared family environment has only weak effects on mental traits and disorders (Reiss et al. 1991; Plomin et al. 2000). By contrast, cohort and case-control studies of the same outcomes often point to just the opposite conclusion, that the shared family environment has very powerful effects. This discrepancy between the results of heritability studies and epidemiologic designs raises interesting methodological issues that are a central focus of this chapter.

In accord with our stance throughout this section of the book, we will focus on the basic principles of the heritability design. We limit discussion to heritability studies of twins, which we will use as a prototype. We also limit discussion to a categorical disease outcome. Henceforth we refer to this design simply as a twin study, although there are other kinds of both twin and heritability studies. (For a wider perspective on heritability and twin studies, see Gottesman 1991; Torrey et al. 1994; Plomin et al. 2000; Purcell 2002; Purcell and Sham 2002.) We first describe the twin study, a type of natural experiment (chapter 10) and explain how it can estimate the contributions of genetic and environmental causes of a disorder. Then we compare the twin studies to risk factor designs. We propose a reason that these approaches can yield different results for the effect of shared family environment.

Prototypical Twin Study

The twin study we use as a prototype begins by identifying affected probands who are members of a twin pair. The design requires affected probands from both monozygotic (MZ) and dizygotic (DZ) twin pairs. The presence or absence of the disorder in the co-twins of these affected probands is assessed. A co-twin who also has the disorder is concordant with the affected proband, whereas a co-twin without the disorder is discordant with the affected proband.

The co-twins' outcomes are used to compute concordance and discordance proportions for MZ twins and for DZ twins.[1] The MZ concordance in the sample is the percentage of MZ probands whose co-twin is concordant for the disorder. Similarly, the MZ discordance is computed as the percentage of MZ probands whose co-twin is discordant for the disorder. Since twin pairs are either concordant or discordant, the concordance and discordance of MZ pairs must sum to 100 percent, or in terms of proportions must sum to one. The DZ concordance and DZ discordance are computed in the same way and, likewise, sum to one. As will be seen, these concordance and discordance proportions are used to determine the relative roles of genetic and environmental contributions in the development of a disease. As shown in table 31.1, this basic approach has been used to investigate a wide range of psychiatric disorders, including panic disorders (Kendler et al. 1993), autism (Bailey et al. 1995), drug abuse (Tsuang et al. 1996), and schizophrenia (Cannon et al. 1998).

Causal Components

The twin study conceptualizes the causes of interindividual variation in disease in terms of three broad components: genes, shared environment, and unique environment. Like a family history (or familial aggregation) study, a twin study evaluates the contribution of the genetic component as a whole. It does not attempt to differentiate the effects of specific genes. A twin study attempts to move a step beyond the family history study, however, by separating the contributions of genes from those of the environment.

To illustrate this strategy most simply, we will follow an approach often used in behavioral genetics: we will assume an additive polygenic model in which many genes contribute to disease. The greater the number of disease-causing alleles inherited by an individual, the greater the disease risk. (This model is

---

[1] Twin studies nowadays use more sophisticated statistical techniques, such as correlations, rather than simple concordance measures. In addition, there are different methods (e.g., pairwise versus probandwise) to calculate concordance. Nonetheless, the logic behind twin analyses is the same, regardless of the particular statistical methods used. We will discuss concordance estimates calculated as described in the text throughout for clarity.

Table 31.1 Heritability Studies

Sources	Study Description and Selected Findings
Kendler et al. (1993)	*Study*: Investigated genetic hypothesis of panic disorder.
	Twin pairs (N = 1,033 female twin pairs): Population-based ascertainment.
	Finding: The concordance for panic disorder was 24% and 11% in MZ and DZ twin pairs.
Bailey et al. (1995)	*Study*: Investigated genetic hypothesis of autism.
	Twin pairs (N = 44 sets of twins and triplets): Clinic-based ascertainment.
	Finding: The concordance for autism was 73% and 0% in MZ and DZ twin pairs.
Tsuang et al. (1996)	*Study*: Investigated genetic hypothesis of drug abuse and dependence.
	Twin pairs (N = 3,372 male twin pairs): Military record registry ascertainment.
	Finding: The concordance for drug abuse was 26% and 16% in MZ and DZ twin pairs.
Cannon et al. (1998)	*Study*: Investigated genetic hypothesis of schizophrenia.
	Twin pairs (N = 7,873 twin pairs): Population-based ascertainment.
	Finding: The concordance for schizophrenia was 46% and 9% in MZ and DZ twin pairs.

for illustrative purposes; for discussion of polygenic models, see Risch 2000.) Under this polygenic model, the MZ co-twin of an affected proband shares all the disease-causing genes inherited by the proband. Basic Mendelian laws of inheritance tell us that, on average, DZ co-twins share 50 percent of their genes. Therefore, on average, DZ co-twins of affected probands share 50 percent of the disease-causing genes inherited by the proband.

Thus, the twin study can be thought of as defining two different doses of exposure to the disease-causing genes. The MZ co-twin of an affected proband receives a full dose, and the DZ co-twin of an affected proband receives half a dose. Although each disease-causing gene makes a separate contribution, the genetic component can be thought of as a dose of the genetic effect, without our differentiating the specific genes in terms of the strength or nature of their effect.

The twin study conceptualizes shared environment and unique environment in an equivalent way. **Shared environment** comprises the totality of nongenetic causes that are shared by both members of a twin pair—for example, the parenting styles and the socioeconomic status of their parents.[2]

---

[2] As discussed later, this is the conceptual meaning of *shared environment*. As actually estimated in twin studies, *shared environment* refers strictly to environmental factors that make twins more alike.

The members of a twin pair are, by definition, exposed to the same shared environment. The remaining, nonshared environment is referred to as **unique environment**. The unique environment encompasses all the nongenetic disease-causing factors that differ for members of the same twin pair: for instance, they may receive different shares of the maternal blood flow in utero, go to different schools, or have different kinds of friends.

Necessary Assumptions

There are several assumptions necessary to utilize this conceptual schema to separate genetic from environmental effects. One assumption is that there is no assortative mating. This means that we assume people do not select their spouses in a way that increases their genetic similarity—for example, by choosing a spouse on the basis of a shared disorder. Assortative mating is difficult to measure and probably more common than is recognized for traits influencing mental health (Merikangas 1982). Assortative mating increases the genetic similarity of DZ twins. Under this condition they would share, on average, more than half their genes.

A second assumption is that there are no interactions among genes (epistasis), among environments, or between genes and environments; we will return later in the chapter to discuss the implications of this assumption.

A third, the **equal environment** assumption, is that MZ twin pairs share their environment to the same degree as DZ twin pairs. We will revisit this assumption later in the chapter and show that its meaning is much more subtle than it appears on first impression. For now, note that, although this assumption is often reasonable, there are many ways in which it can be violated at every stage of the life cycle. During the prenatal period, for example, MZ twin pairs differ from DZ twin pairs in their patterns of sharing the placenta, the main source of sustenance (Moore and Persaud 1993). For this and other reasons, MZ twin pairs tend to share some in utero exposures more and others less than do DZ twin pairs (Torrey et al. 1994). In childhood, parents may treat MZ twins more similarly than parents treat DZ twins, simply because they look more similar (Hopper 1999). In any study, one needs to consider whether the conclusions are affected by violations of the equal environment assumption.

Heritability Analysis

The basic premise of a heritability analysis is that variation in the occurrence of disease within a population can be explained by the variation among individuals in their genes, shared environment, and unique environment.[3] The purpose of a heritability analysis is to estimate what proportion of the total

---

[3] The variance actually comprises not only additive genetic factors, shared environment, and unique environment, but also dominance genetic factors and the covariances among the factors. However, models cannot look at all of these factors simultaneously and typically drop genetic dominance and gene/environment covariance from consideration. See Plomin et al. (2000) for further discussion.

variation in a disease within a given population can be explained by the variation in each of these three components. Since its premise is that the total variation in disease within a population represents the sum of the contributions of these three components, the proportions (or percentages) of variation that they explain must add up to one (or 100 percent).

As an example, consider a well-designed twin study that investigated heritability of drug abuse (table 31.1; Tsuang et al. 1996). This study used MZ and DZ twin pairs ascertained from military records of the U.S. Department of Defense. For abuse of one or more illicit drugs, the authors estimated that the contributions to the total variance were 20 percent for genetic factors, 74 percent for unique environment, and 6 percent for shared environment.

We will explain next how the twin data were used to arrive at these estimates. Note, however, that the results suggested that shared environment makes little contribution to the variance. Yet risk factor studies suggest that shared environment, such as shared access to drugs, can be very important in explaining variation in drug abuse (Anthony and Helzer 1995).

Procedures of Heritability Analysis

Although different approaches may be used to estimate the proportions of variance attributable to each of the three causal categories, the principles underlying all of them are essentially the same. The three components of the variance are symbolized by h^2 for genetic, c^2 for shared environmental, and e^2 for unique environmental factors. The term **heritability** is sometimes used to refer to h^2. It is important to note that in the prototypic twin design these components of variance—genetic factors, shared environment, and unique environment—are not directly measured. Rather, their influences are estimated from an examination of the patterns of concordance and discordance among pairs of MZ and DZ twins, as summarized in figure 31.1.

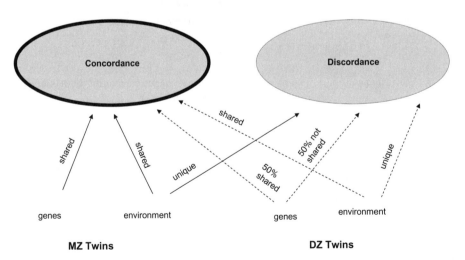

Figure 31.1 Sources of concordance and discordance in MZ and DZ twin pairs.

Within MZ twin pairs, because the twins share all their genes, genetic factors can contribute only to concordance. Any disease-causing gene present in the proband must also be present in the co-twin and increase the probability that the co-twin also has the disorder. Similarly, a premise of the analysis is that shared environmental factors can contribute only to concordance. Any disease-causing shared environmental factor that is present for the proband is by definition also present for the co-twin. Unique environmental factors, on the other hand, can contribute only to discordance. Any disease-causing unique environmental factor that is present for the proband is by definition absent for the co-twin.

Within DZ twin pairs, the situation is different for genetic factors. DZ twins share, on average, only half of their genes.[4] Therefore, any disease-causing gene can contribute either to concordance (if the twins share the implicated gene), or to discordance (if alleles of the gene are unshared). Genes, on average, will contribute to concordance half of the time and to discordance half of the time. In regard to shared and unique environment, the situation for DZ twins is the same as for MZ twins. By definition, shared environment can contribute only to concordance, and unique environment can contribute only to discordance.

Based on these differences, twin studies enable us to estimate the proportion of total variance attributable to genetic and environmental influences (see table 31.2). The analysis begins by estimating the genetic contribution. Heritability (h^2) is estimated as twice the difference in concordance between MZ and DZ twins. The concordance for MZ twins reflects all the contribution of genes and all the contribution of shared environment to the total

Table 31.2 Partitioning of Variance into Genetic, Shared Environmental, and Unique Environmental Causes

Component	Computation
Heritability (h^2)	2 (MZ concordance – DZ concordance)
	Example: MZ concordance = 0.26
	DZ concordance = 0.16
	2 (0.26 – 0.16) = 0.20
Shared environment (c^2)	MZ concordance – genetic component (heritability, h^2)
	Example: 0.26 – 0.20 = 0.06
Unique environment (e^2)	100% – MZ concordance
	Example: 1 – 0.26 = 0.74

Note: The method presented in this table does not illustrate current approaches to twin analyses. It is a distillation of more complex methods, used here to show the logic of the design.
MZ concordance reflects 100% of the genetic and 100% of the shared environment effects.
DZ concordance reflects 50% of the genetic and 100% of the shared environment effects.
Assumption: Variance reflects effects of genes, shared environment, and unique environment.

[4] Note that this assumes no interaction among genes (epistasis). Epistasis will decrease DZ genetic concordance but will not influence MZ concordance.

variance, whereas the concordance for DZ twins reflects half of the contribution of genes and all the contribution of shared environment. Hence, the difference between the MZ and the DZ concordance will be equal to one-half the genetic contribution to the total variance: $h^2 = 2 \times$ (MZ concordance minus DZ concordance).

To estimate the contribution of the shared environment (c^2), we rely on the fact that shared environment and genes together account for all the MZ concordance. The shared environment effect is what remains after subtraction of the genetic effect from the MZ concordance: $c^2 =$ MZ concordance minus h^2.

The contribution of unique environment (e^2) to the total variance is estimated by the MZ discordance. Only unique environment can contribute to discordance for MZ twins. The MZ discordance and the MZ concordance must sum to one. Consequently, $e^2 =$ MZ discordance = 1 minus MZ concordance. It should be noted that, although this formulation interprets MZ discordance as the effect of unique environment, the MZ discordance also reflects the effects of methodological errors, for instance, misclassification of disease.

For an example of how this is done, we return to the twin study of drug abuse (table 31.1; Tsuang et al. 1996). Table 31.2 shows how the contributions of genes, shared environment, and unique environment could be estimated from the results of this study. The MZ concordance is 26 percent, and the DZ concordance is 16 percent. Based on these concordance figures, the heritability is computed as $2 \times$ (MZ concordance minus DZ concordance) = $2 \times$ (26 percent − 16 percent) = 20 percent. The shared environmental effect is computed as MZ concordance minus h^2 = 26 percent − 20 percent = 6 percent. The unique environmental effect is computed as 100 percent minus the MZ concordance = 100 percent − 26 percent = 74 percent.

Although this basic logic underlies all twin studies, the statistical methods used to calculate the variance components are nowadays more sophisticated than simply examining the relationships among concordance proportions. Because our purpose here is only to clarify the premises of twin studies and to show how these premises can influence the interpretation of the results, we will not discuss these refinements (for a good discussion, see Plomin et al. 2000). Instead we proceed to compare the twin and risk factor designs.

Comparison of Twin and Risk Factor Studies

There are some fundamental similarities between twin and risk factor studies. First, like the risk factor study, the twin study is based on the premise that different kinds of causes (or in epidemiologic parlance, different sufficient causes) can lead to the same disease. Each of the three broadly defined causal factors can contribute to the occurrence of the disease being investigated. The premises are not identical, however, since twin studies are compelled to assume that there is no interaction among the three broadly defined causal factors, whereas risk factor studies do not require this basic assumption. We will return to explain this difference and its implications later in the chapter.

Second, like risk factor studies, twin studies are designed to explain inter-individual variation within specific populations. A heritability analysis does not seek to explain variation in disease rates across populations.

Third, heritability estimates, like risk ratios, are context dependent. For the same outcome, the proportion of the variance due to genes, shared environment, and unique environment will differ across populations. All else being equal, heritability will be lower in more genetically homogenous populations. This effect is seen most easily from an extreme example. If everyone in the population had the same genes, then the genetic factors, however crucial for the disease, would not explain variation in disease risk. Similarly, environmental factors will explain a smaller proportion of the variance in environmentally homogenous groups.

In theory, a study of twins could be conducted as a risk factor study. As we have shown for family history studies (see chapter 30), the risk factor approach can be adapted to a context where genetic cause is very broadly defined as encompassing all genetic factors. In addition, the risk factor approach can be adapted to compare the effects of different doses of such a broadly defined factor. Taking this approach in a twin study, we could simply compare the disease risk in the MZ co-twins (exposed to a full dose of genetic causes) to the disease risk in the DZ co-twins (exposed to half a dose of genetic causes). A risk difference could be computed: MZ co-twin risk minus DZ co-twin risk. It could be interpreted as the effect on disease risk of the extra half a dose received by the MZ co-twins.

In practice, as we have described, twin studies analyze the data from a very different vantage point. Rather than examining the effect of the genetic component on the disease risk, they use a heritability analysis to apportion the variance in disease risk among three causal components. With heritability analysis, the twin study parts company with risk factor epidemiology. What are the corollaries of this divergence?

The Meaning of "Genetic" and "Environmental"

One of the most important corollaries is that the terms *genetic* and *environmental* have a different meaning in twin and risk factor studies. The same effect that is considered genetic in a twin study may be considered environmental in a risk factor study.

At the heart of the problem is that environmental factors in a heritability analysis are not measured directly. Instead, shared environment is a residual cause of variation; that is, it is whatever is left of MZ concordance after subtracting the genetic effects. Similarly, causes of MZ discordance are labeled unique environment without any direct measures of these risk factors.

As a consequence, some factors that epidemiologists have considered environmental factors are implicitly considered genetic factors by behavioral geneticists. To illustrate this point, we refer again to our analysis of a twin study of substance abuse shown in table 31.2. As is the convention, our heritability analysis was conducted under the assumption of equal environment (i.e., MZ and DZ twins share their environments to the same degree). Yet genetic differences between DZ twins may well have led them to different peer groups, resulting in different exposures to drugs. As a result of such genetic effects on the environment, DZ twins may have shared their environments to a lesser degree than MZ twins. Similarly, because of genetic factors, MZ twins may be treated more similarly. Under these conditions, the environmental sharing of MZ and DZ twins are clearly not equal. However, the equal environment assumption as defined in heritability studies may not have been violated. The effects of genes that operate by means of changes in environment are considered in the heritability model to be genetic effects. Within the terms of the twin study design, the analysis of heritability was entirely legitimate.

Nonetheless, this environmental effect would have appeared as a risk factor in a study that directly measured it. For example, a cohort study might compare children who have different peer groups with respect to the risk of drug abuse in adulthood. The peer group would be considered as an environmental risk factor within the context of the study. Thus, the shared environment in a twin study is what would have been shared had there not been any genetic influences on the sharing of environment. In any risk factor study of shared environmental factors, by contrast, we would conceptualize shared environment as what was actually shared by the co-twins. This subtle difference proves crucial to interpretation. However, it is not usually made explicit in heritability analyses.

In the language of behavioral genetics, the effects of many types of gene-environment correlations are considered genetic effects. These correlations include many ways in which genetic factors influence environments. The mediational effects of the environment are discounted when they have a genetic antecedent (Dickens and Flynn 2001; Rutter 2004; Rutter and McGuffin 2004). However, such environmental effects may be effective targets for intervention, despite their genetic origins.

Conversely, in a risk factor study where genetic effects are not measured, confounding by genetic factors may be unrecognized, and genetic effects may be mistaken for environmental effects. If genetic propensity causes both a disease outcome and an environmental exposure, the environmental exposure may be misidentified as a cause. In our hypothetical example of a cohort study of peer groups and drug abuse, a genetic factor with effects on both peer group and drug abuse could be an unmeasured confounder.

To recapitulate, we have suggested that a twin and risk factor study conceptualize and measure the contributions of genes and environments in different ways. These differences can lead to discrepant conclusions about genetic and environmental effects from the two types of studies.

The Result for Shared Environment

Another, closely related corollary of the divergent analytic strategies of twin and risk factor studies is that interactions between genes and environment have different implications for their results. In fact, the validity of the twin study depends on the assumption of no interaction. Herein lies a key to understanding the perplexing differences in the results of twin and risk factor studies on shared environment.

Before explaining the assumption of no interaction, we will reiterate what we mean by interaction, using an example of an interaction between genes and environment. An interaction between genes and environment means that the genetic effect depends on the environment and vice-versa. In part II, we used the example of neural tube defects to illustrate an interaction between genes and environment. In that case, it was hypothesized that a genetic variation increasing the need for folate, coupled with an insufficiency in maternal folate intake, led to neural tube defects. As another example, closer to the realm of behavioral genetics, consider a report from the Dunedin cohort described in chapter 9 (table 9.1; Caspi et al. 2002). The results suggested an interaction between childhood maltreatment and a polymorphism of *MAOA*, a gene related to monoamine oxidase, a neurotransmitter-metabolizing enzyme. The combination of childhood maltreatment and the *MAOA* polymorphism was associated (in males) with higher rates of antisocial and violent behavior in young adulthood. It appeared that the genetic variant had an effect under specific environmental conditions, and the effect of the environment was similarly modified by genetic factors.

The Assumption of No Interaction

Currently, most causal theories of human disease postulate an important role for interactions between genetic and environmental causes. Such interactions are thought to arise in almost every domain of human disease, including cancers, cardiovascular diseases, and autoimmune disorders. Gene-environment interactions may be especially germane to neuropsychiatric disorders (Rutter and McGuffin 2004). They are also thought to influence the distribution of normal traits, including mental and behavioral traits. Like other researchers, most twin researchers subscribe to these theories.

Notwithstanding current theories, in a prototypical twin study we assume no interactions among the component causes of genes, shared environment, and unique environment. More precisely, what we assume is that such interactions do not contribute to variation in the occurrence of a disease within a population.

The fact that the heritability analysis assumes no interaction does not by itself set the twin study apart from other designs. Risk factor researchers frequently assume no interaction between genes and environment, in order to limit the required sample size and simplify the analysis of the data. The effects for the factor examined are therefore the average effects in a population (see chapter 27). Researchers in many other contexts also tend to assume no interaction between genes and environment. Making this assumption does not necessarily undermine a study.

In the context of a heritability analysis, however, the assumption can undermine the validity of the estimate of shared family environment. We explain next why we are compelled to make the assumption of no interaction in a twin study and why it undermines this result.

Implications for Shared Environment

We will begin with a scenario where a heritability analysis can produce the correct result despite the presence of interaction between genes and environment. Consider the example of phenylketonuria (PKU), a disease associated with mental retardation. We use this example because it is exceptional and commonly employed in both behavioral genetics (e.g., Plomin 1990) and epidemiology (e.g., Rothman and Greenland 1998) to illustrate this point.[5]

PKU is caused by recessive inheritance of any of multiple mutations in phenylalanine hydroxylase, leading to an inability to metabolize phenylalanine, an amino acid ubiquitous in the ordinary diet of human populations. PKU is therefore the result of an interaction. It requires the combination of an environmental factor and a genetic factor: the ingestion of phenylalanine in the presence of this phenylalanine hydroxylase mutation. However, the cause of interindividual variation in this disease is solely attributable to the genetic variant because, under ordinary circumstances, ingestion of phenylalanine is universal. In a twin study, we would correctly find that the heritability of this disorder is close to one.

PKU represents a scenario where the environment is known to play an important role. The disease can be prevented in children with two copies of a phenylalanine hydroxylase mutation by modifying their diet. Yet the heritability result would still be correct, in the sense that natural variation in the environment does not explain any variation in disease risk within the population.

In other instances, however, the environmental factors that play a role in disease causation will vary within the population. We described earlier a report of a possible interaction between childhood maltreatment and a genetic polymorphism in the *MAOA* gene; childhood maltreatment does show substantial variation within populations. When this is the case, the interaction between genes and environment will contribute to interindividual variation.

When a gene-environment interaction contributes to interindividual variation, heritability analysis cannot meaningfully apportion the contributions of genes, shared environment, and unique environment. To see why, note that in any interaction the same proportion of variance is explained by both partners in the interaction. If, for example, 80 percent of the variance in a disorder is attributable to a genetic effect and this genetic effect works in tandem with an environmental effect, then that variance is also attributable to the environmental effect. If we were to sum their contributions, we would obtain 80 percent + 80 percent = 160 percent.

One way to make this more understandable is to think about the proportion of the disease that would be prevented through the removal of each partner in the interaction. If the interaction is necessary for expression of, say, 80 percent of the variation of the trait, then removing the genetic factor will prevent 80 percent of the disease. Removing the environmental factor will similarly prevent 80 percent of the disease. Therefore, each factor can legitimately be considered as contributing to 80 percent of the cases of disease.

---

[5] It should be noted, however, that the simple twin design of concern here would not be used to study a disorder like PKU. Because inheritance of PKU is recessive, a heritability model as explained in this chapter would not be an appropriate method of analysis. The heritability analysis described here is based on an underlying polygenic model, not single-gene inheritance. We will overlook this nuance in the presentation and simply treat PKU as if the genetic effect were additive.

At the same time, however, removing both factors will also prevent just 80 percent of the disease (it will not prevent 160 percent).

It may also help to recall our discussion of attributable proportions in part II. We applied exactly the same reasoning to explain why the sum of population attributable proportions can be more than 100 percent for risk factors that interact with one another.[6]

Let us return to our example of the *MAOA* polymorphism and antisocial and violent behavior, but now consider childhood maltreatment as an adverse family environmental factor that varies across twin pairs but is the same for both twins of any one pair. In a MZ twin pair, when the proband has both the genetic factor and is exposed to an adverse family environment, the MZ co-twin will also have both factors, so the interaction will always contribute to MZ concordance. In a DZ twin pair, on the other hand, when the proband both has the genetic factor and is exposed to the adverse family environment, only 50 percent of DZ co-twins will have both factors—that is, if the DZ proband and co-twin inherit the same allele of the gene. So the interaction will contribute to DZ concordance on average in 50 percent of pairs. Thus, the interaction between the genetic factor and the childhood maltreatment contributes twice as much to MZ as to DZ concordance, mimicking a purely genetic effect.

Since the interaction effect mimics a genetic effect in the heritability analysis, it will be counted as part of the genetic contribution to the variance. By contrast, it will not be counted as part of the shared environmental contribution to the variance. Recall that c^2 (shared environment contribution) is obtained by subtracting h^2 (genetic contribution) from the MZ concordance. Consequently, the interaction has already been included as part of the genetic contribution, or h^2, before the shared environmental contribution is estimated. The same argument can be made for many shared environmental factors, social, biological, and psychological.

It can also be shown that interactions between unique (e.g., birth order) and shared environmental factors (family environment) are attributed to unique environment for similar reasons. Further discussion of this point can be found in Schwartz and Susser (in press).

Interaction in Risk Factor Studies

Readers may be wondering at this point why, if the assumption of no interaction damages the analysis of shared family environment in a heritability study, it does not do the same damage in a risk factor study. We have explained that in a heritability analysis the contributions of the three categories of cause are constrained to sum to one. As a result, the effect of an interaction is assigned to just one of the causal categories. If the effect were assigned to both of the

---

[6] Among epidemiologic measures, population attributable proportion is most analogous to estimates derived from a heritability analysis. Attributable proportions, however, are usually estimated for risk factors specifically defined and directly measured (e.g., exposure to nutritional deficiency), rather than for components broadly defined and indirectly measured, such as genes, shared environment, and unique environment.

partners in an interaction, the contributions of the three causal categories to the variance would sum to more than one.

By contrast, in the risk factor approach the effect of an interaction can be assigned to both of the partners in the interaction. We are not apportioning variance and face no constraint about the sum of the contributions. When we estimate population attributable proportion, the risk factor measure most analogous to heritability estimates, we can and often do find that the population attributable proportions for different risk factors sum to more than one.

When we compute a risk ratio, we can examine the average effect of a risk factor across categories of the other factor. Alternatively, if both factors have been measured, we can estimate both their separate and joint effects. For further explanation, see chapter 27 or the more in-depth discussion of interaction in part VIII.

Conclusion

Our purpose in this chapter has been to illuminate the elementary logic behind the twin design and place it in the context of risk factor epidemiology. Heritability and risk factor studies are similar in the kinds of questions they can and cannot aspire to answer. They are both suitable for answering questions about the causes of interindividual variation in a trait or disorder, or in other words, why one individual in a given population has a higher disease risk than another. Neither design is meant to answer questions about variation across societies or over time.

With respect to the shared environment, twin and risk factor designs have approached the estimation of the magnitude of effect in different ways and have sometimes also reached very different conclusions. For psychiatric disorders, in particular, heritability results often suggest a small role for shared environment, whereas risk factor results suggest a large one.

Recent developments in twin designs create a hybrid of risk factor and heritability approaches (Hopper 1999). These designs incorporate explicit measures of environmental factors into twin studies and can therefore examine gene-environment correlations and interactions more effectively. Caution is still warranted, however, because the detection of shared environment is plagued by problems of low power (Hopper 1999) and masked interactions even in these new designs. Nonetheless, the incorporation of explicit measures of the environment in twin designs opens a new realm of possibilities for the integration of genetic and risk factor epidemiology.

References

Anthony JC and Helzer JE (1995). Epidemiology of Drug Dependence. In Tsuang MT, Tohen M, and Zahner GEP, eds., *Textbook in Psychiatric Epidemiology*. New York: Wiley.

Bailey A, Le Couteur A, Gottesman I, Bolton P, Simonoff E, Yuzda E, and Rutter M (1995). Autism as a Strongly Genetic Disorder: Evidence from a British Twin Study. *Psychol. Med.* 25:63–77.

Cannon TD, Kaprio J, Lonnqvist J, Huttunen M, and Koskenvuo M (1998). The Genetic Epidemiology of Schizophrenia in a Finnish Twin Cohort. A Population-Based Modeling Study. *Arch. Gen. Psychiatry* 55:67–74.

Caspi A, McClay J, Moffitt TE, Mill J, Martin J, Craig IW, Taylor A, and Poulton R (2002). Role of Genotype in the Cycle of Violence in Maltreated Children. *Science* 297:851–854.

Dickens WT and Flynn JR (2001). Heritability Estimates versus Large Environmental Effects: The IQ Paradox Resolved. *Psychol. Rev.* 108:346–369.

Gottesman I (1991). *Schizophrenia Genesis: The Origins of Madness.* New York: Freeman.

Gottesman I and Shields J (1982). *Schizophrenia: The Epigenetic Puzzle.* Cambridge: Cambridge University Press.

Hopper J (1999). Why "Common Environmental Effects" Are So Uncommon in the Literature. In Spector T, Sneider H, and MacGregor A, eds., *Advances in Twin and Sib-Pair Analysis.* Cambridge: Cambridge University Press.

Kendler KS, Neale MC, Kessler RC, Heath AC, and Eaves LJ (1993). Panic Disorder in Women: A Population-Based Twin Study. *Psychol. Med.* 23:397–406.

Merikangas KR (1982). Assortative Mating for Psychiatric Disorders and Psychological Traits. *Arch. Gen. Psychiatry* 39:1173–1180.

Moore KL and Persaud TVN (1993). The Placenta and Fetal Membranes. *The Developing Human: Clinically Oriented Embryology.* Philadelphia: Saunders.

Plomin R (1990). *Nature and Nurture: An Introduction to Human Behavioral Genetics.* Pacific Grove, CA: Brooks/Cole Publishing.

Plomin R, DeFries J, McClearn GE, and McGuffin P (2000). *Behavioral Genetics*, 4th ed. New York: Freeman.

Purcell S (2002). Variance Components Models for Gene-Environment Interaction in Twin Analysis. *Twin. Res.* 5:554–571.

Purcell S and Sham P (2002). Variance Components Models for Gene-Environment Interaction in Quantitative Trait Locus Linkage Analysis. *Twin. Res.* 5:572–576.

Reiss D, Plomin R, and Hetherington EM (1991). Genetics and Psychiatry: An Unheralded Window on the Environment. *Am. J. Psychiatry* 148:283–291.

Risch NJ (2000). Searching for Genetic Determinants in the New Millennium. *Nature* 405:847–856.

Rothman KJ and Greenland S (1998). *Modern Epidemiology*, 2nd ed. Philadelphia: Lippincott-Raven.

Rutter M (2004). Pathways of Genetic Influences on Psychopathology. *Eur. Rev.* 12:19–33.

Rutter M and McGuffin P (2004). The Social, Genetic and Developmental Psychiatry Centre: Its Origins, Conception and Initial Accomplishments. *Psychol. Med.* 34:1–15.

Schwartz S and Susser E (2006). The Myth of the Heritability Index. In MacCabe J, O'Daly O, Murray RM, McGuffin P, and Wright P, eds., *Beyond Nature and Nurture in Psychiatry: Genes, Environment and their Interplay.* Oxfordshire, England: Taylor and Francis Books.

Torrey EF, Bowler AE, Taylor EH, and Gottesman II (1994). *Schizophrenia and Manic-Depressive Disorder.* New York: Basic Books.

Tsuang MT, Lyons MJ, Eisen SA, et al. (1996). Genetic Influences on *DSM-III-R* Drug Abuse and Dependence: A Study of 3,372 Twin Pairs. *Am. J. Med. Genet.* 67:473–477.

Genetic Linkage Studies

32

Susan E. Hodge, Habibul Ahsan, Gary A. Heiman, and Ezra Susser

This chapter describes the basic concepts and methods of genetic linkage studies. (Readers already familiar with genetic linkage may proceed directly to the next chapter.) Genetic linkage studies aim to establish the location on the genome, and ultimately the identity, of genes with major effects on disease (Ott 1999). One of the first successful applications of the method was to a neuropsychiatric disorder, Huntington's disease (for a current review, see Tobin and Signer 2000). In 1983, Gusella and colleagues localized, through linkage analysis, a disease gene locus on chromosome 4 and within the next decade the same researchers identified and cloned the disease-causing gene. Linkage methods have subsequently led the way to the identification of genes for several other neuropsychiatric conditions. Notably, linkage studies have identified genes for highly familial forms of Alzheimer's disease (Heston et al. 1991; Schellenberg et al. 1992; Rocchi et al. 2003; Pastor and Goate 2004) and, as previously described (chapter 28), were important in the discovery of the *APOE4* allele as a risk factor for Alzheimer's disease.

We first describe what linkage means and how investigators go about detecting linkage. Then we discuss the causal paradigm of the genetic linkage study and contrast linkage with association studies. Finally, using the example of dystonia, we show how linkage can be interwoven with other designs in the search for genetic causes.

The Concept of Linkage

The concept of genetic linkage is rather different from concepts discussed so far, and quite distinct from the concept of genetic association. The terms *linkage* and *association* are easily confused. In ordinary English, they are more or less interchangeable: we can say, "cigarette smoking has been linked to lung cancer," or equivalently, "cigarette smoking and lung cancer are associated." But, as we will explain, these statements have different meanings in a genetic context.

Genetic linkage refers to a relationship between two loci (i.e., genetic locations) on chromosomes in the human genome. The first locus is the (putative)

disease locus. We do not know where this locus is situated in the genome. In addition, when studying complex diseases, we may not know how the disease is inherited.

The second locus is the **marker locus**, where a unique stretch of DNA sequence is known to be located. The chromosomal locations and allelic forms of genetic markers are known, from the genetic map constructed by the Human Genome Project (Kent et al. 2002; Karolchik et al. 2003; Wheeler et al. 2003). Genes that show considerable allelic variation, making them suitable for use as markers in a linkage study, are referred to as **polymorphic markers**. The marker locus, unlike the disease locus, has known inheritance, and we can usually trace how its alleles are transmitted within a pedigree. This is what gives linkage analysis its power.

In a linkage study, we hypothesize that these two loci are on the same chromosome. If in fact they are on the same chromosome and are close enough together on it, they are *linked* loci.

More precisely, by "close enough" we mean that the two loci experience recombination *less than 50 percent* of the time. **Genetic recombination** refers to the crossing-over (exchange) of genetic material between sister chromatids (homologous pairs from two parents) during meiosis (see, e.g., Jorde et al. 1999; Nussbaum et al. 2001). Geneticists define the **recombination fraction** (often denoted as θ) as the proportion of meioses in which recombination occurs between two loci. This recombination fraction θ, although a probability, also serves as a measure of distance between the two loci in question. Thus, $\theta = 0$ implies that the two loci are extremely close, and θ in the range of 0.001 to 0.01 is considered "tight linkage." The upper limit of θ is not 1.0, as one might expect, but rather 0.5 (50 percent). A θ of 0.5 corresponds to the independent assortment of Mendel's Second Law. When θ equals 0.5, the two loci are unlinked, by definition, whether they are on two different chromosomes, or are on the same chromosome but are far apart on that chromosome.

To test the hypothesis that a disease locus is linked to a marker locus, linkage studies examine the pattern of cosegregation (or coinheritance) of the disease with an allele of a polymorphic marker within a pedigree (or sibship). Cosegregation refers to a situation in which affected individuals in the pedigree share the same allele at the marker locus more often than expected by chance; similarly, unaffected individuals also share (other) alleles at the marker locus more often than expected by chance (see figure 32.1). When a study includes multiple pedigrees or families, the cosegregation is examined within each pedigree; then, eventually, the results may be combined across the pedigrees.

Note that the cosegregation of two linked loci within a pedigree results entirely from their physical proximity on the chromosome, not from any underlying causal process. The marker alleles are not themselves causal genes. A positive finding from linkage analysis implies the existence of a major disease-causing gene located near the marker locus on the chromosome.

An important point, not intuitively obvious, is that it does not matter which allele of the marker gene cosegregates with the disease within a pedigree, just

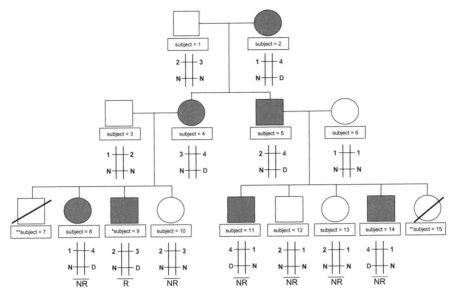

Figure 32.1 The transmission pattern of alleles of a marker locus and a putative disease locus in a hypothetical three-generational pedigree with 15 family members. 1, 2, 3, 4 = alleles of marker locus. D, N = disease (D) and normal (N) alleles of a putative disease locus. *Subject 9 = crossing over between 3-N and 4-D chromosomal segments in meiosis leading to this person. **Subjects 7 and 15 = deceased; no information on disease status or genotype. N, NR = recombinant (R) and nonrecombinant (NR) pattern in grandchildren defined by coinheritance of grandparental disease and marker alleles. Note that allele 4 of marker locus cosegregates with allele D of disease locus, except in subject 9, where because of crossing over between 3-N and 4-D during maternal meiosis, allele 3 cosegregates with D.

that *some* allele consistently cosegregates within any one pedigree. This is because the marker allele does not cause disease, but simply provides a clue to the location of the disease-causing allele. For example, consider the study of Huntington's disease, which originally showed it to be linked to the *G8* locus on chromosome 4 (table 32.1; Gusella et al. 1983). Within some pedigrees, allele *A* of *G8* cosegregated with Huntington's disease; within others, allele *B* of *G8* cosegregated with Huntington's disease. Since the *G8* locus was serving only as a marker of location, it did not matter which allele at that locus happened to be cosegregating with Huntington's disease. This is what we mean by saying that linkage describes a relationship between loci, not between alleles.

The following analogy might help to clarify the concept of linkage. If we were giving someone directions to our house, we might say, "We live near the Lutheran church on the corner." We have nothing to do with the church; it serves merely as a landmark for locating our house. If the church were subsequently converted from, say, Lutheran to Catholic, that change would be irrelevant for our driving directions. It is the location of the church near our

Table 32.1 Examples of Linkage Studies

Sources	Study Description and Selected Findings
Gusella et al. (1983)	*Description*: Performed a linkage analysis with 12 polymorphic markers among two multiplex families (one American and one Venezuelan) of Huntington's disease.
	Finding: Found significant evidence for linkage on chromosome 4. The maximum LOD score was 8.6.
Brzustowicz et al. (2000)	*Description*: Performed a genome-wide scan in 22 multiplex families with schizophrenia.
	Finding: Found highly significant evidence for linkage on chromosome 1 *1q21–q22* region. The maximum heterogeneity LOD score was 6.5.

house, not its denomination, that matters in this context. Analogously, what matters in a linkage study is the location of a marker gene near the disease-causing gene, not the specific allele (or alleles) that happens to cosegregate with the disease in one or more pedigrees.

By contrast, as previously described (chapter 29), a genetic association study may seek to establish a causal relationship between an allele and a disease, often an allele that has a modest effect on disease risk. Clearly, both linkage and association designs are essential tools for elucidating the genetic causes of psychiatric illnesses, but they are applicable in different contexts and answer different questions (see chapter 33).

Detection of Linkage

Most genetic linkage studies collect information on extended pedigrees of affected and unaffected people. Neither unrelated individuals nor pedigrees of only unaffected people are informative for linkage studies. The minimum requirements for linkage analysis include data on disease status and on family relationships within a pedigree, as well as a source of genomic DNA for genotyping marker alleles.

Imagine a three-generation pedigree with 15 family members. Of those 15 people, say that 7 are affected and all 7 inherited the *A* allele at the marker locus, 6 are unaffected and all 6 inherited the *B* allele, and the remaining two are deceased or uninformative. The important information in this example is the consistent cosegregation, in this particular pedigree, of the *A* allele with affectedness and, likewise, the consistent cosegregation of the *B* allele with being unaffected. The *A* allele does not contribute to disease susceptibility; in the next pedigree to enter the study, disease might cosegregate with the *B* allele.

A similar but slightly more realistic scenario is depicted in figure 32.1. Again, the scenario is a three-generational pedigree with 15 family members, of whom 7 are affected, 6 are unaffected, and 2 are deceased and uninformative. We have a more polymorphic marker, with four possible alleles, 1, 2, 3, or 4. Six of the 7 affected family members inherited the 4 allele at the marker locus, along with the D disease allele. Because of a recombination event, the other affected family member (subject 9) inherited the 3 allele, along with the D allele. This pattern would still offer strong evidence for genetic linkage. However, the farther the marker allele is from the disease locus, the more recombination events there will be, and the weaker the cosegregation or linkage of the 4 allele with the D allele.

Genetic linkage studies typically examine a large number of marker loci in this way, to determine whether any of them show evidence of linkage. Genotyping markers on all chromosomes and at multiple sites more or less evenly spaced on each chromosome is referred to as a **genome scan**. Performing a genome scan raises questions of multiple testing. When one examines many loci, there is a higher danger that one of them may happen to cosegregate with the disease by chance alone, not because of linkage. This fact becomes important for interpretation of the results.

A study of schizophrenia offers an example of this type of approach to linkage (table 32.1; Brzustowicz et al. 2000). Notwithstanding the prevailing view that schizophrenia is related to multiple genetic and nongenetic risk factors with small effects, it is plausible that within particular multiply affected pedigrees there may be a major genetic cause (see chapter 33). With this in mind, the authors collected 22 pedigrees, each of which included multiple family members with schizophrenia or schizoaffective disorder. After genotyping the family members on 381 marker loci throughout the genome, the authors examined the cosegregation of alleles at each of the loci with the disease within the pedigrees. They found suggestive evidence that one particular marker locus on the long arm of chromosome 1 might cosegregate with the disease. This suggested that within some of these pedigrees, there might be a major susceptibility gene located in the same chromosomal region.

Another approach to linkage detection relies upon collecting **affected sib pairs** rather than extended pedigrees. If the disease of interest is linked to the marker, then the two affected siblings are likely to share alleles **identical by descent** more often than predicted by Mendelian principles.[1] Affected-sib-pair methods of linkage detection evaluate how many of the affected sib pairs share alleles at the marker locus of interest. A proportion significantly greater than expected provides evidence of linkage. Affected sib pair methods

---

[1] Two individuals share alleles identical by descent (IBD) if those alleles are derived from the same original piece of DNA in a common ancestor. For example, say we are examining a locus with four alleles, a, b, c, and d. Consider Family 1, where the father has genotype ab and the mother has cd, and say they have two children, one ac and the other ad. Those two children share their a alleles IBD because both a alleles were inherited from the same original a allele in the father. Now consider Family 2, where the father has ab and the mother has ac, and they have two children, one ac and the other ab. In this case, the two children do not share their a alleles IBD, because the first child inherited the a from the father, whereas the second child inherited the a from the mother.

are inherently less informative than methods using whole pedigrees (Hodge 2001), but these methods can be useful in some contexts.

Lod Scores

For statistical analyses of linkage data, a *lod score* is used to assess the extent of cosegregation within families or extended pedigrees. *Lod* is an acronym for *log of the odds*. However, strictly speaking, it is not the odds that are used, but the likelihood ratio; and the lod score is actually the log of this likelihood ratio.

In statistical parlance, the likelihood is proportional to the probability of observing the data that have been collected by a study, if a specified hypothesis were true. For example, one might toss a coin three times and get heads each time. Under the hypothesis that the coin is fair (i.e., probability of head = .5), the likelihood of observing this result is proportional to $.5 \times .5 \times .5 = .125$.

To obtain the likelihood ratio used in a linkage analysis, we compute the probability of the observed family (whether extended pedigree, nuclear family, or affected sib pair), first under the hypothesis of linkage, then under the hypothesis of no-linkage. The probability of the observed data under the hypothesis of linkage goes in the numerator, and the probability of the observed data under the hypothesis of no-linkage goes in the denominator. The resultant ratio is the likelihood ratio. A likelihood ratio greater than one means that the data collected had a higher probability of being observed under the hypothesis of linkage than under the hypothesis of no-linkage. (The linkage hypothesis is specified at a particular value of the recombination fraction θ; and the no-linkage hypothesis is specified at $\theta = 1/2$.)

To obtain the lod score, we take the log (to the base 10) of this likelihood ratio. The log of a number greater than one is always positive. Thus, a positive lod score means that the likelihood ratio is greater than one and represents evidence in favor of linkage. (For a further elementary explanation of the principles involved in linkage analysis, see Ott 1999; see also Nussbaum et al. 2001.)

But how strong must that evidence be? A lod score of 3.0 historically has been taken as representing proof of linkage between the indicated disease and the indicated marker locus, at that value of recombination fraction (so long as the finding is also confirmed independently by another group). Note that a lod of 3.0 corresponds to a likelihood ratio of 1000 to one; in other words, the likelihood of linkage is 1000 times greater than the likelihood of no linkage.

Students often confuse the lod scores used in linkage studies with the more familiar *p*-values used in association studies. However, these are quite different concepts. A lod score indicates the relative likelihood of observing the study data under two specified hypotheses. By contrast, as explained in chapter 23, the *p*-value gives the probability of observing either the study data or other data more deviant from the null hypothesis; this probability is calculated under the assumption that the null hypothesis (i.e., no linkage) is true. For further discussion of these points, see Vieland and Hodge (1998) or Ott (1999, chap. 3).

To get a practical feeling for what a lod of 3.0 implies, reconsider the imaginary pedigree of 15 family members already described, in which the 7 affected members all received the A allele at the marker locus, and 6 unaffected members all received the same B allele. The probability of observing this outcome would be reasonably high under the hypothesis of linkage but very low under the hypothesis of no linkage. A family like this could alone yield a lod score as high as 3.0.

The likelihood ratio can also be less than one, in which case the lod score is negative. A negative lod score provides statistical evidence against linkage. Consider the same 15-member pedigree, but this time say that of the 7 affected individuals, 3 get the A and 4 get the B allele; also, among the 6 unaffected people, 3 get the A and 3 get the B. This family would yield negative lod scores and would provide strong evidence against linkage between the disease and that marker.

Causal Paradigm

Genetic linkage methods were originally developed for studying diseases with a single, genetic origin, where the gene is necessary and sufficient to cause disease. These diseases exhibit Mendelian transmission. Huntington's disease, for example, is a dominantly inherited trait with a single mutant allele that is both necessary and sufficient for disease.

In the past 15 years, linkage studies have extended well beyond this original application, to other circumstances in which genes play (or may play) a major but not necessarily decisive role in disease etiology. The method may be apt whenever the gene in question has (or may have) a powerful effect on disease risk within one or more pedigrees selected for study. Linkage detection depends upon consistent cosegregation of the marker allele and the disease within families. Genes that do not exert a major effect on disease within a pedigree do not cosegregate very consistently.

A gene may have a relatively modest influence on disease overall but play a major role in the disease in some families. This can occur if a particularly pathogenic allele of the disease gene occurs in the severely affected families and alleles of more modest effect occur more frequently in the population. This phenomenon is an example of **genetic heterogeneity** (see chapter 33). In such situations, a linkage study can be an effective method for detecting the gene. Evaluating linkage within families reduces heterogeneity. Several strategies are available for this situation, depending on the context and on what is already known about the disease (Risch and Baron 1982; Hodge et al. 1983; Ott 1983; Greenberg and Doneshka 1996).

Linkage may not be the most effective method to detect genes that are hypothesized to have a modest effect on disease risk (Greenberg 1993; Bray and Owen 2001), such as the common genetic polymorphisms described in chapter 29. In these contexts, a genetic allele is usefully conceptualized as a risk factor that is neither necessary nor sufficient to cause disease. Nonetheless, even in these contexts genetic linkage studies can play a key role. As previously described (chapter 28), the late-onset form of Alzheimer's disease was linked to the chromosome *19q13* region, where the gene for apolipoprotein E (*APOE*) is located, and this ultimately led to the identification of the *APOE4* allele as a genetic risk factor for the disease.

Linkage Disequilibrium

Ordinary linkage studies assume that the loci being studied are in **linkage equilibrium** with each other. This means that there is no association between any allele at one locus and any allele at the other locus. (For example, if the disease allele, call it *D,* at the disease locus occurs in 2 percent of the population, it also occurs in 2 percent of individuals who have allele *A* at the marker locus—neither more frequently nor less frequently than 2 percent.) This is why, in a linkage study, we do not care *which* marker allele is cosegregating with the disease within a pedigree, only that *some* allele is cosegregating with the disease. This is also why in one pedigree, allele *A* at the marker locus may cosegregate with the disease, whereas in the next pedigree, it may be allele *B* that cosegregates with the disease.

However, some loci are in **linkage disequilibrium** (LD), which means that a particular allele of one locus and a particular allele at the other locus occur together more frequently than one would expect by chance. LD can (but does not necessarily) occur between loci that are very close together (i.e., very small θ). LD may arise because the relevant mutation at the disease locus occurred relatively recently in genetic history. A new mutation can induce LD, and then subsequent recombination over the generations undoes the LD. Or LD may arise because a certain **haplotype** confers a selective advantage. (For more details on LD, consult a basic medical genetics text, such as Jorde et al. 1999, or Nussbaum et al. 2001, or a population genetics text, such as Hartl and Clark 1997, or Cavalli-Sforza and Bodmer 1999.) For our purposes here, the point is that the existence of LD can benefit some kinds of association studies.

Specifically, in contrast to what we said earlier, when there is LD, disease allele *D* at the disease locus may occur more frequently together with, and be coinherited with, allele *A* at the marker locus. In this case, an association study may detect this association between these two alleles. The association would be due not to a causal effect of allele *A* on disease, but to LD. Since LD generally occurs between only closely linked loci, by indirect reasoning we would conclude that the two loci are linked. Thus, we can sometimes locate disease genes by exploiting LD.

Though we have been at pains to differentiate linkage and association, in this context the two concepts are integrated. On the one hand, LD resembles association, in that one tests whether a particular allele is associated with the disease. On the other hand, LD resembles ordinary linkage, in that no causal relationship is necessarily expected between the allele and the disease.

Example of Dystonia

In practice, genetic linkage studies are often used in conjunction with other designs in the search for genetic causes. We will illustrate how these approaches can be interwoven, using the example of dystonia, a neuropsychiatric condition characterized by twisting movements and abnormal postures (Fahn 1988). In this instance, linkage studies successfully identified a disease gene and also provided clues to a better understanding of the disease spectrum.

For many years, the cause of dystonia was controversial. While some cases of dystonia were known to be due to brain trauma or side effects of certain medications, many cases had no known cause and were classified as idiopathic (Fahn 1988). For this latter group, some researchers and clinicians hypothesized that dystonia was a psychogenic condition (Cleveland 1961; Goetz et al. 2001). Studies of psychiatric symptoms were conducted among individuals with dystonia. The logic behind these studies was that, if dystonia were psychogenic, it would be associated with psychiatric symptoms. Although the results were somewhat inconsistent, the psychiatric studies generally found a higher prevalence of affective and obsessive-compulsive symptoms in individuals with dystonia than in those without (Jahanshahi and Marsden 1988; Bihari et al. 1992; Wenzel et al. 2000).

At about the same time as the earliest psychiatric studies were being conducted, other studies were investigating whether dystonia was an inherited disorder. A study examining all dystonia patients seen in a 25-year period in the greater Indianapolis area hospitals identified six families in which two or more members had dystonia, suggesting that some cases of dystonia could be inherited (Zeman and Dyken 1967). At that time, however, genetic tools were not yet in place to follow up the study of familial aggregation with effective methods to identify a disease gene.

In 1988, a family history study (Bressman 1998) reported that age-adjusted risks for dystonia in first- and second-degree relatives of dystonia patients were 15.5 percent and 6.5 percent, respectively, and concluded that dystonia was most likely inherited as an autosomal dominant with reduced penetrance. The next year, the first reports of genetic linkage appeared. In a large French-Canadian family, the primary dystonia gene (*DYT1*) was mapped to a region on the long arm of chromosome 9 (Ozelius et al. 1989). One year later, linkage to the same region was found in 12 Ashkenazi Jewish families (Kramer et al. 1990).

Next, the gene was localized to a small region of only 150,000 base pairs on chromosome 9 (Ozelius et al. 1992a; Ozelius et al. 1992b). This work took advantage of linkage disequilibrium. In several families, alleles of markers at loci near each other on chromosome 9 formed a haplotype, that is, alleles of markers close to each other on the same chromosome that are inherited together because they are in linkage disequilibrium. The haplotype was associated with the disease in each of the families. Thus, it could be inferred that the gene was in linkage disequilibrium with the haplotype and was located in the region of the haplotype.

In 1997, the *DYT1* gene (also called *TOR1A*) was identified, and the same mutation, a deletion of three base pairs, was found in Jewish and non-Jewish families (Ozelius et al. 1997). In addition to *DYT1*, two other dystonia genes (*DYT6* and *DYT7*) have been mapped to chromosomes 8 and 18 (Leube et al. 1996; Almasy et al. 1997).

Although many cases of dystonia are now considered to be genetic, comorbidity of dystonia with affective disorders and obsessive-compulsive disorders remained a mystery. Genetic findings in dystonia refuted the hypothesis that dystonia is solely a psychogenic or conversion disorder. Possibly the comorbidity represents an emotional reaction to the chronic debilitating physical disorder. But an intriguing alternative explanation is **pleiotropy**: both the involuntary movements and the psychiatric symptoms may be the result of the same underlying genetic abnormality.

To investigate this possibility, researchers compared individuals who carried the *DYT1* dystonia mutation but were free of dystonia symptoms (i.e., the nonmanifesting carriers) with individuals from the same families who did not carry the *DYT1* mutation (i.e., noncarriers) (Heiman et al. 2004). In this comparison, no one exhibited symptoms of dystonia. Also, because all the individuals were from families with dystonia, the psychological impact of having a relative with dystonia was similar for all. Results of the comparison revealed that the prevalence of early-onset recurrent major depression was about fivefold higher in nonmanifesting carriers than in noncarriers. This effect was not due to the carriers' knowing their carrier status. Thus, recurrent major depression might indeed be another manifestation of mutations in the *DYT1* dystonia gene and might appear even in the absence of dystonia symptoms.

What this example shows is that it is not sufficient to understand and utilize any one of the genetic designs alone. They may all be required in a program of research, and hybrid study designs are often created. Keeping the varying designs within an integrated conceptual framework is all-important.

Conclusion

Genetic linkage studies have had remarkable success in the discovery of genetic causes of diseases in which a genetic abnormality is necessary for the disease to occur. However, their usefulness is by no means limited to this purpose. In the pursuit of genetic risk factors, linkage remains a cornerstone of the process of discovery, and it has already played a key role in the identification of risk factors such as the *APOE4* allele. But in this context linkage is more likely to be used in combination with other methods. In this chapter, we used the example of dystonia to illustrate the application to a single problem of linkage analysis, linkage disequilibrium analysis (via haplotypes), and an association study. In the next chapter, we propose a schema for the discovery of genetic risk factors, which incorporates genetic linkage as a critical first step.

References

Almasy L, Bressman SB, Raymond D, et al. (1997). Idiopathic Torsion Dystonia Linked to Chromosome 8 in Two Mennonite Families. *Ann. Neurol.* 42:670–673.

Bihari K, Hill JL, and Murphy DL (1992). Obsessive-Compulsive Characteristics in Patients with Idiopathic Spasmodic Torticollis. *Psychiatry Res.* 42:267–272.

Bray NJ and Owen MJ (2001). Searching for Schizophrenia Genes. *Trends Mol. Med.* 7:169–174.

Bressman SB (1998). Dystonia. *Curr. Opin. Neurol.* 11:363–372.

Brzustowicz LM, Hodgkinson KA, Chow EW, Honer WG, and Bassett AS (2000). Location of a Major Susceptibility Locus for Familial Schizophrenia on Chromosome *1q21-Q22. Science* 288:678–682.

Cavalli-Sforza LL and Bodmer WF (1999/1971). *The Genetics of Human Populations.* Mineola, N.Y.: Dover Publications.

Cleveland SE (1961). Personality Dynamics in Torticollis. *J. Nerv. Ment. Dis.* 129: 150–161.

Fahn S (1988). Concept and Classification of Dystonia. *Adv. Neurol.* 50:1–8.

Goetz CG, Chmura TA, and Lanska DJ (2001). History of Dystonia: Part 4 of the MDS-Sponsored History of Movement Disorders Exhibit, Barcelona, June, 2000. *Mov. Disord.* 16:339–345.

Greenberg DA (1993). Linkage Analysis of "Necessary" Disease Loci versus "Susceptibility" Loci. *Am. J. Hum. Genet.* 52:135–143.

Greenberg DA and Doneshka P (1996). Partitioned Association-Linkage Test: Distinguishing "Necessary" from "Susceptibility" Loci. *Genet. Epidemiol.* 13: 243–252.

Gusella JF, Wexler NS, Conneally PM, et al. (1983). A Polymorphic DNA Marker Genetically Linked to Huntington's Disease. *Nature* 306:234–238.

Hartl DL and Clark AG (1997). *Principles of Population Genetics,* 3rd ed. Sunderland, Mass.: Sinauer.

Heiman GA, Ottman R, Saunders-Pullman R, Ozelius LJ, Risch NJ, and Bressman SB (2004). Increased Risk for Recurrent Major Depression in *DYT1* Dystonia Mutation Carriers. *Neurology* 63(4):631–637.

Heston LL, Orr HT, Rich SS, and White JA (1991). Linkage of an Alzheimer Disease Susceptibility Locus to Markers on Human Chromosome 21. *Am. J. Med. Genet.* 40:449–453.

Hodge SE (2001). Model-Free vs. Model-Based Linkage Analysis: A False Dichotomy? *Am. J. Med. Genet.* 105:62–64.

Hodge SE, Anderson CE, Neiswanger K, Sparkes RS, and Rimoin DL (1983). The Search for Heterogeneity in Insulin-Dependent Diabetes Mellitus (IDDM): Linkage Studies, Two-Locus Models, and Genetic Heterogeneity. *Am. J. Hum. Genet.* 35:1139–1155.

Jahanshahi M and Marsden CD (1988). Depression in Torticollis: A Controlled Study. *Psychol. Med.* 18:925–923.

Jorde LB, Carey JC, Bamshad MJ, and White RL (1999). *Medical Genetics,* 2nd ed. St. Louis, Mo.: Mosby.

Karolchik D, Baertsch R, Diekhans M, et al. (2003). The UCSC Genome Browser Database. *Nucleic Acids Res.* 31:51–54.

Kent WJ, Sugnet CW, Furey TS, Roskin KM, Pringle TH, Zahler AM, and Haussler D (2002). The Human Genome Browser at UCSC. *Genome Res.* 12:996–1006.

Kramer PL, de Leon D, Ozelius L, et al. (1990). Dystonia Gene in Ashkenazi Jewish Population Is Located on Chromosome *9q32–34. Ann. Neurol.* 27:114–120.

Leube B, Rudnicki D, Ratzlaff T, Kessler KR, Benecke R, and Auburger G (1996). Idiopathic Torsion Dystonia: Assignment of a Gene to Chromosome *18p* in a German Family with Adult Onset, Autosomal Dominant Inheritance and Purely Focal Distribution. *Hum. Mol. Genet.* 5:1673–1677.

Nussbaum RL, McInnes RR, and Willard HF (2001). *Thompson and Thompson Genetics in Medicine,* 6th ed. Philadelphia: Saunders.

Ott J (1983). Linkage Analysis and Family Classification under Heterogeneity. *Ann. Hum. Genet.* 47(pt. 4):311–320.

Ott J (1999). *Analysis of Human Genetic Linkage,* 3rd ed. Baltimore: Johns Hopkins University Press.

Ozelius LJ, Hewett JW, Page CE, et al. (1997). The Early-Onset Torsion Dystonia Gene (*DYT1*) Encodes an ATP-Binding Protein. *Nat. Genet.* 17:40–48.

Ozelius LJ, Kramer PL, de Leon D, et al. (1992a). Strong Allelic Association Between the Torsion Dystonia Gene (*DYT1*) and loci on Chromosome *9q34* in Ashkenazi Jews. *Am. J Hum. Genet.* 50:619–628.

Ozelius LJ, Kramer PL, Moskowitz CB, et al. (1989). Human Gene for Torsion Dystonia Located on Chromosome *9q32-Q34*. *Neuron* 2:1427–1434.

Ozelius LJ, Kwiatkowski DJ, Schuback DE, Breakefield XO, Wexler NS, Gusella JF, and Haines JL (1992b). A Genetic Linkage Map of Human Chromosome *9q*. *Genomics* 14:715–720.

Pastor P and Goate AM (2004). Molecular Genetics of Alzheimer's Disease. *Curr. Psychiatry Rep.* 6:125–133.

Risch N and Baron M (1982). X-Linkage and Genetic Heterogeneity in Bipolar-Related Major Affective Illness: Reanalysis of Linkage Data. *Ann. Hum. Genet.* 46:153–166.

Rocchi A, Pellegrini S, Siciliano G, and Murri L (2003). Causative and Susceptibility Genes for Alzheimer's Disease: A Review. *Brain Res. Bull.* 61:1–24.

Schellenberg GD, Bird TD, Wijsman EM, et al. (1992). Genetic Linkage Evidence for a Familial Alzheimer's Disease Locus on Chromosome 14. *Science* 258:668–671.

Tobin AJ and Signer ER (2000). Huntington's Disease: The Challenge for Cell Biologists. *Trends Cell Biol.* 10:531–536.

Vieland VJ and Hodge SE (1998). Review of Statistical Evidence: A Likelihood Paradigm, by R. Royall. *Am. J. Hum. Genet.* 63:283–289.

Wenzel T, Schnider P, Griengl H, Birner P, Nepp J, and Auff E (2000). Psychiatric Disorders in Patients With Blepharospasm—a Reactive Pattern? *J. Psychosom. Res.* 48:589–591.

Wheeler DL, Church DM, Federhen S, et al. (2003). Database Resources of the National Center for Biotechnology. *Nucleic Acids Res.* 31:28–33.

Zeman W and Dyken P (1967). Dystonia Musculorum Deformans. Clinical, Genetic and Pathoanatomical Studies. *Psychiatr. Neurol. Neurochir.* 70:77–121.

Designs for the Genomic Era

33

Mary-Claire King, Habibul Ahsan, and Ezra Susser

The sequencing of the human genome has changed the ways in which we search for genetic causes. According to a recent commentary, genomics is the "ambitious study of all the genes in the genome" (Insel and Collins 2003). Genomics offers to genetics and to epidemiology powerful analytic tools and information unprecedented in medical research.

Searches for genetic causes now exploit this richness. Traditional designs are modified to achieve their goals more directly, and new designs are possible. Because the designs are still evolving, often by trial and error, any description of the present state may soon be outdated. We therefore focus on a limited number of themes that should have enduring import. We describe some of the key challenges presented by the use of genomic information and then suggest a strategy to help address these challenges.

Challenges

In the application of genomics to understanding of complex traits, three themes recur: (1) genetic heterogeneity of disease, (2) the role of common alleles in disease, and (3) the vast amount of genomic data available. These phenomena have important implications for the design of studies of complex psychiatric disorders.

Genetic Heterogeneity

The basic premise of genetic analysis is that a phenotype is related to some underlying variation in genotype. Typically, however, the genetic origins of a complex disease are not the same for all or even most families in which susceptibility is inherited. That is, the disease phenotype may be related to many different genotypes, either to different alleles of the same gene (allelic heterogeneity) or to different genes (locus heterogeneity).

Consider the example of the epilepsies. In chapter 30, we described the process by which a genetic cause was discovered for an apparently rare familial form of epilepsy. Examination of the relationships between family history

and various clinical features of epilepsy led to identification of a highly familial form of the disease characterized by temporal lobe seizures with auditory
features (Ottman et al. 1996a; Ottman et al. 1996b; Ottman et al. 1998).
Linkage analysis and physical mapping ultimately revealed that a mutation in
the *LGI1* gene caused this form of epilepsy (Kalachikov et al. 2002).

Soon thereafter, it became clear that several different mutations in the
LGI1 gene can cause this form of epilepsy. To further characterize the
relation between *LGI1* and epilepsy, researchers genotyped members of 15
families with this form of epilepsy (Ottman et al. 2004). Eight families seg-
regated *LGI1* mutations, but 7 did not, suggesting that an indistinguishable
clinical syndrome might be caused by mutations in other genes. In addition,
although most family members carrying a *LGI1* mutation developed the
expected form of epilepsy, some developed different forms of epilepsy or no
epilepsy at all.

Thus, the emerging picture for this illness is one of genetic heterogeneity,
even within the narrow clinical spectrum carefully defined for these studies.
There are many mutations within the known causal gene, possibly other
causal genes yet to be discovered, and some variation in the clinical expression of the known genetic mutations. The genetic heterogeneity underlying
the epilepsies as a whole is far greater. There are many forms of epilepsy,
and the genetic causes of some other forms are similarly heterogeneous
(George 2004).

We expect that genetic heterogeneity is a critical feature of many other
neuropsychiatric disorders. This would also be compatible with what we know
about the evolution of human genetic variation. The oldest human alleles
originated before the first human migrations out of Africa ~50,000 years ago
(Cavalli-Sforza et al. 1994; Rosenberg et al. 2002). These common polymorphisms account for about 95 percent of human variation. The exponential
growth of human populations over the last 10,000 years has resulted in a vast
number of new alleles, each individually rare and specific to one population
(or even one family). Most variants are of this sort. Thus, the paradox: most
human variation is ancient and shared; most alleles are recent and rare.

Genetic heterogeneity has profound implications for discovery of genetic
causes. In particular, it poses a challenge to genetic association studies. In the
presence of genetic heterogeneity, genetic association studies may not reveal
a true association of an allele with disease, because any particular genetic
cause may be present in only a tiny fraction of affected individuals. In an
association study, co-occurrence of an allele and disease in these few cases
will appear to be readily explained by chance. In other words, an ordinary
cohort study, case-control study, or family-based association study may have
an extremely low probability of detecting a true disease-causing gene, even
one with a very major influence on disease risk among the individuals who
carry it.

The genetics of inherited hearing loss illustrates this point. To date more
than 90 genes have been identified with mutations that cause hearing loss
(Petit et al. 2001; Friedman and Griffith 2003). Each gene harbors multiple
deafness-associated mutations. All mutations are recent, and all but one are
individually rare. The one frequent mutation, *GJB2.30delG*, is the exception

that proves the rule, in that the same mutation has occurred multiple times in a mutational hotspot and thus appears on multiple haplotypes. Association studies of individual alleles or haplotypes could not have identified any of the mutations.

Genetic heterogeneity also poses a challenge to linkage disequilibrium studies, described in the previous chapter, in which we test for association of marker alleles with the disease. This is done under the assumption that a true disease allele will be in linkage disequilibrium with markers somewhere in the genome. Genome-wide scans enable us to examine many thousands of markers simultaneously for association with the disease.

As noted already, under genetic heterogeneity the probability of correctly identifying a disease allele is quite low. Since the marker allele will have a smaller association with the disease than will the disease allele, the probability of correctly identifying a marker allele may be lower still. At the same time, when several thousand potential markers are examined, hundreds of them may have a statistically significant association with the disease by chance alone, while the true marker may not have a statistically significant association with the disease, because of genetic heterogeneity.

These challenges are not always insuperable. Furthermore, some diseases present a mixed picture. There may be substantial heterogeneity in critical disease-causing genes, yet common alleles may have a detectable effect. In Alzheimer disease, multiple rare disease-related mutations have been identified, but also the fairly common *APOE4* allele proved detectable.

Genetic heterogeneity does not pose as severe a problem to genetic linkage studies, particularly if large kindreds are available for analysis. Within a single pedigree, the allele causing disease is much more likely to be the same for all cases. Nonetheless, each pedigree may be transmitting a mutation at a different susceptibility locus. Under genetic heterogeneity, therefore, pooling data from different pedigrees may lead to missing the critical gene. Analytic tools that incorporate heterogeneity have been developed to contend with this problem (Ott 1999).

Common Alleles

Genomic technology has opened up a new generation of association studies of common polymorphisms and disease. Genetic studies of psychiatric disorders often focus on such polymorphic alleles. This was illustrated in chapter 29, where we described association studies of the *Val158Met* polymorphism of the *COMT* gene with panic disorder. In many populations, the *Val* and *Met* alleles at *COMT* amino acid 158 are about equally common. A modest association has been suggested between the *Val* allele and panic disorder in women (Hamilton et al. 2002; Domschke et al. 2004).

Determinants of the strength of an observed association between a risk factor and a disease (part II) pertain to genetic, as well as nongenetic, risk factors. In any population, the strength of effect of a risk factor depends upon the frequency of its causal partners, the other factors whose presence is required for the risk factor to produce disease. The causal partners may be environmental or genetic, or both. In a population in which its causal partners are rare, a risk factor will have a small effect; when the causal partners are common, the risk factor will have a large effect. The biological effect of the risk factor is the same, but its ability to cause disease is different.

The implications for intervention, however, are not the same for environmental and genetic causes. This is most obvious for risk factors that have modest effects and are common in the population. A population-wide intervention can be launched to reduce the prevalence of a common environmental risk factor. Although we are always concerned about unforeseen consequences, these interventions have the potential to ameliorate a feature of the world in which we live and in many instances have led to a substantial reduction in the population incidence of disease. This is possible even when the risk ratio is small, because the attributable proportion may still be large (part II).

In contrast, intervention on a genetic risk factor is typically a form of medical treatment of an individual: altering the deleterious effect of a gene involves intervening with the individual carrying the risk allele. The intervention may be an effort to reverse a change in gene expression due to the risk allele, to reverse the downstream consequences of altered gene expression, or to preclude subsequent effects on critical pathways. A major challenge is that the unintended adverse effects of these interventions on the individuals carrying the risk allele may be considerable and may also vary across individuals.

A central focus of pharmacogenomics is to identify persons with a known risk genotype for whom a specific intervention is most beneficial and least likely to produce adverse effects. Meanwhile, the public health question of whether to intervene medically on common genetic risk factors of modest effect will be difficult. The answer will depend, among other things, on the severity of the disease, the variation in disease expression among susceptible individuals because of other modifying factors, and the possible adverse effects of the intervention on the individuals treated. According to this reasoning, the question whether to intervene medically on an endophenotype is even more difficult.

Despite this difficulty, the identification of common allelic variants with modest effects on disease risk can be useful, particularly if the effect turns out to be the result of a heightened response to a modifiable environmental exposure. For example, a polymorphism (*C/T 13910*) near the lactase phlorizin hydrolase (*LPH*) gene is associated with the trait of lactose intolerance (Enattah et al. 2002). When individuals with this trait consume dairy products, they can develop gastrointestinal distress, and are sometimes misdiagnosed as having irritable bowel syndrome.[1] The *LPH* polymorphism is relevant here because the lactose intolerant genotype *CC* is expressed as gastrointestinal distress only if an individual continues to be exposed to dairy products after weaning. In a society in which dairy products are not generally available, the association of the *LPH* polymorphism with gastrointestinal distress will be weak. On the other hand, among people exposed to dairy products, the

---

[1] The polymorphism (*C/T-13910*) appears at different frequencies in different European populations, and in each population the polymorphism is associated with the trait. In Africa, however, it appears that different alleles are involved (Mulcare et al. 2004), as one might expect, given genetic heterogeneity.

association will be strong. Since the gastrointestinal distress due to lactose intolerance is virtually precluded by avoiding lactose, removing dairy products from the diets of susceptible individuals would be a successful preventive measure. At the same time, nonsusceptible individuals could continue to use dairy products safely and beneficially. Therefore, this common allelic variant is useful to know, because the critical environmental exposure can be avoided by susceptible individuals. (It is probably not surprising that the Scandinavian ice cream industry was a major supporter of genetic research on lactose intolerance; Sahi 1994.)

Genotypic Data

With modern technology, it is possible to generate a vast amount of genotypic data on the individuals in a study. The human genome comprises three billion nucleotides, and allelic variants have been found at millions of them. Furthermore, it is possible to analyze archived DNA or pathology specimens in order to obtain genotypes even after individuals have died. Methods such as genome-wide scanning have come into widespread use for examining thousands of markers, both polymorphic microsatellite markers and single nucleotide polymorphisms (SNPs). Still more recently developed tools enable the consolidation of these markers into haplotypes, markers close to each other on the same chromosome whose alleles are inherited together because they are in linkage disequilibrium (see chapter 32). With the development of the HapMap (Altshuler et al. 2005), these haplotypes, as well as individual markers, can be used to test association with disease.

In genetic linkage studies, the investigator generally has no prior hypothesis as to which markers will be associated with the gene. In association studies using the candidate gene approach, one may narrow the field to genes thought to play a role in the biological pathways leading to the disease, but even this narrower field may entail testing a large number of potential disease alleles (Carlson et al. 2004). In a focused gene-based approach, one may also test an association of disease with all allelic variants of a single candidate gene considered jointly (Neale and Sham 2004). Linkage disequilibrium studies may be either genome-wide and hypothesis-free or based on candidate genes and therefore prior hypotheses.

When hundreds or even thousands of loci are examined, many statistical associations with disease will result from chance alone. False positive associations will likely far outnumber true associations. In this sense, the vast number of comparisons may exceed our capacity to interpret them.

The nature of the search for genetic causes compounds the dilemma. The true associations we seek to find are not necessarily the strongest statistically, for reasons we have discussed. Genetic heterogeneity, prevalence of the risk allele in the population, and interactions with unknown modifiers (whether genetic or environmental) will all affect the apparent association between gene and disease.

Statistical tools for adjustment for multiple comparisons do not fully resolve this dilemma. The Bonferroni adjustment is frequently used to address the problem of multiple statistical comparisons. Using the Bonferroni method, one divides the statistical significance level for observed positive findings by the total number of comparisons made. By reducing the number of false positive findings this method provides an adjustment of the statistical significance level for inference. This method can lead to discarding true positive findings. Several alternative approaches have been introduced (e.g., Benjamini and Hochberg 1995; Malley et al. 2002; Westfall et al. 2002) that improve upon the Bonferroni in some respects, but none of these methods can indicate which of the statistical associations reflect true associations.

Therefore, we need other means to discriminate among statistically promising associations. One approach is to prioritize genes for further scrutiny with functional criteria based on the biology of the disease. In the next sections, we present some designs that incorporate these considerations.

A Strategy to Find Genetic Causes

Historically, the process of gene discovery often included three steps: (1) familial aggregation studies suggested that genetic causes could be important, (2) heritability or adoption studies estimated the contribution of genetic causes to familial aggregation, and (3) genetic linkage studies enabled mapping and ultimately identification of a disease-causing gene. Although not always followed, this sequence provided a useful schema with which to approach research in genetic epidemiology.

Genetic influences on most complex traits have been established. Increasingly, for gene discovery efforts, family history and heritability studies are used mainly to define phenotypes more precisely. (These studies are also being used for purposes other than gene discovery; see chapters 30 and 31). The path to gene discovery is shortened. The path from gene discovery to disease prevention is equally important and often less tractable.

In the genomic era, therefore, we make some modifications of the schema. We propose that the search for genetic causes can be conceptualized in terms of three steps: (1) identifying the critical genes, (2) determining how the aberrant genes cause disease, and (3) drawing the implications for prevention. As with the traditional schema, researchers will not always follow this sequence, but it provides a useful framework for approaching the process. Below we describe these steps, and indicate how epidemiologic and genetic thinking can be integrated into the process.

The approach we describe has revealed genes important to many common, complex human diseases, including several neuropsychiatric disorders (Online Mendelian Inheritance in Man [OMIM]). As noted earlier, in the context of genetic heterogeneity, genes responsible for complex traits often harbor a large number of disease-causing mutations, each one of which is individually rare. With the increasingly powerful tools of modern genomic analysis, identifying such alleles for mental disorders will be possible.

The framework we suggest is not the approach most frequently used at present for mental disorders, where genetic studies often focus on endophenotypes rather than the disorders per se, or on identifying common polymorphisms with modest effects rather than critical genes with strong effects. The framework we suggest and such common allele approaches are not mutually exclusive and are sometimes complementary. Rare severe mutations may occur in genes that also harbor more common variants. Thus, detection of highly penetrant and individually rare mutations may provide clues for discovery of common alleles of modest effect.

Identifying the Critical Genes

A valid and reliable definition of the phenotype is an indispensable platform for successful gene discovery. This pertains whether the phenotype is a disease, an endophenotype, or some other trait. Family history studies and heritability studies offer important contributions to the definition of phenotypes. Making use of these studies, we can reduce the genetic heterogeneity underlying the phenotype, and improve the correspondence between variations in genotype and the occurrence of the phenotype.

Once a useful phenotype is defined, the search for genetic causes can be undertaken with a fair chance of success. We propose starting with a search for genes with strong effects, using natural experiments for this purpose, and then testing for alleles with modest effects in the same genes. In association studies that lack a strong prior hypothesis, the probability of correctly identifying disease alleles of modest effects is very low. Therefore, we suggest that the optimal use of association studies is more often at a later stage in the process.

Families with multiple cases of disease over several generations comprise a classic natural experiment for gene discovery. These families may arise for any of three reasons: a strong genetic effect transmitted through the pedigree, a strong environmental effect that runs in the family, or a large number of cases by chance alone. In such families, if genes exist with strong effects on disease, their position in the genome is likely to be detectable by genetic linkage studies. The critical genes should then be identifiable with tools of modern genomics. The design conforms to a natural experiment, because within these families individuals do not choose their genes (see chapter 10).

Another informative type of natural experiment is a study of linkage disequilibrium in a **founder population**.[2] This is a population descended from a relatively small number of ancestors, and characterized by rapid expansion of population size and by marriage within the group (Sheffield et al. 1998; Peltonen et al. 2000). Founder populations carry many rare alleles specific to their group. Also, linkage disequilibrium is stronger around rare alleles (in any population) because rare alleles are younger, so less recombination has occurred to unlink alleles at neighboring loci (Jorde 1995; Kruglyak 1999).

---

[2] Strictly speaking, natural experiments are cohort not case-control studies (chapter 10). However, in a linkage disequilibrium study, the gene is known to be antecedent to the disease, so it seems reasonable to consider these studies as a variation on the natural experiment.

Therefore, in a founder population linkage disequilibrium studies have a much better chance of correctly identifying an allele near a disease gene, both because genetic heterogeneity is reduced and because linkage disequilibrium is enhanced.

A natural experiment of an environmental exposure yields still another strategy. Consider the example of the Dutch famine described in chapter 10, an historic event in which prenatal exposure to famine was associated with an increased risk of schizophrenia in offspring. If this association reflects a causal relationship between a specific prenatal nutritional deficiency and schizophrenia, then people who developed schizophrenia after prenatal famine will overrepresent this particular environmental cause. They will also overrepresent any genes that interacted with the prenatal nutritional deficiency to cause the disease. The reduced heterogeneity can be utilized to improve the chances of identifying critical genes. Samples of cases that share an environmental exposure identified by other methods could be evaluated in the same way.

Natural experiments may also be aimed at detection of critical *de novo* mutations. For instance, the family of a case with a chromosomal translocation may reveal a critical gene at a chromosomal breakpoint. Since the technology for identifying small deletions and duplications in the genome is advancing rapidly, these designs are likely to play an increasingly important role in gene discovery.

Having found the genomic position of a critical gene, by these or other means, the identification of the gene is the next step. Even with the most advanced methods, this is still difficult. The disease status of some relatives may not be clear, because of an imprecise definition of the phenotype, or variable expression of the genotype. In addition, limited numbers of families or small families may lead to very large genomic regions that are either linked with, or are in disequilibrium with, disease and thus may lead to a very large number of genes to evaluate. It may require years to progress from either a linkage or a disequilibrium result to the actual gene.

We expect that for many complex psychiatric disorders, genes with strong effects will ultimately be identified. Although some psychiatric researchers have come to suspect that such genes may not exist for mental disorders such as schizophrenia, the pattern of results up to this point can be explained by genetic heterogeneity. Most such genes will likely harbor multiple, different disease-associated alleles in different families; other genes will be mutant in only one family. We anticipate that most disease alleles will be individually rare. Whether individual mutations are common or rare, each gene with mutations leading to psychiatric disorder reveals a critical biological component of the disease and opens an opportunity for prevention and treatment.

The steps of our proposed schema may be undertaken for several genes simultaneously. Also, in practice, studies may not always occur in this order, and some results may permit shortcuts. One series of studies, for example, began with a highly informative linkage of chromosome 7 to a well-characterized endophenotype, event-related oscillations. Motivated by the linkage finding, investigators proceeded directly to focused association analysis of both alcohol dependence and major depression with muscarinic acetylcholine receptor (*CHRM2*), a candidate gene from the linked region on chromosome 7 (Wang et al. 2004). The investigators logically chose to skip genome-wide association analysis of alcohol dependence and major depression because the previous linkage studies of the associated endophenotype (event-related oscillations) provided sufficient clues.

How the Aberrant Gene Causes Disease

After identifying a critical gene, we still have to determine the allelic variant of the gene that was a cause of the disease in the cases in whom it was identified. The nature of critical mutations is not always clear. The importance of mutations causing loss of gene function may be relatively straightforward, but the meaning of amino acid differences (whether rare or common) or of alterations in regulatory regions of genes can be extremely difficult to determine. A wide variety of approaches are being developed to address these questions. Gene expression studies, often using high-throughput tools such as microarrays, enable one to determine the effects of the potential disease-causing mutation on other genes. Effects of amino acid substitutions on a protein's capacity to bind critical partners can be assessed with tools from biochemistry. Effects of mutations on protein localization, and on cell structure and critical cellular function, can be assessed by introducing normal and mutant genes into appropriate types of cells. It is now possible to create animal models of mutations of interest from many species. For mutations that may be important for psychiatric traits, it is now virtually routine to develop a mouse model of the appropriate homologous genotype and to evaluate the phenotype at cellular, developmental, and behavioral levels (e.g., see Stefansson et al. 2003). Clearly these experiments require collaborations across disciplines and collectively can lead to more convincing evidence for disease involvement of a gene.

Once we are convinced that we have identified an allele involved in causation of disease, we look for other alleles of the same gene that may be related to the disease in other people. This can entail studies of other familial clusters of cases, in the same and in different populations. Within a given family, or pedigree, we sequence the gene in selected cases to identify candidate alleles, and investigate which, if any, of these alleles are likely to cause the disease within the cluster. All the methods described here can be used for these tests. Often, numerous different allelic variants of the same gene turn out to be causes of the disease, each within different families.

We also examine the relationships between causal alleles and clinical manifestations. These studies are often called **genotype-phenotype correlation studies**. The different causative alleles may be associated with somewhat different clinical features of disease. Conversely, a single clinical subtype may be associated with more than one causative allele. Also, by examining the effects of a single allele within a family, we may find variable expression. That is, among family members with the allele, we may find some with the disease, some with a related phenotype, and some with no disorder at all. (Recall that these same complexities made finding the alleles difficult at the gene discovery step.)

Furthermore, while a critical allele has a strong effect on disease, other alleles of the same gene may have more modest effects. Other associations between alleles and disease within a family may be suggestive but far from definitive, because the familial cluster is small and the association is modest. These effects may be measurable with biological tools, as described above, but their epidemiologic impact cannot be known at this stage.

Drawing Implications for Prevention

Having found a critical gene, and even understanding how it causes disease, we are still far from preventive intervention. To start on this path, we estimate the frequency of the known or hypothesized disease-causing alleles of the gene in various populations. We also test their association with disease in a variety of populations. For this purpose, we use genetic association studies, as described in chapter 29. Note that in this context association studies are initiated with strong *a priori* hypotheses.

The choice of design for these association studies will depend on a number of factors (see chapter 29). For very rare alleles, one may opt for a case-control study, because this approach may be the only way to generate the large numbers of cases required to detect an effect. For less rare alleles, or, in settings for which case-control designs may be susceptible to bias, family-based designs offer the most definitive results, but other association designs may also be appropriate.

Knowing the frequency of the allele and the size of its effect on disease in a given population allows us to estimate the potential benefits of preventive intervention for public health. For example, we can now estimate an attributable proportion. This information is nowhere near sufficient, however, for designing and testing an intervention.

To identify potential points for intervention, we search for modifiable environmental factors that influence the effect of the gene. Most often, the alteration of such environmental exposures presents the best opportunity for ameliorating the effects of the disease alleles. In chapter 30, we illustrated this point for breast cancer and inherited mutations in *BRCA1* and *BRCA2*, with results suggesting that increased physical activity in youth might delay the onset of breast cancer in later decades. We may also develop pharmacologic or other therapeutic interventions that modify the phenotypic effect of a gene, and in turn we may find that other genotypic variations modify the effect of these interventions.

Prior studies of environmental exposures may greatly facilitate this process. For example, previous studies may implicate an environmental exposure with biological effect (e.g., a toxic chemical, a nutritional deficiency, or a virus) as a potential cause of a psychiatric disorder. Then the search for environmental modifiers might usefully focus on previously implicated exposures with the potential for biological synergy with the genetic effect. Currently, there is growing interest in the potential of environmental exposures to influence the expression of genes by means of epigenetic effects, such as DNA methylation (Beaudet 2002).

Conclusion

Epidemiology and human genetics have developed distinct research designs to discover causes. Yet it is ever more apparent that the most important causal pathways include both genetic and nongenetic factors. To understand these pathways to disease and ultimately prevent disease most effectively, epidemiologists and geneticists should be working in partnership. To make this possible, we need a common framework for thinking about causal research. The many points of convergence discussed in this part of the book provide the basis for developing one.

This part of the book has extended our scope to genetic as well as nongenetic causes. The next part reaches further still. We seek a vantage point from which to consider interactions and other relationships between causes, causes at multiple levels of organization, and causes that produce change over time in individuals or in societies.

References

Altshuler D, Brooks LD, Chakravarti A, Collins FS, Daly MJ, and Donnelly P (2005). A Haplotype Map of the Human Genome. *Nature* 437:1299–1320.

Beaudet AL (2002). Is Medical Genetics Neglecting Epigenetics? *Genet. Med.* 4: 399–402.

Benjamini Y and Hochberg Y (1995). Controlling the False Discovery Rate—a Practical and Powerful Approach to Multiple Testing. *J. R. Stat. Soc. Ser. B* 57:289–300.

Carlson CS, Eberle MA, Kruglyak L, and Nickerson DA (2004). Mapping complex disease loci in whole-genome association studies. *Nature* 429:446–452.

Cavalli-Sforza LL, Menozzi P, and Piazza A (1994). *The History and Geography of Human Genes.* Princeton, N.J.: Princeton University Press.

Domschke K, Freitag CM, Kuhlenbumer G, et al. (2004). Association of the Functional *V158M* Catechol-O-Methyl-Transferase Polymorphism with Panic Disorder in Women. *Int. J. Neuropsychopharmacol.* 7:183–188.

Enattah NS, Sahi T, Savilahti E, Terwilliger JD, Peltonen L, and Jarvela I (2002). Identification of a Variant Associated with Adult-Type Hypolactasia. *Nat. Genet.* 30:233–237.

Friedman TB and Griffith AJ (2003). Human Nonsyndromic Sensorineural Deafness. *Annu. Rev. Genomics Hum. Genet.* 4:341–402.

George AL, Jr. (2004). Molecular Basis of Inherited Epilepsy. *Arch. Neurol.* 61: 473–478.

Hamilton SP, Slager SL, Heiman GA, et al. (2002). Evidence for a Susceptibility Locus for Panic Disorder Near the Catechol-O-Methyltransferase Gene on Chromosome 22. *Biol. Psychiatry* 51:591–601.

Insel TR and Collins FS (2003). Psychiatry in the Genomics Era. *Am. J. Psychiatry* 160:616–620.

Online Mendelian Inheritance in Man (OMIM). http//:www.ncbi.nlm.nih.gov/omim.

Jorde LB (1995). Linkage Disequilibrium as a Gene-Mapping Tool. *Am. J. Hum. Genet.* 56:11–14.

Kalachikov S, Evgrafov O, Ross B, et al. (2002). Mutations in *LGI1* Cause Autosomal-Dominant Partial Epilepsy with Auditory Features. *Nat. Genet.* 30(3):335–341.

Kruglyak L (1999). Prospects for Whole-Genome Linkage Disequilibrium Mapping of Common Disease Genes. *Nat. Genet.* 22:139–144.

Malley JD, Naiman DQ, and Bailey-Wilson JE (2002). A Comprehensive Method for Genome Scans. *Hum. Hered.* 54:174–185.

Mulcare CA, Weale ME, Jones AL, Connell B, Zeitlyn D, Tarekegn A, Swallow DM, Bradman N, and Thomas MG (2004). The *T* Allele of a Single-Nucleotide Polymorphism 13.9 Kb Upstream of the Lactase Gene (*LCT*) (*C-13.9kbT*) Does Not Predict or Cause the Lactase-Persistence Phenotype in Africans. *Am. J. Hum. Genet.* 74:1102–1110.

Neale BM and Sham PC (2004). The Future of Association Studies: Gene-Based Analysis and Replication. *Am. J. Hum. Genet.* 75:353–362.

Ott J (1999). *Analysis of Human Genetic Linkage*, 3rd ed. Baltimore: Johns Hopkins University Press.

Ottman R, Annegers JF, Risch N, Hauser WA, and Susser M (1996a). Relations of Genetic and Environmental Factors in the Etiology of Epilepsy. *Ann. Neurol.* 39:442–449.

Ottman R, Lee JH, Hauser WA, and Risch N (1998). Are Generalized and Localization-Related Epilepsies Genetically Distinct? *Arch. Neurol.* 55:339–344.

Ottman R, Lee JH, Risch N, Hauser WA, and Susser M (1996b). Clinical Indicators of Genetic Susceptibility to Epilepsy. *Epilepsia* 37:353–361.

Ottman R, Winawer MR, Kalachikov S, Barker-Cummings C, Gilliam TC, Pedley TA, and Hauser WA (2004). *LGI1* Mutations in Autosomal Dominant Partial Epilepsy with Auditory Features. *Neurology* 62:1120–1126.

Peltonen L, Palotie A, and Lange K (2000). Use of Population Isolates for Mapping Complex Traits. *Nat. Rev. Genet.* 1:182–190.

Petit C, Levilliers J, and Hardelin JP (2001). Molecular Genetics of Hearing Loss. *Annu. Rev. Genet.* 35:589–646.

Rosenberg NA, Pritchard JK, Weber JL, Cann HM, Kidd KK, Zhivotovsky LA, and Feldman MW (2002). Genetic Structure of Human Populations. *Science* 298:2381–2385.

Sahi T (1994). Genetics and Epidemiology of Adult-Type Hypolactasia. *Scand. J. Gastroenterol. Suppl.* 202:7–20.

Sheffield VC, Stone EM, and Carmi R (1998). Use of Isolated Inbred Human Populations for Identification of Disease Genes. *Trends Genet.* 14:391–396.

Stefansson H, Sarginson J, Kong A, et al. (2003). Association of Neuregulin 1 with Schizophrenia Confirmed in a Scottish Population. *Am. J. Hum. Genet.* 72:83–87.

Wang JC, Hinrichs AL, Stock H, et al. (2004). Evidence of Common and Specific Genetic Effects: Association of the Muscarinic Acetylcholine Receptor M2 (*CHRM2*) Gene with Alcohol Dependence and Major Depressive Syndrome. *Hum. Mol. Genet.* 13: 1903–1911.

Westfall PH, Zaykin DV, and Young SS (2002). Multiple Tests for Genetic Effects in Association Studies. *Methods Mol. Biol.* 184:143–168.

COMPLEX CAUSAL
RELATIONSHIPS

Eco-Epidemiology

34

Ezra Susser, Sharon Schwartz, and Alfredo Morabia

The focus of epidemiology on the identification of risk factors emerged in the mid-20th century to address the questions and health concerns most salient at that time. To meet the challenges of the present time, epidemiologists are gravitating toward a broader paradigm that subsumes the identification of risk factors as one important component. This emphasis has stimulated the development of new concepts and methods. The emerging themes resonate with approaches that have a strong tradition in psychiatric epidemiology, are especially appropriate for research on mental disorders, and offer psychiatric epidemiologists the opportunity to help shape the future of epidemiology.

Building Blocks

The building blocks for a broader framework can be found in current trends in epidemiology. We focus here on three recent developments. Many of the proposals for a more integrative epidemiology take up these developments as central themes.

First, epidemiologists increasingly recognize the enrichment that follows from examining the trajectory of health and illness over the life course (Kuh and Ben-Schlomo 2004). The onset of disease in an adult may reflect earlier life experiences in many ways. These include long-deferred effects of an in utero insult, a chain of social and biological experiences initiated by an early childhood exposure, and cumulative exposure to toxic biological or social factors over a long period. The life course perspective has always been influential among psychiatric epidemiologists (Leighton 1959; Rutter 1988), but not in many other domains of epidemiology. This vantage point is now being integrated into the mainstream of epidemiology, and in the process researchers are tracing its historical antecedents (Kuh and Davey Smith 1993), spelling out its implications (see chapter 36), and refining the analytic methods.

Second, epidemiologists increasingly consider multiple levels of causation (Von Korff et al. 1992; Diez Roux 1998; Bingenheimer and Raudenbush 2004). The causes of health outcomes in populations can be sought at macrolevels, as in the distribution of wealth across and within societies; at

415

individual levels, as in individual behavior; and at microlevels, as in the expression of genes in cells. Although disease always occurs in an individual, disease prevention may be directed toward any of these levels. Different approaches are needed to identify the causal processes at each level and, equally important, to examine how a process at one level (e.g., societal cohesion or cellular changes) can manifest at another level (e.g., health behaviors in an individual).

We have proposed that a multilevel perspective has the potential to incorporate the advances made by epidemiology in previous eras and to use them to full advantage (part I). Sketching a history of dominant causal paradigms, we described how epidemiologists shifted their focus among these levels of causation in successive eras and in the process sometimes neglected the contributions of previous eras. But we also found within each era far-sighted epidemiologists who considered multiple levels of causation, which set precedents for this way of thinking.

Third, at least some epidemiologists are engaged in expanding their reach and reversing the long-standing trend toward fragmentation into subspecialties. A broader and more unified framework would sustain the coherence of the discipline and empower each domain by affording it new designs crafted in other domains. In the previous parts of this book, we have emphasized bridging the divide between the epidemiology of mental and physical disorders, and that between studies of genetic and nongenetic causes. It is also true that for at least half a century infectious disease and risk factor epidemiology proceeded largely in parallel, and in these chapters we will indicate points of convergence between them.

An integrated approach to investigating disease and its prevention will necessarily encompass these elements: life course trajectories, levels of causation, and the interconnections among different causes and disease domains. To describe this emergent way of thinking, we have proposed the term *eco-epidemiology* (Susser and Susser 1996; Susser 2004). Calls for integrating risk factor epidemiology within a broader framework have also been articulated by others (e.g., Krieger 1994; Pearce 1996; Levins 1997; McMichael 1999). Whether or not the label eco-epidemiology proves useful, the endeavor toward integration is essential.

Causal Explanation

Proposals for an integrated approach have been embedded in critiques of current practices in epidemiology. These critiques often advocate one or more of the specific themes just outlined. They suggest the need to redress epidemiology's imbalanced focus on causal identification as opposed to causal explanation.

Several interconnected aspects of causal explanation are particularly prominent in these critiques. Many have noted that epidemiologic methods for identifying risk factors overlook the study of other types of causes. We focus on the characteristics of individuals, such as diet and other lifestyle factors, while the historical and social milieus in which risk factors develop and have their effects are given short shrift. To address pressing public health concerns, the identification of risk factors may be necessary, but not nearly sufficient. Even when a powerful risk factor is identified, effective intervention generally requires an understanding of its societal antecedents. To take a classic example, demonstrating the potency of cigarette smoking as a cause of lung cancer was not enough. For prevention, we also had to understand why cigarettes are produced and why people smoke them.

Others have criticized the "black box" nature of much epidemiologic research, with its focus on risk factor disease associations without sufficient consideration of the downstream mechanisms that allow us to understand how the risk factor operates. It is sometimes also alleged that this restricted focus has led to numerous causal inferences that ultimately proved false.

A particularly radical critique is that the development and spread of disease is characterized by nonlinear dynamic relationships that are neither recognized nor measured in risk factor epidemiology (e.g. Philippe and Mansi 1998; Koopman and Lynch 1999). From this perspective, causal explanation lies in the relationships among causes and their contexts rather than in a neat progression from antecedent to cause of interest to mediator to outcome. Infectious disease epidemiologists have long appreciated this gap in causal thinking and are now prominent in filling it.

The Salience of Theory

The imbalanced focus on causal identification over causal explanation is reflected in the secondary role of theory in risk factor epidemiology (Krieger and Zierler 1996). Its strength has been the honing of methods of isolation of specific causes, rather than the development of theories of explanation. The critiques of epidemiology and accompanying broader purview are bringing theory to the fore. In developing an epidemiologic study within this new context, the researcher must make decisions about the point in the life course, level of organization, and types of causes to be investigated. Such decisions are based in prior knowledge and understanding of the disease processes and the context in which they are embedded.

Of course, as emphasized throughout this volume, in a risk factor study we also make choices about design based on prior knowledge and understanding of disease processes. But in designing these studies, one level of organization, the individual, and one phase in the life course, that in which the disease is diagnosed, have been afforded prominence. Perhaps as a result, the rationale for choosing to focus on individual level and temporally proximate causes was not usually articulated. Rather, the rationale for those decisions was hidden in the assumptions underpinning the risk factor paradigm. With greater legitimacy granted to other levels and time periods, the incentive to articulate a theory behind these choices is increased.

Other developments have also contributed to increasing the salience of theory. Some epidemiologic studies are being conducted on a very large scale, collecting data on hundreds of thousands of participants. Together with new technologies, such as enhanced computational power and genome-wide scanning, this scale promotes the simultaneous examination of an enormous number of putative causes. The need for theoretical guidance in choosing among these riches is evident. Otherwise, it is clear that spurious associations and misleading conclusions will increasingly plague epidemiologic research.

Methodological developments within risk factor epidemiology itself, such as a deeper understanding of confounding, reinforce the need for prior theory, even in the process of causal identification. For example, deciding whether or not to adjust for a variable that is associated with the exposure and disease necessitates consideration of the disease process. Under some circumstances, controlling for such a variable is required for a valid estimate; in other circumstances, control will induce invalidity. Valid decisions depend on good theory. It is for this reason, at least in part, that we have organized our presentation of the basic principles of epidemiology around the concept of testing competing hypotheses. The hypotheses may be deduced from current theories or emanate from puzzling findings that help stimulate new theories (Susser and Stein 2002).

The Example of Schizophrenia

To illustrate how far epidemiologists have already moved in the direction of an integrative approach, we use the example of schizophrenia. We briefly describe here how epidemiologists in this field have taken up the three central themes we have outlined, and have shifted their focus toward causal explanation.[1] First, investigations over different phases of the life cycle have illuminated the trajectory of schizophrenia. It now appears that disturbances in brain development before the time of birth, deficits in neurodevelopment during the childhood years, and an extended period of prodromal symptoms in adolescence and young adulthood often precede the onset of the psychotic symptoms required for diagnosis. These features justify the designation of schizophrenia as a neurodevelopmental disorder.

The trajectory of schizophrenia is very different, however, from the disorders that have been traditionally classified as neurodevelopmental. These disorders tend to be evident early in life and persist in a fairly stable form thereafter. By contrast, schizophrenia is largely latent until adolescence and sometimes well into adulthood. The antecedent manifestations of schizophrenia are subtle and as yet are detectable only on average—for instance, by showing differences in average IQ between youth who do and youth who do not develop schizophrenia at a later time. Schizophrenia also tends to have a fluctuating course after onset and may progress over the long term to neurodegenerative disease, to partial remission, or to full recovery. Thus, an individual's trajectory may not be predetermined by early brain development.

The distinctive trajectory of schizophrenia suggests many potential points of intervention, both before and after the onset of the disease as presently

---

[1] Since our aim is to illustrate these themes, rather than to review the epidemiology of schizophrenia, we refer readers elsewhere for a full discussion of the findings and supporting evidence see (Murray et al. 2002).

defined. Investigations have yielded strong though not definitive evidence that potentially modifiable environmental exposures influence the development of the disorder. In utero exposures such as nutritional deficiency, and childhood and adolescent exposures such as cannabis use, have been associated with an increased incidence of schizophrenia. Clinical interventions have been designed for the prodromal period, to delay or even prevent the onset of the full disorder. The course and outcome after onset can be influenced by treatment, family relationships, and also sociocultural environment; for instance, patients tend to have better outcomes in developing than in developed countries.

Second, we are now learning about causes of schizophrenia at many levels (March and Susser, in press). We have greatly extended the identification of individual risk factors for schizophrenia; many of these results were described in previous parts of this volume. At the same time, however, epidemiologists are finding clues to societal-level causes. Especially intriguing is the increased incidence of schizophrenia among certain immigrant groups in northern Europe (e.g., Afro-Caribbeans in the United Kingdom, and Moroccans in the Netherlands); the incidence is even higher in their second-generation offspring born in Europe. Currently, the pattern of results across numerous studies suggests that the social experience of discrimination contributes to this high incidence. Still other studies—though not usually led by epidemiologists—have yielded insights into causes at the cellular level. Recent results from linkage and association studies direct attention to genes that play a role in neurodevelopment (e.g., neureglin, dysbindin, *DISC1*). Postmortem studies implicate genetic influences on abnormal neuronal growth and synaptic connections in schizophrenia.

Third, pursuing these leads, investigators increasingly cross the divide between mental and physical health, and between noninfectious and infectious causes. For instance, when schizophrenia is considered as a neurodevelopmental disturbance with latent effects, investigators use as a referent the investigations of nonpsychiatric disorders that appear to be influenced by the fetal environment. These range from congenital brain disorders, such as neural tube defects, to cardiovascular diseases of adulthood, such as insulin-resistant diabetes. Infectious causes of schizophrenia are being studied both as prenatal determinants and in subsequent phases of the life course.

Finally, investigators are formulating theories that bring various strands together. For instance, some theorize a role for epigenetic processes, such as DNA methylation, which influence the expression of genes without altering the DNA sequence. Since epigenetic effects are believed to be subtle and more variable than ordinary genetic effects, this theory offers an explanation for the highly variable manifestations of schizophrenia over the life course. It also offers an explanation for some of the results from risk factor studies. Among the factors that might influence DNA methylation in offspring are maternal prenatal nutrition (through effects on the in utero environment) and paternal age (through effects on the germ line), both of which have been identified as risk factors for schizophrenia. Furthermore, the theory is compatible with the genetic epidemiology of schizophrenia. This theory has generated specific hypotheses about epigenetic effects that are currently being tested.

On the other hand, the present state of research on schizophrenia also illustrates how far we have yet to go. For instance, we are not systematically investigating the interactions between causes of schizophrenia that are being identified at different levels of organization. Although we have begun to contemplate these questions, we lack research designs tailored to answer them. In this respect, of course, the present state of research on schizophrenia is characteristic of many diseases.

In this genomic era, it will be essential to develop methods to answer these questions. To see why, it is useful to draw an analogy between the transformation of epidemiology during the "Golden Age of microbiology" one hundred years ago and the way in which genomics is transforming epidemiology today. After the discovery of germs and the proof that they could cause diseases, it took many decades to recognize the complex processes that linked infection at the cellular level to disease in an individual, and that linked infection in individuals to epidemic transmission in societies, as required to draw the implications for population health (chapter 2). Similarly, to extract the public health implications of genomics, we need to identify not only the DNA sequences that contribute to human disease, but also the processes that link these cellular-level variations to the development of disease in individuals and to the rates of disease in populations.

Considering Complexity

The following chapters discuss methods to enhance causal explanation, and attempt to adumbrate a broader framework for epidemiology. The chapters are arranged in order of increasing departure from the concepts of risk factor epidemiology and well-established methods. Chapter 35, on mediation and interaction, concerns developments within the risk factor paradigm, developments by which epidemiology has made great progress. However, as we shall see, it provides a cautionary tale for the analysis of more complex models.

The methods described in chapters 36 and 37 are less well developed. Indeed, only nascent methods exist for testing the concepts that best represent current thinking about the development of psychiatric disorders. It seems to us and others (e.g., Krieger 1994; Philippe and Mansi 1998) that our concepts of disease are ahead of our methods. As in the past, necessity is sometimes the mother of invention, with the impetus for the development of new methods deriving from new (or renewed) questions that older methods cannot address.

Finally, it should always be kept in mind that epidemiology is a science of public health. We do not pursue complexity as an end in itself. The purpose of taking account of complex relationships is to reveal otherwise obscured causal pathways and ways of modifying them. Diseases that at one time appear intractably complex can later appear simple when their causes are better understood. Thus, our goal is to arrive at a simpler, more useful understanding of causes, to facilitate prevention and treatment of disease.

References

Bingenheimer JB and Raudenbush SW (2004). Statistical and Substantive Inferences in Public Health: Issues in the Application of Multilevel Models. *Annu. Rev. Public Health* 25:53–77.

Diez Roux AV (1998). On Genes, Individuals, Society, and Epidemiology. *Am. J. Epidemiol.* 148:1027–1032.

Koopman JS and Lynch JW (1999). Individual Causal Models and Population System Models in Epidemiology. *Am. J. Public Health* 89:1170–1174.

Krieger N (1994). Epidemiology and the Web of Causation: Has Anyone Seen the Spider? *Soc. Sci. Med.* 39:887–903.

Krieger N and Zierler S (1996). What Explains the Public's Health?—A Call for Epidemiologic Theory. *Epidemiology* 7:107–109.

Kuh D and Ben-Schlomo Y (2004). *A Life Course Approach to Chronic Disease Epidemiology*. New York: Oxford University Press.

Kuh D and Davey Smith G (1993). When Is Mortality Risk Determined? Historical Insights into a Current Debate. *Soc. Hist. Med.* 6:101–123.

Leighton AH (1959). *My Name Is Legion: Foundations for a Theory of Man in Relation to Culture.* Vol 1. *The Stirling County Study of Psychiatric Disorder and Sociocultural Environment.* New York: Basic Books.

Levins R (1997). When Science Fails Us. *Forest, Trees and People* 32/33:1–18.

March D and Susser E (in press). Taking the Search for Causes to a Different Level: Schizophrenia and Eco-epidemiology. *Am. J. Epidemiol.*

McMichael AJ (1999). Prisoners of the Proximate: Loosening the Constraints on Epidemiology in an Age of Change. *Am. J. Epidemiol.* 149:887–897.

Murray RM, Jones PB, Susser E, van Os J, and Cannon M, eds. (2002). *The Epidemiology of Schizophrenia.* New York: Cambridge University Press.

Pearce N (1996). Traditional Epidemiology, Modern Epidemiology, and Public Health. *Am. J. Public Health* 86:678–683.

Philippe P and Mansi O (1998). Nonlinearity in the Epidemiology of Complex Health and Disease Processes. *Theor. Med. Bioeth.* 19:591–607.

Rutter M (1988). Epidemiological Approaches to Developmental Psychopathology. *Arch. Gen. Psychiatry* 45:486–495.

Susser E (2004). Eco-Epidemiology: Thinking outside the Black Box. *Epidemiology* 15:519–520.

Susser M and Stein Z (2002). Commentary: Civilization and Peptic Ulcer 40 Years On. *Int. J. Epidemiol.* 31:18–21.

Susser M and Susser E (1996). Choosing a Future for Epidemiology: II. From Black Box to Chinese Boxes and Eco-Epidemiology. *Am. J. Public Health* 86:674–677.

Von Korff M, Koepsell T, Curry S, and Diehr P (1992). Multi-Level Analysis in Epidemiologic Research on Health Behaviors and Outcomes. *Am. J Epidemiol.* 135:1077–1082.

35 Causal Explanation within a Risk Factor Framework

Sharon Schwartz and Ezra Susser

Our presentation of epidemiologic methods has distinguished two endeavors: causal identification and causal explanation. Current epidemiologic methods focus on causal identification, determining whether or not the exposure under investigation has a causal effect on the health outcome. Causal explanation, in contrast, describes how and under what circumstances an identified causal factor has an effect. Although methods for assessing it are less developed, causal explanation serves two critical functions. First, it increases our confidence that we have identified a cause; second, it helps us to generalize our findings beyond the particular circumstances of the study.

The first function is necessary because all empirical methods, no matter how carefully hewn and executed, are fallible. After observing an association, we try to rule out noncasual explanations by removing all sources of noncomparability. But it is always possible that differences remain that we did not detect or could not control. Indeed, the more fully we understand noncomparability and its sources, the more apparent it becomes that our current methods for dealing with it are sometimes insufficient. This is true for all epidemiologic study designs, including randomized controlled trials. We can never be sure that we have identified and falsified all plausible alternative explanations for the exposure disease relationship other than a causal one. Even if we did successfully deal with all plausible explanations, others, currently considered implausible, may prove to be correct.

Causal explanation helps to limit the number of alternative explanations through a different route. When we make our hypotheses about the data more specific by stipulating the active ingredients of the exposure, the mechanisms through which the exposure causes the disease, and the conditions under which the exposure has an effect, the number of plausible alternative explanations is decreased. Any alternative would now have to account not only for the exposure-disease association, but also for the explanatory power of the mechanism.

This approach was used in a report from a cohort study of children in New York State (Cohen et al. 1993a; Cohen et al. 1993b; Cohen and Cohen 1996). The analysis suggested that an adverse childhood family environment was a risk factor for suicide in late adolescence and early adulthood. However, the researchers proceeded further (as described in chapter 9) to show that inter-personal difficulties in adolescence mediated the effect. Any alternative explanation for the family environment–suicide association would have to account for the relationship among all three variables. Thus, the greater specificity winnowed the explanatory field.

But causal explanation plays a second critical role: it allows us to generalize beyond the specific instance of the study in which we tested our theory. Every study employs particular measures of the exposures and diseases that we want to study. These numeric representations inevitably measure both more and less than we intended. For example, check lists of stressful life events usually capture variation in recall, as well as the actual experience we want to measure. On the other hand, the measure will miss stressful events that are not enumerated.

In addition, in each study we test our hypotheses among a particular group of people within a particular social, historical, and material context. We have described the British birth cohort of 1946 as an exemplar of a cohort study's producing important results across the life course (chapter 10). We also emphasized that the cohort bears the imprint of the particular social movements under way at that time.

We want the knowledge generated by our studies to have meaning outside the confines of the study particulars. One way to accomplish this goal is to identify the mechanisms through which the exposure affects the disease, and the circumstances under which its effects are activated. We refer to the former as **construct validity** and to the latter as **external validity** (Shadish et al. 2002).

Construct Validity: Identifying Mediators

As already noted, when we accept a risk factor as a cause, we are satisfied that there is no other plausible explanation for the exposure-disease association. Of course, the list of alternatives is limited by our knowledge and imagination, so it is never exhaustive. Nonetheless, if we have identified the major rival hypotheses and ruled them out, we judge the exposure to be a cause, at least for the time being. When we reach this conclusion, the next logical question arises: what is it about the exposure that caused the disease?

To address the question of how the exposure works, we need to identify the active ingredients of the exposure and understand the chain of causation through which they lead to disease. Construct validity addresses questions about these mediational processes. Such knowledge allows us to see the range of measures of the exposure and outcome over which the causal relationship extends. Thus, knowledge about construct validity helps us generalize beyond the specific measures of our study.

For example, studies about the relationship of stress to depression are often conducted by measuring specific stressful life events. Much work has been done to understand what it is about stressful life events that make them pathogenic for depression. In one theory (Brown 1998), humiliation is among the central pathogenic elements. This theory would suggest that life events that involve humiliation but were not assessed in a given study could also cause depression. Thus, understanding this mechanism helps generalize the results beyond the specific measures of life events used in a given study. Furthermore, understanding this mechanism may lead us to a broader view of the outcome. If other outcomes, perhaps dysthymia, were found to be related specifically to life events involving humiliation, the finding would suggest that these outcomes could be branches of the pathogenic process associated with depression.

Within observational risk factor studies, epidemiologists test mediation with the same statistical procedures used to assess confounding (see part VI). We estimate the exposure-disease relationship adjusted for the hypothesized mediator (e.g., humiliation in our current example, or interpersonal difficulties in the preceding example) and compare the crude and adjusted effect estimates. An appreciable decrease from the crude to the adjusted estimate indicates that the mediator accounts for at least part of the exposure-disease relationship.

To make this process more concrete, consider the ongoing example in this book, the relationship between maternal overweight and schizophrenia spectrum disorders in the Prenatal Determinants of Schizophrenia Example (PDSE) study. In examining the hypothesis that there is a causal relationship between maternal overweight and these disorders, the researchers would be careful to minimize or adjust for differences between the exposed and unexposed on third-variable risk factors, on loss to follow-up, and on disease ascertainment. Then, if they found a relationship between maternal overweight and schizophrenia spectrum disorders, as in the PDSE, they might consider it to be plausibly causal.

However, there is always the possibility that, despite the researchers' care, the relationship is spurious. In addition, there might be something peculiar to the women in this study, in this location, at this time period, that made maternal overweight a risk factor for schizophrenia that would not apply outside this study's unique constellation. To curtail these objections, the researchers could address the next logical problem: identifying the mechanisms through which maternal overweight could cause schizophrenia spectrum disorders in the child.

One possible mechanism is that maternal overweight disrupts fetal development through its influence on gestational diabetes. This is plausible because maternal overweight is associated with gestational diabetes and gestational diabetes affects fetal development. The researchers might then examine maternal medical records to determine the occurrence of gestational diabetes.

Other mechanisms are possible. For example, at the time of the PDSE, physicians were concerned that excessive maternal weight gain could be detrimental. They often recommended restrictive diets or amphetamine use (or both) to overweight women to limit their weight gain during pregnancy. It is possible that maternal overweight did indeed lead to schizophrenia spectrum disorders in this study, but only because it initiated a particular physician response. If this mechanism were operative, the relationship between maternal overweight and schizophrenia spectrum disorders would not reside in a biological consequence of maternal overweight. The researchers might then examine maternal records on dietary restriction and amphetamine to evaluate this alternative explanation.

Suppose that adjustment for gestational diabetes, but not dietary restriction or amphetamine use, yielded an estimate that was smaller than the crude. This result would indicate that gestational diabetes was indeed a plausible mechanism to explain the exposure-disease relationship. This result would greatly increase our confidence in maternal overweight as a cause of schizophrenia spectrum disorder in the PDSE, and as a cause that would have an effect outside the specific circumstances of the PDSE.

Several issues are notable from this example. First, mediational processes cannot be tested unless the researchers have hypotheses about and measures of them. The more that is known about the disease under investigation, the easier it is to posit mediational processes. Nonetheless, we can usually formulate some hypotheses about mediation, even if they are tentative. As previously noted (chapter 8), we can enhance the opportunities for studying mediation in a cohort study by collecting comprehensive information and archiving biological specimens for future use when the disease processes are more fully understood. In the PDSE, extensive information was collected from maternal records in the original birth cohort study and biological specimens were archived. As a result, some of the analyses described here are feasible and under way.

Second, this example shows that whether a variable is considered a mediator or a confounder is sometimes a matter of theory, not data. In the scenario we have described, we hypothesized that the link between maternal overweight and schizophrenia was gestational diabetes. Amphetamine use was treated as a confounder, a third-variable alternative explanation, because it did not lie on the causal path of interest between the exposure and disease (see figure 35.1). But we could also have hypothesized that the link between maternal overweight and schizophrenia was amphetamine use. If so, amphetamine use would be a mediator, not a confounder.

In general, when a variable is a consequence of the exposure, the distinction between a mediational and a confounding effect depends upon the researchers' theory. This distinction is critical, nonetheless. The same methods are used to assess confounding and mediation, but similar results yield divergent interpretations. To the extent that adjustment for a confounder decreases the association of the exposure and the disease, the confidence we have in our causal theory is diminished. The viability of the confounding variable as an alternative explanation for the association is enhanced.[1] In contrast, when adjustment for a mediator decreases the effect estimate for the exposure-disease relationship, our confidence in the causal theory increases. This data pattern supports a plausible mechanism through which the exposure may work. Our theory, being more specific in its predictions, has passed a more difficult test.

---

[1] Of course, confounders can also suppress a relationship between the exposure and disease. However, under such circumstances it would hide the association rather than pose an alternative explanation for the association.

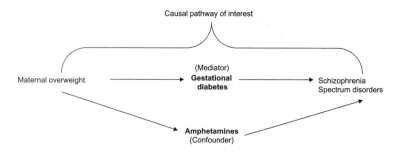

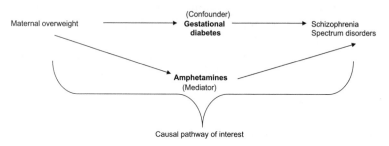

Figure 35.1 Theory dependence of confounding versus mediation.

Testing for mediation is therefore vital to causal explanation. But such tests of mediation warrant caution. The addition of this variable requires consideration of a new class of potential confounders, those that apply to the relationship between the mediator and the disease. To the extent that there are uncontrolled confounders of that relationship, adjusting for the mediator may produce a biased estimate. Adjustment for a mediator that is measured with error may also result in a biased estimate of the mediational effect (Weinberg 1993; Greenland et al. 1999; Cole and Hernan 2002; McNamee 2003; Greenland 2003).

Similar problems arise in the control of confounders. In the methods used most commonly in epidemiology and described in the statistics sections of this book, we deal with confounders through design and statistical adjustment. In so doing, we usually think about confounding as caused by individual risk factors. But confounding is based on the totality and balance of all risk factors between the exposed and unexposed. Unless we fully understand the interplay among these potential confounders, which we virtually never do, our adjustment may be insufficient or even misleading. A variable may meet all of the criteria for a potential confounder, adjustment may lead to an estimate that is appreciably different from the crude, yet the adjusted association may be less valid than the crude (Lieberson 1985; Greenland and Robins 1986; Weinberg 1993; Greenland et al. 1999). This lesser validity occurs because the exposed may have an excess of one risk factor, while the unexposed may have an excess of another. When we adjust for one and not the other, the delicate equilibrium is disturbed (Greenland and Morgenstern 2001).

Drawing causal diagrams of the relationships among the theory's influential variables helps identify these potential problems (Susser 1973). There is a substantial and growing epidemiologic literature on the application of these methods, particularly under the rubric of directed acyclic graphs (DAGs). These graphs depict causal relationships among both measured and unmeasured variables, using arrows to indicate the direction of the posited effects. Drawing the diagram forces us to think through the elements in our causal model. When DAGs are drawn before we begin our studies, they can provide a guide to the information we need to adequately address our causal questions. Note, however, that the DAGs are only as valid as the postulated relationships they represent—that is, only as good as our theory.

When we formulate our conceptual models, the distinction between natural and artifactual confounding becomes important. When confounding is created by a methodological artifact, such as selection bias, there is no true relationship between the exposure and the confounder. Therefore, removal of the exposure from the population will not influence the prevalence of the confounding causal factor. In contrast, if the exposure is associated with the cause in the population—that is, it is a natural confounder—removal of the exposure may have an effect on the prevalence of the confounder. The impact will depend upon the linkages between the exposure and the confounder in the population.

Drawing the relationship between the exposure and confounding variables may help identify the impact of the exposure's removal. For example, if the exposure and confounder are caused by the same antecedent, removal of the antecedent may be the best way to improve public health since it will remove the effect, at least in part, of two causes of the disease at once. Indeed, a failure to remove the antecedent may lead to the confounding cause's substituting for the exposure. This substitution could happen, for instance, in an investigation of methamphetamine addiction as a cause of psychosis. If cocaine use were a confounder of the methamphetamine-psychosis relationship because they shared the antecedent cause of a thrill-seeking personality, focusing on removing methamphetamine from the environment may simply lead to an increase in cocaine use.

Figure 35.2A shows a simple DAG depicting the mediational hypothesis described for the relationship between maternal overweight and

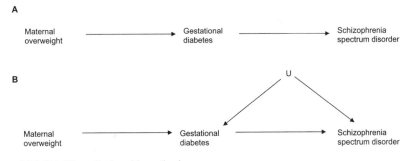

Figure 35.2 DAGS mediational hypothesis.

schizophrenia spectrum disorders. For this model, adjustment for gestational diabetes would provide an indication of its mediational effect. However, there may be some unmeasured cause of both schizophrenia spectrum disorders and gestational diabetes, perhaps some underlying genetic vulnerability, which could confound the gestational diabetes–schizophrenia spectrum relationship (see figure 35.2B). If so, adjustment for gestational diabetes would give a biased estimate of the mediational effect. In fact, it can be shown that adjustment for gestational diabetes could induce an association between maternal overweight and schizophrenia spectrum disorder by linking them in another pathway (Cole and Hernan 2002).

Rules have been developed for determining the variables that should be controlled to obtain valid estimates of the exposure-disease relationship (see, e.g., Weinberg 1993; Greenland et al. 1999; Greenland and Brumback 2002; Cole and Hernan 2002; Greenland 2003). In addition, some epidemiologists have proposed new methods, such as Robin's g-estimation, to deal with these situations more effectively (Cole and Hernan 2002).

Despite these caveats, examining mediational effects, when thoughtfully done, can greatly enhance the generalizability of the study's results. External validity is another element of causal explanation that plays a complementary role.

External Validity: The Identification of Causal Partners

External validity is the extent to which the causal effect found in a study is generalizable across characteristics of persons, places, and time periods (Shadish et al. 2002). Our expectations about external validity are somewhat paradoxical. On the one hand, we often question the applicability of our findings to populations that differ from those in the study. We always consider the possibility that populations are unique in their constellation of causal factors. For example, a concern has been raised that most epidemiologic research on cardiovascular disease has been conducted among white men. Examining the applicability of these findings to women and nonwhites is considered an important research issue. At the same time, the consistency of our findings across populations is often seen as an indication of the validity of our study results. As discussed in part I, consistency is one of the standards by which causal inferences are often assessed.

A resolution to this paradox requires an understanding of the origins of variation between populations. A central tenet of the risk factor paradigm is that causes act in concert with their causal partners to produce disease. Elaborating the implications of this tenet can give us some insight into variation across populations. The joint action of causal partners is variously referred to as **synergy**, **interaction**, and **effect modification**. To avoid confusion, in this section we will reserve the terms synergy and interaction for the joint action of causal partners and use the terms **effect modification**, and *statistical interaction* for statistical representations of this joint action.

One of the important consequences of synergy is that the prevalence of an exposure's causal partners influences the size of the exposure's effect. We explained this in detail in chapter 4, but briefly review the conclusions here. In general, the more common the causal partners, the larger the effect size; the more rare the causal partners, the smaller the effect size. The potential biological role of the cause remains constant, but its activation depends on its causal partners. A cause's strength, defined in epidemiologic terms (e.g., the size of the risk ratio), hinges on the frequency with which its potential effects are activated. For example, if a cause is very common in a population, but its causal partners occur in only one percent of the population, then only one percent of the people with the exposure will get the disease from that exposure. However, if the causal partners are ubiquitous, then all of the people with the exposure will get the disease.

Thus, we would expect the strength of a cause to differ across persons, places, and time periods when the prevalence and distribution of the causal partners differ. If all the causal partners of an exposure were identified, we would have an explanation for the disease that would be universally applicable and indicate the populations where this cause would and would not be potent. Of course, in practice we never know all of the causal partners.

We often make the reasonable, but not always correct, assumption that if a risk factor acts as a cause in one population it will act as a cause in another. Even when this assumption is correct, it does not imply that the magnitude of the effects should be constant. Researchers sometimes contend that the causal effect of the exposure is secure because the effect size they have found is identical to the effect size another researcher found in a different setting. Finding precisely the same effect for an exposure in different settings is not required for an effect to be causal. Indeed, we should expect to see at least some variation across settings because of variation in the distribution of causal partners.

It may not even be necessary that a cause lead to any disease at all in a different setting. A commonly used example of this phenomenon (discussed previously) is phenylketonuria (PKU). In this disease, a genetic anomaly prevents the metabolism of the amino acid phenylalanine. An accumulation of phenylalanine in the blood is toxic to the brain and causes mental retardation. Consequently, there is a synergistic relationship between the genetic anomaly and the consumption of food containing phenylalanine. This genetic anomaly would have no effect in populations where phenylalanine is absent in the diet. If we did not know that phenylalanine was a causal partner of the PKU gene, we would note that there is an effect of the gene that is population-specific. Once we know the causal partner, we can make a more universal statement: across populations and time periods, the PKU gene will be a cause of disease in the presence of phenylalanine.

External validity, then, is about specification of the conditions under which the cause does and does not act, through which we approach a universally applicable understanding of the disease development. Thought of in this way, generalizability is a step in the process of causal explanation, one that entails the identification of an exposure's casual partners. It follows that assessing the interaction among causes, or synergy, is vital for our understanding of generalizability.

Assessing Synergy in our Studies

The assessment and detection of synergy has an interesting history in epidemiology. Typically, as described in chapter 27, we consider our data to support a synergistic relationship between two risk factors if the disease risk among those with both risk factors is higher than would be expected if each risk factor were working independently. So, for example, if two risk factors each have a risk ratio of 3.0, then, assuming no synergistic effect, we might expect a risk ratio of 9.0 among those with both factors, because the effect of each risk factor would be unaffected by the other.

This approach to interaction is conceptually problematic. Our question may be framed as follows: is the effect of the joint presence of both of these factors greater than what one would expect from their independent effects alone? The answer depends on what one would expect. Each measure of effect—risk difference, risk ratio, odds ratio, or other—has a different expectation of the results under an assumption of independence. When risk ratios are being used, as in our example, the assumption is that, absent interaction, risks multiply in their effects. This situation is sometimes referred to as a **multiplicative model**. When risk differences are used, the assumption is that, absent interaction, risks add in their effects; hence, we have an **additive model**.[2]

This problem was at the core of a debate in psychiatric epidemiology about vulnerability factors for depression. Brown and Harris (1978a; 1978b) claimed that certain vulnerability factors (such as intimacy problems) interact with life events in causing depression. Tennent and Bebbington (1978) challenged this assertion, contesting that there was no evidence of interaction between these variables. Table 35.1 shows the data that produced these conflicting interpretations.

Brown and Harris analyzed the data under the assumption that risks add in their effect. Under this premise, the data indeed showed that the effect of both life events and intimacy problems was greater than what would be expected from the effects of life events and intimacy acting independently of each other. The proportion of people with neither life events nor intimacy problems who developed depression was one percent, the baseline risk. The proportion was 10 percent for those with only life events, an increase of 9 percent over the

Table 35.1 Data for Brown and Harris Example: Proportion of Respondents Developing Depression

Severe Life Event or Major Difficulty	Intimacy Problems	
	Yes	No
Yes	32%	10%
No	3%	1%

Source: Brown and Harris (1978, p. 585).

[2] Note that when one is estimating main effects, ratio measures or difference measures can be used without implying a specific model of joint effects.

baseline risk. The proportion was 3 percent for those with only intimacy problems, an increase of 2 percent over the base line risk. Under this additive model, if there were no interaction we would expect a risk of 12 percent for those with both risk factors, an increase of 11 percent (9 percent + 2 percent) over the baseline of one percent. In the data, however, the risk for those with both life events and intimacy problems was 32 percent, clearly much more than the expected 12 percent. Brown and Harris therefore concluded that interaction was evident because the outcome among those with both risk factors was greater than the additive effects of each of them in isolation.

Tenent and Bebbington (1978) reanalyzed these data under the assumption that risks multiply in their effects. This assumption derived from their use of a log linear model, a statistical procedure that tests interaction on the premise that independent risks multiply in their effects. Under this premise, the data show that there was no interaction. In these data women with only life events had a risk that was 10 times the baseline risk (10 percent versus one percent). Women with only intimacy problems had a risk that was 3 times the baseline risk (3 percent versus one percent). If there were no interaction between intimacy problems and life events, one would expect women with both life events and intimacy problems to have a risk of depression that is 30 times the baseline risk (10 * 3 = 30), quite close to the actual risk in women who had both risk factors (32 percent). Therefore, Tennent and Bebbington concluded from these same data that there was no interaction between life events and intimacy problems.

Each of these alternative interpretations is consistent with the premises of the mathematical models that were used. There is evidence of statistical interaction if we assume, as did Brown and Harris, that, absent interaction, risk factors add in their effects. There is no evidence of statistical interaction if we assume, as did Tennet and Bebbington, that, absent interaction, risk factors multiply in their effects. It is, however, entirely illogical to claim that our data can simultaneously support and not support synergy. Next we offer an exit from this conundrum. We begin by describing the proposed method and then discuss its derivation.

An Additive Model with a "Twist"

Darroch (1997) and Rothman and Greenland (1998) grappled with this problem and concluded that the additive model, with a "twist," allows the best representation of synergy. An additive model assumes that risks add in their effects. Thus, positive deviations from additivity—or superadditivity—indicate the presence of synergy. The twist is that risks do something slightly less than add; therefore, although superadditivity does indicate synergy, a failure to find superadditivity does not necessarily imply the absence of synergy.

The twist originates from redundancy among causes. That some individuals can develop disease from either one of the two exposures under study alone leads to a phenomenon labeled **parallelism**. As will be further explained, this redundancy reduces the measure of the exposures' combined effect. What we see as the combined effect reflects the balance of synergy, which is the interaction of two causal partners in causing disease, and parallelism, which is the substitutability of two risk factors in causing disease. Thus, the results of our mathematical models for detecting deviations from additivity represent the balance between the subadditivity of parallelism and the super-additivity of synergy.

Consider the routes to depression in the Brown and Harris example. Suppose that there is no synergy between life events and intimacy problems. Some people may develop depression from a constellation of causes that includes life events but not intimacy problems. Others develop depression from a constellation that includes intimacy problems but not life events. Still others could develop depression from either of these two constellations. When individuals in the latter group are exposed to both life events and intimacy problems there is a "competition" between them to cause depression.

Now suppose that there is synergy. This implies that there is yet another group of individuals who develop depression only from a constellation that includes both stressful life events and intimacy problems. Next we discuss the implications of this approach for the detection of synergy.

Estimating Synergy

Our measures of effect imply assumptions about our expectations in the absence of synergy. Difference measures assume that risks add, whereas ratio measures assume that risks multiply. Similarly, each mathematical model that we use to analyze our data implies a different underlying assumption about whether risks add or multiply. For example, linear regression assumes that risks add and therefore provides a direct way to assess deviations from additivity. In contrast, logistic regression assumes that risks multiply.

For several reasons, we generally analyze our data according to multiplicative models such as logistic regression (see part VI). This practice poses a dilemma for the assessment of synergy if we think that synergy should be assessed under an additive model. However, under some circumstances there are resolutions to the dilemma.

First, if there is positive interaction on a multiplicative scale, there will be positive interaction on an additive scale. Supermultiplicativity implies super-additivity. Therefore, if we enter an interaction term in a multiplicative model and it is positive, the results support synergy.

Second, when we use a multiplicative model we can nonetheless translate the estimates to assess interaction on an additive scale by calculating an **interaction contrast** (Rothman and Greenland 1998). To illustrate how this is done, we return to the interaction between a serotonin transporter gene polymorphism and life stress in causing depression, as reported from the Dunedin birth cohort (Caspi et al. 2003) described in chapters 27 and 29. In the analysis we discuss here, the authors contrasted people with the short (s) allele (s/l or s/s) and without the s allele (l/l) in terms of their susceptibility to depression after four or more life events. Accordingly, we consider individuals with either the $s/1$ or s/s genotype as having the susceptible genotype. In accordance with data displayed in table 35.2, we will calculate the interaction contrast, comparing the effects of four or more life events among those with and without the susceptible genotype.

Table 35.2 Data from Dunedin Example: Percentage of Individuals in Each Category Meeting Criteria for Depression

4+ Life Events	S Genotype	
	Yes	No
Yes	33%	17%
No	10%	10%

Source: Caspi et al. (2003).

The disease prevalence among those with neither the susceptible genotype nor life events was 10 percent; among those with only the susceptible genotype, 10 percent; among those with only life events, 17 percent; and among those with both life events and the susceptible genotype, 33 percent. In this instance the interaction contrast would be .33 − .17 − .10 + .10 = .16. The interaction contrast thus equals the risk among those with both factors (.33), minus the risk among those with one (.17), minus the risk among those with the other (.10), plus the baseline risk (.10). Since the interaction contrast here is greater than zero (.16), it indicates the presence of synergy in this population.

In this example, the risks required for the computation were directly provided by the report. However, in a cohort study we can compute the interaction contrast, regardless of the form in which the results are analyzed and presented. Suppose we analyzed the data under a logistic regression model. The baseline odds of disease would be derived from the intercept. The odds ratios from the logistic regression would then be used to obtain the odds of disease under the other conditions. Finally, the odds would be converted to risks (odds $= p/(1 - p)$).

When we cannot estimate the baseline risk of disease, as in a case-control study, we can calculate an **interaction contrast ratio** by using odds ratios. For illustration, we computed the odds ratios for the Dunedin study from the prevalence estimates given (see table 35.2). In this instance, the interaction contrast ratio would be 4.4 − 1.8 − 1 + 1 = 2.6. The interaction contrast ratio is the odds ratio for those with both factors (4.4), minus the odds ratio for those with one factor (1.8), minus the odds ratio for those with the other factor (1), plus one.[3]

The interaction contrast ratio divided by the odds ratio in those exposed to both risk factors can be interpreted as the proportion of disease among those with both risk factors that is attributable to the interaction. In this instance, we would estimate that 59 percent (2.6/4.4) of the disease among those with four or more life events and the susceptible genotype is attributable

---

[3] The odds for those exposed to both factors is .33/.67; for those exposed to only life events, .17/.83; for those exposed to only the *s* allele, .10/.90; and for those exposed to neither, .10/.90. Therefore, the odds ratios for those exposed to both risk factors versus those exposed to neither is 4.4; for those exposed to only life events versus those exposed to neither, 1.8; and for those exposed to only the *s* allele versus those exposed to neither, 1.

to the interaction between these factors. Several methods have been developed to calculate *p*-values and confidence intervals around these estimates (see, e.g., Hosmer and Lemeshow 1992; Assmann et al. 1996; Rothman and Greenland 1998).

From Synergy to Its Mathematical Representation

To show how epidemiologists (e.g., Darroch 1997; Rothman and Greenland 1998) reached the conclusion that an additive model, with a twist, provides the best representation of synergy, we begin with a very simple situation, one based on the Brown and Harris example. We want to test the hypothesis that recent stressful life events and intimacy problems exhibit a synergistic relationship in causing depression for at least some people.

Since our theory of depression is multicausal, we do not hypothesize that this is the only way to get depression, nor do we hypothesize that intimacy problems and stressful life events are monogamously paired. Intimacy problems may also cause depression when paired with other risk factors (e.g., death of a parent in childhood), and, similarly, stressful life events may also cause depression when paired with other risk factors (e.g., genetic vulnerability). This conceptual model is illustrated in figure 35.3. Because of our interest in these two risk factors, we posit four different causal pies leading to depression: (1) life events, intimacy problems, and other causal partners; (2) life events and causal partners other than intimacy problems; (3) intimacy problems and causal partners other than life events; and (4) causal partners that include neither intimacy problems nor life events.

If our hypothesis is correct, there are some people who become depressed by means of the first causal pie. For these people, intimacy problems represent

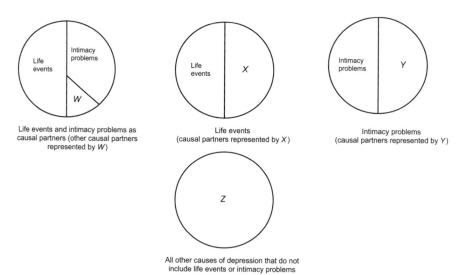

Figure 35.3 Causes of depression: theory about life events and their interaction with intimacy problems.

a context that activates the deleterious effect of stressful life events and vice-versa. Our goal is to determine whether such people exist in the study population.

As a first step, we need to categorize people according to their capacity to develop depression when exposed to the risk factors under investigation (see the left-hand section of figure 35.4). We categorize people who would develop disease if, and only if, they were exposed to both life events and intimacy problems as synergistic types. What makes someone a synergistic type is the presence of W, the stand-in for all the additional causal partners necessary for life events and a lack of intimacy to interact and cause depression. These are the people we want to be able to detect.

Those who would develop depression if exposed to life events, even without intimacy problems, are categorized as life events–susceptible people. Those who have X, the stand-in for all causal partners of life events other than a lack of intimacy, are placed in this category. Similarly, those who would develop depression if exposed to intimacy problems, even without life events, are categorized as intimacy problem–susceptible people. Those who have Y, the stand-in for all causal partners of intimacy problems other than life events, are placed in this category. We categorize as doomed those with all of the causal partners needed to become depressed from causes other than the risk factors under investigation (Z). We categorize as immune people who will not incur depression even if they are exposed to life events or intimacy problems. These people do not have W, X, Y, or Z.

Now we introduce one more category, and it constitutes the twist. There are some people who have both X and Y, and therefore are susceptible to

"Type" Person Is:	CAUSAL PARTNERS PERSON HAS	CAUSE PERSON IS SUSCEPTIBLE TO	DISEASE EXPERIENCE IF EXPOSED TO:			
			LIFE EVENTS	INTIMACY PROBLEMS	BOTH	NEITHER
SYNERGYSTIC	W	Life events / Intimacy problems — W	No disease	No disease	D+	No disease
LIFE EVENT susceptible	X	Life events — X	D+	No disease	D+	No disease
INTIMACY PROBLEM susceptible	Y	Intimacy problems — Y	No disease	D+	D+	No disease
DOOMED	Z	Z	D+	D+	D+	D+
IMMUNE		NONE	No disease	No disease	No disease	No disease
PARALLEL	X / Y	Life events or Intimacy problems — X / Y	D+	D+	D+	No disease

Figure 35.4 Assessing interaction between life events and intimacy problems.

getting the disease from either stressful life events or a lack of intimacy. Indeed, if they are exposed to both of these risk factors, there will be a competition between life events and lack of intimacy for causing the disease. Such people are parallel types.

To avoid confusion, note that types are not fixed characteristics of individuals. A person's type is defined only in relation to a particular cause under investigation at a particular moment. It is merely a designation of the causes to which they have been exposed, other than the exposures under study. Thus, in our model, people with *W* are synergistic types only with regard to the interaction of stressful life events and lack of intimacy. If we were investigating the relationship among other risk factors (e.g., genetic variants), these same people would be considered a different type. Furthermore, at a different moment in time individuals may be exposed to new factors and become unexposed to others. This change in exposure would change their type.

The right-hand section of figure 35.4 indicates, for individuals of each type, whether or not they would develop the disease if they were exposed to the risk factors under investigation. For example, people who are life event–susceptible types (row 2), will get the disease if they are exposed to life events, regardless of exposure to intimacy problems. The immune types (row 5) never develop the disease.

By looking down the columns, we can then examine for each exposure condition what types of people will develop the disease. As shown in the column labeled *life events,* individuals who are exposed to life events but not intimacy problems will develop disease if they are one of three types: life event–susceptible, doomed, or parallel. Individuals who are exposed only to intimacy problems, but not life events (the next column), will develop disease if they are intimacy-susceptible, doomed, or parallel. Individuals exposed to both life events and intimacy problems will develop disease if they are any type other than immune. Finally, individuals who are exposed to neither intimacy problems nor life events (the final column) will develop disease only if their type is doomed.

We want to find a mathematical model that will allow us to detect the presence of synergistic types, people for whom life events and intimacy problems work together to cause depression. Types, however, are not observable; we do not know the causal partners necessary for different exposures to have an effect, nor can we measure all of these factors: *W, X, Y,* and *Z* represent a large number of unknown exposures. What we can observe is the exposure and disease experience of the people in our study. We can categorize people by the exposure condition and compute the risk for each condition. As summarized in figure 35.5 and as already outlined here, we also know how different types would respond under different exposure conditions. It is from this combination of empirical observations and hypothetical responses that we try to discern the presence of synergistic types.

We can think of each column in figure 35.5 as representing a different exposure group in a cohort study, with each group defined by its exposure experiences. The group with neither life events nor intimacy problems can be considered the counterfactual for each of the other exposure groups. The disease risk of the people in this column (the last column in the figure) is used

Disease risk	Among those exposed to both life events and intimacy problems	Among those exposed only to life events	Among those exposed to intimacy problems	Among those exposed to neither life events nor intimacy problems
Observation	Proportion diseased among those exposed to both	Proportion diseased in those exposed only to life events	Proportion diseased in those exposed to only intimacy problems	Proportion diseased among those exposed to neither
Numeric representation	R_{12}	R_1	R_2	R
Types contributing to this risk	Synergistic, doomed, life event susceptible, intimacy problem susceptible, parallel	Doomed, life event susceptible, parallel	Doomed, intimacy problem susceptible, parallel	Doomed

Relationship Between Observed Risk and Unobserved Types

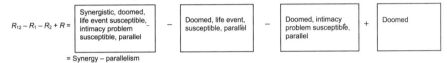

$$R_{12} - R_1 - R_2 + R =$$ Synergistic, doomed, life event susceptible, intimacy problem susceptible, parallel $-$ Doomed, life event, susceptible, parallel $-$ Doomed, intimacy problem susceptible, parallel $+$ Doomed

= Synergy – parallelism

Figure 35.5 Relationship between observed risk (proportion with disease) and unobserved types.

to represent the disease risk that each of the other exposure groups would have had if they were exposed to neither of the risk factors under investigation. Therefore, analogous to ensuring comparability of the exposed and unexposed in a cohort study, comparability of all three exposure groups with the unexposed group must be ensured. In other words, the distribution of types in the different exposure groups should be the same. That is, the proportion of life events–susceptible, intimacy-problem-susceptible, doomed, synergistic, and immune types should be the same across exposure cohorts. When this is so, the proportion of types in each exposure group equals the proportion of types in the sample as a whole. Under this condition, the disease risk in the unexposed group represents what the disease risk would have been in each of the other groups, absent the exposure.

Assuming we have such comparable groups, the pattern of exposure-disease relationships in our data can tell us something about the presence or absence of interaction. As noted, although we know neither the types nor the distribution of types for any of the exposure groups, we do know the following:

1. Among those exposed to both life events and lack of intimacy, the proportion of diseased people (R_{12}) equals the total proportion of synergistic, doomed, life event–susceptible, intimacy-problem-susceptible, and parallel types in the sample;
2. Among those exposed to life events but not intimacy problems, the proportion of diseased people (R_1) equals the total proportion of doomed, life event–susceptible, and parallel types in the sample;
3. Among those exposed to intimacy problems but not life events, the proportion of diseased people (R_2) equals the total proportion of doomed, intimacy-problem-susceptible, and parallel types in the sample;
4. Among those exposed to neither of these risk factors, the proportion of diseased people (R) equals the proportion of doomed types in the sample.

Based on the pattern of disease experience among the exposed and unexposed we cannot fully isolate the synergistic types to estimate their proportion. However, we can estimate the difference between the proportion of synergistic and parallel types. This result is obtained by simple subtraction after we have delineated the types contributing to the diseased among each exposure combination. As illustrated at the bottom of figure 35.5, the disease risk (proportion) among those with both factors (R_{12}), minus the risk among those with only life events (R_1), minus the risk among those with only intimacy problems (R_2), plus the risk among those with neither exposure (or the baseline risk) (R), equals the proportion of synergistic types minus the proportion of parallel types.

To illustrate how this approach works, we apply it to the data from Brown and Harris (1978a). As we saw in table 35.1, the risk among those exposed to both a severe life event and intimacy problems was .32; the risk among those with a severe event but no intimacy problems was .03; the risk among those with intimacy problems but no severe event was .10; and the risk among those with neither risk factor was .01. In this instance, then, the proportion of synergistic types minus the proportion of parallel types is represented by .32 (the risk among those with both risk factors) − .10 (the risk among those with one) − .03 (the risk among those with the other) + .01 (the risk among those with neither) = .20. Since this estimate is appreciably greater than zero, the hypothesis that stressful life events and intimacy problems work in a synergistic manner to produce depression for at least some people in this population would be supported. Note, however, that this estimate may be an underestimate of the proportion of individuals who developed the disease because of synergy, since it is for synergy minus parallelism.

We can now ask what mathematical model best corresponds to the argument we have just laid out. It turns out that it is the additive model, albeit the correspondence is imperfect. If risks add, then in the absence of synergy the additional risk (i.e., the risk above baseline) conferred by both factors ($R_{12} - R$) should equal the sum of the additional risks conferred by each alone ($R_1 - R$) + ($R_2 - R$). Therefore ($R_{12} - R$) − ($R_1 - R$) − ($R_2 - R$) should equal zero. We can state this more simply as $R_{12} - R_1 - R_2 + R$. If this equation is greater than zero, there is an indication of synergy. Therefore, superadditivity indicates the presence of synergy.

What makes the correspondence less than perfect is the possible presence of parallel types. Among the group with both factors of interest (i.e., stressful life events and intimacy problems) there may be some people for whom either risk factor alone would be sufficient to complete a sufficient cause for the disease. These people have more risk factors than necessary for the disease to develop. Parallel types are likely to occur when social forces, such as socioeconomic status, are linked to disease through multiple pathways. Such factors are likely to lead to a myriad of causal partners that can work with many different risk factors to cause disease. When this happens, parallel types will arise. If the resulting subadditivity of parallelism is similar in magnitude to the superadditivity of synergy, the risks will appear to be additive. Therefore, we may tend to underestimate synergy in this situation.

This approach to assessing interaction is appealing because it begins with our conceptual model and deduces the mathematical model that best represents it. Statistics are used appropriately as a tool to test our causal theories rather than as a template that constrains them. Nonetheless, it provides a cautionary tale in our search for causal explanation. There are many situations in which our results may be indeterminate, even when we are trying to detect synergy between only two risk factors. This is because, although superadditivity indicates the presence of synergy, a lack of superadditivity does not necessarily imply absence of synergy. As is the case in all epidemiologic studies, the effects that we estimate are average effects. In the presence of contravening effects, synergy will be difficult to detect. Parallelism is one such contravening effect. In addition, so far we have made the assumption that the factors under investigation do not increase the risk of disease in some individuals while decreasing the risk of disease in others. In other words, we have assumed there is no antagonism in this population. This may not always be a reasonable assumption. For example, it is possible that, for some children, specific types of parent-child interactions may enhance psychological functioning, whereas for others these same types of interactions would be detrimental. The presence of antagonism is another contravening effect that can also lead to indeterminacy.

Nonetheless, this approach helps us to detect synergy that our usual approaches based in multiplicative models would miss. Our multiplicative models detect only synergy that produces such large deviations from additive effects that they are also greater than multiplicativity. Using an additive model with a twist, through interaction contrasts, or interaction contrast ratios, allows us to detect more subtle evidence of true synergy.

Conclusion

Causal explanation enhances our research endeavors both by increasing our confidence in the causal effect of our risk factors and by delineating the extent to which the results of our study apply to other populations. Within the risk factor paradigm, construct validity and external validity form the basis of causal explanation. Construct validity helps us to identify the active ingredients of our exposures and the mechanisms through which they work so that we can see effects beyond the specific measures we have chosen. The identification of causal partners is at the heart of external validity. Identifying the causal partners of the exposure under investigation specifies the conditions under which the exposure will and will not have an effect. In populations and time periods in which these causal partners are virtually ubiquitous, we would expect the cause to be frequently activated and thus appear as a strong cause. In populations and time periods in which these causal partners are virtually absent, we would expect the cause to be infrequently activated and to be a weak cause. The biology is the same; the activation is different.

The detection of both mediation and synergy, however, is at the edge of what our methods can currently tell us. Such detection requires the acceptance of assumptions that may be limiting and may not conform well to the ways that diseases develop. However, examining the fit between our conceptual and mathematical models is an important step toward understanding the complexity of disease development. Once we have identified mechanisms and causal partners within our observational designs, we can sometimes test them more definitively in prevention trials and intervention studies.

References

Assmann SF, Hosmer DW, Lemeshow S, and Mundt KA (1996). Confidence Intervals for Measures of Interaction. *Epidemiology* 7:286–290.

Brown GW (1998). Genetic and Population Perspectives on Life Events and Depression. *Soc. Psychiatry Psychiatr. Epidemiol.* 33:363–372.

Brown GW and Harris T (1978a). Social Origins of Depression: A Reply. *Psychol. Med.* 8:577–588.

Brown GW and Harris T (1978b). *Social Origins of Depression: A Study of Psychiatric Disorder in Women.* New York: Free Press.

Caspi A, Sugden K, Moffitt TE, et al. (2003). Influence of Life Stress on Depression: Moderation by a Polymorphism in the *5-HTT* Gene. *Science* 301:386–389.

Cohen P and Cohen J (1996). *Life Values and Adolescent Mental Health.* Mahwah, N.J.: Erlbaum.

Cohen P, Cohen J, and Brook J (1993a). An Epidemiological Study of Disorders in Late Childhood and Adolescence—II. Persistence of Disorders. *J. Child Psychol. Psychiatry* 34:869–877.

Cohen P, Cohen J, Kasen S, Velez CN, Hartmark C, Johnson J, Rojas M, Brook J, and Streuning EL (1993b). An Epidemiological Study of Disorders in Late Childhood and Adolescence—I. Age- and Gender-Specific Prevalence. *J. Child Psychol. Psychiatry* 34:851–867.

Cole SR and Hernan MA (2002). Fallibility in Estimating Direct Effects. *Int. J. Epidemiol.* 31:163–165.

Darroch J (1997). Biologic Synergism and Parallelism. *Am. J. Epidemiol.* 145:661–668.

Greenland S (2003). Quantifying Biases in Causal Models: Classical Confounding vs. Collider-Stratification Bias. *Epidemiology* 14:300–306.

Greenland S and Brumback B (2002). An Overview of Relations among Causal Modelling Methods. *Int. J. Epidemiol.* 31:1030–1037.

Greenland S and Morgenstern H (2001). Confounding in Health Research. *Annu. Rev. Public Health* 22:189–212.

Greenland S, Pearl J, and Robins JM (1999). Causal Diagrams for Epidemiologic Research. *Epidemiology* 10:37–48.

Greenland S and Robins JM (1986). Identifiability, Exchangeability, and Epidemiological Confounding. *Int. J. Epidemiol.* 15:413–419.

Hosmer DW and Lemeshow S (1992). Confidence Interval Estimation of Interaction. *Epidemiology* 3:452–456.

Lieberson S (1985). Making It Count: The Improvement of Social Research and Theory. Berkeley: University of California Press.

McNamee R (2003). Confounding and Confounders. *Occup. Environ. Med.* 60:227–234.

Rothman KJ and Greenland S (1998). *Modern Epidemiology,* 2nd ed. Philadelphia: Lippincott-Raven.

Shadish WR, Cook TD, and Campbell DT (2002). *Experimental and Quasi-Experimental Designs for Generalized Causal Inference.* Boston: Houghton Mifflin.

Susser M (1973). *Causal Thinking in the Health Sciences: Concepts and Strategies of Epidemiology.* New York: Oxford University Press.

Tennant C and Bebbington P (1978). The Social Causation of Depression: A Critique of the Work of Brown and His Colleagues. *Psychol. Med.* 8:565–575.

Weinberg CR (1993). Toward a Clearer Definition of Confounding. *Am. J. Epidemiol.* 137:1–8.

Causal Explanation Outside the Black Box

36

Sharon Schwartz, Ana V. Diez Roux, and Ezra Susser

In part I, we sketched the history of epidemiology as a succession of paradigms, each designating the legitimate problems and methodologic standards for its era. As paradigms mature, the methods and tools become more refined and specialized. The field is consolidated, with greater agreement about basic terminology and perspective. Schools are formed and textbooks written that help shape and disseminate the norms throughout the field. Risk factor epidemiology matured in all these ways during the latter half of the 20th century.

This approach to studying the causes of disease emerged in the mid-20th century in tandem with a change in the health profile of the developed countries: a fall in the rate of infectious diseases (Winslow 1943), concurrent with a rise in the rate of chronic diseases such as cancers and cardiovascular diseases (Morris 1957). Risk factor studies were devised as a means to find the causes of these chronic diseases. In the quintessential application, case-control and cohort studies done in the 1940s and 1950s proved a causal connection between cigarette smoking and lung cancer (U.S. Public Health Service 1964). The methods were also shown to be useful for other cancers (MacMahon et al. 1970; Beebe et al. 1971), cardiovascular diseases (Kagan et al. 1962; Morris et al. 1966), birth defects (Record and McKeown 1949; Record and McKeown 1950), and many other diseases.

By the 1960s, it was widely accepted that risk factor studies were capable of identifying causes of chronic diseases. Meanwhile, infectious diseases continued to decline.[1] Living standards and access to health care among the poor were improving; the waning of social inequalities in health was anticipated.

Over the ensuing decades, risk factor methods were widely adopted, continually refined, and increasingly dominant. An influential textbook of the 1980s neatly encapsulated modern epidemiology (Rothman 1986) and was almost exclusively concerned with methods for studying risk factors. The

---

[1] There was also some hope that developing countries would eventually progress in the same direction. A few landmark achievements, such as the worldwide eradication of smallpox (Fenner 1988), and many other smaller ones (Brockington 1985) suggested that it was at least possible to bring the infectious diseases under control in these countries.

study of infectious diseases and societal causes were now at the periphery of the discipline.

As in previous eras, the dominant approach was not the only one. Throughout, epidemiologists continued other kinds of investigations, studying differences in disease rates across countries and time periods, documenting social inequalities in health, modeling infectious disease epidemics, and relating fetal and child experiences to adult-onset disorders. Indeed, these themes were prominent in the work of many of the progenitors of risk factor methods, who sought to promote the study of risk factors, but not to grant them exclusivity (e.g., Morris 1957; Susser 1973). Also, as previously described (chapter 1), psychiatric epidemiology developed along somewhat different lines. Risk factor methods were not fully taken up, and social antecedents and developmental origins remained central to thinking about the causes of mental disorders, if not always to investigating them. These exceptions notwithstanding, the risk factor approach overshadowed all others in the mainstream of epidemiology.

But shortly thereafter, historical conditions began to conspire against this approach. The emergence of new infectious diseases and the reemergence of others caught epidemiology by surprise. The AIDS epidemic, in particular, required reconsideration of the tenacity of infectious disease. Inequalities in health persisted, impervious to explanation by study of risk factors alone (Link and Phelan 1995). In retrospect, perhaps the paradigm blurred our vision, for all along, infectious diseases remained a scourge in developing countries (Dubos 1965), and continuing health inequalities within developed countries were well documented (Susser et al. 1985). As with the proverbial search under the lamplight for the missing key, we tend to construct problems to be amenable to illumination by our methods. As the risk factor paradigm consolidated, its new, cutting-edge tools demanded application and therefore consideration of the types of problems for which the tools can be used.

For a circumscribed range of questions, risk factor methods were increasingly effective, but researchers had difficulty answering questions outside this range. Consider the following questions pertaining to schizophrenia:

1. Why is the incidence of schizophrenia higher among people born in urban than among those born in rural areas?
2. How can a prenatal insult express its effects decades later as schizophrenia?
3. Is the incidence of schizophrenia declining, and, if so, what is responsible for this decline?

None of these questions focuses exclusively on why one individual but not another develops schizophrenia. The first question is about differences in the rate of disease between populations. The second is about the unfolding of disease over the life course of an individual. The third is about the rise and fall of disease rates in societies. To answer these questions, our studies must include the social contexts in which individuals reside, the development of individuals over their life course, and the historical changes in societies.

Until recently, however, in studies of risk factors these phenomena were typically considered stable background not in the domain of investigation.

Risk factor methods had been carefully fashioned for another purpose: to show associations between the characteristics of individuals and their diseases. Risk factor studies most often examined factors that varied among individuals in a given population as causes of diseases, and limited attention to one phase of the life course and one historical period. Restricting the focus to temporally proximate individual-level factors makes sense in our quest to correctly identify risk factors. In general, the more proximate two characteristics are in terms of level of organization, as well as temporality, the fewer third-variable alternative explanations for their co-occurrence. Therefore, characteristics of individuals, closer to disease onset, are more easily isolated from associated causes than are more distal variables. The restriction comes at a cost, however, and the narrowed focus has been characterized by one critic as "imprisoned by the proximate" (McMichael 1999).

In this chapter, we discuss approaches that could be used to answer questions that often fall outside the range of risk factor studies. Some of these approaches are accommodated by extension of the scope of risk factor designs. Others are still embryonic, and their full development is a central challenge for epidemiology and, specifically, psychiatric epidemiology in the current era. We focus on the three domains corresponding to the questions above: differences in disease rates across populations, the context of the life course, and the rise and fall of disease rates over time.

Differences in Disease Rates across Populations

Within the risk factor paradigm, to explain differences in disease rates across populations we can look for differences in the prevalence and distribution of risk factors across these populations. In a rigorous application of this approach, researchers compared the rates of mental disorder and other behavioral outcomes among children in inner London and the Isle of Wight (Rutter et al. 1976; Rutter 1989). Although the disorder rates were considerably higher in London, the same risk factors were important within each community. Thus, the excess risk in London could be partly explained by the higher prevalence of these risk factors.

Also, to explain differences in the effect of a risk factor across populations we can look for differences in the prevalence of its causal partners. Weaker effects derive from a lower prevalence of causal partners; stronger effects derive from a higher prevalence (part II). For example, studies indicate that negative stressful life events increase the risk of depression when these life events are combined with certain vulnerability factors (e.g., a lack of material resources to cope with the events; Turner and Lloyd 1999; Turner et al. 1999). In addition, some, although not all, studies suggest that negative stressful life events have a stronger effect on depression in lower socioeconomic groups than in higher ones. If true, this difference in effect may be explained by the pervasiveness of vulnerability factors (e.g., lack of material resources) among people in lower socioeconomic groups.

Thus, differences between populations can be explained, at least in part, by differences in the distribution of causes that differentiate healthy from ill individuals within a population. This type of analysis makes sense. It seems logical to attribute differences between groups of individuals to differences in the characteristics of the individuals who comprise the groups. The reasoning is as applicable to mental disorder as to any other disease. Mental disorder, like all disease, is an attribute of an individual. However, many epidemiologists have begun to question the sufficiency of this approach (e.g., Krieger 1994; Pearce 1996; Marmot 1998; Beaglehole and Bonita 1998; Davey Smith and Ebrahim 2001; Kaufman and Kaufman 2001). These critics contend that, although diseases, including psychiatric disorders, are characteristics of individuals, causes need not be. Causes that are characteristics of populations can also be usefully examined. Indeed, finding that populations differ on the prevalence of risk factors or their causal partners begs the question why this difference came to be (Krieger 1994).

This is essentially the problem that researchers confronted after finding a difference in risk factors between London and the Isle of Wight in the study mentioned. Their result led them to pose a further question: why were the risk factors more common in London? As the authors recognized, to answer this question would require a different kind of investigation.[2]

Although not amenable to studies that compare individuals within a community, such a question might be answered by examination of differences between communities. In other words, the cause of the prevalence and distribution of risk factors may be addressed by examination of causes that are upstream from the individual. For example, community differences in the supervision that children receive may be explained by differences in the availability of child care, the length of the school day, the quality of playground facilities, or the accessible pool of well-paid jobs with flexible hours. These causes are characteristics of a community and not of an individual within a community. To fully understand differences in the prevalence of risk factors, and ultimately disease rates, between communities, we need to study these characteristics of communities.

So far, we have explained why it is useful to understand the characteristics of populations as antecedents of risk factors, but the importance of studying the characteristics of populations goes well beyond this application. There is something unique about the causes of disease rates, something not captured in variation among individuals within a population. We will explain later in the chapter that the causes of incidence, a characteristic of a population, and the causes of becoming a case, a characteristic of individuals within a population, may be distinct (Rose 1992).

For simplicity, we will use the generic term **social fact** (Durkheim 1964) to refer to any characteristic of a population or social group. The social group may be as large as a society or as small as a village or even a household. In accord with previous parts of this book, we will reserve the term risk factor to refer to an exposure or characteristic that varies among individuals within a population and influences their disease risk.

---

[2] In this study, the authors actually looked beyond the individual characteristics of children, to identify causes in the family, a very small social group. The families were, however, embedded in the larger social group of the community, the implications of which will be discussed.

Social Facts in the Era of Risk Factor Epidemiology

During the apogee of risk factor epidemiology, social facts were rarely investigated as causes in their own right. For optimal use of risk factor methods, epidemiologists increasingly narrowed their designs to study the characteristics of individuals as the main variables of interest. In addition, when social facts were included (usually as confounders) in risk factor studies, they were often poorly conceived and measured. It follows from the nature of risk factor studies, in which the individual is the unit of analysis, that variables are measured by observations made on individuals.

In some circumstances, it can be reasonable to use observations of individuals to measure social facts to which they were exposed. For example, if we can determine that an individual resides in an impoverished neighborhood, we know that he or she was exposed to that social fact. In practice, however, the observations made on individuals were too crude to serve the purpose. Following the same example, studies in the United States that considered neighborhood poverty as a potential confounder sometimes measured it merely by determining whether an individual resided in a low-income census tract, without clearly articulating the construct being measured and without recognizing the limitations of census tracts as proxies for neighborhoods. As a result, the measures were of limited value even for control of confounding.

A further problem was that investigators did not always recognize that the same observation can have a dual meaning as a social fact and a risk factor. An individual's age, for example, signifies his or her belonging to a generation with a shared historical experience, which is a social fact. It also signifies duration of life experience and biological development, which are individual risk factors. Similarly, an individual's gender, occupation, education, religion, sexual orientation, income, and many other variables can have dual meanings. Each of these variables can signify belonging to a group with certain shared characteristics that differentiate it from other groups. At the same time, each can signify an individual characteristic that differentiates an individual from other individuals in the population. Of necessity, in a particular study we may take such a variable to represent an individual risk factor. Nonetheless, we need to be aware of its dual meaning, because the social fact it also measures may pose alternative explanations for our results. Conversely, if we take the variable to represent a social fact, we need to be aware that it also measures a risk factor.

During this period, studies that directly measured the characteristics of social groups and examined the associations between the characteristics and disease rates of social groups were seen as tainted by the **ecologic fallacy** (Robinson 1950; Morgenstern 1982; Schwartz 1994; Susser 1994a; Susser 1994b). The ecologic fallacy is the bias that can occur in the estimate of the effect of a risk factor when group-level variables (e.g., average income and average disease risk for neighborhoods) are used as substitutes for information on the exposure and disease experience of individuals. In some instances, such studies were in fact searching for risk factors, and the ecologic fallacy applied. In other instances, however, they were studying social facts as causes, and their purpose was simply not comprehended by critics.

Within the framework of risk factor epidemiology, the usefulness of study-ing social facts is not at all self-evident. First, if social facts are merely ante-cedents of more proximate individual-level variables, which indeed they must be if disease resides in individual bodies, then why do we insist that social facts are so central? And further, how is it possible that the causes of incidence, the proportion of people in a population who develop disease, can be different from the causes of cases of disease, of which the incidence is composed?

Levels of Organization

We begin with a short discussion of what we mean by levels of organization. This concept is central to sociology. Similar concepts have been developed in neuroscience and other disciplines.

The basic premise is that phenomena can be organized into a hierarchy of ascending complexity. Each level can be thought of as a more complex whole that comprises less complex parts. The interaction of the parts leads to the emergence of a whole that has properties unique to it. That is, despite the fact that the whole was created from the parts, the whole has properties distinct from the properties of the parts. For example, water can be thought of as a whole that emerges from the interaction of hydrogen and oxygen molecules. It is a new level of organization because water has properties, such as liquidity, that characterize the whole (i.e., water) but are not applicable to the parts (hydrogen and oxygen molecules; Levins 1998). Although our discussion here is about individuals as the parts and social groupings as the whole, this example shows that the idea is much more general. Our understanding of the relationship of cells to organs (and neurons to the brain) is informed by these same ideas (e.g., Diez Roux 1998). If we could trace the process by which a biological change at the cellular or molecular level leads to a disease, we would likely find emergent phenomena (i.e., wholes created from parts) at many intermediate levels between the cell and the individual (see part VII; Weinberger et al. 2001).

The relationship between the whole and the parts is assumed to be dynamic in that the whole can influence the functioning and meaning of the parts just as the parts influence the whole. This approach is nonreductionist in that it assumes the whole cannot be fully understood from examination of the parts, because characteristics of the whole are distinct from characteristics of the parts.

With respect to social groups, we see a hierarchy of complexity as we move from smaller to larger units. A family is a small social grouping of a few individuals, a community comprises many families, a society comprises many communities, and so forth. Furthermore, social groups can be created around many and diverse characteristics, such as geographic location, stigmatized conditions, or social norms.

In investigation of causes of disease, it is most useful to focus on a social grouping that is carefully chosen because of its relevance to the particular question at hand. For example, we may hypothesize that the average income of a neighborhood has different consequences for the disease being investi-gated than the income of the individuals in that neighborhood. This may be so even though the neighborhood income is defined in terms of the income of the individuals in it. The average income of the neighborhood has consequences and characteristics unique to it, such as the frequency of garbage pickup, the number and quality of local hospitals, or the presence or absence of toxic waste. All of these neighborhood characteristics may have an influence on the health of an individual in the neighborhood, over and above the influence of an individual's income. To reinforce this distinction, note that the neighborhood income may be stable even while the income of each individual within the neighborhood changes. As one generation ages and the next grows up, the individuals living in the neighborhood will change, and the distribution of the income among these individuals will change, but the neighborhood income will not necessarily change.

In addition, the meaning and consequences of individual income may be determined in part by the income of the neighborhood in which the individual resides. Living in a rich neighborhood may exacerbate the deleterious effects of an individual's low income through invidious comparisons with rich neighbors and exclusion from local social networks. Alternatively, living in a rich neighborhood may mitigate some of the consequences of low income, since everyone shares neighborhood amenities like the availability of safe parks and modern libraries. Thus, the causes of incidence (i.e., the proportion of people in a neighborhood with a disease) and the causes of cases (i.e., why particular people within a neighborhood became diseased) may be different. This distinction flows from the premise that wholes and parts can have different characteristics (Rose 1992).

Causes of Incidence versus Causes of Cases

The term causes of incidence refers to the social facts that influence the amount of disease in a population and the reasons for differences between populations. The term causes of cases refers to the factors that cause one individual but not another within the same population to have a disease. One way to understand how the causes of incidence and those of cases may differ derives from the very framework that we used to examine causation in risk factor epidemiology. We have said that a cause is something that makes a difference, that without the cause the disease would not have occurred when and how it did. We operationalized this concept as the difference between the outcome among people who have experienced the cause and the outcome in these same people in the absence of the cause. We isolate the risk factor by allowing it to vary while assuming that all else is equal. That is, we assume a certain static background stage on which the effects of the cause appear.

Anytime we look for a cause of disease, we assume some background conditions that we hold constant and therefore leave unexamined. For example, in a study of the risk factors for stroke we typically hold constant universals of the human body, such as the inability of the brain to function without sufficient blood flow to bring oxygen to it. The invariant background conditions remain assumed and uninvestigated. No one would suggest doing otherwise.

But many other factors will also be relegated to the invariant background. To understand how the causes of incidence and the causes of cases can be different, it is useful to examine what other kinds of phenomena are considered to be invariant. When the risk factors for stroke are studied in a particular population, which they always must be, certain social facts are made invariant. This is because populations are usually not composed of random groupings of unrelated individuals, but rather composed of individuals who are members of social groups, individuals tied together by some common features.

The social phenomena that define individuals into a group, and all other characteristics of the group, are invariant for group members. Living in a democracy is a social fact shared by a population with a certain kind of political system. It may not impact all individuals in the same way, just as individual risk factors may not impact all individuals in the same way. Nonetheless, the exposure to the social fact is ubiquitous and invariant among the population.

Note that invariant does not mean constant over time, but only constant across people. Historical changes transform the invariant background, as when a country changes from a democracy to a dictatorship. Then the invariant background changes for everyone in the group, although, of course, not all are affected by the change in the same way.

In studies examining causes of disease for individuals within a population, the factors shared by the population cannot be identified as causes. This is true even if not a single case of the disease could occur without exposure to these shared factors. The reason is that these shared phenomena, though having an impact on individuals, are not characteristics of individuals. They are *social facts,* the multifaceted rules, norms, and ways of being that constrain the actions and behaviors of individuals (Durkheim 1964). Clearly, social facts do not cause disease in a disembodied way; they cause disease through mediating factors that, at some point in the causal chain, become biologic phenomena. Nonetheless, they are not reducible to individual-level phenomena; they may cause disease through a large number of interactive pathways that cannot be fully itemized.

Although not reducible, social facts sometimes offer the most useful explanations for the incidence of disease. The amount of disease in the society may best be explained by the background risk conferred by social facts that both shape the distribution of risk factors and interact with them to lead to disease. Thus, the study of social facts has the potential to illuminate apparently mysterious differences in the incidences of disease between societies and other social groups.

A simple example in psychiatric epidemiology is the incidence of alcoholism. What cannot be detected in a study of individuals within a society are such causes as the availability of alcohol in the society, the norms about drinking, the prevalence of advertising, and the ubiquity of socializing in bars. These phenomena are characteristics of societies; therefore, individuals within the society will not differ on them. Individuals will, of course, vary in terms of how they are influenced by these social variables. People will vary in the extent to which they take advantage of the availability of the alcohol, adhere to the norms about drinking, live in neighborhoods with many liquor stores and bars, submit to the pressures of advertising, and participate in normal socializing practices. They will also vary in genetic vulnerability to alcoholism. Nonetheless, the social context constrains and helps shape the pattern of alcohol use of all individuals in the society.

Suppose two societies have disparate rates of alcoholism primarily because they have different laws regulating the sale of alcohol. Although this social fact causes the rates of alcoholism to differ between the societies, it will not explain any of the interindividual differences in alcoholism within either society. Thus, the causes of between-group variation can be quite different from the causes of within-group variation.

It is of course true that the availability of alcohol in and of itself cannot lead to alcoholism without working through the behavior of individuals. The alcohol has to enter the body to make a difference. However, the availability of alcohol influences the alcoholism rate through many pathways and through interaction with numerous risk factors. Rather than measure and consider all of these interacting risks, it may be simpler to consider the social fact itself— in this instance, the law regulating the sale of alcohol. Social phenomena may be useful as loci for intervention precisely because of the multiple linkages and distance from the onset of the disorder. They also may provide critical information about generalizability by defining the conditions under which risk factors may and may not have effects.

The same reasoning can be extended to other levels of social organization. In a given society, certain social experiences may be shared by men and others by women. The disease rates for men and for women may be influenced by these shared social experiences. Comparisons *between* men and women may reveal these social facts, but comparisons *within* gender groups will not. Similarly, shared social experiences vary by religion, occupation, or ethnicity.

Studying Social Facts

The literature examining the effects of social facts on disease, such as the impact of economic inequality within a society, of neighborhood characteristics, and of societal change (see, e.g., Wilkinson 1996; Diez Roux et al. 1997; Davey Smith 1997; Marmot and Wilkinson 1999; Berkman and Kawachi 2000), has grown tremendously in recent years. The study of such social facts poses unique challenges for epidemiology even when the conceptual hurdles have been overcome.

The determination of the influence of social facts on disease requires, as a first step at least, studies that measure these variables. As noted earlier, risk factor studies generally rely on observations made on individuals to measure group-level variables, and these variables are often grossly misspecified. For instance, in a risk factor study researchers may recognize the need to take into account the influence of neighborhood social cohesion but may lack any direct, reliable, and valid measure of it. They may, therefore, resort to measuring the variable by asking the study participants questions about the frequency of social interactions with their neighbors. This measure would be at best a very crude proxy.

Once the variables are precisely conceptualized and measured, we need to isolate their effects from other associated causes of disease. In particular, individual-level variables often serve as alternative competing hypotheses for the effect of a group-level variable. This is especially true of social facts measured as aggregate variables, that is, derived from the average of individual-level variables.

The potential confounding can be readily seen in our previous example of average neighborhood income. The disease risk could differ in a rich versus a poor neighborhood as a result of the effects of individuals' incomes on their disease risks. To gauge the contribution of average neighborhood income to the difference in neighborhood disease risks, we must differentiate the effect of this social fact from the effect of individual income.

But this is difficult to do with conventional risk factor methods. One problem is that most of our statistical techniques treat the individuals in the study as independent of each other. Clearly, when studying group phenomena, we assume exactly the opposite. The hypothesis is that the individuals within groups are not independent precisely because they belong to a group. The very phenomena that make individuals into a group create dependencies among the members.

The isolation of the group-level variable can be assisted by the use of analytic models such as multilevel analyses. With the growth of interest, or perhaps renewed interest, in the impact of social variables on disease has come the increased use of statistical techniques that take into account the interdependencies of individuals nested within groups. Such models facilitate the simultaneous assessment of the causes of between- and within-group variation and the interactions between them. These techniques have been used to examine the effects on disease of neighborhood characteristics such as average income, over and above the effects of individual income (e.g., Diez Roux et al. 1997).

Multilevel approaches have clear applicability to many questions that arise in psychiatric epidemiology. Among the most obvious are questions about differences across sociocultural environments—for example, the worse prognosis of schizophrenia in high- as opposed to low-income countries, and the epidemic of anorexia nervosa in high- but not low-income countries. But the study of any variation in disease rates across populations may benefit from consideration of multiple levels of causation.

The Context of the Life Course

Just as individual disease risk evolves within a social context, it evolves within a temporal context, as well. Over the life course, biological and social experiences become embodied in the individual (Krieger and Davey Smith 2004). Thus, what has happened before always sets part of the context for what happens now.

This context comprises the full span of the previous life course. Numerous pathways allow distal events in the life course to influence the present disease risk (Kuh and Ben-Schlomo 2004). Even intrauterine exposures may have latent effects that are expressed in adult neuropsychiatric diseases. They may do this by programming a pattern of neuroendocrine response over the life course, by epigenetic effects such as DNA methylation (see chapter 34), by a brain insult that is expressed in different manifest forms across the life cycle, depending upon the developmental context and other factors, or by other pathways. Childhood exposures can cause permanent bodily changes that modify the effects of later exposures. Ongoing exposure over a long period of time may have a cumulative effect on disease risk. Furthermore, remote past experiences can influence current behavior and other factors which determine the constellation of an individual's current exposures.

By systematically considering the context of the life course, we enrich our thinking about the causal pathways that may explain an observed association between an exposure and a disease. Consider the association, reported in some studies (e.g., Davidson et al. 1999), between lower IQ in adolescence and increased risk of schizophrenia in young adulthood. First, an intrauterine exposure with latent effects may be a common cause of both. Second, early social adversity may become embodied by early childhood in lower IQ, and lower childhood IQ may increase susceptibility to later childhood exposures that increase the risk of schizophrenia. Third, lower IQ in adolescence may be an early manifestation of the disease. At present we do not diagnose schizophrenia until the appearance of psychotic symptoms, but in the future we may identify an underlying disease pathophysiology that enables us to diagnose it at an earlier phase. These are but a few of the hypotheses that can be formulated and tested when we extend our thinking to encompass the events from conception onward.

The life course perspective also has practical implications for control of confounding that pertain to almost any investigation. Consider the approaches to the control of confounding by socioeconomic status in a study of an adult disease. Commonly, one adjusts for current socioeconomic status. An adult's disease risk may, however, be no less influenced by the socioeconomic status of his or her family of origin during infancy, childhood, and adolescence, than by the socioeconomic status achieved in adulthood. These effects originating from socioeconomic status in different phases of the life course may operate either irrespective of or in interaction with one another (Davey Smith et al. 2000). In a typical cycle, family socioeconomic status around the time of birth is embodied in the infant's birthweight; family socioeconomic status during childhood is embodied in physical and cognitive growth; and, finally, these factors together have been shown to influence the risk of adult diseases. It follows that adjustment for adult socioeconomic status can leave considerable residual confounding.

We can make exposure and disease relationships that unfold over the life course accessible to investigation by extending the ordinary purview of risk factor designs. In part III, we described several examples of cohort studies that encompassed a broad span of the life course. Cohorts followed over the life course allow us to study the effects of exposure from before birth up to late life, the relation of biological and social maturation to health and disease, and the early manifestations and subsequent progress of disease. These investigations yield valuable insights in the study of psychiatric disorders in particular, since they may emerge insidiously, change their manifest forms over the life course, and express latent effects of early life exposures.

Similar to distal social facts, exposures that are distal in the life course sometimes have manifold implications for disease risk and operate via many pathways not easily itemized. Some studies suggest, for example, that early cognitive development may, through a variety of pathways, influence the risk of several adult diseases (Kuh et al. 2004). Other studies suggest that, even earlier in the life course, in utero exposures may have an adverse effect on fetal development with implications for diseases throughout the life course (e.g. Susser et al. 1996; St. Clair et al. 2005). If these relationships prove true, approaches to prevention of adult diseases might usefully focus on in utero and childhood, in addition to adult, exposures.

Life course cohorts are generally limited in their purview, however, to the life history of individuals within a particular social and historical context. Indeed, a strength of the design is that it holds historical change in the society invariant; that is, everyone in the cohort study is followed through the same historical period. But the relationships investigated in these cohort studies vary across societies and across time. Historical change modifies biological, as well as social, development, as illustrated by the declining age at menarche in many societies during the 20th century. These historical effects cannot ordinarily be detected in a life course cohort.

The Rise and Fall of Disease Rates over Time

The consideration of the temporal context is also central to understanding societal patterns of disease. The past historical experience of a population is reflected in its members' biological states, their exposures, and their social relationships. To illustrate the practical implications of this broad assertion, we will discuss the analysis of secular trends.

The rise and fall of disease rates in a population reflect both contemporary and historical societal change. In the analysis of a secular trend, therefore, we begin by attempting to determine whether its causes are to be sought primarily in contemporary or in historical events. The effects of contemporary societal change on secular trends in disease are referred to as **period effects**. A period effect changes the disease rate of a population during a limited time period around the time of its occurrence. An example would be the effect of the Great Depression on health disorders in the United States during the 1930s. The varying effects of past historical change on successive generations are referred to as **cohort effects**. Individuals within an age group share exposures over the life course that are common to their age group or generation, and these exposures are assigned to them as a whole group. People raised in a certain location during a certain historical time period share norms, exposures to technology, language, and values that are unique to, define, and differentiate their generation from the generations that came before and those that come after. In popular culture in the United States, we acknowledge these influences when we refer to "baby boomers" or "generation X."

These historical exposures differ across generations and cause variation in current disease rates across generations. Changes in exposures that have latent effects on disease produce the clearest examples of cohort effects. An early life exposure that is shared by some age groups but not others and influences disease risk in adult life will be manifest as a cohort effect. In other words, different early experiences shared by successive generations can produce different patterns of disease in these generations in adulthood. Such effects are best appreciated by analyses that compare age-specific disease rates among successive generations defined by their time of birth. For example, people born in 1901–1910, 1911–1920, and 1921–1930 might be compared with respect to their mortality rates at age 50–59. By comparing an array of successive generations, this approach enables us to detect the deferred effects of a change in exposure that occurred at some point in the life cycle antecedent to the age-specific disease rates being examined.

Cohort effects are virtually always present to some degree. A generation at a certain age carries the cumulative effects of all its prior exposures. Since successive generations reach a given age at successively later points in history, they necessarily differ somewhat on their cumulative experience up to that age. The term generation effects would be a better descriptor, since these effects are not captured by the cohort research design, but the term cohort effects is by now conventional.

Age-Period-Cohort Analysis

The methods for isolating these effects from one another are referred to as *age-period-cohort analysis*. Age effects also must enter the analysis because individuals age at the same time as history unfolds. The term **age effects** refers to the disease risk change that is intrinsic to an individual human life, because of biological development, and to the accumulation of exposure to environment with age through the life course.

The central difficulty in the analysis of a secular trend is that age, period, and cohort effects are so inherently interwoven that analyses cannot entirely disentangle them. Within a given time period, being a different age means belonging to a different generation. Within a given generation, being a different age means being in a different time period.

One approach to analyzing a secular trend is a period analysis (figure 36.1A). We compare age-specific disease rates across successive periods of time in order to detect a period effect. The comparison across time periods will always be confounded, however, by cohort effects. In successive time periods, the persons in a particular age group belong to different generations.

An alternative approach is a cohort analysis. We compare age-specific disease rates across successive generations (figure 36.1B). The comparison across generations will be confounded by period effects. In the successive generations, persons in a given age group are observed at different time periods.

Furthermore, we cannot observe the effect of an individual's age on disease risk without confounding by either period or cohort effects. When we compare the disease rates of different age groups within a time period, cohort effects

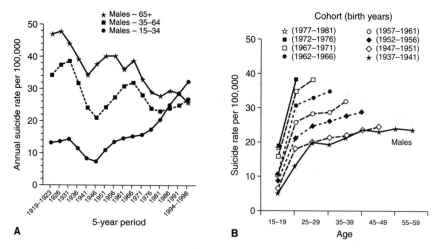

Figure 36.1 Example of age, period, and cohort effects: suicide rates in Australia. (A) This figure displays annual rates of suicide in Australia for three age groups from 1919–1998. There are clear period effects reflected in the figure. Higher rates in the Great Depression years and lower rates during World War II are seen in all age groups. During 1919–1966, there is also a consistent age effect. After 1966, the picture becomes confusing. (B) This figure displays suicide rates for eight Australian birth cohorts. There is a clear generational effect, with the oldest cohort (1937–1941) experiencing the lowest rates of suicide, and with progressively higher rates experienced by each succeeding birth cohort at any given age. This generational effect produces the confusing picture after 1966 in (A). Adapted from Snowdon and Hunt (2002) with permission from Blackwell Publishing.

are uncontrolled. When we compare the disease rates at different ages over the life course of a generation, period effects are uncontrolled.

Thus, age, period, and cohort effects are so intertwined that one of them is uncontrolled in any form of analysis. The problem arises because an individual's age at the time of any observation is defined by the time interval between the date of birth and the date of observation. On one hand, the date of birth places the individual in a generation. On the other hand, the date of observation places the individual in a time period. Consequently, the individual's disease risk at a given age necessarily reflects both cohort and period effects.

These difficulties should not deter us, however, from seeking the causes of changing patterns of disease. A salient effect can often be detected by careful reasoning and graphic display of disease rates. If a period effect predominates, we may see a pattern resembling that shown in figure 36.1A. If a cohort effect predominates, we may observe a pattern resembling that shown in figure 36.1B. The analysis of peptic ulcer rates over the 20th century is recognized as a classic example (Susser and Stein 1962; Levenstein 2002; Langman 2002; Sonnenberg et al. 2002; Marshall 2002; Susser and Stein 2002a; Susser and Stein 2002b). It is an example particularly germane to psychiatric epidemiology.

The Example of Peptic Ulcer

Peptic ulcer disease was first described at the turn of the 19th century and included in British mortality statistics throughout the 20th century. Even before World War II, peptic ulcer appeared to be increasing at a rapid rate. Like cancer and cardiovascular disease, it was reputedly a prime "disease of civilization." Unlike cancer and cardiovascular disease, however, the epidemic of peptic ulcer was widely believed to be due to psychological factors (Davey Smith 2005). Many studies reported associations between psychological stress and peptic ulcer.

By the 1960s, it had been demonstrated that British mortality rates for peptic ulcer exhibited cohort effects (Susser and Stein 1962). At a given age, the rates were highest for generations born in the late 19th century but were declining across successive generations born in the early 20th century onward. This analysis showed that the rate of peptic ulcer was not rising as generally believed but in fact declining. During the middle of the 20th century, the generations born in the late 19th century were at their peak age of risk, leading to the impression that the disease was increasing and associated with the stresses of the time.

The parsimonious interpretation was that the earlier-born generations shared some exposure in childhood or young adulthood that led them to develop high rates of peptic ulcer as they aged. This notion was clearly incompatible with the prevailing notions about psychological stress and other factors, however, and at the time the cohort effects were largely disregarded. Much later, in the 1980s, *Helicobacter pylori* was finally identified as a major cause of peptic ulcer (Marshall et al. 1984; see chapter 2). The discovery was made with methods dating back to the era of infectious disease epidemiology. It then became apparent that the cohort effects had offered an early clue to this undetected cause. In a current theory, infection with *H. pylori* was once ubiquitous in early life; such early infection carried a low risk for peptic ulcer as a generation aged, and it perhaps conferred a degree of immunity. Among subsequent generations born in the late 19th century, with sanitary conditions improving, infection was often deferred until late childhood, and such delayed infection carried a high risk of peptic ulcer as these generations aged. Among still later generations, born in the 20th century, with living conditions further improved, most people were not infected at all and carried no risk of peptic ulcer from this source. Although alternative theories have been advanced, neither the cohort effect itself nor the causal role of *H. pylori* are in dispute.

A number of observations follow from this example. First, the risk factor paradigm blurred the vision of epidemiologists, delaying the discovery of an important cause with preventive implications. Second, the methods of the previous infectious disease era, then neglected, were still directly relevant, underscoring the importance of incorporating rather than disregarding the advances of previous eras. Third, after discovering a major cause, we should avoid the temptation to revert to thinking about only a single level of causation, or a single cause at any given level of causation. At the societal level, we need to understand the effects of hygiene, sanitation, crowding, and other social facts on the transmission and prevalence of *H. pylori*. At the individual level, we need to understand the relation of *H. pylori* infection to the risk of peptic ulcer in individuals, and as noted earlier, the context of the life course is crucial to understanding this relationship. Also, the relation of *H. pylori* infection to individual risk of peptic ulcer may be modified by other factors, and it is not the definitive cause of all cases. There may well be some role for psychological risk factors (Levenstein 2002). Finally, the pursuit of complexity—detecting distal societal causes by studying cohort effects—opened a path (although not one taken) that led toward a single cause: early exposure to the *H. pylori*. Indeed, among the hypotheses put forward to explain the generation effects, one was a specific undetected early life exposure (Susser 1967). Thus, the consideration of historical trends, other levels of causation, and development over the life course, need not make the end result more complicated, but instead might help to simplify it.

Epidemiology and the Analysis of Historical Change

Questions about changing patterns of disease stimulated the emergence of epidemiology in the 19th century, and answering these questions has been central to public health mission of epidemiology ever since. In the post–World War II era, when Jeremy Morris (1957) first articulated the new shape of epidemiology, he listed seven uses of epidemiology. The study of historical change in disease was at the top of the list and was also the first chapter in his book.

This perspective has not always been sustained. The study of historical change in disease is sometimes referred to as descriptive epidemiology, as though historical change does not require analysis and interpretation. Nothing could be further from the truth. The analysis of secular trends is not only one of the most important, but also one of the most complex, endeavors of analytic epidemiology.

Currently, we can at the very least pose the analytic questions in a clear way. This in itself would illuminate some current controversies about changing disease rates for psychiatric disorders and steer investigators toward research designs that address the pertinent questions. Without understanding the interrelationships among age, period, and cohort effects, we cannot correctly interpret recent secular trends reported for autism, attention deficit disorder, schizophrenia, suicide, depression, and other disorders.

Yet it is also true that the approaches for analyzing historical change have not been developed at the same pace as the risk factor methods. Although statistical modeling has been applied to facilitate age-period-cohort analysis, it does not dispose of the logical conundrum (Clayton and Schifflers 1987a; Clayton and Schifflers 1987b). Advancing the analysis of historical change is one of the greatest challenges for epidemiology in the 21st century.

Further Challenges

We have described the difficulties of implementing rigorous risk factor studies in some detail in previous parts of this volume, and of course the approaches described in this chapter face difficulties, as well. Group-level data are often not available on a sufficient number of groups or on the specific characteristics that our theories suggest are salient. For example, in the United States, many studies on neighborhood effects define neighborhoods in terms of census tract categorizations. But usually a census tract does not fully correspond to what the researchers have in mind as neighborhood. These data are widely used, however, because of their easy availability and the dearth of alternatives. Similarly, data on early antecedents are frequently available in only crude form. Not all populations maintain good enough morbidity and mortality data for the analysis of secular trends.

Nonetheless, an increasing number of studies examine causal factors defined at levels of organization above the individual. Also more common are studies examining exposures that are distal in the history of the individual, the evolution of disease over the life course, and the links between in utero and childhood experiences and adult diseases. In psychiatric epidemiology in particular, a developmental perspective is well entrenched.

We believe that as epidemiologic research becomes more inclusive it is important to continually integrate the knowledge derived from studies of risk factors and studies of other kinds of causes. We will gain most from our studies if we keep in mind the causes that are present but not detectable in the design we have chosen. Each type of study offers valuable insights for other types. In the studies of child psychopathology in London and the Isle of Wight, investigations of risk factors and family-wide causes led to the formulation of hypotheses about community and societal causes. In the studies of peptic ulcer, the analysis of secular trends offered a clue to a bacterial cause of disease.

But even with all these approaches at hand, we still have more to do in developing methods to search for causes. Although multilevel methods can capture the effects of different levels of organization, and studies of early antecedents capture the history of the individuals, the models used are still more analogous to a snapshot than a video. In these studies, new types of variables, previously neglected, have come under consideration. However, the ways in which the variables can be examined still constrain us.

The effects of these variables are separated out from each other, albeit with limited possibilities for the modeling of static interactions. The dynamic aspects of the association, the ways in which the whole, the group, changes the behavior, attitudes, activities, and risks of the parts (the individuals), and the ways in which the parts alter and produce the whole are still not captured. For example, in looking at the influence of children on the family, multilevel models can examine the effects of family characteristics, child characteristics, and their interaction on the development of psychopathology in the child. Such models cannot, however, show the ways in which the child characteristics both shape and are shaped by the characteristics of the family. They do not allow for the prediction of how the family will change over time and what contributions the child characteristics make to this change. It is this dynamic interplay that is generally omitted from these models.

Perhaps even more important, the dynamic interplay is not yet incorporated fully into our thinking about causes. Once this happens, we may conceive research designs that bring into relief the dynamic phenomena we want to investigate. As always, statistical modeling can supplement but not substitute for a well-developed research question with a design crafted to answer it.

In the next chapter, we discuss some tentative steps toward consideration of this interplay in thinking about causes and designs. Ultimately, we believe, this line of thinking will help identify causes of disease that are currently beyond our reach. Some of what now seems inexplicable about the occurrence of diseases may then be explained and, if possible, modified.

References

Beaglehole R and Bonita R (1998). Public Health at the Crossroads: Which Way Forward? *Lancet* 351:590–592.

Beebe GW, Kato H, and Land CE (1971). Studies of the Mortality of A-Bomb Survivors. 4. Mortality and Radiation Dose, 1950–1966. *Radiat. Res.* 48:613–649.

Berkman L and Kawachi I, eds. (2000). *Social Epidemiology*. Oxford University Press.

Brockington F (1985). *The Health of the Developing World*. Lewes, Sussex, U.K.: Book Guild.

Clayton D and Schifflers E (1987a). Models for Temporal Variation in Cancer Rates. I. Age-Period and Age-Cohort Models. *Stat. Med.* 6:449–467.

Clayton D and Schifflers E (1987b). Models for Temporal Variation in Cancer Rates. II. Age-Period-Cohort Models. *Stat. Med.* 6:469–481.

Davey Smith G (1997). Socioeconomic Differentials. In Kuh D and Ben Schlomo Y, eds., *A Life Course Approach to Chronic Disease Epidemiology*, 242–273. Oxford: Oxford University Press.

Davey Smith G (2005). The Biopsychosocial Approach: A Note of Caution. In White P, ed. *Biopsychosocial Medicine: An Integrated Approach to Understanding Illness*, pp. 77–102. New York: Oxford University Press.

Davey Smith G and Ebrahim S (2001). Epidemiology—Is It Time to Call It a Day? *Int. J. Epidemiol.* 30:1–11.

Davey Smith G, Gunnel D, and Ben-Shlomo Y (2000). Life-Course Approaches to Socio-Economic Differentials in Cause-Specific Adult Mortality. In Leon DA and Walt G, eds., *Poverty, Inequality and Health*, 88–124. Oxford: Oxford University Press.

Davidson M, Reichenberg A, Rabinowitz J, Weiser M, Kaplan Z, and Mark M (1999). Behavioral and Intellectual Markers for Schizophrenia in Apparently Healthy Male Adolescents. *Am. J. Psychiatry* 156:1328–1335.

Diez Roux AV (1998). On Genes, Individuals, Society, and Epidemiology. *Am. J. Epidemiol.* 148:1027–1032.

Diez Roux AV, Nieto FJ, Muntaner C, Tyroler HA, Comstock GW, Shahar E, Cooper LS, Watson RL, and Szklo M (1997). Neighborhood Environments and Coronary Heart Disease: A Multilevel Analysis. *Am. J. Epidemiol.* 146:48–63.

Dubos RJ (1965). *Man Adapting.* New Haven: Yale University Press.

Durkheim E (1964). *The Rules of Sociological Method,* 8th ed. New York: Free Press of Glencoe.

Fenner F (1988). *Smallpox and Its Eradication.* Geneva: World Health Organization.

Int. J. Epidemiol. (2002) 31:13–33. See "Reprints and Reflections" collection of articles one peptic ulcer.

Kagan A, Dawber TR, Kannel WB, and Revotskie N (1962). The Framingham Study: A Prospective Study of Coronary Heart Disease. *Fed. Proc.* 21:52–57.

Kaufman JS and Kaufman S (2001). Assessment of Structured Socioeconomic Effects on Health. *Epidemiology* 12:157–167.

Krieger N (1994). Epidemiology and the Web of Causation: Has Anyone Seen the Spider? *Soc. Sci. Med.* 39:887–903.

Krieger N and Davey Smith G (2004). "Bodies Count," and Body Counts: Social Epidemiology and Embodying Inequality. *Epidemiol. Rev.* 26:92–103.

Kuh D and Ben-Schlomo Y (2004). *A Life Course Approach to Chronic Disease Epidemiology.* New York: Oxford University Press.

Kuh D, Richards M, Hardy R, Butterworth S, and Wadsworth ME (2004). Childhood Cognitive Ability and Deaths up until Middle Age: A Post-War Birth Cohort Study. *Int. J. Epidemiol.* 33:408–413.

Langman M (2002). Commentary: Peptic Ulcer, Susser and Stein and the Cohort Phenomenon. *Int. J. Epidemiol.* 31:27–28.

Levenstein S (2002). Commentary: Peptic Ulcer and Its Discontents. *Int. J. Epidemiol.* 31:29–33.

Levins R (1998). Dialectics and Systems Theory. *Sci. Soc.* 62:375–399.

Link BG and Phelan J (1995). Social Conditions as Fundamental Causes of Disease. *J. Health Soc. Behav.* 35(spec.):80–94.

MacMahon B, Cole P, Lin TM, Lowe CR, Mirra AP, Ravnihar B, Salber EJ, Valaoras VG, and Yuasa S (1970). Age at First Birth and Breast Cancer Risk. *Bull. World Health Organ.* 43:209–221.

Marmot M (1998). Improvement of the Social Environment to Improve Health. *Lancet* 351:57–60.

Marmot M and Wilkinson R, eds. (1999). *Social Determinants of Health.* Oxford: Oxford University Press.

Marshall B (2002). Commentary: Helicobacter as the "Environmental Factor" in Susser and Stein's Cohort Theory of Peptic Ulcer Disease. *Int. J. Epidemiol.* 31:21–22.

Marshall BJ, McGechie DB, Francis GJ, and Utley PJ (1984). Pyloric Campylobacter Serology. *Lancet* 2:281.

McMichael AJ (1999). Prisoners of the Proximate: Loosening the Constraints on Epidemiology in an Age of Change. *Am. J. Epidemiol.* 149:887–897.

Morgenstern H (1982). Uses of Ecologic Analysis in Epidemiologic Research. *Am. J. Public Health* 72:1336–1344.

Morris JN (1957). *Uses of Epidemiology.* Edinburgh, Scotland: Livingstone.

Morris JN, Kagan A, Pattison DC, and Gardner MJ (1966). Incidence and Prediction of Ischaemic Heart-Disease in London Busmen. *Lancet* 2:553–559.

Pearce N (1996). Traditional Epidemiology, Modern Epidemiology, and Public Health. *Am. J. Public Health* 86:678–683.

Record RG and McKeown T (1949). Congenital Malformations of the Central Nervous System: I. A Survey of 930 Cases. *Br. J. Soc. Med.* 3:183–219.

Record RG and McKeown T (1950). Congenital Malformations of the Central Nervous System: II. Maternal Reproductive History and Familial Incidence. *Br. J. Soc. Med.* 4:26–40.

Robinson WS (1950). Ecological Correlations and the Behavior of Individuals. *Am. Soc. Rev.* 15:351–357.

Rose G (1992). *The Strategy of Preventive Medicine.* New York: Oxford University Press.

Rothman KJ (1986). *Modern Epidemiology.* Boston: Little, Brown.

Rutter M (1989). Isle of Wight Revisited: Twenty-Five Years of Child Psychiatric Epidemiology. *J. Am. Acad. Child Adolesc. Psychiatry* 28:633–653.

Rutter M, Tizard J, Yule W, Graham P, and Whitmore K (1976). Research Report: Isle of Wight Studies, 1964–1974. *Psychol. Med.* 6:313–332.

Schwartz S (1994). The Fallacy of the Ecological Fallacy: the Potential Misuse of a Concept and the Consequences. *Am. J. Public Health* 84:819–824.

Snowdon J and Hunt GE (2002). Age, Period and Cohort Effects on Suicide Rates in Australia, 1919–1999. *Acta Psychiatr. Scand.* 105:265–270.

Sonnenberg A, Cucino C, and Bauerfeind P (2002). Commentary: The Unresolved Mystery of Birth-Cohort Phenomena in Gastroenterology. *Int. J. Epidemiol.* 31:23–26.

St. Clair D, Xu M, Wang P, et al. (2005). Rates of Adult Schizophrenia following Prenatal Exposure to the Chinese Famine of 1959–1961. *JAMA* 294:557–562.

Susser E, Neugebauer R, Hoek HW, Brown AS, Lin S, Labovitz D, and Gorman JM (1996). Schizophrenia after Prenatal Famine. Further Evidence. *Arch. Gen. Psychiatry* 53:25–31.

Susser M (1967). Causes of Peptic Ulcer: A Selective Epidemiologic Review. *J. Chronic Dis.* 20:435–456.

Susser M (1973). *Causal Thinking in the Health Sciences: Concepts and Strategies of Epidemiology.* New York: Oxford University Press.

Susser M (1994a). The Logic in Ecological: I. The Logic of Analysis. *Am. J. Public Health* 84:825–829.

Susser M (1994b). The Logic in Ecological: II. The Logic of Design. *Am. J. Public Health* 84:830–835.

Susser M and Stein Z (1962). Civilisation and Peptic Ulcer. *Lancet* 1:115–119.

Susser M and Stein Z (2002a). Civilization and Peptic Ulcer. 1962. *Int. J. Epidemiol.* 31:13–17.

Susser M and Stein Z (2002b). Commentary: Civilization and Peptic Ulcer 40 Years On. *Int. J. Epidemiol.* 31:18–21.

Susser MW, Watson W, and Hopper K (1985). *Sociology in Medicine,* 3rd ed. New York: Oxford University Press.

Turner RJ and Lloyd DA (1999). The Stress Process and the Social Distribution of Depression. *J Health Soc. Behav.* 40:374–404.

Turner RJ, Lloyd DA, and Roszell P (1999). Personal Resources and the Social Distribution of Depression. *Am. J. Community Psychol.* 27:643–672.

U.S. Public Health Service (1964). *Smoking and Health: Report of the Advisory Committee to the Surgeon General of the Public Health Service.* Washington, D.C.: U.S. Government Printing Office.

Weinberger DR, Egan MF, Bertolino A, Callicott JH, Mattay VS, Lipska BK, Berman KF, and Goldberg TE (2001). Prefrontal Neurons and the Genetics of Schizophrenia. *Biol. Psychiatry* 50:825–844.

Wilkinson RG (1996). *Unhealthy Societies: The Afflictions of Inequality.* London: Routledge.

Winslow CEA (1943). *The Conquest of Epidemic Disease.* Princeton, N.J.: Princeton University Press.

Dependent and Dynamic Processes

Sharon Schwartz, Ana V. Diez Roux, and Ezra Susser

With recent advances, epidemiology has begun to overcome some of the limitations critiqued in previous chapters. Social epidemiology, with the inclusion of distal social facts, and life course epidemiology, with the inclusion of risk factors distal in personal history, have been reinvigorated and have made substantial inroads into mainstream epidemiology. The investigation of genetic, alongside nongenetic, causes is now commonplace, and genetic epidemiology is increasingly central to the discipline. But this response has been developed through accommodation. The inclusion of these new factors stretches current epidemiologic methods but does not radically transform them.

In the most modest accommodations, the basic designs and statistics of risk factor epidemiology are used, but applied to a wider range of exposures. For example, in some instances individuals in several neighborhoods are compared, with those living in low-income areas designated exposed and those in high-income areas designated unexposed. Similarly, individuals in a study may be coded as exposed or unexposed in accordance with a low or normal birth weight.

Stretching the paradigm further are studies that employ multilevel modeling to examine both neighborhood- and individual-level effects within the same studies, or that use longitudinal data to construct trajectories over part of the life course. In genetic epidemiology, designs are adapted to incorporate gene biology (see part VII). But even in these approaches the most fundamental premises of risk factor epidemiology remain intact. It is assumed that disease etiology will be uncovered through the isolation of exposures in individuals who are the units of analytic interest (Frohlich et al. 2001).

This approach is in accord with the triumvirate of established scientific method—isolation, reductionism, and linearity. These elements are used to simplify all kinds of scientific problems, and in epidemiology they allow us to see clearly and to identify causal factors. Reductionism as a tool, if not a philosophy, has been extremely successful (Lewontin and Levins 2000). As attested by the many discoveries of risk factors and the resulting benefits to public health, incomplete causal explanation does not negate the utility of reductionism and isolation.

We can, however, strive for more complete causal explanations and for insight into complex causal processes. Following this path may lead us to powerful and modifiable causes that cannot be seen with current designs. This in turn would guide us to useful public health interventions.

Recently, established scientific method itself has come under multidisciplinary scrutiny. In physics, biology, demography, developmental psychology, and sociology (e.g., Levins and Lewontin 1985; Gleick 1987; Berk 1988; Mainzer 1997; Holland 1998; Ollman 1998; Philippe and Mansi 1998; Wachs 2000), new ways of thinking challenge the primacy of traditional standards. These approaches cluster under the rubric of complexity theories but come in many forms—nonlinear dynamics, chaos theory, neural networks, systems theory, and dialectics. These theories, well rooted in the past, have become a movement within science as a cross-disciplinary approach with effects percolating into many fields, including epidemiology.

Although critiques of current epidemiologic methods frequently invoke concepts derived from a complexity framework (e.g., Krieger 1994; Pearce 1996; Koopman and Lynch 1999), applications of these approaches to epidemiologic problems are scarce. Broader application awaits both conceptual and methodological development. We therefore simply describe the broad outlines of this approach to explore and envision its potential for psychiatric epidemiologic research. We also draw attention to some nascent examples on the horizon.

No Man Is an Island

In risk factor studies, disease states of individuals are the center of analytic interest, and disease rates in populations are understood as representing the average of individual disease risks. The causes of disease rates in the population are analyzed in terms of the characteristics of the parts, the individuals who become diseased.

When population parameters are taken into consideration, as in multilevel analyses, the study outcome is still located in the individual. In addition, the effects examined are generally unidirectional. We study the effects of the context on the individual net of individual characteristics. We also assume a generally linear effect of exposure on disease and therefore expect large changes in disease rates to result from large changes in exposure prevalence.

In contrast, perspectives that come under the general rubric of complexity share in common a focus on the whole. The characteristics of the whole, the dynamic interrelationship between the whole and the parts, and the ways in which the whole emerges from interactions among the parts take center stage. For example, questions might be asked about why, at a particular moment in time, a disease emerged as a large-scale problem in a society, when previously it was under control. Interrelationships among individuals are examined to explain the emergence of this societal-level phenomenon. In turn, the effect of the emergent societal-level phenomenon on the individuals and their relationships would be assessed (Waldrop 1992; Holland 1998;

Ollman 1998). Thus, instead of cause and effect being considered in terms of temporal sequencing, cause and effect are seen as interchangeable and simultaneous. Outcomes in individuals are assumed to be dependent; the outcome in one individual is assumed to have impact on the outcome in other individuals. At the same time, these outcomes shape, and are shaped by, the context in which they occur. Large and sudden changes in the whole are expected to arise from small changes in the parts and the relationship among the parts.

The transformation of Hushpuppies from a shoe style on the brink of extinction to a "hot ticket item" is an example used in Malcolm Gladwell's (2000) *The Tipping Point: How Little Things Can Make a Big Difference,* a book popularizing this way of thinking. Without any intent, effort, or campaign, in the United States the sales of Hushpuppies increased from 30,000 to 420,000 pairs a year over a brief period. This fad apparently began from the quirky fashion sense of a few teenagers in downtown Manhattan. Other people began to imitate their behavior. From a small change among individuals and their interactions, a large and rapid change in the group arose. Thus, the fad initially spread through the social networks and contexts in which these individuals moved until a "tipping point" was reached, after which the growth in sales was exponential. Wearing Hushpuppies became, so to speak, a raging epidemic.

These ideas were presaged within epidemiology in the early 20th century, particularly in the work of William Heaton Hamer (1906), Edward Halford Ross (1911), and Sir Ronald Ross (1928), who developed mathematical models to describe patterns of disease transmission in malaria. The distinguishing notion of these models for epidemiology is the presumed dependency among individuals in creating disease rates, and the importance of nonlinear dynamics. From this perspective, studying individuals as isolated units provides satisfactory answers to the prediction of neither individual risk nor population patterns (Koopman and Lynch 1999). Sophisticated models of disease transmission have been developed to account for these effects (Anderson and May 1991), but they are only beginning to make an appearance in applied epidemiologic contexts (Halloran 1998).

This appearance is most notable in the arena of infectious disease and the consideration of social networks. In infectious diseases, the dependency of disease occurrence among individuals is inescapable. Although risk factors for infectious disease can often be identified with the methods described in this book, such as risky sexual behaviors for HIV, the magnitude of the risk for individuals, the average risk for a population, and the prediction of disease rates cannot be accomplished without consideration of the dependencies among individuals.

In infectious disease, these dependencies are sometimes studied in terms of the interconnections among individuals in social networks. Much early work on social networks collected information on the number and types of contacts of individuals in the study, called an *egocentric* approach (Berkman and Glass 2000). Each individual would be asked to describe his or her social network. This approach is akin to the addition of social networks to existing risk factor methods.

Newer approaches examine mixing across groups and the implications for disease transmission, for example, sexual mixing of age or serostatus groups in studies of HIV (Service and Blower 1995). They may also examine the social network patterns that form social groups, rather than the social networks of single individuals. It is from this pattern of networks that disease risk can best be estimated. Koopman and Lynch (1999) provide a compelling example. Suppose that there are two social networks where each individual in the network is in contact with two other individuals. Despite the fact that each individual has the same number of contacts, the disease rate in the two social networks would differ drastically according to the interconnectedness of the networks. If the triads were unconnected, disease would not spread, or spread less rapidly, than if the triads were connected. The patterning of the connections helps determine the disease rate.

Some rudimentary effects of network relationships are partly captured in such statistics as the basic reproductive rate. In Giesecke (2002), the basic reproductive rate is defined as "the average number of individuals directly infected by an infectious case . . . when he/she enters a totally susceptible population." This type of statistics, which allows for the dependency of disease among individuals, can be used to model the growth of disease spread in populations, rather than simply document disease presence or absence. It maps epidemics as emerging from the interrelationships among individuals and defines a tipping point beyond which an epidemic will be on the path to an exponential increase or to fading out. These measures provide a starting point for the development of useful models.

Application to Psychiatric Disorders

The application to infectious disease makes a compelling argument for the inclusion of complexity approaches in psychiatric epidemiology. Many prevalent infections (e.g. HIV, syphilis) have profound neuropsychiatric manifestations, and infectious agents have been implicated as causes of schizophrenia, among other mental disorders. Clearly any study of infectious causal agents warrants consideration of these methods.

But parallels between infectious diseases and psychiatric disorders and behavioral risk factors make an equally compelling argument for a broader consideration of these methods, as well. The notion of contagion itself may apply, although in an altered form, to many psychiatric disorders. Individual behaviors are obviously influenced by norms, learning, contact, and feedback from others. Norms are social facts that exist before the members of the group and exist after the members leave the group (Durkheim 1964). Thus, norms shape the behaviors of the individuals in the group. At the same time, the behaviors of the individuals and their interactions can reinforce and strengthen, challenge, weaken, and change the norms. The relationship is not one of a simple temporal sequencing from cause to effect, but rather a simultaneous process in which causes and effects are ontologically indistinguishable and interpenetrating.

As discussed in the previous chapter, individual risks for alcoholism depend not only on risks that are defined at the level of the individual, but also on group-level factors (e.g., norms about drinking, the number of bars in the neighborhood). But the relationship between the group- and individual-level factors is not static with a unidirectional causal effect. Rather the dynamic interplay among the behaviors of the individuals, their effects on the norms, the responses to the normative changes, and their feedback influence both the pattern of disease rates and individual risks. The methods used to track infectious disease patterns are applicable, and have begun to be applied, to the spread of substance abuse (Anthony 1992). Many of the underlying processes of psychiatric disorders, emotional liability, stress responses, symptom recognition, and the use of addictive agents, have a learned component. In addition, causal factors implicated in the development of psychiatric disorders, such as social support, life events, parenting styles, and social statuses, emerge from interactions with others. Causal explanations for psychiatric disorders would be more complete to the extent that complexity perspectives were considered—the patterned distribution of causal factors, the interrelationships among individuals, and the dynamic relationship between group characteristics and individual behaviors.

The contagion of emotions, psychiatric symptoms, and even syndromes has long been recognized in psychiatry and allied fields (Eaton 2001). This point was brought home in a particularly dramatic way after the September 11, 2001, terrorist attack on the World Trade Center in New York City. A study of schoolchildren 6 months after the attack (described in chapter 14; Hoven et al., 2005) suggested a powerful impact on mental disorders among the hundreds of thousands of children who were highly exposed as defined by the study (e.g., a relative was in the vicinity of the attack and the child had trouble getting home). Given the constant communication about the event in its aftermath, and the general fear that it generated among the population of the city (together with the anthrax bioterrorism that followed it), it seems implausible that the responses of each of these children developed independently. Using current methods, however, studies were able to consider the children only as separate units, each with his or her own exposure.

In addition, a complexity approach is echoed in psychiatry in the conceptualization of how our thoughts, behaviors, and feelings—the defining features of psychiatric disorders—emerge from the physicality of our brains. Neurons, the parts of which our brains are composed, are studied as a system of communication with bidirectional feedback loops among individual neurons, as well as among and between the neural pathways in which the neurons function. This interaction gives rise to emotions and thoughts, which in turn influence behaviors. These emergent properties also interact with and feed back to the system, influencing the functioning of the individual neurons, as well as their interactions. Cause and effect are merged; temporal ordering and isolation are not primary considerations. The system itself, and its emergence from the interaction and structuring of the parts, is the unit of analytic interest. Thus, the disturbed thoughts, emotions, and behaviors denoting the presence of psychiatric disorders are assumed to emerge from a complex system of interacting genetic and biologic factors, the components of which are at a cellular or molecular level. And, of course, their expression in individuals interacts with the social context in which they arise and are expressed.

Steps toward the Future

Current epidemiologic methods provide the basis for the identification of many important causes of disease in individuals and of disease rates in populations. But there is little consideration of process, nonlinearity, and interpenetration of causes and effects. To identify causes, we isolate them in time and space, often assume independence among individuals, and examine neat, temporally ordered chains of causes and effects. In reality we know that things are not that simple. There are contingencies and feedback loops that make our neatly drawn causal lines seem a childlike representation of the world.

As we consider more complex approaches, our first task is to distinguish those problems for which the simplicity of current methods is useful from those problems for which current methods are too simple. Current epidemiologic methods are best suited to detect causes when the effect is powerful (Philippe and Mansi 1998). Thus, it is not surprising that these are precisely the types of causes on which we tend to focus.

One of the insights of the counterfactual approach is that the distinction between small and large effects lies in the prevalence of the causal partners of the cause under investigation. (As previously explained in part II, when the factors that interact with a cause are common, the effect is large; when the factors that interact with a cause are rare, the effect is small.) In a given population, small and large effects may differ in their impact on that population, but they may not differ in the biologic importance for the disease process. Indeed, necessary ubiquitous causes will often have no apparent effect at all. Their role cannot be seen through isolation. Causal explanation is necessary for their detection. New approaches, perhaps deriving from complexity, are required to detect such causes. Because they are ubiquitous, their detection may guide us to preventive interventions that have a powerful impact on the health of populations. We saw in the previous chapter that our current methods are also insufficient for answering questions about changes in the patterns and rates of disease over time. This observation also pertains to patterns across place. These questions may also be ripe for complexity approaches. Interconnections among individuals, learning, norms, and social interactions are likely to be necessary components to explain these patterns.

This way of thinking may also be required to explain biological processes within individuals. It is seen in schizophrenia research, for example, where many investigators have been led to recast the biology of schizophrenia in terms of subtle deficits that reverberate over many interconnections and feedback loops from whose interactions the disease emerges. We described one such theory about genetic origins of schizophrenia in part VII (Weinberger et al. 2001).

All this suggests that progress in understanding the etiology of psychiatric disorders may not lie solely in more rigorous application of current methods—more stringent attention to confounding and bias, the tools of isolation—but rather require more attention to construct validity and external validity, the tools of explanation. The key may lie in the uncovering of process and interactions. For us to see such processes, new approaches may be warranted.

There is much in complexity theories that can be applied to these types of questions. But considerable conceptual, methodological, and statistical work needs to be done before it is accessible to routine epidemiologic analyses. Nonetheless, we can begin by posing the problem in a clear enough way that we can later get an answer. What is considered in the system is larger than what is considered for creating isolation, but something is always left out, in the background, and beyond the system. The challenge is to examine enough to get reasonable answers, but not to encompass so much that we create only confusion. What we end up with is always a crude approximation, a cleaned up version of a messy reality. It is the detection of a pattern that has utility for understanding. New approaches may help us to detect new patterns that may provide more powerful tools to explain the etiology of psychiatric disorders. The ultimate test of this way of thinking will be whether it leads us toward useful public health interventions.

Meanwhile, what we can do is acknowledge the existence of multiple levels of organization and enrich the range of causes that we consider. At a minimum, we should know the levels that we are excluding, the factors we are placing in the background, and the phenomena we are potentially missing. Such sensitization should alert us to problems that require new approaches and, it is to be hoped, inspire their development.

References

Anderson RM and May RM (1991). *Infectious Diseases of Humans Dynamics and Control*. Oxford: Oxford University Press.

Anthony JC (1992). Epidemiological Research on Cocaine Use in the USA. *Ciba Found. Symp.* 166:20–33.

Berk R (1988). Causal Inference for Sociological Data. In Smelser NJ, ed., *Handbook of Sociology*, 155–172. Newbury Park, Calif.: Sage.

Berkman L and Glass T (2000). Social Integration, Social Networks, Social Support, and Health. In Berkman L and Kawachi I, eds., *Social Epidemiology*, 137–146. New York: Oxford University Press.

Durkheim E (1964). *The Rules of Sociological Method*, 8th ed. New York: Free Press of Glencoe.

Eaton W (2001). *The Sociology of Mental Disorders*, 3rd ed. Westport, Conn.: Praeger Publishers.

Frohlich KL, Corin E, and Potvin L (2001). A Theoretical Proposal for the Relationship between Context and Disease. *Sociol. Health Illn.* 23:776–797.

Giesecke J (2002). *Modern Infectious Disease Epidemiology*, 2nd ed. London: Arnold.

Gladwell M (2000). *The Tipping Point: How Little Things Can Make a Big Difference*. Boston: Little, Brown.

Gleick J (1987). *Chaos: Making a New Science*. New York: Viking.

Halloran ME (1998). Concepts of Infectious Disease Epidemiology. In Rothman KJ and Greenland S, eds., *Modern Epidemiolog*, pp. 529–554. Philadelphia: Lippincott Williams & Wilkins.

Hamer WH (1906). *The Milroy Lectures on Epidemic Disease in England; the Evidence of Variability and of Persistence of Type*. London: Bedford Press.

Holland JH (1998). *Emergence: From Chaos to Order*. Reading, MA: Addison-Wesley.

Hoven CW, Duarte CS, Lucas CP, et al. (2005). Psychopathology among New York City School Children Six Months after September 11th. *Arch. Gen. Psychiatry.* 62:545–552.

Koopman JS and Lynch JW (1999). Individual Causal Models and Population System Models in Epidemiology. *Am. J. Public Health* 89:1170–1174.

Krieger N (1994). Epidemiology and the Web of Causation: Has Anyone Seen the Spider? *Soc. Sci. Med.* 39:887–903.

Levins R and Lewontin RC (1985). *The Dialectical Biologist.* Cambridge, MA: Harvard University Press.

Lewontin R and Levins R (2000). Let the Numbers Speak. *Int. J. Health Serv.* 30:873–877.

Mainzer K (1997). *Thinking in Complexity: The Complex Dynamics of Matter, Mind, and Mankind,* 3rd ed. Berlin: Springer.

Ollman B (1998). Why Dialectics? Why Now? *Sci. Soc.* 62:338–357.

Pearce N (1996). Traditional Epidemiology, Modern Epidemiology, and Public Health. *Am. J. Public Health;* 86:678–683.

Philippe P and Mansi O (1998). Nonlinearity in the Epidemiology of Complex Health and Disease Processes. *Theor. Med. Bioeth.* 19:591–607.

Ross EH (1911). *The Reduction of the Domestic Mosquitos: Instructions for the Use of Municipalities, Town Councils, Health Officers, Sanitary Inspectors, and Residents in Warm Climates.* London: Murray.

Ross R (1928). *Studies on Malaria.* London: Murray.

Service S and Blower SM (1995). HIV Transmission in Sexual Networks: An Empirical Analysis. *Proc. R. Soc. Lond. B Biol. Sci.* 260:237–244.

Wachs TD (2000). *Necessary but Not Sufficient: The Respective Roles of Single and Multiple Influences on Individual Development.* Washington, DC: American Psychological Association.

Waldrop MM (1992). *Complexity: The Emerging Science at the Edge of Order and Chaos.* New York: Simon & Schuster.

Weinberger DR, Egan MF, Bertolino A, Callicott JH, Mattay VS, Lipska BK, Berman KF, and Goldberg TE (2001). Prefrontal Neurons and the Genetics of Schizophrenia. *Biol. Psychiatry* 50:825–844.

Appendix A

Our Approach to Epidemiologic Concepts and Methods

Sharon Schwartz and Ezra Susser

Throughout this book, we have sought to present epidemiologic concepts and methods in a way that is relevant and accessible to investigators studying psychiatric disorders, particularly those interested in causal hypotheses. Teaching epidemiology, we have found it is easiest to convey methods when they are tightly tied to a few central organizing principles. We therefore developed such organizing principles in the first parts of the book and presented epidemiologic methods with reference to these principles in the subsequent parts.

Although this book is about epidemiologic approaches, we integrated insights from many other disciplines. Influenced by our cross-disciplinary training in sociology (SS), psychiatry (ES), and epidemiology (SS and ES), we drew from the work of methodologists in epidemiology, psychology, sociology, human genetics, and other disciplines. These disciplines converge and overlap around the central theme of this book—uncovering causes of mental health problems.

We have emphasized that the investigation of causes demands a far broader scope than the study of risk factors. Nonetheless, a large part of the book concerns the designs used to study risk factors. This appendix explains how we arrived at our particular approach to the presentation of these designs. It is intended for readers already familiar with epidemiology. Researchers for whom this book is an introduction to epidemiologic methods may safely skip it or postpone its reading until it becomes germane.

Our Approach to Risk Factor Designs

Our approach to the risk factor designs can be viewed as an attempt to integrate epidemiologic methods as articulated by Rothman and Greenland (1998) into the validity typology presented by Shadish and co-workers (2002). Since the Shadish et al. typology is widely used by other disciplines, especially the social sciences, one advantage of this approach is that it facilitates linking epidemiology to other disciplines. However, such integration required that both Rothman and Greenland and Shadish et al. be adjusted, altered, and adapted to make a coherent whole. Here we make it clear how much we have borrowed from these two sources, and we explain the ways in which we departed from them. Although many of the changes may seem subtle, we think that they have implications for decisions that researchers make in how they conduct their studies, analyze their data, and interpret their results.

Our departures from Shadish et al.'s validity typology derive from its application to the outcomes and designs of central concern to epidemiology. Epidemiologic outcomes are frequently dichotomous, as opposed to the continuous outcomes of psychological quasi-experiments. More centrally, viewing epidemiologic designs as proxies to quasi-experiments often underestimates their utility. For example, Shadish and colleagues' discussion of case-control studies as a type of "quasi-experimental design that uses a control group but no pretest," leads to a more pessimistic assessment of this design than an epidemiologic perspective would suggest.

Our departures from Rothman and Greenland's approach derive mainly from our viewing epidemiology's central task as theory testing rather than effect estimation; on this point our perspective is more in line with Shadish et al. In addition, our reading of their work is refracted through our prior training in sociology (SS) and psychiatry (ES). This refraction has led us to some insights deriving directly from their work that they might wish to reject. Our understanding of the reasons behind our points of departure greatly benefited from comments of Sander Greenland on earlier drafts of the introductory chapters and this appendix.

Adaptations of Shadish et al. (2002)

We kept the essentials of the Shadish et al. (2002) validity scheme by organizing the tasks of epidemiologic research into a series of loosely hierarchical questions: (1) How large and reliable is the association between the exposure and the disease? (2) Is the association between the exposure and disease, as measured, plausibly causal? (3) Which constructs are reflected in the causal effect? (4) How generalizable is the effect over persons, times, and settings? Although the language is adapted for the epidemiologic context, these questions correspond closely to the Shadish et al. validity scheme.

We also kept as an ongoing underlying theme, what Shadish et al. (2002, p. 16) refer to as a "falliblilist version of falsification." This means that the researcher's continual task is to "rule out" plausible alternatives to hypotheses while recognizing that each assessment is fallible. Increased understanding can be gained from this process, despite this fallibility.

The first adaptation we made was to label the first question in Shadish et al.'s validity scheme *association* rather than *statistical conclusion validity*. We did so to limit the introduction of unfamiliar terms. Association is familiar to epidemiologists and has the same meaning in epidemiology as in Shadish et al. We considered any factors that would decrease the precision of our estimate or cause biases toward the null value as threats to finding an association.

Second, we carved temporality out from internal validity for special attention. In quasi-experimental designs, the issue of temporality is of minor concern, as Shadish et al. note, because in such designs the cause is manipulated and occurs before the outcome. In epidemiologic studies, temporal order is a concern so central and problematic that it warrants separate attention.

To accommodate this alteration, we employ the term *sole plausible explanation* to refer specifically to internal validity concerns other than temporality. This is in accord with Shadish et al.: "We use the term internal validity to refer to inferences about whether observed covariation between A and B reflects a casual relationship from A to B in the form in which the variables were manipulated or measured. To support such inference, the researcher must show that A precedes B in time, that A covaries with B (already covered under statistical conclusion validity) and that no other explanations for the relationship are plausible." (Shadish et al. 2002, p. 53). Thus, temporality and sole plausibility are the two components of internal validity in Shadish et al. These three central components of causal identification—association, temporal order, and sole plausibility—date back to John Stuart Mill (1843) and have been used in a similar way in epidemiology (e.g., Susser 1973; Susser 1991).

We did not use the term *internal validity* in this text. We wanted to avoid the implication that temporality is not a component of internal validity. In addition, *internal validity* has different and varied meanings in epidemiology that diverge from Shadish et al.'s definition.

Third, some adaptations were required to place particular threats to validity in the context of observational epidemiologic studies where, unlike quasi-experiments, the exposures are not manipulated. For example, it was not clear where to place nondifferential and differential misclassification. Since Shadish et al. did not focus on dichotomous variables, this type of problem was not discussed explicitly. In deciding how to categorize various threats, we give priority to their consequences for answering the four questions of causal inference. We grouped all measurement problems that generally bias toward the null, including nondifferential misclassification, under problems of identifying an association, because they mask associations. Differential misclassification is mentioned twice—as causing difficulties for finding an association (when it causes bias toward the null) and also as posing a plausible alternative explanation for an exposure disease relationship (when the misclassification exaggerates the effect.)

Similarly, it was not clear where to place certain other measurement problems. Disease detection bias could have been legitimately considered under either sole plausibility (one component of internal validity under Shadish et al.) or under construct validity. In Shadish et al. confounding is at the heart of both internal and construct validity. The distinction is that "internal validity confounds are forces that could have occurred in the absence of the treatment and could have caused some or all of the outcome observed" (Shadish et al. 2002, p. 95), whereas construct confounds are part of the treatment and could not have occurred in absence of the treatment.

In observational epidemiology, we study nonmanipulated exposures; consequently, this distinction is often blurred. In particular, disease detection bias is a confound that occurs because the measurement error in the disease is linked with the exposure. In this sense, it would not have occurred without the exposure. On the other hand, the measurement error in the disease could have occurred from the same biases and caused the appearance of the disease even in the absence of the exposure.

Ultimately, we decided to include disease detection biases under sole plausibility for two reasons. First, disease detection bias is an alternative explanation for the relationship between the exposure and disease as they are measured. Second, we wanted to differentiate disease detection bias from construct validity, to highlight those aspects of construct validity that are relatively neglected in epidemiology and well developed in psychiatric epidemiology. In our view, the gap between our constructs and the operationalization of those constructs has not been given enough consideration in epidemiology. To draw attention to this issue, we gave centrality in construct validity to the identification of the active ingredient of the exposure and the factors that give rise to it. We discussed construct validity as the separation of the aspects of our measures that are essential to the meaning we had in mind, from those that are not.

It is important to distinguish our definition of construct validity from the notion of the resemblance of a measure to a gold standard. For example, we might use a *DSM* diagnosis of depression as the gold standard and some more easily applied symptom scale score as a proxy to it. The construct validity issue, however, is the extent to which the gold standard itself captures our concept of depression. This issue requires an iterative relationship among theory, research, and measurement. Probing the mechanisms in our studies refines the construct.

We think that these adaptations are within the spirit of Shadish et al. As they note, their list of specific threats to validity is "not divinely ordained." "Threats are better identified from insiders' knowledge than from abstract and non-local lists of threats," they acknowledge (2002, p. 473). Indeed, this is why we prefer to present a few key principles rather than a long list of specific threats. The principles provide a guideline to think through potential threats to validity that may or may not apply in particular situations.

Adaptations of Rothman and Greenland (1998)

We find the concept of exchangeability, introduced to us through the work of Greenland and Robins (1986), extremely useful in presenting epidemiologic methods within an integrated framework. Exchangeability, rooted in the counterfactual, provides the logical connection between confounding, a central concept in epidemiology, and the logic of causal inference. Once introduced, the notion, like many well-thought-out ideas, seems quite obvious and clear. Confounding is the difference between the comparison in our study (i.e., the exposed and unexposed) and the comparison of true interest (i.e., the exposed and the counterfactual). A good proxy for the counterfactual is when the disease risk in the unexposed represents the disease risk in the exposed had they not been exposed. Therefore, confounding is the imbalance in risk factors for disease, other than the exposure, between the exposed and the unexposed.

This notion parallels the aspect of sole plausible explanation in Shadish et al.'s discussion of internal validity. Indeed, Shadish et al. explicitly ground internal validity in counterfactual thinking. However, with some exceptions (e.g., Lewis 1973), Shadish et al. and Rothman and Greenland invoke different literature. Shadish et al. ground their presentation of counterfactual thinking in the work of Mackie (1974), brought into psychology by Meehl (1977). Rothman and Greenland depend more on the statistical literature (Rubin 1990). Shadish et al. explicitly set Rubin's work in the background as being of critical importance to students of causal thinking but more relevant to statistical rather than the conceptual issues that are their main concern. Here our own perspective is more in line with Shadish et al. This emphasis leads to several differences between Rothman and Greenland's and our application of the counterfactual.

In Rothman and Greenland's model, and as explicated earlier in Greenland and Robins (1986), people in the population are divided into four "types": *susceptible positives* and *negatives, immune,* and *doomed. Susceptible positives* and *negatives* are people who have the causal partners required for the exposure to have an effect either causing (susceptible positive) or preventing (susceptible negative) the disease. The *immune* are people who do not have a full complement of risk factors necessary to cause disease. The *doomed* are those who have a full complement of risk factors to cause disease from a sufficient cause other than one that includes the exposure of interest.

Among the exposed, disease occurs in the susceptible positives and the doomed. Among the unexposed, disease occurs in the susceptible negatives and the doomed. Therefore, for the exposed and unexposed to be exchangeable, the sum of the susceptible negative and doomed in the unexposed must equal the sum of the susceptible negative and doomed in the exposed. Under these conditions, the disease risk in the unexposed will represent the disease risk in the exposed had they not been exposed.

Through the connection to the counterfactual, the fundamental meaning and effects of confounding are greatly clarified by their contributions. Confounding becomes a concept that has meaning that is dependent neither on criteria nor on statistical tests that only imperfectly detect its presence. This realization makes it clear that confounding is not about single risk factors for disease but about the relationship and balance among the totality of risk factors that differ between the exposed and unexposed. Rothman and Greenland's approach offers a useful way to think through practical problems in murky situations where the imperfect rules may provide misleading direction.

We think exchangeability can be used more broadly, however, to include not only the unequal distribution of true causes of disease, but also the unequal distribution of methodological artifacts. For example, the maldistributions of follow-up time and disease ascertainment also pose threats to the validity of causal inference. They are alternative explanations for an apparent exposure-disease association. We find it most compelling to have a parsimonious model—one that unites all the ways in which an apparent association between an exposure and disease as measured in our data can be caused by factors other than a causal relationship between the exposure and the disease.

We think that this more expansive application is alluded to in Maldonado and Greenland (2002) and in Miettinen (1985). Nonetheless, Rothman and Greenland make it clear in their textbook (and in personal communication with Greenland) that their notion of exchangeability, and correspondingly confounding, applies only to true risk factors for disease (for reasons that will be explained). Therefore, to avoid confusion, we use a different term, *full comparability,* to refer to our expanded notion, and we reserve the term *confounding* to refer to a subtype of noncomparability that derives from differences between the exposed and unexposed on other causes of disease, so that our use of this term is more in line with Rothman and Greenland.

We prefer the unified concept of noncomparability because the maldistribution of true causes of disease and the maldistribution of artifacts cause the same types of problems—they provide alternative explanations for a relationship between the exposure and disease in our data. They all relate to Shadish et al.'s second question: given that there is an association between the exposure and the disease, is that association plausibly causal? To answer this question it is necessary to face all plausible explanations for the association other than the exposure of interest. Any factor that links the exposure as measured with the disease as measured is a candidate. Thus, the maldistribution of true causes of disease (i.e., confounders) and the maldistribution of artifacts (e.g., differences in follow-up time or disease detection) serve the same function in our schema. This notion ties the whole enterprise of causal inference more closely to the counterfactual and is true to Shadish et al.'s schema.

Why then do Rothman and Greenland separate out maldistribution between the exposed and the unexposed on true causes of disease from the maldistribution on methodological artifacts? We think that there are several reasons. First, Rothman and Greenland seem to group biases according to their "cure" rather than their harm. For example, confounding and selection bias are categorized separately because their harm cannot always be cured in the same manner. In their discussion of selection bias they state that "some forms of selection bias (selection confounding) can be controlled like confounding; other forms can be impossible to control without external information that is rarely (if ever) available" (Rothman and Greenland 1998, p. 355). However, selection bias and confounding cause the same harm (i.e., cause the appearance of an association between the exposed and unexposed that is not causal). For selection bias that can be cured in the same manner as confounding, the hybrid label *selection confounding* is applied. This approach is particularly awkward because selection causes the exposed and unexposed to differ on true risk factors for disease and, in this sense, leads to confounding.

The focus on the cures is also seen in the inclusion of surrogates or proxies that are associated with causes of disease but are not themselves causes of disease under the rubric of confounders.[1] Surrogates or proxies do not cause confounding. Nonetheless, their control may improve the validity of the esti-

---

[1] This insight was provided by Ulka Campbell.

mate of the effect by controlling for the effect of the causes for which they are a proxy.

A similar rationale lies behind the separation of differential misclassification from confounding. Rothman and Greenland note that even when the cause of differential misclassification can be identified and controlled like a third-variable confounder, the resulting adjusted effect estimate still suffers from the effect of nondifferential misclassification. Thus, the adjusted effect estimate is likely to be biased toward the null. Rothman and Greenland specifically admonish researchers against controlling for differential misclassification as they do confounders, with the warning that the adjusted effect estimate may be more biased (albeit toward the null) than the nonadjusted effect estimate (away from the null). This is an important point. However, in terms of addressing the questions that we pose to assess our causal ideas, biases toward and away from the null play different roles. Once we see an association, we then ask if it is causal. To provide a plausible alternate explanation for the exposure-disease relationship, the misclassification must bias away from the null. We can control for it and see what happens to the effect estimate. If the adjusted estimate is no longer appreciably different from the null value, differential misclassification is a plausible explanation for the relationship. This does not mean, however, that we should necessarily accept the adjusted estimate as the true estimate, or the one more accurate than the unadjusted. Rather, the analysis helps probe our causal idea and suggest that an identified alternative explanation is plausible.

We suspect that underlying this specific difference is a more general difference in perspective on the goal of epidemiologic studies. Rothman and Greenland state that the "overall goal of an epidemiologic study is accuracy in estimation: to estimate the value of the parameter that is the object of measurement with little error" (Rothman and Greenland 1998, p. 116). Thus, the goal is to have a true estimate of the exposure effect in the study. Our perspective, which we think we share with Shadish et al., is somewhat different. We consider the estimates in our data to be the imperfect tools we use to reach our goal of testing our theories of disease causation. What we want from our studies is evidence that will lead us to change the belief in our causal ideas. Of course we cannot do this with data that are not trustworthy, but the precise or true estimate of the effect is the means, not the end goal, of the study.

We see our effect estimates as ephemeral and context dependent. The risk ratio can change according to characteristics of persons, places, and settings. As Rothman and Greenland's scheme makes abundantly clear, the risk ratio is dependent on the prevalence and distribution of the causal partners of the exposure. Again, it is critical for our tools to be as accurate as possible, but the tool and the goal are, for us, separate.

This distinction is reflected in a subtle difference in the definition of *internal validity* in Rothman and Greenland and in Shadish et al. For Rothman and Greenland, "Precision . . . corresponds to the reduction of random error" (p. 116), and "internal validity implies validity of inference for the source population of study subjects" (p. 118). For Shadish et al., *statistical conclusion validity* addresses the issue of inferences about the association between the exposure and the disease, and *internal validity* is the extent to which casual attributions are correctly made for an exposure-disease association.

Precision in Rothman and Greenland encompasses only random measurement error. Internal validity includes all systematic errors, whether they serve to mask or exaggerate an association. For Shadish et al., statistical conclusion validity includes random measurement error, but also systematic errors that would bias toward the null. Internal validity, therefore, is only about alternative explanations for an association (other than the exposure causing the disease) that the data suggest. The underlying difference is whether the central concern in internal validity is validity of the effect estimate or the validity of the causal inference.

Our understanding of external validity, though generally consistent with both Rothman and Greenland and Shadish et al., is also influenced by the difference in goal between effect estimation and theory testing. We agree with Rothman and Greenland that external validity is not about the generalization of the study findings to some target population. As they state, "Scientific generalization amounts to moving from time- and place-specific observations to an abstract 'universal' hypothesis" (p. 124). However, we think that the way to reach this universal hypothesis is through the specification of the range of persons, places, and settings over which the risk factor has an effect. This specification amounts to identifying the causal partners of the risk factors. If a risk factor is shown to have a causal effect in any context, even a very limited idiosyncratic one, then it is a cause in the sense that if the context were re-created the disease would occur. We find the identification of contexts critically important both for public health and understanding of disease causation.

Conclusion

We think that organizational schema are not about truth and falsehood, but about utility. As a framework for understanding the logic of risk factor designs, Shadish et al.'s validity scheme, we believe, meets this standard. It is a parsimonious tool for guiding us along the often concealed path toward informative studies. It has been successfully used in psychology, sociology, and intervention studies in public health, and we think that it can serve as a useful organizing scheme in psychiatric epidemiology, as well. Nonetheless, the specific application to epidemiology makes the contribution of Rothman and Greenland essential. We think that their approach represents a clear distillation of epidemiologic principles that provides the localization for which Shadish et al. advocate. It is our hope that the integration of these two disciplinary traditions will aid researchers in improving the validity of their studies and ultimately in enriching their search for causes.

References

Greenland S and Robins JM (1986). Identifiability, Exchangeability, and Epidemiological Confounding. *Int. J. Epidemiol.* 15:413–419.
Lewis D (1973). Causation. *J. Philos.* 70:556–567.

Mackie JL (1974). *The Cement of the Universe: A Study of Causation.* New York: Oxford University Press.

Maldonado G and Greenland S (2002). Estimating Causal Effects. *Int. J. Epidemiol.* 31:422–429.

Meehl P (1977). Specific Etiology and Other Forms of Strong Influence: Some Quantitative Meanings. *J. Med. Philos.* 2:33–53.

Miettinen OS (1985). *Theoretical Epidemiology: Principles of Occurrence Research in Medicine.* New York: Wiley.

Mill JS (1843). *A System of Logic.* London: Parker.

Rothman KJ and Greenland S (1998). *Modern Epidemiology,* 2nd ed. Philadelphia: Lippincott-Raven.

Rubin DB (1990). Formal Modes of Statistical-Inference for Causal Effects. *J. Stat. Plan. Inference.* 25:279–292.

Shadish WR, Cook TD, and Campbell DT (2002). *Experimental and Quasi-Experimental Designs for Generalized Causal Inference.* Boston: Houghton Mifflin.

Susser M (1973). *Causal Thinking in the Health Sciences: Concepts and Strategies of Epidemiology.* New York: Oxford University Press.

Susser M (1991). What Is a Cause and How Do We Know One? A Grammar for Pragmatic Epidemiology. *Am. J. Epidemiol.* 133:635–648.

Appendix B

*Application of Survival Analysis to Prenatal Determinants
of Schizophrenia Example (PDSE) Data*

Michaeline Bresnahan and Ezra Susser

We apply the Kaplan-Meier method of survival analysis (Kaplan and Meier 1958) to the data of the Prenatal Determinants of Schizophrenia Example (PDSE) study. Recall that the PDSE is a birth cohort in which we examine exposure to high maternal body mass index as a risk factor for schizophrenia spectrum disorder in offspring (see tables 10.6–10.8). Cases are ascertained by a health plan treatment registry (and subsequently diagnosed). The cohort under observation is enumerated by a health plan membership registry.

We will use the Kaplan-Meier approach to calculate the risk for the exposed group in the PDSE. The exposed comprise 912 of the 12,090 cohort members. The same procedure could be applied to compare the risk in the unexposed group.

The procedures are outlined in a summary table, table B.1, and illustrated in more detail in a display table, table B.2. Throughout the following explanation, it is useful to keep in mind that risk and survival are connected. Over any given time interval, the survival probability is the complement of the disease risk. That is, the probability of surviving disease-free is equal to one minus the probability of developing disease. (Strictly speaking, these are conditional survival probabilities and conditional disease risks: conditional on having reached the given interval).

Step 1. Divide the risk period into many small time intervals. We use time intervals equal to one day, because in the PDSE the health plan membership and treatment registry data are provided according to calendar date. For each one-day interval, a cohort at risk is defined by those who remain members of the health plan and disease-free at the beginning of the interval. For example, as shown in table B.2, there were 912 people at risk on the first day, 802 people at risk on day 1332, and 346 people at risk on the last day. The cohort at risk declines across the intervals because some people drop out of the health plan and others develop the disease.

The cases for each one-day interval are those ascertained by the health plan on that day according to the treatment registry. As shown in table B.2, there were 13 days on which a case of schizophrenia spectrum disorder was ascertained. The one-day intervals are small enough that, in each interval, either no cases or only one case was ascertained.

Step 2. Compute a result for each interval. In the Kaplan-Meier approach, the result we compute is a survival probability. We begin by calculating a risk for each one-day interval (step 2A in table B.1). The risk in the interval can be observed

Table B.1 Summary Table for Kaplan-Meier Survival Analysis: PDSE Exposed Group

Step Number	Action
1	Divide total follow-up period into 6,209 one-day intervals.
2A.	Estimate the interval risk for each of the 13 informative intervals in which a case occurred. Interval risk = N cases / N cohort at risk.
2B.	Estimate interval survival probability for each of the 13 informative intervals in which a case occurred. Interval survival probability = 1 – interval risk.
3A.	Multiply the interval survival probabilities of the 13 informative intervals to obtain survival probability for total period. Cumulative survival probability for total period = $0.9988938 \times 0.9987531 \times \ldots \times 0.9974684 = 0.9799442$.
3B.	Estimate risk for total period (6,209 days) = 1 – cumulative survival probability for total period = $1 - 0.9799442 = 0.0200558 = 0.0201$

Note: Disease risk computed from the informative intervals.

directly, since within the interval there is no attrition. The risk is simply the proportion of people in the cohort at the beginning of the interval who develop disease during the interval. We then calculate the survival probability as one minus this risk (step 2B in table B.1). For example, as shown in table B.2 for day 1,332, the risk is $1/802 = 0.0012469$, and the survival probability is $1 - 0.0012469 = 0.9987531$.

In the vast majority of one-day intervals, no case occurred, and the survival probability is one. These intervals are uninformative because an interval with a survival probability of one has no impact on the overall survival probability, as will be explained. So we need to compute the survival probability for only the 13 informative intervals in which a case did occur.

Step 3. Combine the results across the intervals. In the Kaplan-Meier approach, this step has two parts. To obtain the overall survival probability (step 3A in table B.1), we multiply the survival probabilities for the 13 informative intervals, as shown in table B.2. We disregard the survival probabilities for the other intervals, because an interval with a survival probability of one can have no impact on the result of the multiplication. To obtain the disease risk (step 3B in table B.1), we subtract the overall survival probability from the number one. Using this method, we estimate the risk of schizophrenia spectrum disorder in the exposed group to be 0.0201. This disease risk applies to the entire period (6,209 days), even though the last case occurred well before the end of the period.

Reference

Kaplan EL and Meier P (1958). Nonparametric Estimation from Incomplete Observations. *J. Amer. Stat. Assoc.* 53:457–481.

Table B.2 Display Table for Kaplan-Meier Survival Analysis: PDSE Exposed Group

01/01/81

One-day interval	Day 1	138	1,332	1,368	1,440	1,744	2,044	2,191
Cases N	0	1	1	1	1	1	1	1
Cohort N	912	904	802	798	783	751	714	701
Interval survival probability	1.000000	0.9988938	0.9987531	0.9987469	0.9987229	0.9986684	0.9985994	0.9985735
Cumulative survival	1.000000	0.9988938	0.9976483	0.9963981	0.9951256	0.9938005	0.9924086	0.9909929

One-day interval	2,208	2,212	2,527	4,088	4,968	5,550	Day 6,209
Cases N	1	1	1	1	1	1	0
Cohort N	697	696	662	499	438	395	346
Interval survival probability	0.9985653	0.9985632	0.9984894	0.9979960	0.9977169	0.9974684	1.0000000
Cumulative Survival	0.9895712	0.9881494	0.9866567	0.9846794	0.9824313	0.9799442	0.9799442

Note: Follow-up period divided into 6,209 one-day intervals. Displayed are the first and last day, and 13 days in which cases occurred. Double lines indicate intervals not shown in the table (e.g., days 2–137). For all days not shown, no case occurred so that the interval risk is 0, and the interval survival probability is 1. The risk for a one-day interval = N cohort at risk (e.g., the interval risk for day 1,332 = 1/802 = 0.00124688). The survival probability for a one-day interval = 1 − interval risk (e.g., the interval survival probability for day 1,332 = 1 − 0.00124688 = 0.9987531). The cumulative survival probability on a given day = the product of interval survival probabilities up to and including the specified day (e.g., cumulative survival on day 139 = p(survived day 1) × p(survived day 2 | survived day 1) × . . . × p(survived day 138 | survived day 137) × p (survived day 139 | survived day 138) = 1 × 1 × . . . × 0.9988938 × 1). The cumulative survival probability at the end of the study (day 6,209) = 0.9799442. The risk for the entire period (6,209 days) = 1 − 0.9799442.

480

Glossary

This glossary reflects the use of terms in this textbook. Many of these terms are defined variously across other texts. When we use these terms they have the meanings provided below.

additive model A mathematical model that assumes that risks add in their effects on disease.

adoption study A study using adoptees as a natural experiment to separate genetic from nongenetic causes.

affected pedigree member design A type of nonparametric linkage analysis approach that tests for nonrandom cosegregation of a disease and marker loci by evaluating whether diseased individuals within a family are more similar with respect to a marker locus than expected by chance.

affected sib pairs An analysis of pairs of siblings, both of whom are affected with the disease of interest, to find genetic markers of the disease.

age effects Changes in disease risk that are intrinsic to an individual human life because of biological development and the accumulation of exposures through the life course.

antecedent A cause of the exposure of interest. By exposure we mean any variable being investigated to determine if it is a cause.

artifactual confounder A variable that contributes to artifactual confounding.

artifactual confounding An imbalance of causes of disease (other than the exposure) between exposed and unexposed individuals that does not exist, or exists to a different degree, in naturally occurring populations. Artifactual confounding derives from the nonrandom selection of the people we study from a naturally occurring population, self-selection, selection of an inappropriate unexposed group for comparison, or loss to follow-up.

ascertainment bias Misclassification of disease that is different for the exposed and unexposed.

association   An association between exposure and disease means the co-occurrence of exposure and disease in a population beyond what would be expected by chance.

attributable proportion (attributable fraction)   An estimate of the proportion of disease that could have been prevented through the elimination of a specific cause within a designated context.

balancing the odds   Imposing the same constraints on the selection of controls and cases in a case-control study.

behavioral genetics   A discipline that specializes in studying the genetic causes of mental traits and disorders.

case-base (case-cohort) study   A case-control study in which controls are sampled from the full underlying cohort defined at the beginning of the study.

case-control study   A comparison of cases and controls best understood as a condensed version of a cohort study in which study subjects are selected according to their disease (or other outcome) status.

case-only design   A study design that uses only cases (i.e., people with the outcome under study) and can be used to assess gene- environment or gene-gene interaction.

case-parent triad   A variant of the case-control design in which the alleles carried by the parents of the cases are used to determine the odds of exposure that would be expected in controls.

case-unaffected sibling control   A case-control study in which controls are the unaffected siblings of the cases.

causal criteria   Guidelines, such as those developed by Sir Austin Branford Hill (1965), "Environment and Disease: Association or Causation?" (*Proc. R. Soc. Med.* 58:295–300), often used to help assess the causal effect of exposures.

causal explanation   Descriptions of how causes work. In this book, causal explanation comprises construct validity (the identification of the active ingredients of the exposure) and external validity (the identification of the causal partners of the exposure under study).

causal identification   The determination of whether or not an exposure under investigation has a causal effect on the outcome under study.

causal partner   When two or more risk factors are involved in a causal pathway, we refer to them as causal partners. A causal partner is a variable that works in concert with the exposure under investigation to cause disease.

censoring   When observation is discontinued before the event is observed to occur, resuting in incomplete follow-up for an individual.

clinical cohort   A cohort study that examines the determinants of the course or outcome of a disorder rather than its onset; also called a "natural history" study.

cohort effects The varying effects of past historical change on successive generations.

cohort study A study in which disease-free individuals are selected and categorized based on their exposure status and followed to determine disease onset.

comorbidity The co-occurrence of two or more disorders in the same individual. At a population level, disorders are comorbid when they co-occur among the same individuals more often than would be expected because of chance.

competing risk A condition that precludes developing the disease being studied (e.g. death).

complex disease In the context of genetics, disease that is influenced by contributions from multiple genetic factors, multiple environmental factors, or both.

concurrent case control study A case control study using incidence density sampling.

concurrent odds ratio An odds ratio calculated from a case control study using concurrent (also called incidence density) sampling of controls.

conditional probabilities The probability of one condition, given another specified condition (e.g., probability of disease, given exposure).

confidence interval A range of plausible values for a true population parameter, which depends on the point estimate, its variability, and the sample size.

confounding When the exposed and unexposed differ on risk of disease for reasons other than the exposure.

construct validity The extent to which variables measure the intended concepts.

counterfactual Consideration of what would have occurred under different circumstances. Usually used in epidemiology to refer to the disease experience of an exposed cohort under conditions of nonexposure.

cumulative incidence Another term for average risk in a cohort.

dependent nondifferential misclassification Errors in the classification of exposure that are linked to errors in the classification of disease.

differential attrition When attrition in a cohort results in a different relationship between exposure and disease in the cohort remaining under observation than in the initial cohort.

differential misclassification Misclassification of the disease that depends on the exposure status, or misclassification of the exposure that depends on disease status.

disease locus The location on the genome of a gene associated with a disease.

disease odds ratio   The odds of disease in the exposed divided by the odds of disease in the unexposed. The odds are the probability of disease divided by its complement.

double-blind   A situation in which neither the field research team nor the participants know which participants are in the exposed versus the unexposed groups.

eco-epidemiology   For studying causes in epidemiology, a proposed rubric that incorporates different levels of causation, individual development over the life cycle, and historical change. Study designs and statistical approaches for carrying out epidemiologic investigations from within this rubric are in nascent stages.

ecologic fallacy   The bias that can occur in the estimate of the effect of a risk factor when group-level variables are used as substitutes for information on the exposure and disease experience of individuals.

ecologic studies   Studies in which the units of analysis are groups rather than individuals.

effect measure modification (statistical interaction)   Heterogeneity of an estimate of the effect of one exposure across presence (or absence) or level of another.

end-of-study case ascertainment   A study in which we attempt to identify all the cases that occurred at any time during the risk period by means of a single assessment at the end of the risk period.

endophenotypes   Postulated intermediate outcomes that are on the pathway between the genetic determinant and the disease.

epidemiology   The study of the determinants of health and disease in human populations.

equal-environment assumption   In twin studies, the assumption that monozygotic and dizygotic twin pairs share their environment to the same extent.

exposure   A variable being investigated to determine whether it is a cause.

exposure odds ratio   The odds of exposure in diseased individuals divided by the odds of exposure in nondiseased individuals.

external validity   The extent to which the associations in a study apply across varied persons, places and time periods.

family-based genetic association studies   A collection of strategies for matching cases and controls on family of origin and thus ancestry.

family history (family aggregation study)   Studies of the aggregation of psychiatric disorders within families.

founder population   A population descended from a relatively small number of ancestors, and characterized by rapid expansion of population size and by marriage within the group.

full comparability Exposed and unexposed are equal on all factors influencing disease and its detection, other than the active ingredient of the exposure itself.

functional polymorphism A variation in DNA sequence associated with an altered protein function.

genetic association studies A rubric of study designs (e.g., case-control) that are used to examine association of a disease status with respect to the presence or absence of a genetic factor.

genetic heterogeneity When a disease is caused by different genes, or by different mutations of the same gene, in different families (or individuals).

genetic linkage studies Studies that seek to identify putative disease loci by examining cosegregation of known marker loci with disease phenotype within pedigrees.

genetic recombination The crossing over of genetic material between sister chromatids during meiosis.

genome scan The genotyping of markers on all chromosomes and at multiple sites more or less evenly spaced along the chromosomes. A genome scan may apply to both linkage and association studies.

genotype-phenotype correlation studies Studies that examine the relationships between allelic causes and clinical manifestations.

haplotype A set or "string" of alleles that occur close together on the same chromosome.

heritability The proportion of outcome variance that is attributable to inherited genetic effects.

historical cohort study A cohort study in which the measures of exposure and outcome are based on existing data. Also known as a retrospective cohort study.

historical cohort with concurrent follow-up A cohort study in which the exposure assessment is based on historical data but the study outcomes are determined in the course of the investigation.

identical by descent Two individuals share alleles *identical by descent* if those alleles are derived from the same original piece of DNA in a common ancestor.

incident cases New cases of outcome that arise over a specific time interval.

incidence density odds ratio An odds ratio calculated from a case control study using incidence density sampling of controls.

incidence density sampling A procedure for sampling controls, in which controls are selected among subjects free of disease at the time of occurrence of the cases. This type of sampling is used in concurrent case-control studies.

incidence rate (disease rate)   The number of new cases of disease per observed unit of person-time.

incidence rate ratio (rate ratio)   The ratio of the incidence rate in the exposed and unexposed.

interaction contrast   The observed risk among individuals exposed to two risk factors, minus the observed risk among individuals exposed to each plus the baseline risk.

interaction contrast ratio   The risk ratio observed for individuals exposed to two risk factors, minus the observed risk ratios among individuals exposed to each risk factor plus the baseline risk.

INUS   An acronym developed by J. L. Mackie (1974), *The Cement of the Universe: A Study of Causation* (New York: Oxford University Press) describing causes of interest as Insufficient but Nonredundant components of Unnecessary but Sufficient causes (*INUS causes*). In this text we use the term Insufficient but Necessary components of Unnecessary but Sufficient causes.

joint probabilities   The probability of two conditions occurring at once (e.g., probability that an individual is both exposed and diseased).

lifetime prevalence   The proportion of individuals in a population that have ever had the disease.

linkage disequilibrium   Association between alleles at one locus and alleles at another locus (i.e., a particular allele of one locus and a particular allele at the other locus occur together more frequently than one would expect by chance).

linkage equilibrium   Lack of association between alleles at one locus and alleles at another locus.

LOD score   The log of the ratio of the probability of the data under the hypothesis of linkage to the probability of the data under the hypothesis of no-linkage.

loss to follow-up   Members of a cohort who are not observed until the end of the study.

marginal probabilities   The presence or absence of only one condition (e.g., proportion diseased).

marker locus   The location on the genome of a unique identified stretch of DNA sequence.

matching   Comparisons selected to have the same value on a third variable (unexposed matched to exposed or controls matched to cases).

mediator   A cause that links the exposure to the disease (also referred to as an *intervening* or *intermediate variable*).

mendelian randomization   Term used to denote an approach for using genetic association studies to help differentiate valid from artifactual findings on environmental risk factors.

misclassification   The designation of measurement error in dichotomous or other discrete variables.

multiplicative antagonism   When the joint effect of two variables is smaller than the multiplication of their individual effects. Also called negative multiplicative interaction.

multiplicative interaction   When the joint effect of two variables is greater (or less) than the multiplication of their individual effects.

multiplicative model   A mathematical model that assumes that risks multiply in their effects on disease.

multiplicative synergy   When the joint effect of two variables is greater than the multiplication of their individual effects. Also called positive multiplicative interaction.

natural confounder   A variable that contributes to natural confounding.

natural confounding   An imbalance of causes of disease (other than the exposure) between exposed and unexposed individuals in naturally occurring populations.

natural experiment   A study in which people are selected into the exposed or unexposed by some event that is largely or entirely outside their own control. The event is *natural* in the sense that it is not created by the investigator.

necessary cause   A factor without which the outcome cannot occur.

nested case-control study   A case-control study developed within a defined cohort (thus *nested*) from which both the cases and controls are selected.

noncomparability   Exposed and unexposed are not equal on all factors influencing disease and its detection (other than the active ingredient of the exposure itself).

nondifferential misclassification   Misclassification of exposure that is independent of disease status and misclassification of disease that is independent of exposure status.

odds   A probability divided by its complement [e.g., probability of disease / (1 − the probability of disease)].

odds ratio   The ratio of two odds. The exposure odds ratio is the ratio of exposure odds in the diseased and non-diseased. The disease odds ratio is the ratio of the disease odds in the exposed and unexposed.

ongoing case registry ascertainment   A study in which the researcher continually monitors the treatment experience of the cohort during the risk period by means of a case registry.

parallelism   When an individual can develop disease from each of two exposures acting independently of each other in a context where these exposures are under investigation for potential synergistic effects.

penetrance   The risk of developing disease over a defined period, given the presence of the allele of interest. Reduced penetrance means that risk in less than one.

period effects   The effects of contemporary societal change on secular trends in disease.

period prevalence   The proportion of individuals who have had the disease over some past time interval.

periodic case ascertainment   A study in which the cohort is evaluated for the outcome at two or more time points during the risk period.

person-time   The amount of time from an individual's entrance into a study until he/she develops the disease, reaches the end of the study, is lost to a competing risk, or is lost to follow-up.

phenotype   The observable trait or disease for which one seeks a genetic cause.

pleiotropy   When a single gene (or gene pair) produces diverse phenotypic effects.

point estimate   A scalar or one-dimensional estimator for a parameter of interest.

point prevalence   The proportion of individuals who have the disease at the time that the study is conducted.

polymorphic markers   Genetic markers with considerable allelic variation.

population attributable proportion   Proportion of disease that could have been eliminated in this population through removal of the risk factor.

population cohort   A cohort that is assembled from a naturally occurring population (also called a *general population cohort*).

population stratification   A form of confounding based on differences in allelic frequencies and disease risk between populations.

power   The probability of rejecting the null hypothesis when the alternative hypothesis is true.

precision   The amount of sampling error in an estimate.

prevalence   A measure of extant disease.

proportional hazards regression   A regression technique used to assess the impact of one or more categorical and continuous predictor variables on event times.

prospective population cohort study   A cohort study in which both the exposure and the outcome data are collected in the course of the investigation from people free of disease at outset.

***p*-value**   The probability of obtaining the observed data (or data that were even more extreme), assuming that the null hypothesis is true.

random measurement error   Nonsystematic error in the measurement of variables.

randomized controlled trial   A study design in which the researcher randomly assigns exposure.

recall bias   Recall of exposure that depends on case status.

recombination fraction   The proportion of meioses in which recombination occurs between two loci.

reconstructed cohort   A study in which cases and controls are used to define their relatives as exposed or unexposed and these relatives become the cohort in which disease risk is assessed.

relative risk   The ratio of the risk in the exposed to the risk in the unexposed (also called *risk ratio*).

reliability   The replicability of measures across repeated tests, testers, and time periods; or the proportion of variation in repeated measurements that is due to true subject-to-subject variability.

restriction   Limiting a study to persons in a particular category of a potential confounder.

risk   The probability of developing the disease over a time period. Measured as average risk in a population.

risk difference   The difference between the risks in the exposed and the unexposed.

risk factor   Characteristic of an individual that influences disease risk in a population.

risk factor epidemiology   Epidemiologic methods designed specifically to examine causes of disease that are characteristics of individuals.

risk period   The time period during which disease outcomes are identified in a cohort study.

risk ratio   The ratio of the risk in the exposed to the risk in the unexposed (also called *relative risk*).

schizophrenia spectrum disorders   A group of disorders related to schizophrenia that are thought to coaggregate in families. As defined in the Prenatal Determinants of Schizophrenia Example, this group includes schizophrenia, schizoaffective disorder, schizotypal personality disorder, delusional disorder, and psychotic disorder NOS (not otherwise specified).

segregation analysis   Analysis of pedigree data for various modes of inheritance mutant allele frequency, and peretrance probabilities.

selection bias   In a case-control study, selection bias occurs when controls are selected who do not represent the ratio of exposed to unexposed in the source population that gave rise to the cases.

sensitivity   The proportion of people who have a trait that are correctly classified as having the trait.

sensitivity analyses   Analyses conducted to examine the robustness of data patterns to errors related to bias or chance.

shared environment   In twin studies, the totality of nongenetic factors that are shared by both members of a twin pair.

significance level   The criterion chosen for rejecting the null hypothesis, corresponding to the maximum type I error rate.

socialfact   Rules, norms, and ways of being that constrain the actions and behaviors of individuals.

sole plausible explanation   After consideration of all the alternative explanations for the observed association between the exposure and the disease, the only currently plausible explanation is that the exposure is a cause of the disease.

source population   The exposed and unexposed people eligible for participation in a study.

sources of noncomparability   Factors that lead to noncomparability between the exposed and unexposed—other risk factors for the disease, observation time, and disease labeling errors. We refer to these sources of noncomparability as *confounding, unequal attrition,* and *differential misclassification,* respectively.

special exposure cohort   Cohorts developed around an identified exposure for which an unexposed group is selected for comparison. In these types of cohort studies, the exposed and unexposed do not come from the same naturally occurring population.

specificity   The proportion of people who do not have a trait that are correctly classified as not having the trait.

standard deviation   A quantity that gauges the typical distance of measurements from their mean in a population.

standard error   A quantity that gauges the typical distance of an estimator from its mean value over repeated experiments of the same size.

statistical interaction (effect measure modification)   Heterogeneity of an estimate of the effect of one exposure across presence (or absence) or level of another.

statistical power   The probability of accepting a specific hypothesis posed as an alternative to the null, when this alternative hypothesis is true.

study population   The people who actually enter the study.

sufficient cause   A factor or set of factors that inevitably produces the outcome.

survival curve   A plot of the proportion of subjects who remain event-free as a function of time.

synergy   The joint action of causal partners in causing an outcome.

temporal priority   The exposure is present before the onset of the disease (or other outcome) under investigation.

third variable   Some variable or set of variables other than the exposure and disease of interest.

time-to-event analysis (failure-time analysis)   Methods of statistical analysis designed to make inferences about the occurrence and timing of an event, taking into account incomplete follow-up (censoring) on a subset of subjects.

traditional odds ratio   An odds ratio calculated using information from individuals still under observation at the end of a study period.

twin studies of heritability   A study design using differences between monozygotic and dizygotic twins to estimate genetic influences on a trait.

type I error   An error that occurs when a test statistic leads us to reject the null, when in fact the null hypothesis holds true in the population.

type II error   An error that occurs when a test statistic leads us to fail to reject the null hypothesis, when the alternative hypothesis is true in the population.

unequal attrition   Attrition in a cohort that is unequal for the exposed and unexposed groups.

unique environment   In twin studies, the totality of nongenetic factors that are not shared by the members of a twin pair.

unwell controls   Controls selected to have a disease other than the disease under investigation.

well controls   A control group in which people with disorders other than the disease under study are excluded.

Index

Page numbers followed by *f*, *t*, and *n* refer to figures, tables, and notes respectively.
Page numbers in bold refer to terms bolded in the text and defined in the Glossary.